District Nu
Clini

District Nursing Manual of Clinical Procedures

Edited by

Liz O'Brien
RN, BSc (Hons) Specialist Practice District Nursing, BSc (Hons), DPSN, FETC
Service Manager for Community Nursing
Surrey

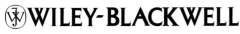
A John Wiley & Sons, Ltd., Publication

This edition first published 2012 © Blackwell Publishing Ltd

Blackwell Publishing was acquired by John Wiley & Sons in February 2007. Blackwell's publishing program has been merged with Wiley's global Scientific, Technical and Medical business to form Wiley-Blackwell.

Registered office: John Wiley & Sons, Ltd, The Atrium, Southern Gate, Chichester, West Sussex, PO19 8SQ, UK

Editorial offices: 9600 Garsington Road, Oxford, OX4 2DQ, UK
The Atrium, Southern Gate, Chichester, West Sussex, PO19 8SQ, UK
111 River Street, Hoboken, NJ 07030-5774, USA

For details of our global editorial offices, for customer services and for information about how to apply for permission to reuse the copyright material in this book please see our website at www. wiley.com/wiley-blackwell.

The right of the author to be identified as the author of this work has been asserted in accordance with the UK Copyright, Designs and Patents Act 1988.

Library of Congress Cataloging-in-Publication Data
District nursing manual of clinical procedures / edited by Liz O'Brien.
      p. ; cm.
  Includes bibliographical references and index.
  ISBN 978-1-4051-1459-2 (pbk. : alk. paper)
  I. O'Brien, Liz, 1962–
  [DNLM: 1. Nursing Care. 2. Nursing Process. WY 100.1]

  362.14–dc23
                          2011042665

A catalogue record for this book is available from the British Library.

Wiley also publishes its books in a variety of electronic formats. Some content that appears in print may not be available in electronic books.

Set in 9.5/11 pt Minion by Toppan Best-set Premedia Limited
Printed and bound in Malaysia by Vivar Printing Sdn Bhd

1   2012

Contents

Contributors

Edited by

Liz O'Brien, RN, BSc (Hons) Specialist Practice
District Nursing, BSc (Hons), DPSN, FETC
Service Manager for Community Nursing, Surrey
      (CHAPTERS 1, 4, 8, 9, 10, 11, 12, 13 and 15)

Contributors

Maureen Benbow, MSc, BA, RGN, HERC
Senior Lecturer,
University of Chester   (CHAPTER 15)

Elissa Bradshaw, RN, BSc
Clinical Nurse Specialist/Biofeedback,
St Mark's Hospital   (CHAPTER 3)

Jennie Burch RN (Adult), MSc, BSc (Hons)
Enhanced Recovery Nurse Facilitator,
St Mark's Hospital   (CHAPTER 3)

Brigitte Collins, RN, BSc (Hons), MSc GI Nursing
Lead Nurse, Biofeedback Therapy,
St Mark's Hospital

     (CHAPTER 3)

Jackie Daly, RGN, RMN, DN CERT
Continuing Care Nurse Assessor,
Croydon Borough Team,
NHS South West London   (CHAPTER 4)

Lisa Dougherty OBE, RN, MSc, DClinP
Nurse Consultant Intravenous Therapy,
The Royal Marsden Hospital NHS Foundation Trust
     (CHAPTER 14)

Patricia Evans, MCSP, Grad Dip Phys
Clinical Physiotherapist/Specialist Biofeedback,
St Mark's Hospital   (CHAPTER 3)

Rachel Gilbert, RN, BSc (Hons), PG Dip Public Health
Senior Lecturer,
University of the West of England   (CHAPTER 11)

Sarah Hart, RN
Formerly Clinical Nurse Specialist, Infection Control
The Royal Marsden Hospital NHS Foundation Trust
London   (CHAPTER 6)

Jill Kayley, MSc RN DN Certificate
Independent Nurse Consultant – Community IV
Therapy   (CHAPTER 7)

Rosie Lake, RGN, RCNT, Dip Nursing (Part A),
ENB A97
Lead Back Care Adviser,
Portsmouth Hospitals NHS Trust,
Queen Alexandra Hospital   (CHAPTER 9)

Rachel B Leaver, MSc, BSc (Hons), PGCE, RN
Lecturer Practitioner – Urological Care,
University College London Hospitals and
London South Bank University   (CHAPTER 13)

Kathy Martyn, MSc Nutriton BSc (Hons) Biological
Sciences, BEd. (Hons), PGDpN SRN
Principal Lecturer, Nutrition,
INAM University of Brighton   (CHAPTER 10)

Lesley Maskell, MSc, PGCEA, RGN, DN
Independent Learning and Development Advisor
     (CHAPTER 1)

Amanda Mayo, MSc, BSC, RGN, NiP
111 Lead – London
Harmoni   (CHAPTER 8)

Eleanor McGill, RN, D/Nurse Cert, Dip Nursing
Community Liaison Nurse,
Croydon Health Services NHS Trust   (CHAPTER 4)

Chrissie Nicholls RGN
Practice Nurse,
Croydon, Surrey   (CHAPTER 5)

Pam Phipps, RGN, C&G 7307, ENB A97
Back Care Adviser,
Portsmouth Hospital NHS Trust,
Queen Alexandra Hospital   (CHAPTER 9)

Marilyn Prentice
Former diabetes specialist nurse
Croydon Health Services NHS Trust   (CHAPTER 2)

Jo Robinson, EN, RGN, DN, Diploma Nursing
(Palliative Care), BSc (Hons)
Community Nursing; PGcert Clinical Governance;
MSc Health Science Clinical Service Manager,
Community Nursing Services East Solent NHS Trust.
The Turner Centre, St James' Hospital   (CHAPTER 9)

Heather Short, MEd, BSc (Hons),
PGCE, Dip/DN, RGN
Senior Lecturer,
University of the West of England   (CHAPTER 11)

Anne Spence, RN, DN, SPT, BSc (Hons)
Clinical Nurse Specialist in Palliative Care,
St Christopher's Hospice   (CHAPTER 12)

Greta Thornbory, TD, MSc OH RGN SCPHNOH
DipN OH PGCEA
Self-employed Occupational Health and Education
Consultant

Fran Williams, RN, BSc, MA
Consultant Practitioner Safeguarding Adults,
Solent NHS Trust, The Turner Centre,
St James' Hospital
(CHAPTER 9)

Sue Woodward RGN, MSc, PGCEA
Lecturer, Florence Nightingale School of Nursing
and Midwifery,
King's College London   (CHAPTER 3)

Keri Wright, RN, DN, DipHE, BSc (Hons), MA
Senior Lecturer, School of Health and Social Care,
University of Greenwich   (CHAPTER 1)

Foreword

The home is a special place for nursing.

It is special for the person receiving care, because it is their environment, and, unlike in hospital, they are in control. Inviting a health professional into their home is an act of trust for the individual. They trust that they will not be judged on the basis of their environment, their style of living or their family. In hospital, they are a patient, and with the best will in the world, ward staff can only know the patient to a superficial degree, based on what he or she chooses to tell them or show them. At home, the individual can only be themselves, and the nurses who treat them there see them as they are.

Home is also a special place for the nurse to practice. Community nurses are privileged to be invited into people's lives and homes. They have to be adaptable, professional, inventive and highly-skilled to deliver complex care in these very diverse environments. And the demands on their skills are growing all the time. Technology, demographics, economics and patient choice are all increasing the pressure to keep people at home rather than in hospital, no matter how serious, complex or unstable their condition.

The Queen's Nursing Institute carried out a survey of patients' and carers' experience of nursing in the home in 2011, resulting in a major new report, 'Nursing People at Home – the issues, the stories, the actions'. The findings underline the importance of nursing in the home, and the degree to which many thousands of frail and older people depend on it. They also reminded us of the challenges of a changing workforce, with community teams increasingly made up of less experienced nurses, and more dependent on assistants. It was clear from people's responses that patients can tell the difference between more and less experienced nurses; between those who are sure of their skills and those who are nervous about them; and between those with what they called 'professional poise' and those who lacked it. Overall, the report also shows that patients want three things of their community nurses: they want them to be competent, confident and caring.

This manual, the first of its kind focused on district nursing, provides the means to build competence and confidence in nurses new to the community, or developing their skills. The comprehensive and evidence-based content provides essential information for competence in key areas of district nursing. With knowledge, evidence and professional consensus, put into practice, comes confidence, the second vital ingredient in successful community nursing. The third, caring, resides in the individual practitioner, and completes the picture of the poised professional that patients want to see when they invite community nurses into that very special place – their home.

Rosemary Cook CBE, Hon D Lett, MSc, PG Dip, RGN
Director, The Queen's Nursing Institute
December 2011

Preface

The idea for a nursing manual of clinical procedures written specifically for district nurses first began in 2002. The purpose of the manual is to provide community nursing staff with an up-to-date text that is evidence based, practical in its approach but moreover, reflective of the uniqueness and reality of the individual environment in which care takes place, the patient's home. 'This unique setting demands a workforce with specialist knowledge and skills' (Queen's Nursing Institute, 2011. page 10). I also felt it was important to promote the development of clinical practice and actively support the recognition of the complexity of care, procedures and treatments provided by district nurses and their teams.

The clinical procedures in this manual are only a small proportion of those performed by community nurses, but as the current evidence base for district nursing procedures is not extensive and as the first text of its kind, the manual represents a strong starting point for this branch of the nursing profession. Through background evidence and inclusion of comprehensive procedure guidelines it covers a number of key areas highlighted by the Queen's Nursing Institute as being important to patients: communication, knowledge, competence, empathy and compassion (Queen's Nursing Institute, 2011). It also covers a number of the key areas that community nurses, especially junior nurses, often struggle with or find difficult when, unlike in a hospital setting, they are on their own in a patient's home. For example, when making decisions regarding some of the more technical procedures such as nasogastric tube placement and feeds, wound management and the use of syringe pumps.

I envisage that this book will evolve through successive editions to be as successful, thorough and evidence based as *The Royal Marsden Manual*.

I would like to take this opportunity to thank Beth Knight at Wiley-Blackwell, not only for her enthusiasm for my manuscript proposal, but also for her continued advice and support and unwavering belief in my ability to complete this journey and ultimately for giving me the opportunity to do it. Thanks also to Catriona Cooper and all at Wiley-Blackwell's. I would also like to thank the chapter authors for their patience and help with the completion of the manual and those who helped by reading, reviewing and providing feedback on the chapters – Anna Marie Stevens, Clare Shaw and Sue Brooker.

Finally, a special thank you to Lisa for her continued generous support and advice.

Liz O'Brien
2012

Queen's Nursing Institute (2011) *Nursing People at Home: The issues, the stories, the actions*. Queen's Nursing Institute: London.

Assessment and communication (general principles)

Introduction

There is wide recognition that patient assessment by community nurses is central to the provision of high-quality care and that assessment in the home care setting is a complex process requiring a wide range of knowledge and skills (McIntosh 2006). The nursing process was the forerunner of modern day care management; however, as patient care becomes more complex, its continued use as a problem-solving approach has been questioned (Crow *et al.* 1995; Lawton *et al.* 2000).

This chapter explores the assessment process carried out by community nurses to help them plan patient care, the importance of communication in relation to assessment and the issue of consent in community nursing.

Background evidence

Assessment

Assessment is a patient-focused, interactive process that enables the nurse to gain knowledge about a patient in order to identify problems and plan the care interventions that are best suited to meet the patient's needs (Walsh 1998; Aggleton & Chalmers 2000). It is fundamental to individualised patient care, and therefore how that knowledge is gained, and what objective and subjective knowledge is sought to inform care decisions, is essential (Walsh 1998).

A comprehensive nursing assessment contains multi-faceted dimensions:

- physical
- emotional
- spiritual
- psychological
- cultural
- social.

To complete the four-stage cyclical process requires:

- assessment of patient needs
- planning care that meets the patient's identified needs
- the implementation of planned nursing interventions
- the evaluation of the nursing interventions.

It is essential for the community nurse to expand their knowledge and understanding of the patient's, and where relevant carer's, perspective of their own needs so that they can plan care that maintains and promotes patient independence (Alfaro-Lefevre 2002).

Assessment can be divided into two stages:

1 gathering the information and knowledge about the patient
2 using this information to make decisions about potential patient problems (Barrows & Feltovich 1987; Carnevali & Thomas 1993; Walsh 1998).

The type of information that the nurse collects from the patient can be divided into two main categories (Walsh 1998).

1 Qualitative information – information based on the individual's and the nurse's feelings, thoughts and experiences. This information explores the interpretations and meanings that individuals place on events. For example, how a patient feels about a recent diagnosis of cancer.
2 Quantitative information – information based on tested scientific methods, objective facts and observations. For example, blood results.

District Nursing Manual of Clinical Procedures, First Edition. Edited by Liz O'Brien.
© 2012 Blackwell Publishing Ltd. Published 2012 by Blackwell Publishing Ltd.

2

Both types of information are required to gain a full picture of the individual's health and social care needs. Consequently assessments often involve nurses measuring and recording facts about patient's vital signs, weight and medical history, as well as asking more subjective questions, such as how they feel about having a particular disease or living alone.

Assessing a patient to ascertain needs involves an inductive and deductive approach (Crow *et al.* 1995). The inductive approach involves information being gathered and general conclusions being drawn from this information about needs. The deductive approach entails the nurse making inferences about the information given and then working backwards to gather more information to support or reject the idea.

Factors affecting nursing assessment

As already indicated, in order to plan care delivery the patient's needs must be identified; however, this identification cannot occur between the nurse and patient in isolation. The nursing assessment carried out and the needs ascertained are influenced by external factors, for example:

- type of need
- health need versus healthcare need
- health policy
- nursing versus social care
- professional accountability
- resource issues.

(Walsh 1998)

Identifying patient need

Type of need

Bradshaw's taxonomy of needs (1972) describes four different types of need, as follows.

- Felt need – need that a person feels that they have. This need may not always be expressed.
- Comparative need – a need that is only realised through comparing with other people or groups.
- Normative need – need that a healthcare professional determines an individual to have.
- Expressed need – a need that an individual expresses in some way.

It is important that community nurses recognise the different types of need when carrying out a patient assessment as this will help them assess the patient accurately.

Health needs versus healthcare needs

There is a subtle difference between an individual's health needs and an individual's healthcare needs. Health needs includes those factors that may influence the individual's health, such as housing, socioeconomic status and education. Healthcare needs are those needs that would benefit from the provision of healthcare, such as treatment, rehabilitation or health education (Steven & Raftery 1997). The ideal situation would be for every patient to be able to have all their needs assessed and for care to be available to meet all of these needs. The reality, however, is that limited availability of resources in the area can restrict the care available and the care that is offered to the patient. This can influence the information gathered about a patient. Prior knowledge about the services available allows nurses to explore some needs in depth, as they know that the supply is available to meet that demand. For example, if the community nurse knows that there is a bed free at the local hospice they may be more willing to discuss the possibility of imminent respite/inpatient symptom management (Bryans & McIntosh 1996).

Nursing versus social care

Since the introduction of the Community Care Act in 1993, social services have become responsible for meeting the 'social needs' of people in the community and community nursing has become responsible for meeting the 'nursing needs'. Such an artificial definition has proved problematic and confusion still exists among nurses over how to differentiate between these two needs (Wright 2003). With the Community Care Act, responsibility for the placement of individuals' long-term care in the community moved from the NHS to social services. This meant that clients who had stayed permanently in long-stay wards in hospitals under NHS responsibility began to be moved to nursing homes under social service responsibility (Wright 2002a). Despite this change, the NHS is still responsible for the nursing care element of long-term placements and for assessing every individual entering a nursing home under social service responsibility. However, the local authority and social services do not have the responsibility for all nursing home and residential residents.

The Single Assessment Process (SAP)

The Single Assessment Process (SAP) was introduced in 2001 as a key part of the National Service Framework (NSF) for Older People (DH 2000c) with a requirement for it to be implemented by April 2004. The NSF identified the single assessment as a key way to meet the aim of 'ensuring that older people are treated as individuals and receive appropriate and timely packages of care which meet their needs as individuals, regardless of health and social services boundaries' (DH 2000c: 23).

The fundamental principle of the SAP is that there is an individualised person-centred assessment to which different health and social care professions contribute. The process requires partnership, collaboration and shared communication between all those involved in the assessment, planning and delivery of care to the patient. The intention is for care needs to be assessed thoroughly and accurately without patients needing to discuss their needs with a range of different professionals and without procedures being unnecessarily duplicated by different agencies involved in the delivery of care. To achieve this, the SAP assessment of the patient (Box 1.1) is carried out by one front-line professional, for example a district nurse. If other professionals need to be involved in the package of care, a referral, e.g. for specialist assessment, is made by the initial assessor to ensure that the patient receives a seamless service.

Although originally designed for the assessment of older people, the SAP is increasingly being used by health and social care agencies as a framework for assessing need and delivering services to other adults requiring care.

Some of the benefits of the SAP include:

- increased patient involvement in decision making
- improved use of specialist time
- reduced duplication in the gathering of assessment information
- reduced repetition of information giving by the patient
- improved co-ordination of care to offer a seamless service
- improved outcomes for patients and linking of outcomes to assessment information.

Assessment for end of life care

It is suggested that approximately half a million people die in England each year; however, people find it difficult to discuss this aspect of life openly. Of the total number of deaths it is estimated that:

- 58% occur in hospital
- 18% at home
- 17% in care homes
- 4% in hospices
- 3% elsewhere.

(DH 2008a)

Box 1.1 Single assessment core domains

User's perspective
- Problems or issues in the user's own words
- User's expectations and motivation

Clinical background
- History of medical problems
- History of falls
- Medication use

Disease prevention
- History of blood pressure monitoring
- Nutrition
- Vaccination history
- Drinking and smoking history
- Exercise pattern
- History of cervical and breast screening

Personal care and physical wellbeing
- Personal hygiene, including washing, bathing, toileting and grooming
- Dressing
- Pain
- Oral health
- Foot care
- Tissue viability
- Mobility
- Continence
- Sleeping patterns

Senses
- Sight
- Hearing
- Communication

Mental health
- Cognition including dementia
- Mental health including depression

Relationships
- Social contacts, relationships and involvement
- Caring arrangements

Safety
- Abuse or neglect
- Other aspects of personal safety
- Public safety

Immediate environment and resources
- Care of the home
- Accommodation
- Finances
- Access to local facilities and services

Source: DH 2000c.

3

4

For the community nursing team, 18% of deaths at home is equivalent to 8% of their total caseload; however, in reality, 40% of actual community nursing time is spent on face-to-face contact with those requiring palliative and end of life care (DH 2008a).

Communication, assessment, care planning and symptom management are the fundamental basis for achieving high-quality end of life care (Mahmood-Yousuf et al. 2008; NHS National End of Life Care Programme 2009). To support practitioners and enable them to do this successfully, a number of initiatives and tools have been developed and these are now seen as an integral part of many community nurses' clinical practice. For example:

- the Gold Standards Framework (GSF) (King et al. 2005; Mahmood-Yousuf et al. 2008)
- the Liverpool Care Pathway (LCP) (Taylor 2005; DH 2008a)
- prognostic indicators (Thomas & Free 2008)
- advance care planning (National End of Life Care Programme 2011)
- national guidelines for continuing healthcare (DoH 2009a, 2009b, 2010).

Gold Standards Framework (GSF)

The GSF has been introduced as a National Framework that is aimed at facilitating a consistently high-quality approach within palliative care. The framework focuses on an anticipatory approach to care needs based on three steps for good practice (King et al. 2005).

1 Practitioners, e.g. community nurses and GPs, work in partnership to identify palliative care patients and place them on a GSF register. The register should then be used during multiprofessional GSF meetings to guide discussion and planning for individual patients' current and future needs.
2 Assessment of the patient and, where appropriate, carer's needs.
3 The planning of care and, where necessary, additional support to meet identified needs.

The GSF contains seven key areas known as the '7 Cs':

- Communication
- Co-ordination
- Control of symptoms
- Continuity
- Continued learning
- Carer support
- Care of the dying.

(King et al. 2005; DH 2008a)

To ensure that holistic care is provided, all seven domains must be considered during the initial patient assessment and reassessment stages, and all care needs identified must be met.

The Liverpool Care Pathway (LCP)

The Liverpool Care Pathway for the dying adult patient contains three elements: initial assessment, ongoing assessment and care after death, and is a crucial component of the GSF (Taylor 2005). It is an evidence-based approach to assessment and care that places multiprofessional working, communication, needs identification of both the patient and carer, and clinical decision making at the centre of care (Taylor 2005; Ellershaw 2007; Marie Curie 2009).

Once a multiprofessional diagnosis of the last hours or days of life has been reached and where, for example, two or more of the following symptoms are present, the LCP should be initiated (Taylor 2005).

- The patient is semi or fully comatose.
- The patient is bedbound.
- The patient is able to take only sips of fluid.
- The patient is unable to take oral tablets.

Prognostic indicators

Developed in line with the GSF, prognostic indicators provide clinicians with an insight into the potential prognosis and care needs of patients in advanced disease or those predicted to be in the last six to 12 months of life (Thomas & Free 2008). They include those people who are living with a long-term condition or life-limiting illness such as:

- renal disease
- dementia
- Parkinson's disease
- heart disease
- chronic obstructive pulmonary disease (COPD)
- cancer
- motor neurone disease
- co-morbidities.

(DH 2008a; Thomas & Free 2008)

Prognostic indicators may be used as a predictive guide during relevant patient assessment to help identify current care needs and anticipate others. By using the tool in this way it is suggested that the patient will receive the correct care and support at the right time in a proactive manner (Thomas & Free 2008). They may also be used as a trigger to initiate discussion with the patient, and where relevant significant other(s) regarding their wishes during the final stages of their illness; for example preferred place of care, resuscitation status

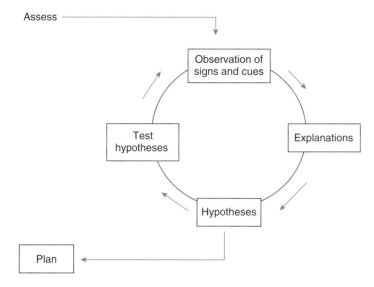

Assess

Figure 1.1 Diagram showing the information processing theory.

and care after death (Reid & Jeffrey 2002; DH 2008b; Lucas & Wells 2009; NHS National End of Life Care Programme 2009; NHS National End of Life Care Programme 2011; Wilson & White 2011).

Decision making

Using the information gathered about a patient during an assessment, nurses are required to plan care. To do this, they first need to establish what the patient's problems or needs are. The process of examining the information and identifying problems requires nurses to make decisions, therefore decision making is a key element of the community nurse's assessment practice and decision-making theory can provide a useful conceptual framework.

Information-processing theory

The inductive/deductive approach is similar to the information-processing theory (Junnola *et al.* 2002). This theory attempts to explain how nurses make decisions about patient problems on the basis of the information presented to them (Carnevali & Thomas 1993). The information-processing theory has the following stages (Figure 1.1).

- Observation of signs and cues.
- Generation of alternative explanations.
- Activating an hypothesis.
- Ascertaining and testing the hypothesis in relation to previous knowledge.
- Defining problems.

The effectiveness of a community nurse's decision making will therefore depend on a number of factors.

- knowledge base
- ability to use different methods to collect new information
- ability to extract the new information – those elements that are relevant to solving the problem
- ability to integrate that information with existing knowledge
- ability to generate hypotheses that will carry forward the decision-making process.

(Junnola *et al.* 2002)

Critical thinking

The thinking process of problem solving, when there is no single solution, is known as critical thinking. Critical thinking is therefore an essential component of decision making for nurses. Kataoka-Yahiro and Saylor (1994: 352) have devised a model of critical thinking for nurses and describe critical thinking as:

> Reflective and reasonable thinking about nursing problems without a single solution and is focussed on deciding what to believe and do.

Among other things, critical thinking involves recognising that assumptions exist, making these assumptions explicit and assessing their accuracy. The process of critical thinking enables the nurse to do the following.

- Raise vital questions and problems, formulating them clearly and precisely.
- Gather and assess relevant information, interpreting it effectively, arriving at well-reasoned conclusions and testing them against relevant criteria and standards.
- Think with an open mind using alternative systems of thought and recognising their assumptions, implications and practical consequences.
- Communicate effectively with others in figuring out solutions to complex problems.

(Paul & Elder 2004)

Patient assessment is a dynamic decision-making process that seeks to establish an accurate picture of an individual's condition and through critical thinking enables the community nurse to make decisions about the care the patient requires (Figure 1.1). Possessing key information is a crucial component of any decision making and in order to gather the appropriate information required to accurately assess a patient's condition the community nurse needs to have well-developed communication skills. Careful observation of verbal and non-verbal cues is also required (Hedberg & Larsson 2003).

Communication

There are two main types of communication relevant to assessment.

- Therapeutic communication – seen as communication with patients and families.
- Inter- and intra-professional communication – occurs between other professionals and nurses involved in the assessment process.

(Barr 2001).

Therapeutic communication

For an assessment to be accurate, and the most appropriate needs identified, the nurse must ensure that assessments are individualised (Aggleton & Chalmers 2000). Individualised care means that the patient's personal-subjective dimension is taken into account in the decision-making and information-gathering processes (Jenny & Logan 1992). The interaction between the patient and nurse is seen to be at the heart of nursing and is the vehicle through which nursing care can be delivered (Luker *et al.* 2000; Wright 2002a). This interaction is commonly known as the nurse–patient

relationship. The development of a nurse–patient relationship includes the following stages:

- involvement
- knowing the patient
- nurse–patient relationship.

(May 1991; Radwin 1996; Luker *et al.* 2000; Wright 2002b)

Involvement

May (1991) suggests that becoming involved with patients is part of the process of getting to know patients. Involvement in this sense is seen as the result of encounters between the nurse and the patient in which the nurse obtains knowledge about the patient. During these encounters nurses view patients not simply as objects of clinical attention, but also as individuals who place their own interpretation and meanings on events. Becoming involved with patients is therefore a process that leads towards a greater understanding of the patient as an individual. Involvement has been shown to have other fundamental features relating to the interaction that occurs between a patient and a nurse.

- **Knowledge** – gaining knowledge about patients, understanding their personality, their lives and their potential needs.
- **Reciprocity** – while nurses gain information about the patient they also respond by giving information about themselves. This is thought to allow patients to see that the nurse is actually a person with a life, too. This exchange is thought to offer a 'connection between the nurse and the patient that is both particular and meaningful' (May 1991: 554). The degree of reciprocity is bound by the norms of appropriate behaviour in the course of a nurse–patient relationship (NMC 2008a).
- **Investment** – the knowledge and exchange of information between the nurse and patient is constituted through a particular investment of nursing skills to meet clinical and social objectives. For example, getting to know the patient and becoming involved has a purpose of meeting nursing care needs.

The degree of involvement between the patient and community nurse needs to be balanced. An over-focus on reciprocity by the nurse can cause stress and unsatisfying care for the patient. Whereas an under-focus can lead to less satisfying care for both patient and nurse. As nurses begin to become involved with their patients they must therefore balance the degree of reciprocity and exchange that takes place between them.

Knowing the patient

Knowing the patient is described as a process of understanding and treating the patient as a unique individual (Radwin 1995). The nurse is thought to use their knowledge of the patient to make care choices (Hedberg & Larsson 2003). When the nurse knows the patient, interventions are chosen so that the patient is treated as a unique individual. Knowing the patient is said to have three main concepts:

- the nurse's experience with caring for patients
- chronological time
- a sense of closeness between the patient and the nurse.

(Radwin 1996)

Knowing the patient is thought not only to benefit the decision-making process, but also the achievement of positive patient outcomes (May 1993). Care based on knowing allows that care to be personalised, comforting, supporting and healing (Swanson-Kauffman 1986). Patients also feel cared for when nurses provide individualised care, begin to do more things for themselves and are more willing to accept help when needed (Lamb & Stempel 1994). Getting to know the patient is therefore an important concept for nursing assessment and a precursor to developing a professional relationship (Hedberg & Larsson, 2003).

Nurse–patient relationship

The interactions between a nurse and a patient should be based on accepting the individuality and uniqueness of the patient. Once established a nurse–patient relationship becomes the vehicle through which all other therapeutic care is delivered (Luker 1997; Wright 2002b). Within the community setting, where nurses visit patients in their own homes, the development of a nurse–patient relationship can become more complicated (Luker *et al.* 2000). When visiting patients at home, community nurses often become involved with the patient's relatives and/or carers and this involvement creates another dimension to the relationship developed. Therefore community nurses must be aware of the relationships between the patient and carer/relatives as well as developing and being aware of their own relationships with the patient and carer/relative (Luker *et al.* 2000; Wright 2002b).

The nurse–patient or family relationship is described as a partnership (Munro *et al.* 2000). In this conceptualisation the nurse moves from being an expert provider of care to a patient and family, to being a partner with the patient and family. In a partnership relationship the patient and family participate as much as they are able in the planning and delivery of care. Working in partnership with patients and their families has been found to offer benefits to both the patient and the care they receive. These include the following.

- **Empowerment** – the ability of the patient or family to act on their own through increased control, confidence and competence.
- **Emotional support** – as the nurse works with the patient and family and assists them in implementing the goals required of the partnership, both the patient and family have more opportunities to be supported emotionally. Working in partnership allows the nurse to show acceptance and understanding of the patient and family and can lead to further support through caring.

(Gallant *et al.* 2002)

Partnerships develop from the nurse–patient relationship and the interactions that take place between the nurse and the patient. Two main attributes are required within the nurse–patient relationship for a partnership to develop (Gallant *et al.* 2000):

- power sharing
- negotiation.

Therapeutic communication skills

Effective communication is beneficial for patient care and has been found to increase the rate of patient recovery, reduce pain and increase the concordance with treatment regimens (Stewart 1996; Fallowfield & Jenkins 1999).

Communication skills have been identified as a core skill in nursing (DoH 2000b) and have been described by Wallace (2001: 86) as the 'primary medium of care'.

Egan (1994) identified three core components that he felt needed to be conveyed within a therapeutic relationship.

- **Genuineness or congruence** – being genuine refers to nurses being themselves in the relationship, being authentic and sincere.
- **Warmth** – this has also been described as unconditional positive regard. Being warm towards a patient is showing acceptance and respect for them as a unique individual and being non-judgemental.
- **Empathy** – empathy is seen as being able to perceive accurately the feelings of another person and to communicate this understanding to them.

These core components can be conveyed through both non-verbal and verbal behaviours.

8

Non-verbal communication

Information and messages can be conveyed to other people either consciously or unconsciously through the use of body language. Non-verbal behaviour has a number of different functions.

- Supporting or complementing the verbal meaning of speech, for example pointing directions at the same time as verbally explaining.
- Regulating the flow of the interaction, for example touching someone to get their attention or backing away to end a conversation.
- Signalling specific meanings that are understood by members of one's own culture, for example hand signals.
- Conveying idiosyncratic habits, for example fidgeting with a paperclip when talking or touching one's hair.
- Expressing emotion. This is usually through facial expressions, but can also be conveyed through body posture and distance.

Non-verbal communication is dependent on a number of different variables, for example the context in which it occurs, the individual's personal style and preference, and the personality of the person involved (Burnard 1997; Wallace 2001). For example, an individual may always run their fingers through their hair before speaking. This may be a personal habit of the person and not, for example, an indication of anxiety. Non-verbal communication cannot therefore be used to 'read' what a person is saying, but should be used as clues to what the person may be 'saying'. Any interpretation taken from a patient's non-verbal actions should always be clarified with the patient (Burnard 1997).

Non-verbal behaviour can also be used to convey to a patient that you are listening to what they are saying, for example nodding of the head or using verbal sounds, such as 'Hmm' or 'Yes'. These behaviours are used as minimal prompts to convey to the patient that you are listening and attentive in order to encourage them to continue (Hough 1998).

Verbal communication skills

Verbal communication is thought to be the most common communication method between patients and nurses (Wallace 2001). The skills required for effective verbal communication can assist the nurse in gaining information from the patient as well as communicating and clarifying understanding back to the patient. According to Hough (1998) verbal skills can be categorised as follows:

- questions
- reflection
- selective reflection
- empathy building
- clarifying
- silence.

Questions

Questions can be used for a number of reasons, for example:

- to explore an issue
- to gain further information
- to clarify information and meanings
- to encourage patients to talk.

(Hough 1998)

However, asking too many questions can reduce the amount of active listening that takes place (Hough 1998). Questions can be asked for the nurse's benefit in order to get the facts straight in their own mind and also to understand the patient's subjective experience. There are several types of questions that can be asked, such as closed, open, leading, confronting or funnelling (Burnard 1997; Hough 1998).

Reflection

This is a process of reflecting back or paraphrasing the last few words that the patient has used to encourage them to say more; it is also a way of conveying to the patient that the nurse has actively been listening to what they have said. Skilful reflective responses are those that stay within the patient's internal frame of reference. This means listening to and understanding the issues from their viewpoint (Benner & Wrubel 1989).

Selective reflection

Selective reflection is similar to reflection, except that a specific aspect of what the patient has said or indicated through their non-verbal behaviours is picked up and reflected on. The nurse's reflective response can then include something the patient said from anywhere in the patient's response and not just from the end. Selectively reflecting responses back to patients allows throwaway comments that patients make to be explored (Burnard 1997). Often these remarks contain the real feelings and issues that patients have and require the nurse to acknowledge them and focus in on this issue. The nurse needs to be attentive to what the patient is saying using free-floating attention to be able to pick up on these casual comments and know when to intervene to focus in on these points.

Empathy building

This involves the nurse making statements to the patient to convey that they acknowledge the patient's feelings and that what they are experiencing has been understood. Such feelings may not necessarily be expressed overtly by the patient, but are being implied. This process often involves the nurse listening to the meaning of what the patient is saying and not just to what is being said. Sometimes the interpretation by the nurse of the message being conveyed can be wrong and the patient rejects the empathy-building statement. If this happens, it is suggested that the nurse stops this approach and pays more attention to listening (Burnard 1997).

Clarifying

This can involve checking for understanding by asking the patient or by summarising the conversation to clarify understanding of what has been said so far (Hough 1998). This method can be useful to focus the discussion on particular topics especially if the patient has identified a number of different topics in a short space of time. Clarifying enables the nurse to stay with what the patient is saying and also to ensure effective interpretation of what the patient has said.

Silence

Silence can be a difficult skill to develop and involves more than being quiet. Silence requires nurses to be physically and emotionally present with the patient attending to everything they 'say'. Silence allows patients time to collect their thoughts or to experience a strong emotion or feeling. Breaking the silence inappropriately can intrude on this process. A great deal can be communicated through silence, although it can be uncomfortable at first and requires practice and a conscious effort on the part of the nurse to stay with the patient throughout this period.

Verbal communication refers not just to the words that people say and the meanings these have (linguistics), but also to the way that the words have been said. The way in which words are communicated is referred to as paralinguistic communication (Burnard 1997) and includes elements such as:

- timing
- volume
- pitch
- accent.

Like non-verbal behaviours, paralinguistic aspects of communication could serve as indicators as to how the patient is feeling, but has not expressed in words (Burnard 1997). However, again such indicators should only be used as clues to what the patient is saying and must be validated with the patient. Therefore, nurses can pick up communication clues from non-verbal and paralinguistic communications as well as from the words that the patient uses.

To communicate effectively nurses need to 'hear' what is being communicated by the patient and be able to communicate this understanding back (Kruijver *et al.* 2000). 'Hearing' involves:

- listening to what is said by patients and families
- observing and listening to what is not said through interpreting skills
- communicating understanding of what is said
- responding to the patient's communication.

Barriers to communication

There are a number of ways that communication can be impeded, for example:

- not listening
- blocking
- cultural differences
- disability.

(Barr 2001)

Not listening

Listening can be impeded by the following distracting factors.

- External factors such as noise, interruption and physical discomfort.
- Response rehearsal when the nurse becomes preoccupied with what will be said in reply.
- Fact finding, when too many questions are asked in search of details and facts, instead of listening to the overall message.
- Being judgemental and making mental judgements about the speaker's behaviour.
- Problem solving. Concentrating on trying to solve the patient's problems in your head will prevent listening.
- Tiredness and stress.
- Illness and pain.
- The nurse having had similar experiences to those described by the patient.

(Barr 2001)

Blocking

Nurses can prevent patients from sharing their experiences or how they are feeling by using blocking behaviours. Blocking is when a nurse actively moves the topic of conversation away from a patient's disclosures or expressed feelings (Booth *et al.* 1996). Blocking behaviours can be either conscious or unconscious. Conscious blocking can occur for a number of reasons such as stress, inability to deal with the patient's issues at that present time and not knowing what to say to the patient. Unconscious blocking is normally through a nurse not having the communication skills needed to allow the patient to express their feelings (Kruijver *et al.* 2001; Wilkinson *et al.* 2002).

Cultural differences

The meanings of unspoken and spoken language are learnt through a process of socialisation (Barr 2001). This process of socialisation varies in different countries, geographical locations and communities. There are also differences between social classes and ages (Wallace 2001). Therefore different body language and words may have different meanings depending on the patient's and nurse's experience of socialisation. For this reason it is vital that meanings are clarified with patients during assessment to ensure that a shared understanding of the issues under discussion are defined (Kruijver *et al.* 2001).

The spoken word is the communication tool most often used by nurses within nurse–patient interaction. Different spoken languages between the nurse and the patient can cause difficulties in communicating, assessing needs and in the development of a relationship (Kruijver *et al.* 2001; Wallace 2001). Nurses can use channels other than the spoken word, for example using body language and gestures. However, to be able to assess the patient's needs accurately an interpreter will be needed (Barr 2001). An interpreter could be from a central translating service or a member of the family. However, it is important to recognise that the latter may have implications on how freely the patient will communicate. For example, if a young son is the interpreter, a mother may feel inhibited in disclosing her true feelings and issues to her son as well as the nurse.

Disabilities

Certain disabilities can prevent a patient from using all aspects of communication. For example, aphasic patients who are unable to communicate verbally may rely on non-verbal and written communication to express themselves. Similarly, a patient may be able to verbalise, but due to a neuromuscular condition may not be able to convey effective non-verbal behaviours. Nurses need to be aware of how certain conditions could affect a patient's communication, for example:

- developmental immaturity such as a patient with a learning disability

- sensory loss such as hearing or visual impairments
- neuromuscular difficulties affecting mobility and speech such as multiple sclerosis (MS) or motor neurone disease (MND)
- cerebral trauma, infection or disease, such as cerebral tumours, dementia or Alzheimer's disease
- emotional difficulties or mental health problems, such as clinical depression, stress or anxiety.

Inter- and intra-professional communication

Inter- and intra-professional communication involves conveying messages across different organisations and professions for the benefit of patient care. Such communication within the community occurs within teams and between, for example, community nurses, GPs and practice staff, therapists, hospital, hospice and local authority staff and the voluntary sector. Good communication is an essential component of effective teamwork, which in turn contributes to the quality of care delivered to patients.

The community nurse and patient alone cannot always achieve the assessment and planning of care to meet identified needs. Community nurses may need to refer a patient to other disciplines or organisations in order to meet the needs determined at assessment. The community nurse, with the patient's consent, may also need to discuss issues that have been raised through the assessment process with other specialist community practitioners, for example continence, tissue viability or diabetic specialist nurses. Therefore relationships that the community nurse has with other members of the primary care team and with members of other agencies becomes an important component in the assessment process.

Written communication and record keeping

Effective written communication involves any communication that is expressed in words, either on paper or electronically. This can include:

- paper healthcare records
- electronic health/nursing records
- nursing documentation
- drug administration charts
- referrals
- faxes
- electronic mail.

Like verbal and non-verbal communication, written communication aims to convey a message from a person or group of people to a targeted audience. The written communication documented in the patient's nursing records conveys information to other community nurses and healthcare professionals involved in the patient's care and to the patient and their family.

The NMC (2007, 2009) states that record keeping is an essential part of patient care; it is a tool of professional practice which should assist the care process and not an optional extra. Good records help to protect the welfare of patients by promoting:

- high standards of clinical care
- continuity of care
- better communication and dissemination of information between members of the inter-professional care team
- an accurate account of treatment, care planning and delivery
- the ability to detect problems, such as changes in the patient's condition, at an early stage.

NMC (2009: 6)

Good record keeping is a significant element in ensuring that colleagues have the information they need to provide the necessary and appropriate care for the patient, and the importance of keeping accurate, up-to-date and comprehensive records can never be overstated (Dimond 2005). Failure to maintain such documentation could lead to potential failures in care delivery, which could in turn result in harm being caused to the patient.

Doenges *et al.* (1995) described the goals of documentation as:

- facilitating the delivery of quality patient care
- ensuring documentation of progress with regard to patient-focused outcomes
- facilitating interdisciplinary consistency and the communication of treatment goals and progress.

Therefore when communicating in writing it is important that certain principles are adhered to and the NMC (2007, 2009) advises nurses that patient and client records should:

- be factual, consistent and accurate
- be written as soon as possible after the event, providing current information on the care and condition of the patient
- be written clearly and in such a way that the text cannot be erased
- be written in a way that alterations and additions are dated, timed and signed with the original entry still being clearly visible
- be accurately dated, timed and signed with the signature being clearly identifiable

- not include abbreviations, jargon, meaningless phrases, irrelevant speculation and offensive subject statements
- be readable on any photocopies
- be written wherever possible with the involvement of the patient and their carer
- be written in a way that the patient can understand
- be consecutive
- identify problems that have occurred and the action taken to address them
- provide clear evidence of the care that has been planned, the decisions made, the care delivered and the information shared.

Further advice and guidance on standards for record keeping have been prepared by the Department of Health (1999c) and the Clinical Negligence Scheme for Trusts (CNST) (2005).

Barriers to written communication

There are several barriers to written communication. These barriers can affect both the way that information is presented and the way it is interpreted (Castledine 1998). Barriers can involve the following.

- **Lack of time** by the nurse writing the information will result in badly thought out, unclear and insufficient information being communicated.
- **Jargon and abbreviations** can be misconstrued or not understood by other people reading the information.
- **Written and reading skills** can hinder the clarity of written information given and the ability of individuals, including patients, to read this information. For example, literacy issues.

Data Protection Act 1998

The Data Protection Act 1998 came into force in March 2000 (DH 1998) to protect both the movement and the processing of personal information about individuals. The Act applies to all organisations that collect personal information about individuals but has particular significance for the NHS, which is the largest holder of individuals' most personal information. The Act replaces the previous Data Protection Act (1984), which was devised in response to the large amount of data being held electronically about individuals. The main difference is that the 1998 Act, as well as covering data held on electronic systems, also covers personal data held on other media, including paper. This means that all hand-written information held about patients is now covered within the Act. As community nurses often process large amounts of personal information about patients from various sources, either electronically or manually, it is especially important that they consider whether the way that they are processing this information is in accordance with the principles laid out within the Act (DH 1998). According to Dimond (2005), these principles are designed to ensure that personal data is:

- accurate
- relevant
- held only for the specific designed purposes for which the user has been registered
- not kept for any longer than is necessary
- not disclosed to any unauthorised persons.

There is also a right of subject access whereby the individual should be able, on request and payment of a fee, see what is contained in their records and have it corrected if it is not accurate.

Freedom of Information Act 2000

The Freedom of Information Act grants anyone wide-ranging rights to see all kinds of information held by the government and public authorities that is not governed by the Data Protection Act. It gives the individual the right to ask any public body for all the information they have on a particular subject of choice, and unless there are very good reasons not to, then this information must be provided. Personal information where the applicant is the subject of the information is exempt from the Freedom of Information Act and any individual who wants access to their personal information would need to use the Data Protection Act 1998 as the means of obtaining it (Dimond 2005).

Consent

A patient has a fundamental legal and ethical right to autonomy and self-determination. Ensuring that patients are given this right requires healthcare professionals to obtain agreement from a patient before starting any treatment, physical investigation or providing care for that patient (DCA 2005).

As set out in the Professional Code of Conduct (NMC 2010), nurses have an ethical, legal and professional duty to gain patient consent prior to carrying out any form of patient care. Failure to gain consent could lead to:

- charges of battery in the civil or criminal courts
- claims of negligence if a patient is harmed during a procedure where consent was not gained
- complaints through NHS complaints procedures
- charges of misconduct through the NMC.

Consent must also be obtained from the patient before disclosing confidential information in verbal, written or electronic form, although there are certain exceptions to this rule, for example:

- the patient has given their consent
- disclosure is necessary in the best interest of e.g. the patient or general public
- if not shared with another professional the patient might suffer
- court orders
- statutory duty to disclose information
- public interest
- police
- Data Protection Act 1998 provision.

(Dimond 2005)

By law, the consent obtained from the patient must be valid. There is a fundamental difference between gaining consent from a patient for treatment and gaining valid consent. For consent to be valid:

> It must be given voluntarily by an appropriately informed person who has the capacity to consent to the intervention in question. Acquiescence where the person does not know what the intervention entails is not 'consent'
>
> (DH 2001e: 4)

Therefore, for consent to be valid a patient must:

- be mentally competent to make the particular decision
- have received sufficient information to enable them to make the decision
- be acting voluntarily and not under duress.

Capacity

In order to decide whether a patient has the capacity to give valid consent the following principles apply (DH 2001e).

- The patient must be able to understand and retain information relating to the decision, in particular the consequences of having or not having the intervention in question.
- The patient must be able to use and weigh up this information in the decision-making process.

Adults with capacity

Capacity is related to the retention and understanding of information relating to a particular procedure or planned intervention. An adult over the age of 16 should be assumed to have capacity unless it can be established through appropriate assessment that they lack it (DH 2001e; DCA 2005).

A patient's capacity could differ depending on, for example:

- the intervention being discussed
- the complexity of the decision required
- their health status at the time consent is requested
- fatigue
- shock
- pain
- medication
- anxiety.

For these reasons a patient's capacity to consent must be assessed for each planned intervention. It should not be assumed that a patient incapable of consenting to one procedure is automatically incapable of consenting to another.

Adults without capacity

According to the Mental Capacity Act (DCA 2005), a person lacks capacity if they are unable to make a decision because of an impairment or disturbance in the function of the mind or brain. The individual would be assumed to be incapable of making a decision if they were unable to:

- understand information relevant to the decision
- retain the information
- use and weigh the information as part of the decision-making process
- communicate their decision.

Adults may be permanently or temporarily unable to give valid consent. This could be due to a mental health difficulty, learning difficulty or impaired consciousness. However, people must be given all appropriate help before anyone concludes that they cannot make their own decisions (DCA 2005).

In English law no one is able to give consent to the treatment or examination of an adult patient on his or her behalf (Mental Capacity Act 2007). Therefore parents, relatives or members of the healthcare team cannot consent on behalf of an adult. The principle that must govern the decision about treatment for adults incapable of giving valid consent is whether it is in the 'best interests' of the patient. The decision as to whether or not a procedure or intervention is in the 'best interests' of the patient should be decided by the healthcare professional responsible for carrying out the care intervention or procedure. In making this decision other factors must be taken into consideration:

- the patient's values and preferences when competent
- their psychological health, wellbeing and quality of life

- relationships with family or other carers
- spiritual and religious welfare
- own financial interests.

It is seen as good practice to involve those close to the patient to find out about the patient's views and values before they lost their capacity (DH 2001f). The exception to this is if the patient has previously said that they do not want certain individuals involved.

Young people aged 16–17

For people aged 16 or 17 years the principles for consent remain the same as for adults. Consent must be given voluntarily and must be informed. If the individual is incapable of giving consent then a person with parental responsibility can give consent on their behalf or can override the young person's refusal to give consent. Establishing capacity to consent for 16- or 17-year-olds should follow the same criteria as for adults.

Although legally it is not a requirement for nurses to obtain parental consent in addition to consent from the 16- or 17-year-old, it is seen as good practice to involve those that have parental responsibility in the decision-making process. The exception to this is if the young person has specifically requested that they do not want to involve their parents (DH 2001e).

Sufficient information

Consent is only valid if the patient understands the nature and purpose of the procedure (DH 2001e). However, this information alone is not sufficient to fulfil the practitioner's legal duty of care to the patient. If a practitioner does not give a patient information about the risks of the procedure, such as side effects and potential complications, along with the potential risks of not having the procedure, then the practitioner could be charged with negligence should a patient experience subsequent complications. For example, the patient could claim that the nurse was negligent in not giving certain information about potential complications and had they known about them they would not have consented to the procedure (Sidaway vs Bethlem Royal Hospital Governors and Others 1985).

Voluntary consent

For consent to be valid it must be given voluntarily and freely without pressure or undue influence being placed on the patient to accept or refuse treatment. Pressure may come from family, relatives and healthcare professionals. Community nurses need to be aware of this possibility and, if it is suspected, arrangements need to be made to discuss the proposed care or treatment with the patient individually.

Therefore to ensure that a patient is able to make a balanced judgement on whether to give or withhold their consent, community nurses should inform the patient of:

- any material or significant risks in the proposed treatments
- any alternatives to the treatment
- the risks incurred by not receiving any treatment.

(DOH 2001e)

Some patients may want very detailed information about every possible risk and others may want only the significant risks outlined. Therefore if a patient asks specific questions about their treatment and the risks this should be answered truthfully.

Forms of consent

Valid consent can be implied or given verbally or in writing (DH 2001e).

Implied
Examples of this form of consent are if, having received appropriate information, a patient rolled up their sleeve and proffered their arm to receive a flu vaccination. The inference here being that if the patient was not happy with the amount of information given, or unclear, they would not have voluntarily offered the nurse their arm.

Verbal
A patient can give valid consent verbally (DH 2001f). The patient's records should be used to document the discussion, information given and decisions made (NMC 2008b).

Written
Written consent is often thought to be a more valid form of consent than verbal or implied consent, because it provides physical evidence that a patient has given consent (DH 2001e). Written consent, however, is not proof of valid consent, as it cannot prove that the patient received and understood the information given or that consent was given voluntarily. It is therefore not a legal requirement to gain written consent. Written consent is recommended in the following situations.

- The treatment is complex and risky with the potential for adverse effects.
- Treatment requires a general or local anaesthetic.
- Providing clinical care is not the main purpose.
- The treatment could have significant consequences on the patient's social, employment or personal life.
- Research studies.

- If it is believed that the patient may dispute the care given or they have done in a similar case before.

(DH 2001e, 2001f)

The government has devised a number of standardised consent forms to be used across the country (DH 2001f). These should be available within local work areas. The forms also include a new consent form for when a patient has been assessed to be incapable of giving valid consent. The consent form has a section for recording the rationale for the nurse's decision in terms of capacity and why performing or not performing the procedure is in the patient's best interests.

Refusing and withdrawing consent

Just as a patient has the right to consent to treatment, they also have the right to refuse or withdraw their consent 'for a good reason, a bad reason or no reason at all' (Dimond 2005: 142). The same principles of gaining consent apply to refusing or withdrawing consent. A nurse must establish the patient's capacity to understand the consequences of refusing consent or discontinuing with a treatment. In particular, nurses should bear in mind that factors such as pain, shock and panic may reduce the validity of refusing or withdrawing consent (DH 2001e).

Responsibility for consent

The responsibility for gaining valid consent lies with the practitioner who will be carrying out the nursing intervention (DH 2001f).

Duration of consent

The consent given for a particular intervention remains valid indefinitely unless consent is withdrawn (DH 2001f). Community nurses must ensure that there have not been any changes that could affect the decision made, these could include for example:

- new information about the risks of the intervention
- new treatments that could offer alternatives
- changes to the patient's condition that could affect the likely benefits and risks discussed.

When consent has been gained a long time before the intervention is due to take place, it is seen as good practice to confirm that the patient still wishes to have the intervention performed. This is the case even if there are no changes in the patient's condition or new information to discuss.

Conclusion

The assessment of a patient is a complex process involving a range of nursing knowledge and skills to formulate and plan a patient's care. Assessment involves the community nurse obtaining consent and working in partnership with the patient and other professionals to gather and synthesise information that will enable clinical decisions to be made about the most appropriate care interventions. The SAP has been explored as a means of gathering such information from the patient to decide on their needs and plan care.

The accuracy and effectiveness of a community nursing assessment is reliant on the communication skills of the nurse, the external factors that influence the context in which the assessment is taking place, and the relationship that is developed between the nurse and the patient. This, combined with the multidisciplinary nature of assessment and patient care needs requiring more complex problem solving, means that community nurses must work in partnership with other health and social care professionals (Fonteyn & Cooper 1994).

References and further reading

Aggleton P, Chalmers H (2000) *Nursing Models and Nursing Practice* (2e). Macmillan Press, Hampshire.

Alfaro-Lefevre R (2002) *Applying Nursing Process: promoting collaborative care*. Lippincott, Philadelphia.

Allen D, Bowers B, Diekelmann N (1989) Writing to learn: a reconceptualisation of thinking and writing in the nursing curriculum. *Journal of Nursing Education* 28: 6–11.

Audit Commission (1993) *What Seems to be the Matter? Communication between hospitals and patients*. HMSO, London.

Barr J (2001) Effective communication in primary care. In: Watson N, Wilkinson C (eds) *Nursing in Primary Care*. Palgrave, Hampshire, pp. 139–70.

Barrows H, Feltovich P (1987) The clinical reasoning process. *Medical Education* **21**: 86–91.

Benner P (1984) *From Novice to Expert: excellence and power in clinical practice*. Addison-Wesley, Menlo Park, California.

Benner P, Wrubel J (1989) *The Primacy of Caring: stress and coping in health and illness*. Addison Wesley Menlo Park, California.

Benner P, Tanner C, Chelsea C (1992) From beginner to expert: gaining a differentiated clinical world of critical care nursing. *Advances in Nursing Science* **14**(3): 56–62.

Bolam v Royal Friern Hospital Management Committee (1957) 2 All ER 118.

Bolitho v City and Hackney HA (1997) 4 All ER 771.

Booth K, Maguire P, Butterworth T, Hillier V (1996) Perceived professional support and the use of blocking behaviours by hospice nurses. *Journal of Advanced Nursing* **24**: 522–7.

Bradshaw J (1972) The concept of human need. *New Society* **30**: 640–3.

Bryans A, McIntosh J (1996) Decision making in community nursing: an analysis of the stages of decision making as they related to community nursing assessment practice. *Journal of Advanced Nursing* **24**: 24–30.

Burnard P (1997) *Effective Communication Skills for Health Professionals*. Stanley Thornes, Cheltenham.

Carnevali D, Thomas M (1993) *Diagnostic Reasoning and Treatment Decision Making in Nursing*. Lippincott, Philidelphia.

Carrol J, Johnson E (1990) *Decision Research: a field guide*. Sage, Newbury Park, California.

Castledine G (1998) *Writing Documentation and Communication for Nurses*. Mark Allen, London.

Clinical Negligence Scheme for Trusts (CNST) (2005) *General Clinical Risk Management Standards*. NHS Litigation Authority, London.

Courtney R, Balard E, Fauver S, Gariota M, Holland L (1996) The partnership model: working with individuals, families and communities towards a new vision of health. *Public Health Nursing* **13**: 177–86.

Cowley S, Bergen A, Young K, Kavanagh A (2000) A taxonomy of needs assessment, elicited from a multiple case study of community nursing education and practice. *Journal of Advanced Nursing* **31**: 126–34.

Crow R, Chase J, Lamond D (1995) The cognitive component of nursing assessment. *Journal of Advanced Nursing* **22**: 206–12.

Department for Constitutional Affairs (DCA) (2005) *The Mental Capacity Act*. HMSO, London.

Department of Health (1990) *NHS and Community Care Act*. HMSO, London.

Department of Health (1995) *NHS Continuing Care*. HMSO, London.

Department of Health (1997) *The New NHS: modern, dependable*. HMSO, London.

Department of Health (1998) *The Data Protection Act 1998: protection and use of patient information*. HMSO, London.

Department of Health (1999a) *Saving Lives: our healthier nation*. HMSO, London.

Department of Health (1999b) Ex-Parte Coughlan: Follow-Up Action. HMSO, London.

Department of Health (1999c) *For the Record: managing records in NHS Trusts and health authorities*. Health Service Circular 1999/053. HMSO, London.

Department of Health (2000a) *The National Service Framework for Coronary Heart Disease*. HMSO: London.

Department of Health (2000b) *The National Service Framework for Cancer*. HMSO, London.

Department of Health (2000c) *The National Service Framework for Older People*. HMSO, London.

Department of Health (2000d) *Carers and Disabled Children Act 2000*. HMSO, London.

Department of Health (2000e) *A Plan for Investment, A Plan for Reform*. HMSO: London.

Department of Health (2001a) *Continuing Care: NHS and Social Services responsibilities*. HMSO, London.

Department of Health (2001b) *Guidance on Free Nursing Care in Nursing Homes*. HMSO, London.

Department of Health (2001c) *NHS Funded Nursing Care Practice Guide and Workbook*. HMSO, London.

16

Department of Health (2001d) *Expert Patient Programme: a new approach to chronic disease management for the 21st century*. HMSO, London.

Department of Health (2001e) *Reference Guide to Consent for Examination or Treatment*. HMSO, London.

Department of Health (2001f) *Good Practice in Consent Implementation Guide*. HMSO, London.

Department of Health (2005) *National Service Framework for Long-term Conditions*. DH, London.

Department of Health (2008a) *End of Life Care Strategy: promoting high quality care for all adults at the end of life*. DH, London.

Department of Health (2008b) *High-quality Care For All: next stage review*. DH, London.

Department of Health (2009a) *Fast-track Pathway Tool for NHS Continuing Healthcare*. DH, London.

Department of Health (2009b) *NHS Continuing Healthcare Checklist*. DH, London.

Department of Health (2010) *NHS Continuing Healthcare Practice Guidance*. DH, London.

Dimond B (1995) Exploring the principles of good record keeping in nursing. *British Journal of Nursing* **14**(8): 460–2.

Dimond B (2005) *Legal Aspects of Nursing* (4e). Pearson Education, London.

Doenges M, Moorhouse M, Burley J (1995) *Application of Nursing Process and Nursing Diagnosis* (2e). FA Davis Co, Philidelphia.

Easen P, Wilcockson J (1996) Intuition and rational decision making in professional thinking: a false dichotomy? *Journal of Advanced Nursing* **34**(2): 246–55.

Egan G (1994) *The Skilled Helper* (5e). Brookes/Cole, California.

Ekman P, Friesen W (1969) Nonverbal leakage and cues to deception. *Psychiatry* **32**: 88–106.

Ellershaw J (2007) Care of the dying: what a difference an LCP makes. *Palliative Medicine* **21**: 365–8.

Ellershaw J, Ward C (2003) Care of the dying patient: the last hours or days of life. *British Medical Journal* **326**: 30–4.

Fallowfield L, Jenkins V (1999) Effective communication skills are the key to good cancer care. *European Journal of Cancer* **35**: 1592–7.

Fawcett J (1995) *Conceptual Models of Nursing* (3e). FA Davis Co, Philidelphia.

Fonteyn M, Cooper F (1994) The written nursing process: is it still useful to nursing education. *Journal of Advanced Nursing* **19**: 313–19.

Gallant M, Beaulieu M, Carnevale F (2002) Partnership: an analysis of the concept within the nurse-client relationship. *Journal of Advanced Nursing* **40**: 149–57.

General Medical Council (GMC) 1998) *Seeking Patients' Consent: the ethical considerations*. GMC, London.

Gillick v West Norfolk and Wisbech AHA (1986) AC 112.

Groen G, Patel V (1985) Medical problem solving: some questionable assumptions. *Medical Education* **19**: 95–100.

Hedberg B, Larsson U (2003) Observations, confirmations and strategies – useful tools in decision-making process for nurses in practice? *Journal of Clinical Nursing* **12**: 215–22.

Henderson V (1966) *The Nature of Nursing*. Collier Macmillan, London.

Hennemann E, Lee J, Cohen J (1995) Collaboration: a concept analysis. *Journal of Advanced Nursing* **21**: 103–9.

Holman H, Lorig K (2000) Patients as partners in managing chronic disease. *British Medical Journal* **320**: 527–8.

Hough M (1998) *Counselling Skills and Theory*. Hodder and Stoughton, London.

Hurst K (1993) *Problem Solving in Nursing Practice*. Scutari, London.

Jenny J, Logan J (1992) Knowing the Patient: one aspect of clinical knowledge. *Image* **24**: 254–8.

Junnola T, Eriksson E, Salantera S, Lauri S (2002) Nurses' decision-making in collecting information for the assessment of patients' nursing problems. *Journal of Clinical Nursing* **11**: 186–96.

Kataoka-Yahiro J, Saylor C (1994) A critical thinking model for nursing judgement. *Journal of Nursing Education* **33**(8): 351–6.

King N, Thomas K, Martin N, Bell D, Farrell S (2005) Now nobody falls through the net': practitioners' perspectives on the Gold Standards Framework for community palliative care. *Palliative Medicine* **19**: 619–27.

Kleinmuntz D (1985) Cognitive heuristics and feedback in a dynamic decision environment management. *Science* **31**: 680–702.

Kruijver I, Kerkstra A, Bensing J, van de Weil H (2000) Evaluation of communication training programmes in nursing care'; a review of the literature. *Patient Education and Counselling* **39**: 129–45.

Kruijver I, Kerkstra A, Bensing J, van de Weil H (2001) Communication skills of nurses during interactions with simulated cancer patients. *Journal of Advanced Nursing* **34**: 772–9.

Lamb G, Stempel G (1994) Nursing care management from the client's view: growing as insider expert. *Nursing Outlook* **42**(7): 7–13.

Lawton S, Cantrell J, Harris J (2000) *District Nursing – providing care in a supportive context*. Churchill Livingstone, London.

Lucas A, Wells J (2009) Ethical issues. In: *Oxford Handbook of Palliative Care*. Oxford University Press, Oxford, Chapter 1.

Luker K (1997) Research and configuration of nursing services. *Journal of Advanced Nursing* **6**: 259–67.

Luker K, Austin L, Caress A, Hallett C (2000) The importance of 'knowing the patient': community nurses' constructions of quality in providing palliative care. *Journal of Advanced Nursing* **31**(4): 775–82.

Luker K, Kenrick M (1992) An exploratory study of the sources of influence on the clinical decisions of community nurses. *Journal of Advanced Nursing* **17**: 457–66.

Mahmood-Yousuf K, Munday D, King N, Dale J (2008) Interprofessional relationships and communication in primary palliative care: impact of the Gold Standards Framework. *British Journal of General Practice* **58**(549): 256–63.

Marie Curie (2009) *Liverpool Care Pathway for the Dying Patient: supporting care in the last hours or days of life*. LCP generic version 12. Marie Curie Palliative Care Institute, Liverpool.

May C (1991) Affective neutrality and involvement in nurse–patient relationships: perceptions of appropriate behaviour among nurses in acute medical and surgical wards. *Journal of Advanced Nursing* **16**: 552–8.

May C (1993) Subjectivity and culpability in the constitution of nurse patient relationships. *International Journal Nursing Studies* **30**: 181–92.

McIntosh J (2006) The evidence base for patient and client assessment by community nurses. *Primary Health Care Research and Development* 7: 299–308.

McIntosh J, McCormack D (2001) Partnerships identified within the primary health care literature. *International Journal of Nursing Studies* 38: 547–55.

Mental Capacity Act (2007) The Stationery Office, London.

Munro M, Gallant M, Mackinnon M *et al.* (2000) The Prince Edward Island conceptual model for nursing: a perspective of primary health care. *Canadian Journal of Nursing Research* 32: 39–55.

National Institute for Clinical Excellence (NICE) (2004) *Improving Supportive and Palliative Care for Adults with Cancer.* NICE, London.

Newman C (1991) *The Roper-Logan-Tierney Model in Action.* Macmillan, London.

NHS National End of Life Care Programme (2009) New guide sets the baseline for quality end of life care workforce. Press release, 26 June. NHS NHS National End of Life Care Programme.

NHS National End of Life Care Programme (2011) *Capacity, Care Planning and Advance Care Planning in Life Limiting Illness: a guide for health and social care staff.* NHS National End of Life Care Programme.

Nursing & Midwifery Council (2007) A-Z Advice Sheet – Record Keeping NMC London.

Nursing & Midwifery Council (2008a) *The Code.* NMC, London.

Nursing & Midwifery Council (2008b) *Advice Sheet – Consent.* NMC, London (www.nmc-uk.org/Nurses-and-midwives/Advice-by-topic/A/Advice/Consent; last accessed 1 September 2011).

Nursing & Midwifery Council (2009) *Guidelines for Records and Record Keeping.* NMC, London.

Paul R (1993) The art of redesigning instruction. In: Willsen J, Binker A (eds) *Critical Thinking: how to prepare students for a rapidly changing world.* Foundation for Critical Thinking, Santa Rosa, California.

Paul R, Elder L (2004) *The Miniature Guide to Critical Thinking: concepts and tools.* Foundation for Critical Thinking, Santa Rosa, California.

Pearce v United Bristol Healthcare NHS Trust (1999) 48 BMLR 118.

Pearson A, Vaughan B (1986) *Nursing Models for Practice.* Butterworth-Heinemann, Oxford.

Pritchard P (1995) Learning to work effectively in teams. In: Owens P, Carrier J, Horder J (eds) *Interprofessional Issues in Community and Primary Health Care.* Macmillan, London.

Radwin L (1995) Knowing the patient: a process model for individualised interventions. *Nursing Research* 44: 364–70.

Radwin L (1996) 'Knowing the patient': a review of research on an emerging concept. *Journal of Advanced Nursing* 23: 1142–6.

Redworth F, Watkins D (2000) Multiprofessional working. In: Lawton S, Cantrell J, Harris J (eds) *District Nursing Providing Care in a Supportive Context.* Churchill Livingston, Edinburgh, pp. 59–79.

Reid C, Jeffrey D (2002) Do not attempt resuscitation decisions in a cancer centre: addressing difficult ethical and communication issues. *British Journal of Cancer* 86: 1057–60.

Richardson A (1994) Health needs assessment and resource allocation policy: which comes first? In: Gilman E, Munday S, Somervaille L (eds) *Resource Allocation and Health Needs. From Research to Policy.* HMSO, London, pp. 63–6.

Roberts S, Krouse H (1990) Negotiation as a strategy to empower self care. *Holistic Nursing Practice* 4: 30–6.

Roberts S, Krouse H, Michaud P (1995) Negotiated and non-negotiated nurse-patient interactions. *Clincial Nursing Research* 4: 67–77.

Roper N, Logan W, Tierney A (1985) *The Elements of Nursing: a model for nursing based on a model of living* (2e). Churchill Livingston, Edinburgh.

Roper N, Logan W and Tierney A (1990) *The Elements of Nursing: a model for nursing based on a model of living* (3e). Churchill Livingston, Edinburgh.

Schou K, Hewison J (1999) *Experiencing Cancer.* Open University Press, Buckingham.

Schuster P (2000) *Communication: the key to the therapeutic relationships.* Davis, Philadelphia.

Sidaway v Board of Governors of the Bethlem Royal Hospital (1985) AC 871.

Starhawk M (1987) *Truth or Dare.* Harper and Row, New York.

Steven A, Raftery J (1997) Introduction. In: Steven A, Raftery J (eds) *Health Care Needs Assessment, the Epidemiologically Based Needs Assessment Reviews.* Radcliffe Medical Press, Oxford.

Stewart M (1996) Effective physician-patient communication and health outcomes: a review. *Canadian Medical Association Journal* 152: 1423–33.

Swanson K (1993) Nursing as informed caring for the well-being of others. *Image* 25: 352–7.

Swanson-Kauffman K (1986) Caring in the instance of unexpected pregnancy loss. *Topics in Clinical Nursing* 8(2): 37–46.

Tanner C, Benner P, Chelsea C, Gordon D (1993) The phenomenology of knowing the patient. *Scholarly Inquiry for Nursing Practice: an International Journal* 25(4): 273–80.

Taylor A (2005) Improving practice with the Liverpool care pathway. *Nursing Times* 101(35): 36–7.

Thomas K, Free A (2008) *Prognostic Indicator Guidance.* Royal College of General Practitioners, London.

Tierney A (1998) Nursing Models: extant or extinct. *Journal of Advanced Nursing* 28(1): 77–85.

Tinson S, Hutchinson K (2001) Assessing health needs: putting policy into practice. In: Hyde V (ed) *Community Nursing and Health Care.* Arnold, London, pp. 38–68.

Wallace P (2001) Improving palliative care through effective communication. *International Journal of Palliative Nursing* 7(2): 86–90.

Walsh M (1998) *Models and Critical Care Pathways in Clinical Nursing.* Ballière Tindall, London.

Walsh M (2000) *Nursing Frontiers – Accountability and the Boundaries of Care.* Butterworth-Heinemann, Oxford.

West M, Poulton B (1997) A failure of function: teamwork in primary health care. *Journal of Interprofessional Care* 11(2): 205–16.

Wilkinson S (1991) Factors which influence how nurses communicate with cancer patients. *Journal of Advanced Nursing* 16: 677–88.

18

Wilkinson S, Gambles M, Roberts A (2002) The essence of cancer care: the impact of training on nurses' ability to communicate effectively. *Journal of Advanced Nursing* **40**(6): 731–8.

Wilson J, White C (2011) *Guidance for Staff Responsible for Care After Death (Last Offices)*. NHS National End of Life Care Programme.

Wright K (2002a) The Implications of the Data Protection Act 1998. *Nursing and Residential Care* **4**(8): 376–8.

Wright K (2002b) Caring for the terminally ill: the district nurses' perspective. *British Journal of Nursing* **11**(18): 1180–5.

Wright S (1986) *Building and Using a Nursing Model of Nursing*. Arnold, London.

Wright K (2003) Assessment for long-term care: a snapshot of nursing practice. *British Journal of Community Nursing* **8**(1): 6–14.

Blood glucose monitoring for people with diabetes mellitus

Introduction

Diabetes mellitus is an endocrine disorder caused by the body's inability to produce sufficient insulin. Insulin is produced by the beta cells of the islets of Langerhans in the pancreas, in response to increased levels of glucose in the blood. Insulin is necessary to promote transport and entry of glucose into the cells and other tissues. It also regulates glucose metabolism and lowers the blood glucose level (Williams & Pickup 2003). The two common types of diabetes are classified as type 1 (insulin dependent) and type 2 (non-insulin dependent). Although a family history of diabetes is often found in both types, type 1 is commonly due to autoimmune destruction of the beta cells and patients need insulin to survive. Type 2 diabetes is due to insulin resistance and a defect in insulin secretion; patients do not require insulin to preserve life. Management of type 2 diabetes includes a combination of diet, medication and exercise; the progression to insulin is inevitable for some patients (Wallymahmed & Macfarlane 2005).

The overall aim of diabetes care should be to enable people living with diabetes to achieve a quality of life and life expectancy similar to that of the general population by reducing the complications of the disease (Diabetes UK 2000).

Background evidence

Diabetes is a common long-term condition that affects people of all age groups. It is estimated that more than 95,000 people are newly diagnosed each year in the UK, a further one million adults are thought to have diabetes that is undiagnosed and 3% of the population are living with diabetes (Williams & Farrar 2001). Of those diagnosed, approximately 85% have type 2 diabetes, which is on the increase because of the ageing population, decrease in physical activity and the rising incidence of obesity (Lowey 2005). Worldwide, it is predicted that by 2010 the number of people with diabetes will have doubled since 1997 (Amos et al. 1997).

Healthcare professionals involved in diabetes care have a duty to ensure that patients know how to manage their condition and understand why it is essential to regularly monitor their blood glucose levels. It is recognised that regular monitoring alone will not provide a patient with a good quality of life or reduce the risk of complications. To achieve this patients living with diabetes must:

- have the knowledge, skills and motivation to assess their risks
- understand what they will gain from changing their behaviour and lifestyle and act on that understanding by engaging appropriate behaviours.

(DH 2001)

There is increasing evidence to show that to improve patient outcomes in terms of morbidity and mortality, the careful management of, for example, metabolic control and cardiovascular risk factors, is essential. This can be achieved through the provision of well-organised, integrated diabetes care that incorporates health education (DH 2002; Mold et al. 2008).

Complications arising from diabetes include the following.

- **Microvascular** (damage to the capillaries and small blood vessels):
  - retinopathy
  - neuropathy
  - nephropathy.

District Nursing Manual of Clinical Procedures, First Edition. Edited by Liz O'Brien.
© 2012 Blackwell Publishing Ltd. Published 2012 by Blackwell Publishing Ltd.

- **Macrovascular** (damage to the large blood vessels and arteries):
  - myocardial infarction
  - stroke
  - lower extremity amputation.

The risk of development or progression of complications associated with diabetes increases progressively as the glycosylated haemoglobin (HbA1c) value increases above the normal range for healthy people, which is approximately 4–6% (Barton 2000). The target HbA1c for patients with diabetes is 7.5%, although this will vary depending on the patient. A figure of 6.5% is suggested for patients thought to be at increased risk of developing complications (NICE 2002).

Metabolic control (physiology of blood glucose)

As the level of glucose in the blood rises, the beta cells in the pancreas produce insulin. This decreases the blood sugar by binding with receptors on the cell surfaces, making the cell membranes permeable to glucose in order for:

- muscle cells to use the glucose for energy
- fat cells to metabolise glucose to be stored as triglycerides
- insulin production to enable the liver cell enzymes to convert glucose into glycogen, triglycerides, proteins and amino acids, for use elsewhere in the body
- insulin production to inhibit fat breakdown, which prevents the liver from making ketones.

(Williams & Pickup 2003)

As the blood glucose levels fall in response to insulin production, the alpha cells in the pancreas produce glucagon. This binds with the liver cell receptors to initiate the following chain reaction.

- Stored glycogen is broken down into glucose (glycogenolysis).
- New glucose molecules are converted from amino acids (gluconeogenesis).
- Blood glucose level rises.
- Glucagon, adrenaline, cortisol and growth hormone are released, which helps to inhibit the action of the insulin.

(Williams & Pickup 2003)

Any illness or infection can have an impact on diabetes control. This is due to the interference of biochemical changes that affect the action of insulin

and cause blood glucose levels to rise (Wood 1997) (Table 2.1).

Urine versus blood testing

Glycosuria occurs when the renal threshold for glucose is exceeded, usually 10 mmol/l, but this may vary, as in the following examples.

- During pregnancy, due to a reduced renal threshold for glucose, the blood glucose level will be normal yet glucose will be present in the urine (Owens *et al.* 2005).
- Where the patient's level of fluid intake is low or excessive as this can concentrate or dilute the urine glucose.

Urine glucose testing is suggested as being an unreliable measure as it only approximates the level of glucose over the time that the urine has been produced. It also does not reflect the blood glucose concentration at the time of testing (Tattersall & Gale 1990; American Diabetes Association 2003).

Glycated haemoglobin (HbA1c) is a laboratory blood test that reflects the measurement of glucose exposure over the lifespan of the red blood cell (120 days). It is a weighted measure of average blood glucose control, with 50% of the final value reflecting the final 30 days (Pickup 2003). The HbA1c represents an historical integrated measure of blood glucose and does not reflect the variability in blood glucose concentrations. Therefore the results should not be considered in isolation of additional information derived from blood glucose profiles. It is recommended that a patient's HbA1c should be measured every two to six months (NICE 2002), but this may vary depending on individual hospital or primary care trust's (PCT) protocols.

Capillary blood glucose testing

Capillary blood glucose testing, using a blood glucose meter and capillary blood obtained from a finger-prick sample, is widely used by community nurses to support patient monitoring. This method of testing enables glucose levels to be recorded at a specific moment in time and is therefore an essential aid to:

- assessment of control
- dabetes management
- decision making with regard to treatment titration and changes.

(Burden 2001)

Table 2.1 Biochemical changes present during illness/infection and the associated clinical signs and symptoms

Biochemical changes	Clinical signs
Intercurrent Illness causes increased counter-regulatory hormone excretion that affects the action of insulin and leads to hyperglycaemia	■ Tiredness and lethargy ■ Polydipsia ■ Polyuria/nocturia ■ Dehydration ■ Blood glucose levels >11 mmol/l
Insulin lack and stress hormones together promote fat metabolism to provide energy, but the breakdown of fat is incomplete and leads to the formation of ketone bodies	■ Weight loss ■ Ketonurea ■ Nausea/vomiting ■ Delayed healing
In type 1 diabetes the lack of insulin can increase the risk of developing diabetic ketoacidosis (DKA). It is the hyperglycaemia, dehydration and large amounts of ketones that can lead to life-threatening acidosis	■ Acetone breath ■ Acidotic (Kussmaul) respiration ■ Abdominal pain ■ Nausea/vomiting ■ Confusion and drowsiness
In older adults with type 2 diabetes there is usually some endogenous insulin present, so the risk of DKA is much less. But hyperglycaemia and dehydration can cause hyperosmolar non-ketotic coma (HONK)	■ Marked hyperglycaemia (often >50 mmol/l) ■ Plasma osmolarity raised ■ Confusion ■ Dehydration ■ No ketosis/acidosis
The osmotic diuresis caused by the high blood glucose levels leads to severe dehydration. Electrolytes, e.g. sodium and potassium, shift from within the cells into the circulating plasma and are excreted in the urine	■ Polyuria/nocturia ■ Thirst ■ Low potassium/sodium ■ Weight loss ■ Dry skin ■ Hypotension ■ Tachycardia

Source: Williams & Pickup (2002).

Indications for blood glucose monitoring include:

■ to aid diagnosis of diabetes mellitus
■ to aid diagnosis of hypoglycaemia
■ to aid the management of unstable conditions, e.g. diabetic ketoacidosis and inter-current illness
■ to investigate the effects of the patient's lifestyle, e.g. physical activity, diet or alcohol consumption, on blood glucose levels
■ to monitor blood glucose readings that are incongruent with the clinical status of the patient
■ to aid the titration of drug therapies, e.g. oral hypoglycaemic agents and/or Insulin.

(Burden 2001; Dougherty & Lister 2011)

The frequency of blood glucose monitoring should be determined by presenting clinical, lifestyle and treatment factors. For example:

■ the stability of the patient's diabetes
■ changing or newly commenced insulin regimen
■ type of insulin regimen

■ inter-current problem, e.g. infection, hypoglycaemia
■ type of work undertaken by the patient
■ the patient's level of physical activity/exercise.

The frequency of monitoring should be agreed in partnership with the patient and the healthcare professional responsible for the overall management of their care, for example:

■ community diabetes specialist nurse
■ general practitioner (GP)
■ practice nurse
■ hospital consultant.

To achieve optimal glycaemic control and assess if adjustments to treatment are necessary, it is essential that blood glucose monitoring is carried out at different times over a 24-hour period (Owens *et al.* 2005) (Table 2.2).

Obtaining a capillary blood sample

The recommended site for obtaining a capillary blood sample is the side of the fingertip, this is because it:

Table 2.2 Recommendations for frequency of blood glucose monitoring

Treatment group	Recommended frequency of testing	Suggested usage of strips
Type 2 diabetes – diet and exercise	Not routinely required	N/A
Type 2 diabetes – metformin (+/–glitazone) or glitazone (+/–metformin)	Not routinely required	N/A
Type 2 diabetes –sulphonylurea (+/–other oral anti-diabetic agents)	May require monitoring due to increased risk of hypoglycaemia, e.g. once or twice daily 2–3 times per week at varying times	Up to 30 per month
Type 2 diabetes – combined insulin and oral anti-diabetic therapy	Once daily varying the times of day, i.e. breakfast, lunch, dinner and bedtime. Also timing in relation to meals, i.e. pre- and post-prandial testing	30 per month
Type 2 diabetes – conventional insulin therapy (once or twice daily insulin)	*Stable control* – twice daily 2–3 times per week at varying times	Between 20 and 30 per month
	Less stable control – at least once a day at varying times, to include pre- and post-prandial tests	
Type 1 diabetes or type 2 diabetes on intensive insulin therapy, i.e. multiple daily insulin	Monitor up to 4 times a day.	120 strips per month
	Regular monitoring required to prevent hypoglycaemia and treat hyperglycaemia	
Gestational diabetes	*Diet only* – test once every 2 days (include pre- and post-prandial testing)	Between 50 and 150 strips per month
	Note: some women will require more frequent monitoring	
	Insulin – test at least 4 times a day (include pre- and post-prandial testing)	

Source: Croydon PCT April 2006. Taken from Owens *et al.* 2005.

- allows immediate access to the site
- has a rich blood supply
- improves the ability to completely fill the dosing centre of the test strip.

(McGarraugh *et al.* 2001; Craddock & Hawthorn 2002)

Alternative sites may be considered, e.g. the base or side of the thumb and the forearm. The benefits of using these sites are:

- it allows the fingers to be rested
- the sites are usually free from food and other possible contaminates that could affect results
- it may be the optimum choice for those whose occupation demands a great deal of use of the fingertips, e.g. musicians, computer operators
- it reduces risks to those who are regularly exposed to biohazards, including body fluids, e.g. dental hygienists
- it reduces risks to those working in professions where they are exposed to dirt, e.g. construction workers and mechanics.

(Lock *et al.* 2002)

Blood glucose monitoring training and education

The use of meters by untrained staff can adversely affect the treatment of patients (DH 1996). Therefore it is essential that all community nursing staff involved in blood glucose monitoring receive formal training and understand the importance of a strict quality control (QC) programme (RCN 1993; NMC 2008).

Training should:

- be mandatory (RCN 1993)
- allow the user to understand the applications of the testing (RCN 1993)
- include interpretation of results (RCN 1993)
- enable the identification of variables that contribute to inaccuracy of results (RCN 1993)
- include explanation and discussion of local policy and procedural guidelines
- allow sufficient time for the user to familiarise themselves with the equipment and receive supervision in practice; this should include carrying

out QC procedures and maintenance of the meter.

Recommendations for QC procedures

- QC checks should form part of the maintenance routine with the biochemistry department directly involved.
- QC procedures should aim particularly at maintaining the competence of the equipment user and ensure the reliability of the results being obtained.
- All QC tests must be recorded in the quality control logbook.

(DH 1987)

Types of blood glucose monitoring system

All glucose systems are evaluated for clinical and analytical accuracy before being made available for public use. This is achieved by comparing results obtained from relevant blood samples, e.g. capillary, arterial, venous and neonatal, against two different laboratory reference methods. In addition, clinical studies are supplemented with laboratory evaluation to assess:

- imprecision
- the influence of haematocrit
- operator-dependent steps that may influence the results produced, e.g. insufficient volume of sample and entering an incorrect programme number.

Blood glucose monitoring systems are divided into two categories.

- **Multi-patient use** – this is the only type of system that should be used by healthcare professionals. These can be used with capillary, arterial, venous or neonatal blood samples (Table 2.3).
- **Single individual use** – these are used by people with diabetes for home/self-monitoring and have data management capabilities which allow the patient's and quality control results to be reviewed (Table 2.4).

Limitations of blood glucose meters

When used in accordance with manufacturer's instructions, meters will give a range of acceptable results, e.g. where a laboratory glucose test result is 4 mmol/l, a

Table 2.3 Examples of meters for multi-patient use

Meter type	Manufacturer	Strips used	Quality control
Contour	Ascensia	Ascensia Microfil	Yes
One Touch Ultra	Lifescan	One touch Ultra	Yes
Accu-chek Advantage	Roche	Advantage	Yes
Optium	Medisense	Optium Plus	Yes
Glycomen Glyco	Menarini	Glycomen	Yes

Table 2.4 Examples of meters for single individual use

Meter type	Manufacturer	Strips used	Quality control
Accuchek Active	Roche	Active	Yes
Glucotrend	Roche	Active	Yes
Accuchek Compact	Roche	Compact	Yes

meter could produce a result ranging from 2.8 to 5 mmol/l (Burden 2001). For this reason, meter results should only be used as an assessment guide and not as a single determinant diagnostic tool (Burden 2001).

Contraindications for the use of blood glucose meters

In a number of circumstances it is possible for all blood glucose meters to produce false results and consequently they should not be used (MHRA 2006). It is recommended that a venous blood sample should be obtained for laboratory testing where there is a known or suspected patient diagnosis of:

- severe dehydration
- hypotension
- shock
- peripheral circulatory failure
- hyperosmolar non-ketotic coma (HONK)
- diabetic ketoacidosis (DKA).

Also some meters are not suitable for use with, for example, patients receiving continuous ambulatory peritoneal dialysis. Therefore it is essential that the community nurse is aware of the individual meter's capabilities, prior to using it, and where necessary refers to the relevant meter handbook, community diabetic specialist nurse or manufacturer for advice and guidance.

Maintenance and care of the meter

Maintenance of the meter includes the following.

■ Storage and use of meter – cleaning, temperature range, hazards that may affect use of the meter and changing the batteries.

■ Internal quality control (QC) – how to obtain further supplies of QC solution.
■ Coding/calibration where applicable.
■ Storage and use of strips.

Please refer to the relevant meter handbook for further information regarding individual maintenance requirements.

NB Published evaluation reports are available free of charge to members of the NHS from the relevant manufacturer.

Procedure guideline 2.1 **Guideline for capillary blood glucose monitoring**

Locally agreed policies and equipment for capillary blood glucose monitoring often vary between community provider services. Therefore it is essential that community nurses receive appropriate training and education in specific procedural guidelines, equipment to be used and the manufacturer's instructions prior to carrying out this procedure (RCN 1993).

Equipment

Multi-patient blood glucose meter
Single patient use pricking device/lancet
Test strips (these must be in date and correspond to the programmed code in the meter where applicable)
Control solution (including QC record book)
Sharps bin
Cotton wool or tissues
Non-sterile gloves
Single use disposable apron

Nursing action	Rationale
1 Where appropriate facilities are available, wash hands. Alternatively cleanse hands with antibactericidal alcoholic hand rub (NICE 2003) and apply disposable apron	To prevent the risk of cross-infection/contamination
2 If the patient is known to the service review nursing documentation and current care plan	To update knowledge of patient and maintain patient safety
3 If the patient is unknown to the service a comprehensive assessment must be carried out prior to undertaking the procedure. This should include assessment of the patient's mobility status	To maintain patient safety
4 Explain and discuss the procedure with the patient	To allay any possible anxieties the patient may have and obtain consent for the procedure (Mental Capacity Act 2007)

24

Procedure guideline 2.1 **Guideline for capillary blood glucose monitoring** *(cont'd)*

Nursing action	Rationale
5 Assemble and prepare all equipment on a clean surface, check that: (a) meter is calibrated; (b) test strips match the calibrated code (if applicable); (c) test strips are in date	To prevent disruption to the procedure To prevent contamination of equipment To prevent the risk of erroneous results
6 Cleanse hands with anti-bactericidal alcoholic hand rub (NICE 2003) and apply gloves	To reduce the risk of cross-infection To prevent potential alcohol contamination of the patient's skin
7 Advise the patient to wash and dry their hands thoroughly, if necessary assist them in the procedure. Alcohol-based hand rub should not be used.	To prevent contamination of the result, e.g. from food traces on the finger Alcohol contamination of the patient's skin may produce an inaccurate result
8 Switch meter on, insert strip into meter at the appropriate time and replace cap on the pot of strips	To ensure meter is working correctly and maintain safe storage of strips
9 Select finger to be used to obtain the sample (where possible avoiding the thumb and index finger) ensuring rotation of sites	The thumb and index finger are used frequently to perform daily tasks. Rotation of site will minimise pain and reduce the risk of infection
10 Using appropriate single patient use finger pricking device obtain the sample by pricking the side of the selected finger Wait for 2–3 seconds if a large enough droplet does not form 'milk' the finger to obtain the sample	To prevent the risk of cross-infection (DH 1990) To reduce pain, as the side of the finger is less sensitive than the fingertip Waiting for 2–3 seconds allows the capillaries to open and release blood
11 Apply blood to the test strip according to the manufacturer's instructions Dispose of used lancing device into the sharps bin	To prevent the risk of obtaining an error message and the need to repeat the procedure (this can happen if the strip is dosed with blood before the meter is ready) To prevent the risk of needle-stick injury and cross-infection
12 Apply pressure to puncture site with cotton wool/tissue	To stem bleeding To prevent cross-contamination and ensure patient safety
13 Record result immediately it appears on the meter display screen in the appropriate documentation	To ensure correct result is recorded To maintain patient safety
14 Remove and dispose of test strip and any soiled materials	To prevent the risk of cross-infection
15 Remove and dispose of gloves and apron in accordance with health and safety regulations and local policy	To prevent the risk of cross-infection and contamination
16 If appropriate facilities are available wash and dry hands thoroughly, alternatively apply alcohol based hand rub (NICE 2003)	To prevent the risk of cross-infection

(Continued)

Procedure guideline 2.1 **Guideline for capillary blood glucose monitoring** *(cont'd)*

Nursing action	Rationale
17 Ensure meter has switched off	To preserve the battery life
	Some meters will switch off automatically once the strip has been removed, others will wait for 2 minutes before switching off
18 Complete nursing documentation	To maintain patient safety
	To ensure continuity of care
	To provide baseline findings that may be referred to at a later date if necessary
	To ensure accurate and contemporaneous records are kept
	Documentation should provide clear evidence of care planned, decisions made and care delivered (NMC 2009)

References and further reading

American Diabetes Association (2003) Test of glycaemia in diabetes. *Diabetes Care* **26**: 106–8.

Amos AF, McCarty DJ, Zimmet P (1997) The rising global burden of diabetes and its complications: estimates and projections to the year 2010. *Diabetic Medicine* **14**(Supp 5): S1–85.

Barton S (2000) *Clinical Evidence*, Issue 4. BMJ Publishing Group, London.

Burden M (2001) Diabetes: blood glucose monitoring. *Nursing Times* **97**(8): 36–9.

Craddock S, Hawthorn J (2002) Pain, distress and blood glucose monitoring. *Journal of Diabetes Nursing* **6**(6): 188–91.

Department of Health (1987) *Hazard Notice* (13). Department of Health, London.

Department of Health (1990) *Lancing Devices for Multi-patient Capillary Sampling; Avoidance of Cross Infection by Correct Selection and Use.* Department of Health, London.

Department of Health (1996) *Extra-Laboratory Use of Blood Glucose Meters and Test Strips: Contraindications, Training and Advice to Users.* Medical Devices Agency Adverse Incident Centre Safety Notice 9616, June.

Department of Health (2001) *National Service Framework for Diabetes: Standards.* Department of Health, London.

Department of Health (2002) *National Service Framework for Diabetes.* Department of Health, London.

Diabetes UK Report (2000) *Recommendations for the Management of Diabetes in Primary Care.* Diabetes UK, London.

Dougherty L, Lister S (2011) *The Royal Marsden Hospital Manual of Clinical Nursing Procedures* (8e). Wiley-Blackwell, Oxford.

Lock JP, Szuts EZ, Malomo KJ, Anagnostopoulos A (2002) Whole-blood glucose testing at alternate sites: glucose values and haematocrit of capillary blood drawn from the fingertip and forearm. *Diabetes Care* **25**(2): 337–41.

Lowey A (2005) Drug treatment of type 2 diabetes in adults. *Nursing Standard* **20**(11): 55–64.

McGarraugh G, Price D, Schwartz S, Weinstein R (2001) Physiological influence on one-off finger glucose testing. *Diabetes Technology and Therapeutics* **3**(3): 367–76.

Medicines & Healthcare Products Regulation Agency (MHRA) (2006) Blood glucose meters, press release 18 December (last accessed 1 October 2011).

Mental Capacity Act (2007) The Stationery Office, London.

Mold F, Forbes A, While A (2008) The challenges of managing type 2 diabetes in primary care. *Nursing Times* **104**(7): 32–3.

National Institute for Clinical Excellence (NICE) (2002) *Management of Type 2 Diabetes – Managing Blood Glucose Levels (Guideline G).* Nice, London.

National Institute for Clinical Excellence (NICE) (2003) *Infection Control: Prevention of Health-care Associated Infection in Primary and Community Care (Clinical Guideline 2).* NICE, London.

Nursing and Midwifery Council (2008) *The Code: Standards of Conduct, Performance and Ethics for Nurses and Midwives.* NMC, London.

Nursing and Midwifery Council (2009) *Guidelines for Records and Record Keeping.* UKCC, London.

Owens D, Barnett AH, Pickup J *et al.* (2004) Blood glucose self-monitoring in type 1 and type 2 diabetes: reaching a multidisciplinary consensus. *Diabetes and Primary Care* **6**(1): 8–16.

Owens D, Barnet AH, Pickup J *et al.* (2005) The continuing debate on self-monitoring of blood glucose in diabetes. *Diabetes and Primary Care* **7**(1): 9–21.

Pickup JC (2003) Diabetic control and its measurement. In: Pickup JC, Williams G (eds) *Textbook of Diabetes* (3e), Chapter 34. Blackwell Publishing, Oxford.

Royal College of Nursing (RCN) (1993) *RCN Forum Guidelines on the Use of Blood Glucose Monitoring Equipment by Nurses in Clinical Areas.* RCN, London.

Tattersall RB, Gale EAM (1990) *Diabetes: Clinical Management.* Churchill Livingstone, Edinburgh.

Wallymahmed M, MacFarlane I (2005) The value of group insulin starts in people with type 2 diabetes. *Journal of Diabetes Nursing* **9**(8): 287–90.

Williams R, Farrar H (2001) Diabetes mellitus. In: Health Needs Assessment Series: *The Epidemiological-based Needs Assessment Reviews.* Radcliffe Medical Press, Oxford.

Williams G, Pickup JC (2003) *Handbook of Diabetes.* Blackwell Science, London.

Wood J (1997) Coping with intercurrent infection. *Diabetic Nursing* **26**: 11–13.

Bowel management

Introduction

Bowel management is a fundamental aspect of nursing and yet often receives less attention than other aspects of nursing care. Bowel problems impact significantly on patients' quality of life and effective nursing management of bowel care can make a real difference, but is often relegated to junior nurses, students and healthcare assistants. Nurses are in a very privileged position of being able to physically care for the bodies of others and deal with bodily functions that would normally be considered private (Lawler 1991). Nurses may often engage in this procedure without discussing the subject with patients – as it may be something that neither party necessarily wishes to talk about, possibly due to embarrassment on both sides. Bowel care demands a high level of expertise and nurses are ideally placed to assist patients with this bodily function in a caring and sensitive manner.

Bowel problems of constipation, chronic diarrhoea and faecal incontinence affect significant numbers of people in the UK. It is estimated that constipation affects up to 20% of the population at some point during their life and is more prevalent among females (Kamm 2003). Diarrhoea can be experienced by anyone as a one-off event, but between 4 and 5% of the population are troubled by chronic diarrhoea and watery stools (Thomas *et al.* 2003). This can in turn be associated with faecal incontinence, but faecal incontinence can also occur for a variety of other reasons. Prevalence studies of faecal incontinence report wide variation, but it is generally accepted that this problem affects approximately 5% of the population. All of these problems are more prevalent among certain groups of patients, such as older people or those with neurological problems. Each of these specific bowel problems is addressed within this chapter.

Background evidence

Anatomy and physiology of digestion and absorption

The gastrointestinal tract

The function of the gastrointestinal (GI) tract is to ingest food and fluids, process digestion and absorption, and eliminate waste materials such as faeces. The GI tract runs from the mouth to the anus and includes a variety of organs including the mouth, small bowel (duodenum, jejunum and ileum), large bowel (caecum, ascending colon, transverse colon, descending colon and sigmoid colon), rectum and anus.

Digestion and absorption

The digestion process can be seen as a series of steps. Initially ingestion of food and fluids occurs, generally via the mouth but it may also be via a nasogastric tube for example. The teeth are used to mechanically break down the food and mix it with saliva to form a food bolus. Saliva is produced at a rate of about 1500 ml daily (Black & Hyde 2005) and performs a variety of roles. It helps to keep the mouth healthy and it also contains the enzyme salivary amylase to break down cooked starch and thus it commences chemical digestion (Richards 2005).

The food is then swallowed into the stomach via the oesophagus. Swallowing may be affected by a number of neurological and other conditions, such as stroke, Parkinson's disease or oral tumours. Once swallowed, the food bolus progresses towards the stomach via peristalsis, and the process of digestion is no longer under voluntary control. Peristalsis (muscle contraction to propel food throughout the length of the GI tract) and

District Nursing Manual of Clinical Procedures, First Edition. Edited by Liz O'Brien.
© 2012 Blackwell Publishing Ltd. Published 2012 by Blackwell Publishing Ltd.

segmentation (a backwards and forwards action of the bowel muscles) help to break down the food, mix the food with the secretions and move the food bolus further along the GI tract (Thibodeau & Patton 2007). This is mechanical breakdown of the food.

Once the food reaches the stomach, the stomach begins to mix the food with the various gastric secretions to produce chyme. The stomach can hold approximately 1500 ml and about 3 l of gastric secretions are produced daily, which are reabsorbed later in the GI tract (Black & Hyde 2005). Food generally remains in the stomach for about three to four hours (Thibodeau & Patton 2007). When the chyme reaches the jejunum there is further digestion of proteins, fats and carbohydrates.

Absorption begins in the stomach and continues all the way through the gut to the colon. There are specific areas that absorb the various dietary components. Not much is absorbed from the stomach, except alcohol for example (Tortora & Derrickson 2006); fluids are mainly absorbed from the small bowel and vitamin B_{12} is absorbed via the terminal ileum.

The body also secretes substances into the duodenum to continue the chemical breakdown of the food. The common bile duct and the pancreatic duct enter into the mid-section of the duodenum (McGrath 2005). Bile acids help to neutralise the chyme exiting the stomach (Aspinall & Taylor-Robinson 2002), and emulsify fats to fatty acids, monoglycerides and glycerol (Thibodeau & Patton 2007). Bile also stimulates peristalsis and therefore acts as a natural laxative and, incidentally, as a deodorant for the faeces. Finally, bile is used to excrete toxic substances, poisons, broken-down products of alcohol, drugs and the by-products of red blood cells (Black & Hyde 2005).

The pancreas secretes up to 1.5 l daily of pancreatic juice into the duodenum (Black & Hyde 2005). It contains the digestive enzymes trypsin, pancreatic lipase and pancreatic amylase, which are used to break down protein, carbohydrates and fat. Calcium, magnesium, iron, protein, fats and starch are absorbed in the duodenum (Hinchliff 1981).

The small bowel is able to absorb nutrients via the many folds of intestinal mucosa. The surface area within the small bowel is increased by the mucosal folds and also by the villi (small 'fingers' that line the bowel lumen). It is important to increase the absorptive capacity of the bowel to ensure that we receive adequate nutrition. However, the villi can become damaged, for example as a result of, prolonged starvation, radiation damage, coeliac disease or Crohn's disease (Richards 2005) and this damage may cause weight loss or diarrhoea.

In the last part of the small bowel (the terminal ileum) sodium, potassium, chloride, bicarbonate, bile salts and vitamin B_{12} are absorbed (Stevens & James 2003). Large volumes of fluid are absorbed, not only those fluids that have been ingested but also the majority of the digestive enzymes that were added to the food on its journey through the gut.

The colon

The caecum is the first part of the colon and is a short, blind-ended pouch (Snell 2004). The ileocaecal valve prevents flow of waste back into the ileum. The vermiform appendix joins the caecum and is usually about 9 cm long (Watson 2002). The function of the appendix is uncertain, but it can cause problems and require surgical intervention if it becomes inflamed.

The ascending colon arises from the caecum and lies up the right side of the abdomen (Snell 2004). When the faeces pass along the ascending colon water is absorbed and the faecal output thickens. Additionally sodium, potassium, chloride and glucose are absorbed. The transverse colon continues from the ascending colon following the hepatic flexure and lies from right to left across the abdominal cavity. Within the transverse colon the faeces become thicker and mucus is secreted from the bowel epithelium (Richards 2005). The mucus lubricates the bowel mucosa and protects against contents that may be irritating.

The faeces pass from the transverse colon through the splenic flexure to the descending colon and on to the sigmoid colon, which lies within the pelvis. A problem that occurs predominantly in the sigmoid colon is diverticular disease. Diverticulitis is an acute inflammatory condition that is usually managed conservatively, with dietary manipulation, but surgery may be required as an emergency if the bowel perforates.

As the colon is able to absorb fluids from the waste, only 100–200 ml of faeces is normally passed rectally on each occasion (Tortora & Derrickson 2006). Faeces consist predominantly of water and also indigestible matter from the diet and bacteria (Watson 2002). As the faeces pass through the colon they become more solid and formed and can become hard and pellet-like if they remain within the colon for extended periods of time, resulting in constipation. The colon stores the faeces prior to defecation and faecal material is moved along the colon by peristalsis. Peristalsis within the gut is most active on waking in the morning and in addition a very strong peristaltic wave occurs about three times each day, most strongly in the morning after breakfast, which may result in a bowel motion. Gut motility may also be stimulated and increased following ingestion of food into the stomach, the gastro-colic reflex. Peristaltic

30

activity propels faeces in both directions through the colon, although the bulk of the movement is towards the rectum.

Colonic bacteria are important to health but may also cause problems if the natural balance is altered, for example following some antibiotic treatments. Antibiotics may eradicate various bacteria that the body requires and in doing so can allow other bacteria that are usually present in low volumes to proliferate. This may lead to *Clostridium difficile* diarrhoea for example. Bacterial fermentation is also necessary for the production of vitamin K (Tortora & Derrickson 2007). Additionally, colonic bacteria ferment carbohydrates. This process releases gas such as methane (McGrath 2005). The human body produces about 500 ml of flatus daily (Richards 2005) but this increases with the consumption of high-fibre foods. Often there is an odour associated with flatus, which can be due to gases that include hydrogen sulphide. Most people pass flatus an average of 20 times per day.

Colonic cancer can occur, with symptoms that include rectal bleeding, tenesmus (the desire to defecate with little result) and altered bowel habit. Suspected colonic cancer needs urgent medical review and endoscopic examination to determine if further therapy is required. Additionally, inflammatory bowel disease, which includes ulcerative colitis and Crohn's disease, can affect the GI tract. Ulcerative colitis affects the colon, while Crohn's disease can affect any part of the GI tract. Symptoms of these conditions can include abdominal pain and diarrhoea.

The rectum, anus and defecation

Eventually the faeces move to the rectum. Faeces within the rectum are usually in solid form. The anal canal is approximately 3 cm in length (Marieb 1998), although it may be slightly longer in males. The anal canal is surrounded by two sphincters, the involuntary internal anal sphincter and the voluntarily controlled external sphincter. Both sphincters are usually closed unless defecation is occurring (Tortora & Derrickson 2006). The anus is extremely sensitive and has the ability to differentiate between solid, liquid and gas, as well as to selectively allow gas to pass if there is a combination within the rectum.

Once the amount of faeces within the rectum reaches a certain volume or if the consistency is liquid, as with diarrhoea, the nerves supplying the anal sphincters send a message to the brain and the individual becomes aware of the need to defecate (Norton & Chelvanayagam 2004). Once toilet trained, we have the ability to voluntarily control defecation and if this urge to defecate is ignored it will abate, only to return again a short while later as the next sampling process takes place. There is no exact determination of the ideal number of defecations per week and it is not necessary to have a bowel motion every day. It is generally accepted that the normal limits for bowel frequency are not more than three times per day and not less than once every three days (Norton & Chelvanayagam 2004).

The anal sphincters can become ineffective either because of damage due to trauma, for example during childbirth in women, or because of spinal nerve damage, which may lead to anal incontinence. This can be flatus incontinence through to incontinence of solid or liquid faecal material, both of which can be very distressing. Faecal incontinence may also be due to a number of other reasons and requires investigation to exclude other causes.

Constipation

Constipation is one of the most common digestive complaints and it has been estimated that £46 million is spent each year in England alone on laxatives (DH 2000), but these tend to lose their effect over time. It is more common in women than men, and prevalence increases with age. Reported prevalence rates in the UK vary widely between studies, from 8.2 to 52% of women, and 39% of men (Petticrew *et al.* 1997).

Definition

Constipation is a symptom-based disorder defined as 'unsatisfactory defecation and is characterised by infrequent stools, difficult stool passage, or both. Difficult stool passage includes straining, a sense of difficulty passing stool, incomplete evacuation, hard/lumpy stools, prolonged time to stool or need for manual manoeuvres to pass stool' (American College of Gastroenterology Chronic Constipation Task Force 2005). Stools can be dry and hard, and may be abnormally large, or small. It is a symptom, not a disease, reflecting either slowed colonic transit and/or impairment of rectal emptying (Emmanuel 2004). In view of the difficulty in defining constipation, an international committee has recommended a definition of chronic functional constipation, known as the Rome criteria, which are now in their third edition for use in research studies (Longstreth *et al.* 2006) (Box 3.1).

Classification, categories and causes

Based on the Rome criteria, constipation has been classified on the basis of stool frequency, consistency and

---

Box 3.1 Rome III Criteria for functional constipation

1 Must include two or more of the following:
   a Straining during at least 25% of defecations
   b Lumpy or hard stools in at least 25% of defecations
   c Sensation of incomplete evacuation for at least 25% of defecations
   d Sensation of anorectal obstruction/blockage for at least 25% of defecations
   e Manual manoeuvres to facilitate at least 25% of defecations (e.g. digital evacuation, support of the pelvic floor)
   f Fewer than three defecations per week
2 Loose stools are rarely present without the use of laxatives
3 There are insufficient criteria for the diagnosis of irritable bowel syndrome

Criteria fulfilled for at least 3 months with symptom onset at least 6 months prior to diagnosis.
(Longstreth *et al.* 2006)

Box 3.2 Conditions associated with constipation

Functional bowel disorders
Irritable bowel syndrome

Metabolic conditions
Diabetes mellitus
Hypercalcaemia
Hypokelaemia
Heavey metal poisoning
Hypothyroidism
Hypomagnesaemia
Uraemia

Mechanical obstruction
Colon cancer
External compression from malignant lesion
Rectocele
Strictures: diverticular or postischaemic
Postsurgical abnormalities
Anal fissures
Megacolon

Myopathies
Scleroderma
Amyloidosis

Neuropathies
Spinal cord injury or trauma
Cerebrovascular disease
Parkinson's disease
Multiple sclerosis
Autonomic neuropathy

Miscellaneous conditions
Depression
Eating disorders
Immobility
Cardiac diseases

---

difficulty of defecation. Most cases of constipation are simple, relate to an underlying cause or other risk factor and are easily treated with simple measures. Common factors that contribute to constipation include:

- age
- reduced mobility
- poor dietary and fluid intake, e.g. irregular meals, poor appetite, reduced fibre
- lifestyle
- environment: lack of privacy, poor toilet facilities
- pregnancy
- painful anorectal conditions, e.g. haemorrhoids, anal fissure.

Ageing may not cause constipation as such, but the increasing prevalence of constipation in the older person may reflect changes in mobility, diet, fluid intake and polypharmacy (Pettigrew *et al.* 1997).

However, in some cases, there is no obvious physical or pathological cause; this is known as idiopathic or functional constipation. It may result from a defecatory disorder, such as pelvic floor muscle dysfunction, or a slow gut transit time (Lembo & Cammilleri 2003). Slow transit may be caused by dietary habits, chronic diseases (Box 3.2), polypharmacy or medication (Box 3.3), decreased mobility and altered patterns of fluid intake (Maleki 2002). Patients with functional constipation may require referral to a specialist centre for further

assessment and treatment, when simple interventions have failed to resolve the symptoms.

Disorders of defecation may result in prolonged defecation and feelings of anal blockage requiring manual manoeuvres to aid in the passage of the stool. They can also be caused by painful anorectal diseases such as anal fissures (Box 3.4) or anorectal incoordination (Lembo & Cammillieri 2003).

Assessment of constipation

History

History taking in the main will seek to establish a clear picture of the patient's symptoms, how they are affected

Box 3.3 Medications that have constipation as a side effect

Anticholinergic agents
Tryciclic antidepressants
Calcium channel blockers
Sympathomimetics
Antipsychotics
Diuretics
Antihistamines
Antiparkinsonian drugs
Opiates
Aluminium containing antacids
Iron supplements
Non-steroidal anti-inflammatory agents
Antidiarrhoeal medications

Box 3.4 Indications for referral 'RED FLAGS'

1. Rectal bleeding
2. Persisting change in bowel habit
3. Anaemia
4. Unexplained weight loss
5. Nausea and anorexia
6. Abdominal pain

(NICE 2010)

by them, and what they understand about their constipation. History of dietary habits and fluid intake, as well as a complete list of prescribed and over-the-counter medication (Box 3.3) should be taken. A full medical, surgical, obstetric and psychological history is required and the assessment is then completed by asking about specific bowel symptoms including:

- bowel frequency
- longest time bowels not opened for
- stool form/consistency Bristol Stool Form Scale (Figure 3.1)
- passing blood (on wiping/in toilet)
- mucus
- straining
- urge to defecate (in abdomen/in rectum)
- feeling of incomplete evacuation
- digitation (using a finger to help empty the rectum either per rectum (PR)/per vagina (PV) – to support a rectocele, a protrusion or herniation of the rectum into the vagina; Lembo & Camilleri 2003)
- pain (in abdomen/in rectum; on defecation; relieved by defecation)
- bloating
- impact on daily life and relationships.

(Norton & Chelvanayagam 2004)

A careful, detailed history and physical examination will identify most secondary causes of constipation. It is important to decide if referral to the GP or gastroenterologist is necessary and whether urgent tests are required (Lembo & Camilleri *et al.* 2003; Emmanuel 2004). Most importantly, any history suggestive of colon cancer

should be identified, particularly in those over the age of 50 years, including any 'red flags' (Box 3.4).

Consent
Valid consent must be obtained before starting any treatment, investigation or care for a patient (DH 2001). This designates the right of patients to self-determination and is the fundamental basis of the expectation of best practice (DH 2001).

Physical examination
The aim of a physical examination is primarily to detect:

- masses in the abdomen and the rectum.
- the presence and degree of faecal loading by performing a digital rectal examination (DRE, discussed later)
- faecal impaction
- faecal incontinence.

The rectal examination should also include the assessment of the anal sphincter muscle tone, abnormal perineal descent and/or ballooning during straining.

Treatment of constipation

Initial and primary care management
Most cases of constipation are successfully treated within primary care with simple non-pharmacological measures, for example the review and where possible discontinuation of medication with constipating side effects. Patient education is also an essential part of treatment and an understanding of normal bowel function goes a long way towards dispelling patient-held myths and misconceptions about constipation. For instance, patients may be unaware that a daily bowel motion is unnecessary and that it is normal to have a bowel movement from between three times a day to three times per week (Norton & Chelvanayagam 2004).

THE BRISTOL STOOL FORM SCALE

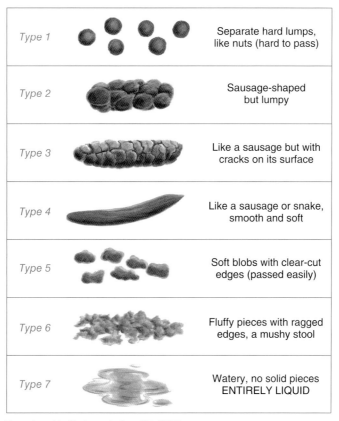

Type 1		Separate hard lumps, like nuts (hard to pass)
Type 2		Sausage-shaped but lumpy
Type 3		Like a sausage but with cracks on its surface
Type 4		Like a sausage or snake, smooth and soft
Type 5		Soft blobs with clear-cut edges (passed easily)
Type 6		Fluffy pieces with ragged edges, a mushy stool
Type 7		Watery, no solid pieces ENTIRELY LIQUID

Reproduced by kind permission of Dr KW Heaton,
Reader in Medicine at the University of Bristol.
© 2000 Produced by Norgine Pharmaceuticals Limited.

Figure 3.1 Bristol stool chart.

Simple measures start with a trial of increased fibre, fluid intake, exercise and lifestyle changes. However, there is little evidence that increasing dietary fibre is effective in the management of severely constipated patients and may induce symptoms such as abdominal distension and flatulence, particularly in those patients with a slow gut transit, i.e. beyond 48 hours (Norton & Chelvanayagam 2004). In addition, there is no evidence that stool consistency and constipation can be affected by increasing fluid intake or exercise (Muller-Lissner *et al.* 2005), but if the patient is dehydrated then increasing fluid intake may help. Lifestyle changes around a toileting routine (Box 3.5) to instil good defecatory habits may also help. These may have been forgotten due to a frenetic pace of life, which leaves little time for unhurried defecation and in which the urge to defecate is often ignored.

If there is little or no response within 2–3 weeks, then laxatives can be administered (Maleki 2002). The lowest effective dose of a laxative should be used, and should be reduced as soon as symptoms begin to resolve. Treatment may begin with a bulk-forming laxative, e.g. Fybogel, but these may exacerbate slow gut transit and cause abdominal cramps and bloating (BNF 2011). If the patient's stool remains hard, then add or switch to an osmotic laxative, e.g. Lactulose. If stools are soft but difficult to pass, or defaecation is incomplete, then a stimulant laxative may be added, e.g. senna or bisacodyl (Dougherty & Lister 2011). Patients should be advised that laxatives can be stopped once the stools become

34

soft and easy to pass. In the older person, faecal impaction is initially treated with suppositories/enemas, but Movicol is also licensed for treatment of faecal impaction (BNF 2011). Digital removal of faeces may rarely be required (RCN 2006).

Biofeedback

Biofeedback is a form of specialist treatment that seeks to normalise bowel function in those with chronic, idiopathic constipation. This is achieved by relaying information about a normally subconscious physiological process to a patient in real time. The patient may learn to change the process of defecation, substituting previous behaviours with correct defecatory patterns (Horton 2004). The success rate of biofeedback therapy in the treatment of intractable constipation has been reported up to 80% in some studies (Glia et al. 1997). Patients with underlying psychological conditions may find psychological counselling a helpful adjunct to biofeedback therapy. Biofeedback is normally carried out in a secondary or tertiary referral centre, is generally a nurse-led area of care and consists of up to four appointments, each session lasting between 30 and 60 minutes. During the clinic sessions patients are instructed in a series of techniques (Chiotakakou-Faliakou et al. 1998; Emmanuel & Kamm 2001; Horton 2004).

Surgery

Surgery for slow transit constipation should only be considered as a last resort when all other measures have failed. The preferred procedure is subtotal colectomy and ileorectal anastomosis. Long-term success has been

demonstrated, with patient satisfaction rates identified between 80 and 100% (Levitt et al. 2011), with complications ranging from diarrhoea, faecal incontinence and recurrent obstruction to pelvic sepsis. Patient selection is paramount. Success is more likely in patients with slow transit constipation in the absence of rectosigmoid outlet delay and psychological disorders.

Laxatives

Poulton and Thomas found in 1999 that community nurses spent up to 10% of their time treating constipation, at an estimated cost of £810,000 per year. The most widely used treatment for constipation is the administration of laxatives. Considering the prevalence of their use, both in the form of over-the-counter as well as prescription-only treatments, it is surprising to note the dearth of information that exists on indications and guidelines for their usage and review of their efficacy (Norton 2006; Petticrew et al. 1997).

While it is suggested that ageing itself does not appear to reduce colonic motility or transit time (Barrett 1993), large numbers of older adults take laxatives even in the absence of symptoms (Harari et al. 1996). Contributory factors include differing expectations and attitudes between the generations; as Norton states 'each of us know what *we* mean when we say we are constipated; however different people mean very different things' (2006: 322). Concomitant conditions such as immobility, frailty and reduced dietary intake, all of which can exacerbate bowel problems, are also prevalent in older people.

Prior to the prescribing of laxatives it is essential to ascertain that constipation is not secondary to an underlying undiagnosed causal factor (BNF 2011: 61). It is also the community nurse's responsibility to understand the properties, effects and contraindications of laxatives that they may be prescribing or administering.

The successful treatment of constipation with laxatives may require a process of trial and error in clinical practice before a suitably effective and tolerable laxative is found. However, a randomised controlled trial into the treatment of constipation and faecal incontinence in stroke patients demonstrated that those patients who received a one-off, nurse-led consultation and assessment, as opposed to prescribed treatment, had significantly improved bowel function (Harari et al. 2004). The implications of this study point to the value of community nurses undertaking a full, accurate assessment of the patients' bowel symptoms and the behaviours that may affect them.

Laxatives are classified into four groups (Table 3.1); however, it is essential to recognise that this classifica-

Table 3.1 Commonly used laxatives

Bulk-forming laxatives	Stimulant laxatives	Faecal softeners	Osmotic laxatives
Bran	Bisacodyl	Arachis oil	Lactulose
Ispaghula husk	Docusate sodium		Macrogols (e.g. movicol)
Fybogel	Senna		Magnesium salts (e.g. Epsom salts)
Normacol			

tion system disguises the fact that some laxatives have more than one property, e.g. docusate sodium is thought to act both as a stimulant and a softening agent (BNF 2011: 61).

Bulk-forming laxatives

Bulk-forming laxatives, as the name suggests, relieve constipation by bulking up faecal mass, which in turn promotes peristalsis. They have a cumulative effect, which can take a few days to develop, and should be introduced gradually, after clearance of any impaction (BNF 2011: 61). They can be used where increasing dietary fibre into the diet alone is difficult (e.g. if a patient has swallowing difficulties or finds dietary fibre unpalatable), but must be taken with plenty of fluid to avoid the risk of intestinal obstruction. Increased bulk will theoretically improve transit time, improve peristalsis and result in a softer stool arriving at the rectum (Norton 2006).

Stimulant laxatives

Stimulant laxatives work by increasing intestinal motility through stimulation of the myenteric nerve plexus, thereby increasing peristalsis. They must be used with extreme caution if faecal impaction is suspected or where there is a potential for bowel obstruction (BNF 2011: 61).

Faecal softeners

Faecal softeners act as a lubricant to help ease the passage of stools. They may be taken in oral form or as an arachis oil enema preparation. They can be used to lubricate and soften impacted faeces.

Osmotic laxatives

Osmotic laxatives, such as lactulose and polyethylene glycol, work by drawing water into the bowel (BNF 2011: 61), so it is important that patients are adequately hydrated. This action allows fluid to be retained in the stool, thereby softening it and making it easier to pass. The additional faecal mass may also stimulate peristalsis.

Enemas

An enema is an amount of liquid that is inserted into the rectum to either (i) stimulate or assist defecation or (ii) administer medication. The following text refers in the main to the use of enemas for producing a bowel movement, rather than medication administration, although the technique to be followed in enema administration would be the same, whichever is being given.

Administration of an enema may cause acute embarrassment to a patient and therefore is not to be undertaken without due consideration and patient preparation. To gain consent, the effects and risks of enema administration, including any specific risks related to a particular product, must be explained to the patient prior to administration. The community nurse should also carry out a risk assessment that incorporates the following.

■ The patient's general condition, sacral skin integrity.
■ Assessment of the patient's mobility and ability to cope and self-care with any potential after effects following the nurse's visit, e.g. if the patient lives alone.
■ Where relevant, the ability and capability of carers.
■ The home environment, e.g. access and proximity of the toilet/commode.
■ Follow-up support and or care that may be necessary on the day of administration, e.g. additional community nurse visits during the day or by the evening or night nursing service.

Enemas that are used in the treatment of constipation fall into two main categories:

■ stimulant/evacuant enemas (Figure 3.2)
■ retention enemas.

Stimulant enemas may be used for the preparation of the bowel prior to some investigations, such as flexible sigmoidoscopy, in preference to orally administered bowel preparation, such as Picolax. Types of enema, their effects, uses and contra-indications are detailed in Table 3.2.

Anecdotally, the use of enemas to treat chronic constipation in practice is reducing as there are now effective and more acceptable oral preparations available, e.g. polyethylene glycol osmotic laxatives (Kyle 2007).

Stimulant/evacuant enemas

The management of chronic constipation may include the administration of a stimulant enema. The most

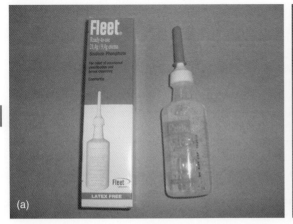
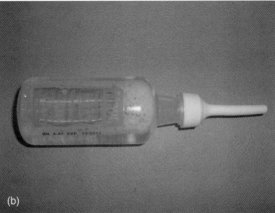

(a)

(b)

Figure 3.2a,b Phosphate (Fleet) enema. Reproduced by kind permission of Fleet Laboratories, UK.

Table 3.2 Types of enema, indications, action and contraindications

Type of enema and dose	Indication for use	Action	Contraindications
Arachis oil 130 ml	Constipation and faecal impaction	Lubricate and soften impacted faeces	Nut allergy
Sodium phosphate, approx 130 ml	Constipation, bowel preparation	Osmotic stimulant laxative	Acute gastrointestinal conditions (see Box 3.7)
Sodium citrate 5 ml or other micro enemas	Constipation	Osmotic stimulant laxative	Acute gastrointestinal conditions

commonly prescribed enemas being sodium phosphate and sodium citrate (Kyle 2007). Stimulant enemas are usually effective within 5–10 minutes (Davies 2004).

Phosphate enemas work by osmosis, drawing water into the rectum and stools therein, causing rectal distension and irritation, stimulating a bowel movement (Davies 2004; Bowers 2006). There is little evidence to support or refute the use of phosphate enemas for the management of chronic constipation; however, they are commonly used, but are not without risk (Bowers 2006; Mendoza *et al.* 2007; BNF 2011: 61) (Box 3.6).

For example, they may cause electrolyte disturbance and the nurse should ensure that the patient remains adequately hydrated (BNF 2011: 61). Because of their potential toxic effects, phosphate enemas are contraindicated in patients with rectal bleeding and acute inflammatory bowel conditions (Davies 2004) and should be used with caution in those with renal impairment, ascites or heart failure (BNF 2011: 61). Hyperphosphataemia is rare, but can occur in both children (Biebl *et al.* 2009) and adults (Carl & Mitchell 2007).

If a phosphate enema has not been evacuated within 30 minutes in patients who are particularly at risk of toxicity (e.g. children and those with impaired renal

---

Box 3.6 Risks associated with phosphate enema administration

- Irritation and rectal mucosal necrosis (especially if the mucosa is lacerated or perforated during enema administration)
- Irritation and blistering of anus and buttocks (especially if the fluid leaks and remains in contact with the skin for a period of time)
- Rectal changes consistent with burns
- Dehydration
- Rarely phosphate toxicity (hyperphosphataemia) and hypo/hypernatraemia

(Knobel & Petchenko 1996; Lambert & Herman 1996; Davies 2004; Bowers 2006)

---

function), it is recommended that the fluid be recovered, even if this means resorting to manual removal of faeces (Lambert & Herman 1996). Where repeated enemas are required for evacuation of impacted faeces, phosphate enemas should not be used due to the increased risks of toxicity following repeated administration (Knobel & Petchenko 1996). They are also contraindicated in patients with renal disease, due to their inability to effectively excrete the phosphate, which again increases the risk of toxicity (Box 3.7) (Nir-Paz *et al.* 1999; Bowers 2006).

Retention enemas

A retention enema is designed to be held within the rectum for a long period of time, even overnight, to soften and lubricate hard, impacted faeces. Many such enemas use an oil-based preparation, such as olive or arachis oil. Arachis or groundnut oil is made from peanuts and therefore should not be given to any patient with a confirmed or suspected nut allergy (Kyle 2007).

Laceration and perforation of the rectum or sigmoid by the enema nozzle is extremely rare but not unheard of (Bell 1990). While the procedure may appear simple and routine, the potential risk of rectal perforation should not be underestimated. The most likely indication that laceration or perforation has occurred is pain at the time of enema administration, usually accompanied by bleeding (Thiele & Zander 2002). The damage caused may then be further compounded by the enema solution causing rectal gangrene, although this appears to be a problem only found with the administration of phosphate solutions (Davies 2004). If pain and/or bleeding occur during or immediately after enema administration, the patient should be urgently reviewed by their GP. Failure to recognise the signs of perforation can lead to delayed diagnosis and treatment, and early diagnosis has been shown to correlate with survival (Paran *et al.* 1999).

Suppositories

A suppository is a solid formulation of a drug or faecal softener, prepared for administration directly into the rectum (Higgins 2007). Once inserted, the patient's body heat will cause the suppository to dissolve into a liquid and the drug to be delivered. Suppositories may be used to either (i) stimulate or assist defecation or (ii) administer medication. The following text refers in the main to the use of suppositories for producing a bowel movement, rather than medication administration, although the technique to be followed in administration would be the same in either case.

Suppositories that are used in the treatment of constipation fall into two main categories:

- glycerin (Figure 3.3)
- bisacodyl.

Box 3.7 Inappropriate use of phosphate enemas

- Patients with renal failure/impairment – increased risk of toxicity
- Patients with dehydration – may be compounded
- Patients unable to take adequate fluid intake to replace that which is lost
- Patients with bowel pathology:
  ○ Intestinal obstruction
  ○ Inflammatory/ulcerative bowel diseases
  ○ Proctitis (may be further inflamed)
  ○ Recent anal/rectal surgery
  ○ Malignancy
  ○ Recent radiotherapy

(Adapted from Bowers 2006)

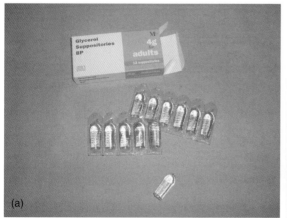
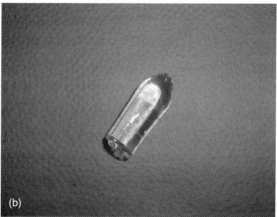

Figure 3.3a,b Glycerin suppository.

Table 3.3 Types of suppository, indications, action and contraindications

Type of suppository and dose	Indication for use	Action	Contraindications
Bisacodyl 10 mg	Constipation, bowel preparation	Stimulant laxative	Intestinal obstruction, acute surgical abdominal conditions, acute inflammatory bowel disease, severe dehydration
Glycerol (glycerin) 1–2 suppositories	Constipation	Lubricant and mild stimulant due to the irritant effect of glycerin	Intestinal obstruction

(BNF 2011)

Suppositories used to treat constipation work as stimulant laxatives (BNF 2011: 61), but glycerin suppositories also produce local lubrication as they dissolve within the rectum.

It is essential that the community nurse remembers that patients requiring help with bowel evacuation who are taking oral laxatives for chronic constipation may have a bowel movement at a time when no one is available to assist or care for them (Davies 2004). Therefore a planned bowel management programme, possibly using suppositories, that takes into consideration the time of day and availability of carers is essential to ensure that the patient's safety and dignity are maintained. Types of suppositories, their effects, uses and contraindications are detailed in Table 3.3.

A suppository is designed with a narrow end (the apex) and a wider, blunted end (the base). They are designed to be inserted apex first, as the curved narrow point helps to ease passage through the anal sphincters and into the rectum. There has been much debate about the correct method of suppository administration since a single small-scale study was published suggesting that the base may distend the anus and prevent it from closing (Abd-el-Maeboud 1991). This study has not been replicated and to date there is insufficient evidence to suggest that a change to practice is necessary. The anal canal is only approximately 2.5–4 cm in length, suggesting that it is shorter than the average nurse's index finger. Therefore, unless the rectum is loaded with hard impacted faeces, there is no reason to believe that it would not be possible to insert a suppository beyond the anal sphincters and into the rectum, allowing the sphincters to close.

Prior to administering a suppository, a digital rectal examination should be performed. If the rectum is loaded with faeces, drug absorption may be affected. Risks associated with suppository administration are low, but particular care should be taken with patients who have had local irradiation or recent surgery to the anus or rectum (Higgins 2007).

Glycerin suppositories may be sufficient to induce bowel evacuation, but bisacodyl suppositories may be used to provide a stronger chemical stimulus if required. Glycerin suppositories are also used as a rescue measure for patients undergoing biofeedback treatment for chronic functional constipation if they have not passed anything per rectum for four or five days.

Diarrhoea

Diarrhoea is a change in normal bowel habit in which normally formed stool passed with a frequency of up to three times daily changes to frequent, multiple, loose-to-watery stools. It may be associated with increased frequency and/or increased liquidity of stools, often with a volume of stool greater than 200 g/day (Thomas et al. 2003). In clinical practice, determining stool weight is necessary only in some cases of chronic diarrhoea.

The severity of diarrhoea can range from an acute self-limited annoyance to a severe life-threatening illness. The duration of symptoms will determine whether it is an acute or chronic episode. For example, it is suggested that diarrhoea lasting longer than four weeks could be classified as chronic (Thomas et al. 2003). Many factors contribute to the development of both acute and chronic diarrhoea (Table 3.4).

Acute diarrhoea is most commonly caused by infection, and is present for less than 3–4 weeks. Large-volume watery diarrhoea usually indicates a small bowel disorder, and frequent small volume stools a colonic or rectal disorder (Kearny 2003). Causes are viral or bacterial infections, bacterial toxins and medication (Table 3.4). Most cases are due to infection through ingestion of contaminated food and/or water.

Table 3.4 Common causes of diarrhoea

Dietary	Excess ingestion of non or poorly ingested carbohydrate:
	sorbitol
	fructose
	Mannitol
	Bran and other fibre supplements
	Excess magnesium: antacids, laxatives, food supplements
	Stimulants such as caffeine
	Food intolerance, e.g. milk or wheat
	Allergy
Infections	Bacterial: *Campylobacter*, *Salmonella*, *Escherichia coli*
	Viral: rotavirus, cytomegalovirus, etc.
Medication	Antibiotics
	Antihypertensives
	Polypharmacy
	Magnesium-containing products
	Non-steroidal anti-inflammatory medications
	Theophyllines
	Antiarrythmics
	Antineoplastic agents
Exercise	Marathon runners' diarrhoea
Intestinal disease	E.g. inflammatory bowel disease, coeliac disease
Functional	Irritable bowel syndrome, anxiety

A similarly affected family member would suggest an infectious origin. If the symptoms of diarrhoea persist beyond 4 weeks, it suggests a non-infectious aetiology and requires further investigation to distinguish between secretory, absorption and inflammatory causes (Thomas *et al.* 2003).

Symptoms suggestive of organic disease include a history of predominantly nocturnal diarrhoea of less than 3 months duration or continuous diarrhoea and significant weight loss. Colonic, inflammatory or secretory forms of diarrhoea, e.g. due to inflammatory bowel disorders such as Crohn's disease or ulcerative colitis, typically present with liquid, loose stools with blood or mucus discharge. Chronic diarrhoea can also be caused by irritable bowel syndrome (IBS) (Thomas *et al.* 2003). Malabsorption syndromes may also result in chronic

diarrhoea and are often accompanied by steatorrhoea (the passage of bulky, fatty, foul-smelling pale stools).

Assessment of diarrhoea

A detailed, careful history is the most important tool to determine the origin of diarrhoea. The setting in which the diarrhoea developed is useful to suggest an origin. Questions should focus on the following factors.

- Travel history: international, domestic and wilderness.
- Foods eaten, which type, liquids drunk and locations where they were consumed.
- Recent hospitalisation or closed community confinement, e.g. nursing home, dormitory, etc.
- Recent use of antibiotics or new medication.
- Exposure to similarly affected people.
- History of shellfish ingestion.
- Exposure to farm animals.
- Presence of systemic disease and other co-morbidities.
- Immune status (i.e. HIV, immunosuppressive therapy).
- Stool form, frequency and volumes passed.
- Onset and duration.
- Other associated symptoms (e.g. weight loss, rectal bleeding, abdominal pain).

The severity of illness is determined from the history and direct examination of the patient. It is vital to find out the appearance of the stools, including the presence of blood, the frequency of bowel movements and the presence of other symptoms such as fever, abdominal pain and dehydration. Most infectious causes of diarrhoea have a self-limited course. Diarrhoea of more than 5 days' duration may indicate a more severe illness or a systemic illness with gastrointestinal symptoms (Lung 2003).

Investigations

If symptoms do not improve within 48 hours, further review and stool investigation, such as collecting samples for microscopy, is advisable. Adults with mild dehydration who are being treated at home may require an early review of their symptoms, but an adult with severe depletion of fluid and electrolytes or a child who develops dehydration should be admitted to secondary care for further investigation and management (Armon *et al.* 2001; BNF 2011: 61).

In patients under the age of 45 years with other typical symptoms of a functional disorder and negative initial tests for infection, IBS may be diagnosed at primary care level without further investigations apart from routine blood tests and the exclusion of coeliac disease (NICE 2008). However, all patients suspected of having IBS should be screened for 'red flag' symptoms (Box 3.4), and atypical and/or severe symptoms should be further evaluated. Adults with a change of bowel habit to looser stools persistent for six weeks or more should be urgently referred under the two-week standard to rule out bowel cancer, even if there is no rectal bleeding (Thomas *et al.* 2003).

Management of acute diarrhoea

As stated above, acute diarrhoea is usually mild and self-limiting, and most people with this condition can be managed at home by replacing fluids. Patients should be assessed for dehydration and advised to ensure that their fluid intake is at least 2 litres per day, and in addition to replace ongoing fluid losses by 200 ml for each loose stool; the frail and older person is particularly at risk (www.cks.nhs.uk). Oral rehydration should continue until the diarrhoea resolves. Diarrhoea can cause loss of electrolytes as well as fluid, and rehydration should replace both fluid and any electrolyte deficit. It should be noted that glucose enhances intestinal absorption of both sodium and water and should be administered when rehydrating a patient (BNF 2011: 61). Commercially produced rehydration solutions for oral rehydration therefore normally contain both salt and glucose.

No special diet is indicated, but fatty foods and foods with high sugar content should be avoided. Antidiarrhoeals (e.g. loperamide) may be used in acute diarrhoea, but should be avoided in the presence of fever or bloody stools and are contraindicated in acute ulcerative colitis (BNF 2011: 61). Antibiotics are rarely indicated, particularly for people with less severe symptoms, as the illness may have resolved before the report is received, and should be reserved for people with positive stool cultures. Ciprofloxacin may occasionally be necessary for those who are at high risk of infection or who present with dysentery (bloody stools). When there is a suspected case of dysentery or *E. coli* infection advice should be sought from the local Health Protection Unit of the Health Protection Agency (Health Protection Agency 2010).

To avoid the risk of re-contamination simple hygiene measures should be advised, for example:

- hand washing
- wiping down any surfaces touched
- no sharing of utensils, towels, etc.

In addition, anyone with acute infective diarrhoea should be excluded from school or work for at least 48 hours after they are symptom-free (Health Protection Agency 2010).

Urgent general practitioner (GP) advice and/or medical review may be required and should be sought if the patient develops blood in the stools, becomes pyrexial, e.g. temperature above 38.5°C, or displays the symptoms of dehydration, including:

- excessive apathy
- dizziness
- dry mouth
- sunken eyes
- the infrequent passing of concentrated urine.

These symptoms, especially with a history of foreign travel, could be suggestive of dysentery. Medical referral should also be made if significant diarrhoea persists for more than 3 days or if signs of other illness are suspected (Health Protection Agency 2010). Cholera is rare in the UK, but should be suspected if the patient has travelled abroad in a country where it is endemic and presents with profuse stools that look like rice water (Health Protection Agency 2008).

Management of chronic diarrhoea

The management of chronic diarrhoea will depend on the underlying cause and a detailed discussion of this specialist area of practice is beyond the scope of this chapter. There may be a role for symptomatic treatment with antidiarrhoeal drugs, such as loperamide or codeine phosphate. Caution should be exercised as these drugs are generally contraindicated in acute colitis as they may cause toxic megacolon (Bell 2004).

Irritable bowel syndrome

An increasingly common problem that can occur with the GI tract is irritable bowel syndrome (IBS). IBS can present with symptoms such as bloating and abdominal pain where no organic cause can be found. Patients present with a variable bowel habit, alternating often between constipation and diarrhoea, although one of these states will usually predominate.

Faecal incontinence

Faecal incontinence is the involuntary leakage of a large amount of either solid or liquid faecal material. It may also involve the passing of flatus uncontrollably, where the volume of faecal material passed is variable and may involve only light soiling of underwear. Nevertheless, these apparently less severe problems may be equally distressing to patients. Faecal incontinence affects approximately 5% of the population living in the community and has many socioeconomic implications (Perry *et al.* 2002). Its prevalence increases with age and it severely impacts on the quality of life of many sufferers and their families, often being cited as the reason for admission to nursing home care (Whitehead *et al.* 2001).

To remain continent, patients need to be able to sense when the rectum is filling and distinguish its contents, to store the faeces for a period of time and prevent unwanted leakage of solid, liquid or gas from the anus. This requires intact anal and rectal sensation, rectal reservoir capacity, and intact internal and external anal sphincters (Wald 1994). The internal sphincter normally remains contracted during rectal filling, but when larger volumes of stool enter the rectum the resulting rectal distension causes reflex relaxation of the internal anal sphincter (Norton & Chelvanayagam 2004). At this time, the external anal sphincter contracts to prevent passive leakage of rectal contents. In addition, the puborectalis muscle within the pelvic floor forms a 'loop' around the junction between the anus and rectum. When contracted, this muscle creates an angle at this junction (the ano-rectal angle), which is also an important element of maintaining continence. During defecation, this muscle relaxes to allow the angle between the rectum and anus to straighten to allow the passage of stool (Norton & Chelvanayagam, 2004).

Faecal incontinence has many causes and contributing factors including:

- impaired puborectalis function resulting in loss of ano-rectal angle pudendal nerve damage (especially in females) resulting in impaired pelvic floor function – this may be caused by:
  - childbirth injury
  - chronic straining at stool
  - nerve root compression
- damage to anal sphincters
- constipation and faecal impaction (may distend anal sphincters) with faecal fluid overflow
- loss of motivation to maintain continence or cognitive decline
- diarrhoea
- inflammatory bowel disease
- previous surgery/tumours/radiotherapy, which may reduce reservoir capacity, cause mucosal damage and/or affect anal sphincter function
- decreased rectal sensation (e.g due to diabetic neuropathy or megarectum)

- neurological disorders affecting spinal nerve roots, spinal cord or cognitive ability.

(Kalantar *et al.* 2002; Norton & Chelvanayagam 2004)

Risk factors associated with the onset of faecal incontinence in women include:

- faecal urgency
- loose stools
- a history of cholecystectomy
- non-obstetric ano-rectal injury.

(Bharucha *et al.* 2006)

Assessment

The problems and associated symptoms of faecal incontinence may be embarrassing for a patient to discuss in depth with a nurse they are meeting for the first time. While it may be possible to glean information about bowel symptoms, the details of the impact of the faecal incontinence on the patient's quality of life is often only identified as the community nurse develops a professional therapeutic relationship with the patient. Therefore assessment should be considered a process rather than a one-off event, and consideration should be given to the number of visits that may be required.

As with the assessment of constipation, assessment of the symptom of faecal incontinence includes a number of elements:

- history taking
- physical examination
- physiological investigation, which may include:
  - ano-rectal physiology studies
  - endo-anal ultrasound of anal sphincters
  - defecating proctogram
  - gut transit studies
  - magnetic resonance imaging (MRI)
  - endoscopy.

(Norton & Chelvanayagam 2004)

Nursing assessment of faecal incontinence should incorporate all of the elements identified in Box 3.8. Use of a bowel diary may help patients to record their bowel movements and incontinence over the course of a week, as relying on recall may bias the accuracy of the assessment.

Until recently, most published assessment tools had been developed by clinicians and tended to focus on physical symptoms and bowel habit; the screening tools failed to focus sufficiently on the elements of faecal incontinence that bothered patients the most, including

42

Box 3.8 Nursing assessment of faecal incontinence

History

- Past medical history (including depression and obstetric history)
- Bowel frequency per day
- Faecal urgency
- Stool consistency (refer to Bristol Stool Form Scale)
- Frequency of bowel accidents/leakage (? Linked to stool consistency or activities)
- Type of leakage (solid/liquid/mucus/wind)
- Amount of leakage (small stain on underwear through to complete bowel evacuation)
- How is the problem currently managed (e.g. change underwear/wear a pad)
- Effect on lifestyle and relationships
- Difficulty emptying bowel (e.g. straining, incomplete evacuation)
- Abdominal pain
- Bleeding
- Passing mucus
- Bloating
- Current medication
- Diet and fluid intake

Examination

- Inspect perineum for soiling and excoriation/incontinence associated dermatitis
- Anal soreness
- Anal closure
- Faecal impaction
- Rectal prolapse
- Any evidence of anal pathology (e.g. anal warts, skin tags, fissure, haemorrhoids)
- Digital examination of rectal contents
- Digital examination of anal sphincters for resting tone, squeeze pressure (referral for more detailed examination may be required)

(Adapted from Norton & Chelvanayagam 2004)

psychological and quality-of-life issues, unpredictability and coping strategies (Cotterill *et al.* 2008). An assessment tool has now been developed to address the shortcomings of previous assessment scales (Cotterill *et al.* 2008) and is currently being evaluated by the International Consultation on Incontinence Modular Questionnaire group (ICIQ). Once adopted this tool will be available via the ICIQ website (www.iciq.net/).

Management of faecal incontinence

One of the most troublesome aspects of faecal incontinence for patients is the unpredictable nature of their defecation (Cotterill *et al.* 2008). Therefore a planned management routine in which the volume of stool produced is reduced and the consistency altered to a more solid form which is then evacuated, often using suppositories/enemas, may be helpful (Norton & Chelvanayagam 2004). This may be achieved through a treatment programme that combines:

- a regular planned toileting regimen/bowel management routine
- dietary manipulation
- pharmacological treatments to control stool consistency (e.g. loperamide) (BNF 2011: 61).
- behavioural techniques.

This type of plan facilitates person-centred care, enables the patient to deal with their bowel management at a time and place that suits them (NICE 2007), and reduces the fear of unpredictable leakage or accidents.

For some people with incontinence, wearing a small pad may be adequate, but others will need specialist review. There are a number of potential treatments and this can include the use of loperamide to alter the consistency of stools (BNF 2011: 61). Treatments range from conservative management with anal plugs or transanal irrigation of the rectum and left colon (Christensen & Krogh 2010) to surgery, which can include insertion of a sacral nerve stimulator or colostomy formation (Parés *et al.* 2008). While research into the causes and management of faecal incontinence is increasing and the methodological quality of studies is improving, there still remains a lack of definitive evidence to support many areas of practice, and treatment is therefore often based on a consensus of expert opinion and small-scale studies (Parés *et al.* 2008).

Pharmacological management

Several drugs are used in the pharmacological management of faecal incontinence to induce constipation, bulk the stools or aid defecation (Box 3.9). These drugs are often used as an adjunct to other behavioural or surgical interventions. Constipating agents are used to reduce the volume of the stool produced and firm up the consistency of liquid stools, although they are not licensed for the treatment of faecal incontinence and there is limited evidence of their effectiveness in the treatment of faecal incontinence (Cheetham 2004). Some patients, particularly those with spinal and other neurological problems, may require bowel evacuation using suppositories, enemas or manual removal of faeces. If constipating agents are used, care must be taken to ensure that the patient does not become impacted.

Box 3.9 Commonly used drugs used to manage faecal incontinence

Constipating agents
- Loperamide
- Codeine phosphate

Bulking agents
- Ispaghula husk
- Bran
- Methylcellulose

Evacuation aids (see also: laxatives and suppositories)
- Glycerin and bisacodyl suppositories
- Enemas

(Adapted from Cheetham 2004)

The use of a constipating agent in combination with an evacuation aid makes bowel evacuation more predictable and enables it to be planned at a time to suit both the patient and carers. This may be a particularly important factor to consider when planning a bowel management programme for patients requiring nursing assistance in the community.

Stool bulking agents supplement non-digestible fibre and therefore remain within the gut and assist in retaining water. This in turn helps to soften the stools, but larger quantities of softer stools are often more difficult to retain and may exacerbate the problem (Cheetham 2004).

Biofeedback

Biofeedback is often used as the first-line management for treatment of faecal incontinence (Norton *et al.* 2003). However, a Cochrane review of the role of biofeedback and/or sphincter exercises did not provide conclusive evidence of the effectiveness of the therapy, although there was some evidence that elements of biofeedback may have some therapeutic effect (Norton *et al.* 2006).

Biofeedback is a means of providing visual or auditory feedback about a bodily function that an individual would not normally be aware of, often achieved through use of visual displays on a monitor of anal sphincter muscle contraction (Norton & Chelvanayagam 2004). Alternatively, a balloon inserted into the rectum is used to increase the patient's perception of rectal distension, and sphincter exercises 'train' the patient to use their abdominal, pelvic floor and anal sphincter muscles correctly to control bowel evacuation (Norton & Chelvanayagam 2004).

Investigators have sought to identify potential predictors for outcome from biofeedback treatment so that appropriate patients may be selected for this therapy and resources therefore targeted towards those who are most likely to benefit. Fernández-Fraga and colleagues (2003) have identified, in an uncontrolled study, that both young age and poor defecatory technique are independent predictors of poor outcome following biofeedback. Norton and Chelvanayagam (2004), however, suggest that patient motivation could also be a significant factor in the outcome from biofeedback.

Electrical stimulation

Electrical stimulation, with or without pelvic floor exercises, has been used to treat urinary incontinence for many years and more recently has also been used to enhance anal sphincter function or sensation in patients with faecal incontinence, although once again there is limited evidence of effectiveness (Hosker *et al.* 2007). It is unclear how frequently this needs to be applied and for how long a period of time in order to be effective, but further research has been called for.

Anal plugs

Anal plugs have been developed for use by patients with faecal incontinence. These can be effective for some, but tend to be better tolerated by patients with poor anorectal sensation (Deutekom & Dobben 2010). Other patients often find the plug uncomfortable to wear, but plugs do allow patients a certain amount of freedom to go about activities of daily living without fear of an episode of faecal incontinence (Norton & Kamm 2001). Many patients will use plugs on 'special occasions', when they need to be sure that they will not have a bowel accident.

The plugs come wrapped in a water-soluble film, which dissolves following contact with moisture within the rectum, and must be lubricated prior to insertion. They may remain in place for up to 12 hours and are removed by using the string to gently pull them out of the anus (Herbert 2008).

Surgery

Surgery may be indicated for patients with intractable and unresolved faecal incontinence that is causing significant impact on quality of life. A number of different surgical approaches may be used (Box 3.10), with variable success rates. A Cochrane review failed to identify sufficient evidence to support alternative surgical procedures and suggests that a combination of conservative and surgical management may be required (Brown *et al.* 2010). Undergoing surgery is often a last resort, is

> **Box 3.10** Surgical approaches to the management of faecal incontinence
>
> - Anal sphincter repairs
> - Post-anal repair
> - Pelvic floor repair
> - Augmentation/replacement of anal sphincter
> - Antegrade continence enema procedures
> - Sacral nerve stimulation
> - Colostomy formation

no guarantee of a cure, results may not last and surgery may need to be repeated.

Digital rectal examination (DRE) and manual removal of faeces (MRF)

Digital rectal examination (DRE) involves observing the perianal area and inserting a lubricated gloved finger into a patient's rectum. Manual removal of faeces (MRF) involves the removal of rectal contents by the insertion of a lubricated, gloved finger into the rectum.

Prior to performing DRE and/or MRF, the community nurse should complete a full holistic assessment that takes account of the patient's normal daily routine, cultural/religious beliefs, environment and access to toilet facilities, availability of carer support if required and usual bowel care routine.

A qualified nurse who has received the relevant training and can demonstrate the required level of competence can perform both DRE and MRF (RCN 2006; NMC 2008). Nurses must have a good knowledge and understanding of:

Normal anatomy and physiology of the gastrointestinal tract

- diseases and disorders of the anus rectum and colon
- assessment of bowel dysfunction
- appropriate use and limitations of laxatives
- procedure for DRE/MRF
- documentation required
- consent
- when to refer to a specialist.

(RCN 2006)

Both of these procedures can also be delegated to carers or patients providing they have been trained and assessed by a qualified nurse as competent in performing the procedure. It is normally inappropriate to delegate these procedures to a close family member, particularly a spouse, as this could have a significant impact on relationships (SCI Centres of the UK & Ireland 2009).

Assessment of the perineal and perianal areas

Prior to performing DRE or MRF it is essential that the community nurse observes the perineal and perianal area for any abnormalities, for example:

- rectal prolapse
- anal skin tags
- anal lesions or swelling: these could indicate anal/rectal malignancy
- skin condition: pressure ulcers or moisture lesions/incontinence associated dermatitis
- gaping anus
- anal warts
- haemorrhoids, particularly position, size and any signs of bleeding
- foreign bodies
- bleeding and the colour of the blood
- the presence, colour and consistency of any discharge.

(RCN 2006)

Any abnormality detected should be clearly documented in the nursing record. The presence of the above may not preclude DRE and/or MRF, but advice should be sought from the local continence advisory service or the patient's GP if the nurse has not encountered the situation before and is unsure whether it is safe to proceed.

Indications for DRE

A DRE may be performed for a number of reasons, but a community nurse is most likely to need to undertake the procedure to assess the presence and consistency of stool in the rectum, possibly before administering suppositories or carrying out MRF (RCN 2006). Specialist nurses and continence advisors additionally carry out DRE to assess anal tone, sensation and the ability to initiate a voluntary contraction (RCN 2006). DRE may also be part of a bowel management programme for a patient with neurogenic bowel dysfunction following spinal cord injury, in which digital stimulation is used to trigger defecation in those whose lesion is above the cauda equina and who still have reflex bowel activity (SCI Centres of the UK & Ireland 2009).

Indications for MRF

Nurses sometimes question the necessity to manually remove faeces or perceive this as undignified for the patient (Woodward 2009). Nevertheless, there will be times when manual removal of faeces is necessary, i.e. for faecal disimpaction or where other techniques have been ineffective, and nurses must ensure they are competent to perform this procedure (NPSA 2004; RCN 2008). For some patients, such as those with spinal

Table 3.5 Causes, recognition and treatment of autonomic dysreflexia

Potential causes	Signs and symptoms	Immediate emergency treatment
Bladder ■ Blocked catheter ■ Distended bladder ■ UTI Bowels ■ Constipation ■ Faecal impaction ■ Anal fissure Wounds ■ Infected pressure sore ■ Boils ■ Ingrown toenails	■ Hypertension ■ Bradycardia ■ Pounding headache ■ Profuse sweating ■ Patient distress and anxiety ■ Flushing or blotching of the face, neck, chest and arms ■ Pallor below level of injury/lesion ■ Nasal congestion ■ Shortness of breath ■ Tightness in the chest ■ Dilated pupils ■ Blurred vision ■ Increase in spasm ■ Seizures	■ Identify cause and where possible remove stimulus ■ Raise the patient's head and lower their feet ■ Monitor blood pressure and pulse ■ In severe hypertension or where the cause cannot be identified administer a vasodilator as prescribed ■ Seek immediate medical advice ■ If symptoms persist the patient must be transferred to hospital

injuries and neurogenic bowel dysfunction, this may be the only appropriate bowel emptying technique (SCI Centres of the UK & Ireland 2009).

Assessment required during MRF
Whether undertaking manual removal of faeces for the first time for a patient or as a regular intervention, the community nurse should observe the patient and their reactions throughout the procedure. This is particularly important for patients with spinal lesions above T6, who may develop signs of autonomic dysreflexia (see Table 3.5). Patients may also become distressed and should be observed for signs of pain and discomfort or bleeding (RCN 2006).

Cautions and contraindications
There will be times when extra care and caution will need to be taken and in some cases both DRE and MRF may be contraindicated. Particular caution should be exercised with patients who have:

■ active inflammatory bowel disease
■ undergone recent pelvic irradiation
■ had recent rectal surgery/rectal or anal trauma
■ spinal injury above T6
■ rectal bleeding
■ previous history of abuse
■ fragile tissue due to age, radiation or malnourishment.

(RCN 2006)

DRE or MRF must never be performed if the patient has not given consent and must be stopped immediately

if they withdraw their consent at any point during the procedure. These procedures may also be contraindicated if instruction has been given by a medical practitioner not to perform the procedure (RCN 2006).

Autonomic dysreflexia
Autonomic dysreflexia (AD) is a rare condition that only occurs in patients with a spinal cord injury at or above T6 and may be triggered by activation of pain receptors or any noxious stimulus below the level of the injury (Brunker 2011). The most prominent feature of AD is a dramatic rise in blood pressure with bradycardia as the sympathetic nervous system 'over-reacts' to the stimulus. Normally blood pressure rises are detected by the baroreceptors, which respond via the autonomic nervous system, lowering blood pressure and keeping it within normal range. However, when there is an injury at T6 or above, inhibitory control is lost and the blood pressure continues to rise until the offending stimulus, such as constipation/faecal impaction or DRE/MRF, is removed. If not treated promptly and correctly, AD may lead to seizures, stroke and even death (Brunker 2011).

Prompt action needs to be taken in situations of AD. The acute management should be to relieve the precipitating cause while managing symptoms and treating potential complications. Most patients will be aware if they are prone to AD and will be able to tell the nurse if they begin to experience symptoms, such as pounding headache. If this occurs, stop the procedure immediately to remove the noxious stimulus and sit the patient upright. If the patient's blood pressure remains high once the stimulus is removed and the patient has been sat up with their legs over the edge of the bed (if possible) then urgent medical treatment with anti-hypertensives will be required (Brunker 2011). Many 'expert' patients will have medication, e.g. sublingual GTN, available to treat an episode of AD, but if the patient's blood pressure does not come down, the community nurse should request an emergency ambulance to transfer the patient to hospital.

community requires the community nurse to have the relevant knowledge, skills and competence. This can be achieved through the provision of ongoing appropriate training and education supported by written procedures, local policies and protocols that reflect best practice and assessment via a locally agreed competency or knowledge skills framework (KSF).

Conclusion

The assessment and safe management of patients living with acute and long-term bowel problems in the

---

Procedure guideline 3.1 **Guideline for digital rectal examination**

Prior to carrying out the procedure, a full assessment must be carried out and consent obtained. Assessment must include identification of exclusion criteria and contraindications.

Equipment

Disposable waterproof protective underpad
Gloves (non-sterile, latex-free)
Disposable plastic apron
Lubricating gel
Toilet paper/Tissues
Bowl
Soap
Wash cloth/wipes
Towel
Bag for disposal of used items
Suitable receiver

Nursing action	Rationale
1 Where appropriate facilities are available wash your hands or alternatively cleanse with 70% alcohol-based hand rub (in accordance with local policy)	To reduce the risk of cross-infection
2 If the patient is known to the service review nursing documentation and current care plan	To update knowledge of patient and maintain patient safety
3 If the patient is unknown to the service a comprehensive assessment must be carried out prior to undertaking the procedure. This should include assessment of the patient's mobility status	To identify potential contraindications and/or cautions To determine if a second nurse is required to assist with the procedure To maintain patient safety
4 Discuss and explain the examination to the patient	Patient information reduces anxiety To gain co-operation and consent Consent is an important and necessary part of good clinical practice. It is the legal means by which the patient gives a valid authorisation for treatment or care (RCN 2006)

Procedure guideline 3.1 **Guideline for digital rectal examination** *(cont'd)*

Nursing action	Rationale
5 Prepare the environment, draw curtains and where necessary obtain patient consent to move furniture	To allow freedom of movement when carrying out the procedure To maintain patient privacy
6 Prepare all necessary equipment	To prevent disruption to the procedure
7 Protect the bed with an appropriate disposable water proof under pad	To protect mattress and bedding from faecal matter/soiling
8 Ask the patient if they wish to use the toilet prior to undertaking the examination	To aid patient comfort and minimise the risk of discomfort during the procedure
9 Where indicated offer the patient assistance with removing all clothing below the waist	To expose the buttock area
10 Help the patient on to their side (normally into the left lateral position) with knees flexed; cover exposed area of body with a blanket/towel	To facilitate examination and allow easy access for digital rectal examination (RCN 2006) To maintain patient privacy and dignity
11 Where appropriate facilities are available wash your hands or alternatively cleanse with 70% alcohol-based hand rub (in accordance with local policy)	To reduce the risk of cross-infection
12 Put on disposable gloves and apron	To prevent contamination. To reduce the risk of cross-infection
13 Observe and examine the perineal and perianal area	To observe for any, abnormalities Any abnormalities identified must be discussed with the patient's GP prior to undertaking the procedure and the findings/outcome documented (RCN 2006) To maintain patient safety
14 Lubricate gloved index finger	To prevent trauma to anal and rectal mucosa by reducing surface friction (Dougherty & Lister 2011)
15 Inform patient that you are about to perform the procedure, then insert the gloved lubricated index finger slowly into the patient's anus and then on into the rectum	To ensure that the patient is relaxed and aware the examination is about to begin To confirm that the patient continues to consent to the procedure being undertaken To gain patient cooperation To minimise patient discomfort (Addison 1999)
16 Undertake assessment of: ■ tone and sensation of the anal sphincter ■ presence and consistency of faeces: with reference to the Bristol Stool Form Scale	To ensure relevant function and faecal loading is assessed (RCN 2006)
17 Verbally explain each step of the procedure to the patient throughout	To offer reassurance To reduce potential anxiety To aid relaxation gain co-operation and minimise patient discomfort

(Continued)

Procedure guideline 3.1 **Guideline for digital rectal examination** *(cont'd)*

Nursing action	Rationale
18 Slowly withdraw index finger from the patient's rectum	The examination and assessment is complete
19 Wipe residual lubricating gel from anal area with toilet paper/tissue	To make the patient comfortable and prevent irritation and soreness
20 Dispose of all used equipment in accordance with locally agreed infection prevention and control policy	To minimise the risk of cross-infection
21 Remove and dispose of gloves in accordance with locally agreed infection prevention and control policy	To minimise the risk of cross-infection To prevent contamination
22 Where appropriate facilities are available wash your hands or alternatively cleanse with 70% alcohol-based hand rub (in accordance with local policy)	To reduce the risk of cross-infection
23 Where necessary apply gloves and wash and dry the area or offer assistance with washing	To make the patient comfortable and prevent irritation and soreness
24 Remove and dispose of gloves in accordance with locally agreed infection prevention and control policy	To minimise the risk of cross-infection To prevent contamination
25 Ask the patient if they would like to use the toilet, commode or bedpan as appropriate (apply gloves as necessary)	Examination may have stimulated the ano-rectal reflex and the urge to defecate To aid patient comfort
26 Where necessary remove and dispose of gloves and apron in accordance with locally agreed infection prevention and control policy	To minimise the risk of cross-infection
27 Where appropriate facilities are available wash your hands or alternatively cleanse with 70% alcohol-based hand rub (in accordance with local policy)	To reduce the risk of cross-infection
28 Where necessary apply disposable apron and help the patient to dress	To enable the patient to continue with their normal activities of daily living To maintain patient comfort and dignity
29 Remove and dispose of apron in accordance with locally agreed infection prevention and control policy	To reduce the risk of cross-infection
30 Where appropriate facilities are available wash your hands or alternatively cleanse with 70% alcohol-based hand rub, (in accordance with local policy)	To reduce the risk of cross-infection
31 Replace any moved items of furniture to their original position	To maintain a safe environment for the patient by restoring any furniture moved to its usual place
32 Verbally discuss the outcome of the procedure with the patient giving further advice as indicated. This should be supported with written information and follow-up visits where appropriate	To reinforce verbal information and support patients understanding

Procedure guideline 3.1 **Guideline for digital rectal examination** *(cont'd)*

Nursing action	Rationale
33 Document the outcome of examination on the community nurse record of visits, this must include: ■ consent ■ stool type ■ findings on examination ■ any further nursing intervention undertaken and the outcome ■ any follow-up action/s to be taken by the community nurse, e.g. follow-up visits, referral to the out-of-hours nursing service liaison/referral to the patient's GP	To maintain patient safety To ensure continuity of care To provide baseline findings that may be referred to at a later date if necessary To ensure accurate and contemporaneous records are kept Documentation should provide clear evidence of care planned, decisions made and care delivered (NMC 2008)

Procedure guideline 3.2 **Guideline for manual removal of faeces**

Equipment

Disposable waterproof protective underpad
Prescribed medication for the emergency treatment of autonomic dysreflexia (where relevant)
Drug administration chart (where relevant)
Sphygmomanometer
Stethoscope
Gloves (non-sterile, latex-free)
Disposable plastic apron
Lubricating gel
Toilet paper/Tissues
Bowl
Soap
Wash cloth/wipes
Towel
Bag for disposal of used items
Suitable receiver

Nursing action	Rationale
1 Where appropriate facilities are available wash your hands or alternatively cleanse with 70% alcohol-based hand rub (in accordance with local policy)	To reduce the risk of cross-infection
2 If the patient is known to the service review nursing documentation and current care plan	To update knowledge of patient and maintain patient safety
3 If the patient is unknown to the service a comprehensive assessment must be carried out prior to undertaking the procedure. This should include assessment of the patient's mobility status	To identify potential contraindications and or cautions Known allergies To determine if a second nurse is required to assist with the procedure To maintain patient safety

(Continued)

Procedure guideline 3.2 **Guideline for manual removal of faeces** *(cont'd)*

Nursing action	Rationale
4 Discuss and explain the procedure to the patient	Information reduces anxiety
	To gain co-operation and consent
	Consent is an important and necessary part of good clinical practice. It is the legal means by which the patient gives a valid authorisation for treatment or care (RCN 2006)
5 For those patients with a spinal injury at T6 or above discuss and document the patient's previous experiences and any history of autonomic dysreflexia	To assess the risk of autonomic dysreflexia
	To aid decision making
	NB A previous history of autonomic dysreflexia significantly increases the risk of further episodes. However this risk should be balanced against the risk of the constipation leading to dysreflexia secondary to not emptying the bowel
6 Prepare the environment, draw curtains and where necessary obtain patient consent to move furniture	To allow freedom of movement when carrying out the procedure
	To maintain patient privacy
7 Prepare all necessary equipment	To prevent disruption to the procedure.
8 Protect the bed with an appropriate disposable waterproof underpad	To protect mattress and bedding from faecal matter/soiling
9 Ask the patient if they wish to use the toilet prior to undertaking the procedure	To aid patient comfort and minimise the risk of discomfort during the procedure
	To reduce the risk of autonomic dysreflexia (where relevant)
10 Where indicated offer the patient assistance with removing all clothing below the waist.	To expose the buttock area
11 Help the patient into the left lateral position with knees flexed; cover exposed area of body with a blanket/towel	To facilitate examination and allow easy access for manual removal of faeces (RCN 2006)
	To maintain patient privacy and dignity
12 Where appropriate facilities are available wash your hands or alternatively cleanse with 70% alcohol-based hand rub (in accordance with local policy)	To reduce the risk of cross-infection
13 Put on disposable apron and gloves	To prevent contamination and reduce the risk of cross-infection
14 Inform patient that you are about to start the examination	To confirm that the patient continues to consent to the procedure being undertaken
	To ensure that the patient is relaxed and aware the examination is about to begin
	To gain patient coperation.
	To minimise patient discomfort (Addison 1999)

Procedure guideline 3.2 **Guideline for manual removal of faeces** *(cont'd)*

Nursing action	Rationale
15 Observe and examine the patient's perineal and perianal area	To detect for any abnormalities To maintain patient safety **NB** Any abnormalities identified must be discussed with the patient's GP prior to undertaking the procedure and the findings/outcome documented (RCN 2006)
16 Lubricate gloved index finger.	To facilitate easier insertion of index finger
17 Some patients will require a local anaesthetic gel applied to the anal area, whether having the procedure performed for the first time or on a regular basis **NB** Contraindications, warnings, precautions and interactions should be read prior to using anaesthetic gel. **Do not apply** if you have documented evidence of anal damage or bleeding or if the patient has a known allergy to any of the ingredients	To reduce sensation and discomfort for the patient Lignocaine may cause anaphylaxis, hypotension, bradycardia or convulsions if applied to damaged mucosa
18 Inform the patient that you are about to insert a gloved, lubricated index finger slowly into the anus and then on into the rectum	To confirm that the patient continues to consent to the procedure being undertaken To ensure that the patient is relaxed and is aware that the procedure is about to begin To gain patient co-operation To minimise patient discomfort (Addison 1999)
19 If faecal matter corresponds to the Bristol stool type 1 remove one lump at a time, placing in a suitable receiver, until no more faecal matter can be felt	To relieve constipation and the patient's discomfort
20 If a solid faecal mass is present (Bristol stool types 2 and 3) push finger into the middle of the mass, split it and remove in small pieces, placing into a suitable receiver, with a hooked finger If faecal mass is too hard or larger than 4cm across and you are unable to break it **stop** and refer to GP	To relieve constipation and the patient's discomfort
21 Verbally explain each step to the patient throughout the procedure	To offer reassurance To reduce potential anxiety To aid relaxation, gain co-operation and minimise patient discomfort
22 Observe and monitor the patient throughout the procedure	To detect signs of distress, pain, bleeding and general discomfort To detect signs of autonomic dysreflexia (where relevant)

(Continued)

51

Procedure guideline 3.2 **Guideline for manual removal of faeces** *(cont'd)*

Nursing action	Rationale
23 **Stop procedure immediately:** ■ if bleeding occurs at the anal area ■ at the first sign or symptom of autonomic dysreflexia (*see* Table 3.5) ■ if the patient withdraws their consent at any point	To maintain patient safety
24 When procedure is completed wipe the area clean using, e.g. toilet paper or damp wash cloth	To aid patient comfort
25 Cover exposed area of the patient's body with a blanket/towel	To maintain patient dignity
26 Place faecal matter into the toilet and flush	To ensure appropriate safe disposal
27 Remove and dispose of gloves and apron in accordance with locally agreed infection prevention and control policy	To reduce the risk of cross-infection
28 Dispose of all used equipment in accordance with locally agreed infection prevention and control policy	To reduce the risk of cross-infection
29 Where appropriate facilities are available wash and dry your hands or alternatively cleanse with 70% alcohol-based hand rub (in accordance with local policy)	To reduce the risk of cross-infection
30 Collect and prepare a bowl of warm water towel and wash cloth/s	To enable cleansing of the patient's buttock and anal area
31 Apply a disposable apron and gloves	To reduce the risk of cross-infection
32 Wash and dry the patient's buttock and anal area or offer assistance	To make the patient comfortable and prevent irritation and soreness
33 On completion of wash discard water and return all patient reusable equipment, e.g. towel, to their normal position	To maintain the patient's home in its normal manner
34 Remove and dispose of gloves in accordance with locally agreed infection prevention and control policy	To reduce the risk of cross-infection
35 Where necessary assist the patient to dress	To enable the patient to continue with their normal activities of daily living To maintain patient comfort and dignity
36 Remove and dispose of apron in accordance with locally agreed infection prevention and control policy	To reduce the risk of cross-infection
37 Where appropriate facilities are available wash your hands or alternatively cleanse with 70% alcohol-based hand rub (in accordance with local policy)	To reduce the risk of cross-infection
38 Replace any moved items of furniture to their original position	To maintain a safe environment for the patient by restoring any furniture moved to its usual place

Nursing action	Rationale
39 Verbally discuss the outcome of the procedure with the patient, giving further advice as indicated. Where possible this should be supported with written information and follow-up visits if appropriate	To reinforce verbal information and support patient's understanding
40 Document the outcome of procedure on the community nurse record of visits, this must include: ■ consent ■ findings on examination ■ stool type ■ result of procedure ■ any further nursing intervention undertaken and the outcome, e.g. following an autonomic episode ■ Any follow-up action/s to be taken by the community nurse, e.g. follow-up visits, referral to the out-of-hours nursing service liaison/referral to the patient's GP	To maintain patient safety To ensure continuity of care Documentation should provide clear evidence of care planned, decisions made and care delivered (NMC 2008)

53

Procedure guideline 3.3 **Guideline for administration of an enema**

Equipment

Disposable waterproof protective underpad/s
Drug administration chart
Prescribed enema
Gloves (non-sterile, latex-free)
Disposable plastic apron
Lubricating gel
Jug with warm water
Bath thermometer
Bedpan or commode if the patient is unable to mobilise to the toilet when required
Toilet paper/Tissues
Bowl (where relevant)
Soap
Wash cloth/wipes
Towel
Bag for disposal of used items

Nursing action	Rationale
1 Where appropriate facilities are available wash your hands or alternatively cleanse with 70% alcohol-based hand rub (in accordance with local policy)	To reduce the risk of infection and maintain patient safety
2 If the patient is known to the service review nursing documentation and current care plan	To update knowledge of patient and maintain patient safety

(Continued)

Procedure guideline 3.3 ***Guideline for administration of an enema*** *(cont'd)*

Nursing action	Rationale
3 If the patient is unknown to the service a comprehensive assessment must be carried out prior to undertaking the procedure. This should include assessment of the patient's mobility status	To identify potential contraindications and or cautions To identify known allergies To determine if a second nurse is required to assist with the procedure To maintain patient safety
4 Discuss and explain the procedure to the patient	Information reduces anxiety To gain co-operation and consent Consent is an important and necessary part of good clinical practice. It is the legal means by which the patient gives a valid authorisation for treatment or care (RCN 2006; NMC 2008)
5 Check the label on the dispensed item against the administration chart and patient information	To confirm details are correct with the GP/medical practitioner's instructions and that the enema is in date To ensure that the correct drug is administered to the correct patient at the correct time via the correct route (NMC 2008) To maintain patient safety
6 Prepare the environment, draw curtains and where necessary obtain patient consent to move furniture	To allow freedom of movement when carrying out the procedure To maintain patient privacy
7 Prepare all necessary equipment, including the close placement of the bedpan or commode at the patient's bedside	To prevent disruption to the procedure To maintain patient safety To ensure that the patient is able to have their bowels open promptly To maintain patient dignity
8 Warm the enema fluid in a jug of water at 40–43°C	To ensure that the patient does not experience an unpleasant cold sensation on insertion Administration of the warm fluid will help to simulate the rectal mucosa (Higgins 2006)
9 Protect the bed with an appropriate disposable waterproof underpad	To protect mattress and bedding from faecal matter/soiling
10 Apply disposable apron	To reduce the risk of cross-infection To reduce the risk of contamination
11 Ask the patient if they wish to use the toilet to empty their bladder prior to undertaking the procedure	To reduce the potential feeling of discomfort during the procedure (Higgins 2006)

Procedure guideline 3.3 **Guideline for administration of an enema** *(cont'd)*

Nursing action	Rationale
12 Where indicated offer the patient assistance with removing all clothing below the waist	To expose the buttock area
13 Help the patient into the left lateral position with knees flexed; cover exposed area of body with a blanket/towel	To facilitate examination. To allow easy insertion of the enema nozzle (RCN 2006) To aid retention of the enema fluid (Kyle 2007) To maintain patient privacy and dignity
14 Where appropriate facilities are available wash your hands or alternatively cleanse with 70% alcohol-based hand rub (in accordance with local policy)	To reduce the risk of contamination and cross-infection
15 Apply gloves	To minimise the risk of cross-infection
16 Inform patient that you are about to start the examination	To confirm that the patient continues to consent to the procedure being undertaken To ensure that the patient is relaxed and aware the examination is about to begin To gain patient co-operation To minimise patient discomfort (Addison 1999)
17 Observe and examine the patient's perineal and perianal area	To detect for any abnormalities. To maintain patient safety **NB** Any abnormalities identified must be discussed with the patient's GP prior to undertaking the procedure and the findings/outcome documented (RCN 2006)
18 Open the enema packaging removing the protective cover from the nozzle	To prepare the enema for administration
19 Lubricate the end of the nozzle with sterile water-soluble lubricant	To minimise patient discomfort as the nozzle enters the rectum
20 Inform the patient that you are about to start the enema administration	To confirm that the patient continues to consent to the procedure being undertaken To ensure that the patient is relaxed and aware the examination is about to begin To gain patient co-operation To minimise patient discomfort (Addison 1999)
21 Gently part the patient's buttocks	To visually expose the anus To ensure that the enema can be administered correctly
22 Displace air from the enema nozzle	Air introduced into the rectum may cause the patient discomfort

55

(Continued)

Procedure guideline 3.3 **Guideline for administration of an enema** *(cont'd)*

Nursing action	Rationale
23 Slowly insert the enema nozzle through the anus into the rectum to a maximum distance of approximately 7–10 cm	The anal canal is approximately 5 cm long, inserting the nozzle beyond this point should ensure that the enema fluid is delivered into the rectum (Kyle 2007)
24 Slowly administer the enema fluid rolling up the container as it empties	To ensure that the full dose of enema fluid is delivered into the rectum To prevent backflow into the container
25 Verbally explain each step of the procedure to the patient throughout	To offer reassurance To reduce potential anxiety To aid relaxation gain co-operation and minimise patient discomfort
26 Once all of the enema fluid has been inserted, slowly remove the nozzle	Withdrawing the nozzle slowly will allow the anal sphincter muscles to close and prevent reflex emptying of the rectum (Kyle 2007)
27 Wipe the patient's perianal area with toilet paper/ damp wash cloth	To remove any excess gel. To promote patient comfort and prevent irritation
28 Cover the patient with a blanket/towel and ask them to remain lying on their left side for the required time, preferably 10–15 minutes, or as long as the patient is able to tolerate	To allow the enema fluid to be retained for the length of time directed by the manufacturer Retention of fluid is often easier if the patient remains lying down (Kyle 2007) To maintain patient dignity
29 Dispose of all used equipment in accordance with locally agreed infection prevention and control policy	To reduce the risk of cross-infection
30 Remove and dispose of gloves in accordance with locally agreed infection prevention and control policy	To reduce the risk of cross-infection and contamination
31 Where appropriate facilities are available wash and dry your hands or alternatively cleanse with 70% alcohol-based hand rub (in accordance with local policy)	To reduce the risk of cross-infection and contamination
32 Apply gloves and disposable apron	In preparation to assist the patient on to the bedpan/ commode/toilet
33 When the patient feels an urge to defecate assist them onto the bedpan/commode/toilet Allow privacy, if the patient's condition allows, while the enema is taking effect, unless they prefer otherwise	To enable bowel evacuation to take place To maintain patient dignity
34 Remove and discard soiled protective pad from bed in accordance with locally agreed policy. Replace if necessary	To reduce the risk of cross-infection To reduce the risk of contamination

Procedure guideline 3.3 **Guideline for administration of an enema** *(cont'd)*

Nursing action	Rationale
35 Once bowel evacuation is complete assist patient to transfer from the bedpan/commode/toilet if required	To maintain patient safety
36 Wash and dry the patient's buttocks and anal area or offer assistance	To ensure that the patient is clean To prevent skin irritation and soreness To enhance patient comfort
37 Remove and dispose of gloves in accordance with locally agreed infection prevention and control policy	To reduce the risk of cross-infection
38 Where necessary assist the patient to dress	To enable the patient to continue with their normal activities of daily living To maintain patient comfort and dignity
39 Remove and dispose of apron in accordance with locally agreed infection prevention and control policy	To reduce the risk of cross-infection
40 Offer the patient the opportunity to wash and dry their hands	Social hand washing is a normal activity following defecation
41 Where appropriate facilities are available wash your hands or alternatively cleanse with 70% alcohol-based hand rub (in accordance with local policy)	To reduce the risk of cross-infection
42 Replace any moved items of furniture to their original position	To maintain a safe environment for the patient by restoring any furniture moved to its usual place
43 Verbally discuss the outcome of the procedure with the patient giving further advice as indicated. Where possible this should be supported with written information and follow-up visits if appropriate	To reinforce verbal information and support patients understanding
44 Document the outcome of the enema on the community nurse record of visits, this must include: ■ consent ■ findings on examination ■ stool type ■ result of procedure ■ any further nursing intervention undertaken and the outcome, e.g. following an autonomic episode ■ any follow up action/s to be taken by the community nurse, e.g. follow-up visits, referral to the out-of-hours nursing service liaison/referral to the patient's GP	To maintain patient safety To ensure that the patient's bowel function can be monitored. To ensure continuity of care To ensure accurate and contemporaneous records are kept To reduce the risk of drug errors Documentation should provide clear evidence of care planned, decisions made and care delivered (NMC 2008)

57

Procedure guideline 3.4 **Guideline for administration of a suppository (management of constipation)**

Equipment

Disposable waterproof protective underpad/s
Drug administration chart
Prescribed suppository
Gloves (non-sterile, latex-free)
Disposable plastic apron
Lubricating gel
Bedpan or commode, if the patient is unable to mobilise to the toilet when required
Toilet paper/Tissues
Bowl (where relevant)
Soap
Wash cloth/wipes
Towel
Bag for disposal of used items

Nursing action	Rationale
1 Where appropriate facilities are available wash your hands or alternatively cleanse with 70% alcohol-based hand rub (in accordance with local policy)	To reduce the risk of infection and maintain patient safety
2 If the patient is known to the service review nursing documentation and current care plan	To update knowledge of patient and maintain patient safety
3 If the patient is unknown to the service a comprehensive assessment must be carried out prior to undertaking the procedure. This should include assessment of the patient's mobility status	To identify potential contraindications and or cautions To identify known allergies To determine if a second nurse is required to assist with the procedure To maintain patient safety
4 Discuss and explain the procedure to the patient	Information reduces anxiety To gain co-operation and consent Consent is an important and necessary part of good clinical practice. It is the legal means by which the patient gives a valid authorisation for treatment or care (RCN 2006; NMC 2008)
5 Check the label on the dispensed item against the administration chart and patient information	To confirm details are correct with the GP/medical practitioner's instructions and that the suppository is in date To ensure that the correct suppository is administered to the correct patient at the correct time To maintain patient safety
6 Prepare the environment, draw curtains and where necessary obtain patient consent to move furniture	To allow freedom of movement when carrying out the procedure To maintain patient privacy

58

Procedure guideline 3.4 **Guideline for administration of a suppository (management of constipation)** *(cont'd)*

Nursing action	Rationale
7 Apply disposable apron	To reduce the risk of cross-infection
	To reduce the risk of contamination
8 Prepare all necessary equipment, including the close placement of the bedpan or commode at the patient's bedside (if relevant)	To prevent disruption to the procedure
	To maintain patient safety
	To ensure that the patient is able to have their bowels open promptly
	To maintain patient dignity
9 Protect the bed with an appropriate disposable waterproof underpad	To protect mattress and bedding from faecal matter/soiling
10 Ask the patient if they wish to use the toilet to empty their bladder prior to undertaking the procedure	To reduce the potential feeling of discomfort during the procedure (Higgins 2006)
11 Where indicated offer the patient assistance with removing all clothing below the waist	To expose the buttock area
12 Help the patient into the left lateral position with knees flexed; cover exposed area of body with a blanket/towel	To facilitate examination
	To allow easy insertion of the suppository (RCN 2006)
	To aid retention of the suppository (RCN 2006)
	To maintain patient privacy and dignity
13 Where appropriate facilities are available wash your hands or alternatively cleanse with 70% alcohol-based hand rub (in accordance with local policy)	To reduce the risk of contamination and cross-infection
14 Apply gloves	To reduce the risk of cross-infection
15 Inform patient that you are about to start the examination	To confirm that the patient continues to consent to the procedure being undertaken
	To ensure that the patient is relaxed and aware the examination is about to begin
	To gain patient co-operation
	To minimise patient discomfort (Addison 1999)
16 Observe and examine the patient's perineal and perianal area	To detect for any abnormalities
	To maintain patient safety
	NB Any abnormalities identified must be discussed with the patient's GP prior to undertaking the procedure and the findings/outcome documented (RCN 2006)
17 Carry out a digital rectal examination (*see* Procedure guideline 3.1, steps 14–19)	To assess content of rectum
18 Open the suppository packaging	To prepare the suppository for administration

(Continued)

Procedure guideline 3.4 **Guideline for administration of a suppository (management of constipation)** *(cont'd)*

Nursing action	Rationale
19 Lubricate the end of the suppository with water soluble lubricant	To minimise patient discomfort as the suppository enters the anal canal and rectum
20 Inform patient that you are about to insert the suppository	To confirm that the patient continues to consent to the procedure being undertaken
	To ensure that the patient is relaxed and aware the procedure is about to begin
	To gain patient co-operation
	To minimise patient discomfort (Addison 1999)
21 Gently part the patient's buttocks	To visually expose the anus
	To ensure that the suppository can be administered correctly
22 Slowly insert the apex of the suppository into the rectum through the anus and ensure it is pushed, by a finger, all the way through the anal canal into the rectum Repeat with a second suppository if prescribed	The anal canal is approximately 5 cm long, so inserting the suppository beyond this point should ensure that the drug contained therein is delivered into the rectum (Kyle 2007)
23 Verbally explain each step of the procedure to the patient throughout	To offer reassurance
	To reduce potential anxiety
	To aid relaxation gain co-operation and minimise patient discomfort
24 Wipe the patient's perianal area with toilet paper/ damp wash cloth	To remove any excess gel
	To promote patient comfort and prevent irritation
25 Remove and dispose of gloves in accordance with locally agreed infection prevention and control policy	To reduce the risk of cross-infection and contamination
26 Cover the patient with a blanket/towel and ask them to remain lying on their left side, preferably for a minimum of 10–15 minutes, or as long as the patient is able to tolerate	To allow the suppository to be retained for the length of time directed by the manufacturer
	To enable the suppository to dissolve into liquid and to take effect
	To maintain patient dignity
27 Dispose of all used equipment in accordance with locally agreed infection prevention and control policy	To reduce the risk of cross-infection
28 Where appropriate facilities are available wash and dry your hands or alternatively cleanse with 70% alcohol-based hand rub (in accordance with local policy)	To reduce the risk of cross-infection and contamination
29 Apply gloves and disposable apron	In preparation to assist the patient on to the bedpan/ commode/toilet

*Procedure guideline 3.4 **Guideline for administration of a suppository (management of constipation)** (cont'd)*

Nursing action	Rationale
30 When the patient feels an urge to defecate assist them on to the bedpan/commode/toilet Allow privacy if the patient's condition allows	To enable bowel evacuation to take place To maintain patient dignity
31 Remove and dispose of soiled protective pad from bed in accordance with locally agreed policy. Replace if necessary	To reduce the risk of cross-infection To reduce the risk of contamination
32 Once bowel evacuation is complete assist patient to transfer from the bedpan/commode/toilet	To maintain patient safety
33 Wash and dry the patient's buttock and anal area or offer assistance	To ensure that the patient is clean To prevent skin irritation and soreness To enhance patient comfort
34 Remove and dispose of gloves in accordance with locally agreed infection prevention and control policy	To reduce the risk of cross-infection
35 Where necessary assist the patient to dress	To enable the patient to continue with their normal activities of daily living To maintain patient comfort and dignity
36 Offer the patient the opportunity to wash and dry their hands	Social hand washing is a normal activity following defecation
37 Remove and dispose of apron in accordance with locally agreed infection prevention and control policy	To reduce the risk of cross-infection
38 Where appropriate facilities are available wash your hands or alternatively cleanse with 70% alcohol based handrub, (in accordance with local policy)	To reduce the risk of cross-infection
39 Replace any moved items of furniture to their original position	To maintain a safe environment for the patient by restoring any furniture moved to its usual place
40 Verbally discuss the outcome of the procedure with the patient giving further advice as indicated. Where possible this should be supported with written information and follow-up visits if appropriate	To reinforce verbal information and support patient's understanding
41 Document the outcome of the suppository on the community nurse record of visits, this must include: ■ consent ■ findings on examination ■ stool type ■ result of procedure ■ any further nursing intervention undertaken and the outcome ■ any follow-up action/s to be taken by the community nurse, e.g. follow up visits, referral to the out of hours nursing service liaison/referral to the patient's GP	To maintain patient safety To ensure that the patient's bowel function can be monitored To ensure continuity of care To ensure accurate and contemporaneous records are kept To reduce the risk of drug errors Documentation should provide clear evidence of care planned, decisions made and care delivered (NMC 2008)

References and further reading

Abd-el-Maeboud KH *et al.* (1991) Rectal suppositories: common-sense mode of insertion. *The Lancet* **338**: 798–800.

Addison R (1999) Digital rectal examination 1 & 2. Practical procedures for nurses nos 33.1 & 33.2. *Nursing Times* **95** (40) & **95**(41) [insert].

American College of Gastroenterology Chronic Constipation Task Force (2005) An evidence based approach to the management of chronic constipation in North America. *American Journal of Gastroenterology* **100**(Suppl. 1): S1–S4.

Armon K, Stephenson T, MacFaul R *et al.* (2001) An evidence and consensus based guideline for acute diarrhoea management. *Archives of Diseases in Childhood* **85**: 132–42.

Aspinall RJ, Taylor-Robinson SD (2002) *Mosby's Color Atlas and Text of Gastroenterology and Liver Disease*. Mosby, London.

Bachoo P, Brazzelli R, Grant A (2004) Surgery for faecal incontinence (Cochrane Review). In: *The Cochrane Library*, Issue 1. John Wiley & Sons, Chichester.

Banwell JG, Graham H, Creasey Avandish M *et al.* (1993) Management of the neurogenic bowel patients with spinal cord injury. *Urological Clinics of North America* **20**(3): 517–25.

Barrett JA (1993) *Faecal Incontinence and Related Problems in the Older Adult*. Edward Arnold, London

Bell AM (1990) Colonic perforation with a phosphate enema. *Journal of the Royal Society of Medicine* **83**(1): 54–5.

Bell S (2004) Investigation and management of chronic diarrhoea in adults. In: Norton, C, Chelvanayagum S (eds) (2004) *Bowel Continence Nursing*. Beaconsfield Publishers, Beaconsfield.

Bharucha AE, Zinsmeister AR, Locke R *et al.* (2006) Risk factors for faecal incontinence: a population-based study in women. *American Journal of Gastroenterology* **101**: 1305–12.

Biebl A, Grillenberger A, Schmitt K (2009) Enema-induced severe hyperphosphatemia in children. *European Journal of Paediatrics* **168**(1): 111–12.

Black PK, Hyde CH (2005) *Diverticular Disease*. Whurr, London.

Bowers B (2006) Evaluating the evidence of administering phosphate enemas. *British Journal of Nursing* **15**(7): 378–81.

British National Fomulary (2011) British Medical Journal Publications, London.

Brown SR, Wadhawan H, Nelson RL (2010) Surgery for faecal incontinence in adults. Cochrane Database of Systematic Reviews 2010, Issue 9. Art. No.: CD001757. DOI: 10.1002/14651858.CD001757.pub3.

Brunker C (2011) Assessment, interpretation and management of altered cardiovascular status in the neurological patient. In: Woodward S, Mestecky A (2011) *Neuroscience Nursing: evidence-based practice*. Wiley-Blackwell, Oxford.

Bycroft J, Shergill I, Choong EAL *et al.* (2005) Autonomic dysreflexia: a medical emergency. *Postgraduate Medical Journal* **81**: 232–5.

Carl I, Mitchell M (2007) Symptomatic hyperphosphataemia following phosphate enema in a healthy adult. *Ulster Medical Journal* **76**(3): 172–3.

Cheetham M (2004) Drug therapy for faecal incontinence. In: Norton, C, Chelvanayagum S (eds) *Bowel Continence Nursing*. Beaconsfield Publishers, Beaconsfield.

Cheetham M, Brazzelli M, Norton C, Glazener CMA (2009) Drug treatment for faecal incontinence in adults (Cochrane Review). In: *The Cochrane Library*, Issue 1. John Wiley & Sons, Chichester.

Chelvanayagam S, Norton C (2004) Nursing assessment of adults with faecal incontinence. In Norton C, Chelvanayagum S (eds) *Bowel Continence Nursing*. Beaconsfield Publishers, Beaconsfield.

Chiotakakou-Faliakou E, Kamm MA, Roy AJ *et al.* (1998) Biofeedback provides long term benefit for patients with intractable, slow and normal transit constipation. *Gut* **42**: 517–21.

Christensen P, Krogh K (2010) Transanal irrigation for disordered defecation: a systematic review. *Scandanavian Journal of Gastroenterology* **45**: 517–27.

Cotterill N, Norton C, Avery KNL *et al.* (2008) A patient-centred approach to developing a comprehensive symptom and quality of life assessment of anal incontinence. *Diseases of the Colon and Rectum* **51**: 82–7.

Davies C (2004) The use of phosphate enemas in the treatment of constipation. *Nursing Times* **100**(18): 32.

Department of Health (2000) *Statistical Bulletin 2000/20 – Prescriptions dispensed in the community, Statistics for 1989 to 1999: England*. Department of Health, London.

Department of Health (2001) *Reference Guide to Consent for Examination or Treatment*. Department of Health, London.

Department of Health (2003) *Essence of Care*. Department of Health, London.

Deutekom M, Dobben AC (2010) Plugs for containing faecal incontinence. Cochrane Database of Systematic Reviews, Issue 3. Art. No.: CD005086. DOI: 10.1002/14651858.CD005086.pub2.

Dougherty L, Lister S (2011) *The Royal Marsden Hospital Manual of Clinical Nursing Procedures, Student edition* (8e). Wiley-Blackwell, Oxford.

Emmanuel A (2002) The use and abuse of laxatives. In: Potter J, Norton C, Cottenden A (eds) *Bowel Care in Older People*. Royal College of Physicians, London.

Emmanuel A (2004). Constipation. In: Norton C, Chelvanayagum S (eds) *Bowel Continence Nursing*, pp. 239–40. Beaconsfield Publishers: Beaconsfield.

Emmanuel A, Kamm MA (2001) Response to a behavioural treatment, biofeedback, in constipated patients is associated with improved gut transit and autonomic innervation. *Gut* **49**: 214–19.

Fernández-Fraga X, Azpiroz F, Aparici A *et al.* (2003) Predictors of response to biofeedback treatment in anal incontinence. *Diseases of the Colon and Rectum* **46**: 1218–25.

Forbes A, Misiewicz JJ, Compton CC *et al.* (2005) *Atlas of Clinical Gastroenterology* (3e). Elsevier Mosby, London.

Fox C, Lombard M (2004) *Gastroenterology* (2e). Mosby, London.

Glia A, Gylin M, Gullberg K, Lindberg G (1997) Biofeedback retraining in patients with functional constipation and paradoxical puborectalis contraction: comparison of anal manometry and sphincter electromyography for feedback. *Diseases of the Colon and Rectum* **40**: 889–95.

Harari D, Gurwitz JH, Minaker KL (1993) Constipation in the elderly. *Journal of the American Geriatric Society* **41**: 1130–40.

Harari D, Gurwitz JH, Avorn J *et al*. (1996) Bowel habit in relation to age and gender. *Archive of Internal Medicine* **156**: 315–20.

Harari D, Norton C, Lockwood L, Swift C (2004) Treatment of constipation and fecal incontinence stroke patients: randomised controlled trial. *Stroke* **35**: 2549–55.

Health Protection Agency (2008) Factsheet on Cholera [online], Available from: www.hpa.org.uk/Topics/InfectiousDiseases/InfectionsAZ/Cholera/choleraCholerafactsheet/ (last accessed 10 August 2011).

Health Protection Agency (2010) Guidance on infection control in schools and other childcare settings. HPA, London.

Herbert J (2008) Use of anal plugs in faecal incontinence management. *Nursing Times* **104**(13): 66–8.

Higgins D (2006) How to administer an enema. *Nursing Times* **102**(20): 24.

Higgins D (2007) Bowel care part 6 – administration of a suppository. *Nursing Times* **103**(47): 26–7.

Hinchliff SM (1981) The normal function of the alimentary tract. In: Breckman B (ed) *Stoma Care*. Beaconsfield Publishers, Buckinghamshire.

Horton N (2004) Behavioural and biofeedback therapy for evacuation disorders. In: Norton C, Chelvanayagam S (eds) *Bowel Continence Nursing*, pp. 251–66. Beaconsfield Publishers, Beaconsfield.

Hosker G, Cody JD, Norton C (2007) Electrical stimulation for faecal incontinence in adults. Cochrane Database of Systematic Reviews 2007, Issue 3. Art. No.: CD001310. DOI: 10.1002/14651858.CD001310.pub2.

Kalantar JS, Howell S, Talley NJ (2002) Prevalence of faecal incontinence and associated risk factors: An underdiagnosed problem in the Australian community? *Medical Journal of Australia* **176**: 54–7.

Kamm MA (2003) Constipation and its management. *British Medical Journal* **327**(7413): 459–60.

Kamm MA, Hawley PR, Lennard-Jones JE (1988) Outcome of colectomy for severe idiopathic constipation. *Gut* **29**: 969–73.

Kearny DJ (2003) Approach to the patient with gastrointestinal disorders. In: Friedman SL, McQuaid KR, Grendell JH (eds) *Current Diagnoses and Treatment in Gastroenterology* (2e). Lange Medical Books/McGraw-Hill, New York.

Knobel B, Petchenko P (1996) Hyperphosphataemic hypocalcemic coma cuased by hypertonic sodium phosphate (fleet) enema intoxication. *Journal of Clinical Gastroenterology* **23**(3): 217–19.

Kyle G (2007) Bowel care part 4 – administering an enema. *Nursing Times* **103**(45): 26–7.

Lambert A, Herman R (1996) Toxicity due to hypertonic sodium phosphate (fleet) enema: approach to the constipated patient. *Canadian Journal of Clinical Pharmacology* **3**(3): 139–44.

Lawler J (1991) *Behind the Screens*. Churchill Livingstone, Melbourne.

Lembo A, Camilleri M (2003) Chronic constipation. *New England Journal of Medicine* **349**: 1360–8.

Levitt MA, Mathis KL, Pemberton JH (2011) Surgical treatment of constipation in children and adults. *Best Practice and Research Clinical Gastroenterology* **25**(1): 167–79.

Longstreth GW, Thompson WG, Chey WD *et al*. (2006) Functional bowel disorders. *Gastroenterology* **130**(5): 148091.

Lung E (2003). Acute diarrheal diseases. In: Friedman SL, McQuaid KR, Grendell JH (eds) *Current Diagnoses and Treatment in Gastroenterology* (2e), pp. 131–2. Lange Medical Books/McGraw-Hill, New York.

Maleki D (2002) Constipation. In: Edmundowicz S (ed.) *20 Common Problems in Gastroenterology*, pp. 180–1. McGraw-Hill, New York.

Mañas M, de Victoria EM, Gil A *et al*. (2003) The gastrointestinal tract. In: Gibney MJ, Macdonald IA, Roche HM (eds) *Nutrition and Metabolism*. Blackwell Publishing, Oxford.

Marieb EN (1998) *Human Anatomy and Physiology* (4e). Benjamin/Cummings Science Publishing, California, US.

McGrath A (2005) Anatomy and physiology of the bowel and urinary systems. In: Porrett T, McGrath A (eds) *Stoma Care*. Blackwell Publishing, Oxford.

Mendoza J, Leqido J, Rubio S, Gisbert JP (2007) Systematic review: the adverse effects of sodium phosphate enema. *Alimentary Pharmacology and Therapeutics* **26**: 9–20.

Metcalf C (2007). Chronic diarrhoea: investigation, treatment and nursing care. *Nursing Standard* **21**: 48–56.

Muller-Lissner S, Kamm MA, Scarpignato C, Wald A (2005) Myths and misconceptions about chronic constipation. *American Journal of Gastroenterology* **100**: 232–42.

National Institute for Health and Clinical Excellence (2007) *Faecal Incontinence*. NICE, London.

National Institute for Health and Clinical Excellence (2008) *Irritable Bowel Syndrome in Adults: diagnosis and management of irritable bowel syndrome in primary care*. NICE, London.

National Institute for Health and Clinical Excellence (2010) *Guidance on Cancer Services: improving outcomes in colorectal cancers*. NICE, London.

National Patient Safety Agenda (2004) *Improving the Safety of Patients with Established Spinal Injuries in Hospital*. NPSA, London.

Nir-Paz R, Cohen R, Haviv Y (1999) Acute hyperphosphataemia caused by sodium phosphate enema in a patient with liver dysfunction and chronic renal failure. *Renal Failure* **21** (5): 541–4.

Norton C (2006) Eliminating. In: Redfern S, Ross F (eds) *Nursing Older People* (4e). Churchill Livingstone, Edinburgh.

Norton C, Chelvanayagum S (eds) (2004) *Bowel Continence Nursing*. Beaconsfield Publishers, Beaconsfield

Norton C, Kamm M (2001) Anal plug for faecal incontinence. *Colorectal Disease* **3**(5): 323–7.

Norton C, Chelvanayagam S, Wilson-Barnett J *et al*. (2003) Randomized controlled trial of biofeedback for fecal incontinence. *Gastroenterology* **125**: 1320–9.

Norton CC, Cody JD, Hosker G (2006) Biofeedback and/or sphincter exercises for the treatment of faecal incontinence in adults. Cochrane Database of Systematic Reviews, Issue 3. Art. No.: CD002111. DOI: 10.1002/14651858.CD002111.pub2.

Nursing and Midwifery Council (2008) *The Code: Standards of conduct, performance and ethics for nurses and midwives*. NMC, London.

Oxford English Dictionary (2007) Oxford University Press, Oxford.

Paran H, Butnaru G, Neufeld D *et al.* (1999) Enema-induced perforation of the rectum in chronically constipated patients. *Diseases of the Colon and Rectum* **42**: 1609–12.

Parés D, Norton C, Chelvanayagam S (2008) Fecal incontinence: the quality of reported randomised controlled trials in the last ten years. *Diseases of the Colon and Rectum* **51**: 88–95.

Perry S, Shaw C, McGrother C *et al.* (2002) Prevalence of faecal incontinence in adults aged 40 years or more living in the community. *Gut* **50**: 480–4.

Petticrew M, Watt I, Sheldon T (1997) Systematic review of effectiveness of laxatives in the elderly. *Health Technology Assessment* **1**(13). NHS Centre for Reviews and Dissemination, York.

Poulton B, Thomas S (1999) The nursing cost of constipation. *Primary Health Care* **9**: 17–22.

Powell M, Rigby D (2000) Management of bowel dysfunction: evacuation difficulties. *Nursing Standard* **14**(4): 47–51.

Royal College of Nursing (2006) *Digital Rectal Examination and Manual Removal of Faeces. Guidance for nurses.* RCN, London.

Royal College of Nursing (2008) *Bowel Care, Including Digital Rectal Examination and Manual Removal of Faeces.* RCN, London.

Richards A (2005) Intestinal physiology and its implications for patients with bowel stomas. In: Breckman B (ed) *Stoma Care and Rehabilitation.* Elsevier Churchill Livingstone, London.

Rolston D (2002) Acute diarrhea in adults. In: Edmundowicz S (ed.) *20 Common problems in Gastroenterology*, pp. 160–76. McGraw-Hill, New York.

Shergill IS, Arya M, Hamid R *et al.* (2004) The importance of sutonomic dysreflexia to the urologist. *British Journal of Urology International* **93**: 923–6.

Snell RS (2004) *Clinical Anatomy for Medical Students* (7e). Lippincott Williams and Wilkins, London.

Spinal Cord Injury Centres of the UK & Ireland (2009) *Guidelines for the Management of Neurogenic Bowel Dysfunction After Spinal Cord Injury.* Coloplast Peterborough.

Spinal Injuries Unit (1999) *Stimulating a Bowel Movement.* Royal National Orthopaedic Hospital, Middlesex.

Stevens P, James P (2003) Anatomy and physiology associated with stoma care. In: Elcoat C (ed.) *Stoma Care Nursing.* Hollister.

Thibodeau GA, Patton KT (2007) *Anatomy and Physiology* (6e). Mosby Elsevier, Missouri.

Thiele J, Zander J (2002) Enema-induced anorectal injuries. *Postgraduate Medicine* **111**(1).

Thomas PD, Forbes A, Green J *et al.* (2003). Guidelines for investigation of chronic diarrhoea (2e). *Gut* **52** (Suppl. v): v1–v15.s.

Thompson WG, Longstreth GF, Drossman DA *et al.* (1999) Functional bowel disorders and functional abdominal pain. *Gut* **45** (Suppl. II): 43–7.

Tortora GJ, Derrickson B (2006) *Principles of Anatomy and Physiology* (11e). John Wiley & Sons, New Jersey.

Tortora GJ, Derrickson B (2007) *Introduction to the Human Body and Essentials of Anatomy and Physiology* (7e). Wiley, New York.

Wald A (1994) Constipation and fecal incontinence in the elderly. *Seminars in Gastrointestinal Disease* **5**(4): 179–88.

Watson R (1997) *Clinical Nursing and Related Sciences.* Ballière Tindall, London.

Watson R (2002) *Anatomy and Physiology for Nurses* (11e). Baillière Tindall, London.

Whitehead WE, Wald A, Norton NJ (2001) Treatment options for fecal incontinence. *Diseases of the Colon and Rectum* **44**: 131–42.

Woodward S (2009) Yes, we can manually remove faeces. *British Journal of Neuroscience Nursing* **5**(5): 196.

4

Discharge planning

Definition

Discharge from hospital to an appropriate setting should be viewed as a process and not an isolated event. It should include the development and implementation of a plan that involves the patient, their significant other(s) and the relevant community/primary care and hospital professionals at all stages (DH 2003a).

Background evidence

A successful co-ordinated discharge from hospital into the community care setting requires organisation, coordination and communication between everyone involved. The process should commence prior to admission, where possible, for example by a community nurse or social services for elective admissions and on admission for all other patients (Salter 2001).

In recent years, UK society has seen an increase in cultural, social and geographical diversity. This, combined with an increase in people living with long-term conditions, advances in technology and a greater focus on value for money has given rise to changing expectations of healthcare provision.

This has resulted in the introduction of government policies and government-led initiatives and targets, which have made the shift from hospital to community care explicit (DH 2002; The Queen's Nursing Institute [QNI] 2006). Example of these include:

- The NHS improvement plan (DH 2004a)
- Modernising nursing careers setting the direction (DH 2006a)
- Our health, our care, our say (DH 2006b)
- Community care delayed discharge act (DH 2003b)
- Commissioning a patient led NHS (DH 2005a)
- Practice based commissioning (DH 2006c).

Therefore it is essential that all community nurses recognise their role and participate in the discharge process and acknowledge the positive impact their contribution makes to the patient journey.

Discharge planning process

The focus of the NHS plan is to provide patient-centred care closer to home and to reduce A&E attendances and the number of unnecessary admissions to hospital (DH 2000a). With evidence to suggest that the pressure for hospital beds continues, patients are sometimes discharged too early with insufficient support; consequently, the risk of readmission in the first two months post discharge is high (Holzhausen 2001).

To reduce these risks and improve individualised care pathways pre-discharge assessment and planning is essential regardless of whether a patient's needs are simple or complex (Sheperd 2001). For those patients who need a higher level of nursing care or support or who have additional social or housing needs (Box 4.1), it is essential that they are identified as early as possible and referred to the appropriate community service prior to discharge (DH 2003a). For an example of a discharge referral form that incorporates the mandatory fields for the single assessment process (SAP), *see* Figure 4.1.

A complex discharge may, for example, be one in which the patient requires:

- a complex, co-ordinated care package involving multidisciplinary/agency planning, assessment and working (Figure 4.2)
- a high level of district nursing interventions, e.g. for multiple nursing complex needs (Figure 4.3 and Box 4.1)
- end of life care

District Nursing Manual of Clinical Procedures, First Edition. Edited by Liz O'Brien.
© 2012 Blackwell Publishing Ltd. Published 2012 by Blackwell Publishing Ltd.

Data marked * must be completed at time of first referral

*Patient surname/ family name	*Patient forename(s)
*Mr, Mrs, Miss, Ms, Dr, Rev, other (circle)	Patient likes to be known as:
*DOB: Age:	
*Gender (as stated by patient)	

*Permanent address	*Address for district nursing team (if different from permanent address)
*Post code	*Post code
*Contact / Home tel No:	*Contact tel no:
Mobile:	Mobile:
Work:	Work:

*Does the patient live alone?   Yes / No (circle)

*Type of accommodation (circle) E.g. house, flat, residential, warden assisted
*Other please state:

Marital status as stated by patient (circle)

Married, Civil partnership, Single, Divorced, Widowed, Living with partner

*Ethnicity (as stated by patient)	
*Religion/spiritual belief (as stated by patient)	
*Preferred language?	
*Interpreter needed?	Yes / No (circle)
* Is a sign language interpreter needed?	Yes / No (circle)
*Written information needed in preferred language?	Yes / No (circle)
* Is Information needed in a different format?	Yes / No (circle)
*If yes please state	

Is patient known to the district nursing service, primary healthcare or social services?
Yes / No (circle) Please state:

Figure 4.1 Example of a district nursing referral form.

NHS no:	Swift no: (if known)	PAS no: (if known)	PCT patient index No: (if known)

Patient surname/ family name	Patient forename(s)	DOB

Planned discharge date: (if appropriate)

*Name of next of kin *Address (if different to patient) *Post code Telephone no(s): *Home: *Mobile: *Work (if relevant): *Is next of kin main carer? Yes / No (circle) *Relationship to patient: *DOB *Any personal health needs identified?	*Name of main carer (if different from next of kin) *Address (if different to patient) *Post code Telephone no(s): *Home: *Mobile: *Work (if relevant): *Relationship to patient: *Please state age if under 18 years: *Any personal health needs identified?
*Name, address & contact details of emergency contact (if different from next of kin/main carer) *Name: *Address: *Contact tel no(s): *Relationship to patient:	*Name, address & contact details of alternative key holder (if appropriate) *Name: *Address: *Contact tel no(s): *Relationship to patient:

Figure 4.1 (*Continued*)

*Name of referrer, relationship to patient, job title, ward & contact details:	*Has the patient/next of kin been informed of referral & given verbal/written consent to share information? **Yes / No** (circle) Comments:

Patient surname/ family name	Patient forename(s)	DOB

*Name of GP:	*Has GP been informed of discharge date? **Yes /No** (circle)

*GP practice name:

*Address

*Post code:

*Tel no:	Fax no:	Email:

* Is the patient permanently registered with this GP?   **Yes / No** (circle) If no please give details

*Name of GP:

*GP practice name:

*Address:

*Post code:

*Tel no: Fax no: Email:

*Has GP been informed of discharge date?   **Yes / No** (circle)

Any risks that visitors should be aware of?	Specials access arrangements?	Are there any pets at the home? What are they & are they friendly?

Figure 4.1 (*Continued*)

*Diagnosis & relevant past medical & surgical history & or disabilities: *State patients/carers understanding of diagnosis/prognosis	*Community nursing needs identified:

Current medication history Concordance aid needed? Yes / No (circle)	Medication administered by: Self Yes / No (circle) Carer Yes / No (circle) *Known allergies? (state)

Drug	Dose & frequency	Route	Drug	Dose & frequency	Route

Does the patient have a central venous / peripheral access device in situ? Yes / No (circle)

Type of device?	Entry site?	Exit site?	Date of placement & external length measurement?	Type & frequency of dressing change?

Daily living activities assessment overview (tick all those relevant)									
Cognitive status		Eating & drinking		Personal hygiene & dressing		Toilet		Mobility	
Orientated		Independent		Independent		Independent		Independent	
Unconscious		Needs help with preparation		Dependent on others		Needs help of 1 / 2 (circle) people		Needs help of 1 / 2 (circle) people	
Needs some prompting		Needs help with eating		Needs help		Commode, bedpan/ urine bottle		Able to transfer independently	
Needs frequent prompting		Special requirements/ meals or wheels (state)		Special requirements (state)		Incontinent of (circle) **Urine** **Faeces** **Both**		Uses mobility aids / transfer equipment	
		Nil by mouth		Uses bath aids		Urethral/supra-pubic catheter insitu		Grab rails fitted	

Figure 4.1 (*Continued*)

Skin integrity
Is the patient nutritionally compromised?   Yes / No (circle) Comments: Pressure sore risk score, e.g. Waterlow score .... Does the patient currently have a wound requiring management and nursing intervention?   Yes / No (circle) Type & grade of wound (state) Site & description of wound (include past & current treatment/s) Dressings/equipment to be supplied on discharge requested?   Yes / No (circle) Number of days to be supplied? ....

*Referral accepted by: District nursing team Yes / No (circle) *If no please state which service referrer has been sign-posted to: *Further action required Yes / No (circle) Comments:	*Referral accepted by: Single point of referral team Yes / No (circle) *If no please state which service referrer has been sign-posted to: *Further action required Yes / No (circle) Comments:

*Confirmed date & time of discharge: Comments: 	*Date & time of community nurse first visit: Comments:
*Details of person completing this form: Name: Job title: Telephone no(s): Date & signature	*Details of person completing this form: Name: Job title: Telephone no(s): Date & signature

Figure 4.1 (Continued)

Box 4.1 Examples of those who may have complex needs

- Those who are frail
- Older adults who live alone
- Patients whose carer may be unable to share the responsibility of meeting increased care needs
- Those for whom the prognosis is limited
- Those who have older adult or young dependants
- Those with mental health needs
- Those who are living with a physical disability

- Those who are asylum seekers or homeless
- Those for whom English is not their first language
- Those who have been a hospital inpatient for an extended period of time
- Those who have limited financial resources

(*The Royal Marsden Manual of Clinical Nursing Procedures*, 2011)

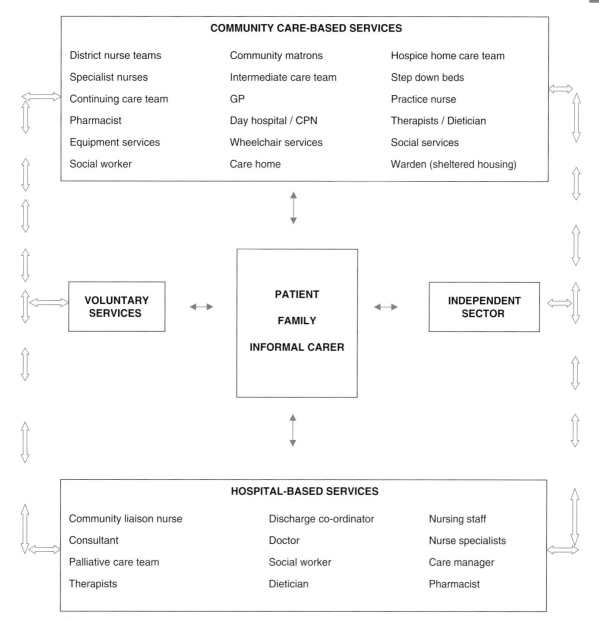

Figure 4.2 Professionals/services that may be involved in a complex discharge.

District nursing complex referral checklist				
CHECK	YES	NO	COMMENTS/ DELIVERY DATE	DATE/SIGN/ DESIGNATION
Has the patient consented to discharge plans/arrangements?				
Is the patient and relatives/carers aware of diagnosis/prognosis?				
Team potential/actual education/training needs identified				
Community nursing • Length of stay in hospital • Is a case conference required? • Has the patient been presented for continuing care funding? (if appropriate) • Is a home assessment necessary? • Date of home assessment • Are home adaptations required? • Is there any identified access problems or risks? • Is the patient independently mobile? • Does the patient have keys? If not how will the patient gain access to his/her home?				
Has a referral been made to social services? If yes: • Date and time band of first visit • Name and contact details of care manager • Has the patient/carer been given contact name and relevant telephone numbers? • Has the patient/carer received a copy of the care plan? • How many visits per day have been agreed and at what time/s?				
Has a referral been made to other primary care professionals for specialist assessment? Include name and contact details) **E.g** • Hospice home care team • Community liaison nurse • Dietician • Community matron • Physiotherapist • Occupational therapist • Community diabetes specialist nurse • Community tissue management team • Intermediate care team				
Equipment reqiured • Has the patient/carer been informed and given their consent? • Variable height bed? • Pressure-relieving aids? • Commode? • Suction machine? • Urine bottle, bed pan [type] • Manual handling aids, e.g. slides, hoist, have any risks been identified? • Which room is equipment to be placed in? • Other specialist equipment? • Is there a lift? (if appropriate) • Narrow stairwell? • Number of flights of stairs?				

Figure 4.3 District nursing complex referral checklist.

Is home oxygen therapy required?				
• Has the medical team faxed appropriate services to order this? • Have any risks been identified and eliminated? e.g non-smoking environment • Oxygen delivery date • Has the patient and/or carer received home O$_2$ training? • What equipment will be provided on discharge and how many days supply?				

Information to be given to referrer
• Name and contact details of named district nurse
• District nurse referral letter to be faxed to the relevant base/single point of referral 5–10 days prior to discharge. This should include confirmed discharge date and time. District nurse should be contacted by telephone if care plan or nursing needs have changed
• Ward staff to provide 5 days supply (or as per local policy), e.g.
  – Dressings
  – Incontinence pads
  – Needles
  – Syringes
  – Urethral catheter and bags
  – IV equipment
  – Medication
• Enteral feeding equipment and feeds
 	
What information has been given to the patient/carer?
• Details of any voluntary groups or self-help groups available in their locality
• Information regarding medication detailing dose, time, specific instructions and side effects in an appropriate language/format
• The date and time band that community services will initially visit and contact details
• The financial cost of for example social services home care provision
• Written information/leaflets explaining their medical/surgical diagnosis in an appropriate language/format
• Information on special precautions, e.g. infection control procedures (if appropriate)				

Source: Dougherty & Lister 2011; DoH (2003a).

Figure 4.3 (*Continued*)

73

- a care package that is led and co-ordinated by a community matron
- discharge to an intermediate care team.

Or it may be one where:

- a patient's length of hospital stay is more difficult to predict
- the stability of a patient's condition is unpredictable.

(DH 2004b)

In all aspects of discharge planning the emphasis should remain focused on the following.

- Care being provided by qualified/trained professionals in the most appropriate environment.
- Realistic multidisciplinary assessment of patient needs.
- Enabling the patient to be as independent as possible.
- Enabling the patient to have increased choice and an active role in the management of their care and

condition through empowerment, for example through referral to the expert patient programme or similar (DH 2006).

- The patient, wherever possible, remaining in their own home.
- Reducing the risk of the patient needing to be transferred to an alternative care environment at a later date.

- What community services are able to provide.
- What the informal caring role will involve.

(DH 2001b, 2005a)

See Table 4.1.

74 Table 4.1 Aims/principles of discharge planning best practice

Aims of discharge planning	Principles of good practice	Rationale
To facilitate the safe transfer of care from hospital to home, or to another care environment	■ Planning should commence on admission or in pre-admission clinics for elective cases ■ Where appropriate and with the patient's consent communication/liaison should commence between community and ward-based nursing staff within 48 hours of admission. Named ward nurse and named community nurse to co-ordinate the discharge process ■ Patient assessment should include the use of the single assessment process (SAP) ■ Planned discharge date should be agreed with patient and all actual and potential professionals/ services documented in the nursing notes. Any changes to the date should be communicated immediately to the relevant professionals ■ Effective and prompt two-way communication between ward staff and all actual and potential community care professionals and agency's involved in care package post discharge throughout the planning process. This should include the patient's GP	■ Patient is discharged to a safe environment of their choice with an appropriate care plan that has been agreed by the patient/carer and primary and social care services ■ Promotes communication and the sharing of appropriate knowledge and information ■ Helps to maintain patient safety and enhance continuity of care ■ A comprehensive assessment will identify actual/potential care needs and those who may be vulnerable or have special needs and prompt early referral to other professionals for a more in-depth specialist assessment ■ This will facilitate integrated care planning ■ Avoids duplication and reduces the amount of times the patient is approached for information ■ Enables ward staff to ask for the patient's consent to share appropriate/relevant information ■ Patient is involved in decision making and is aware of likely length of stay ■ To facilitate the safe efficient transfer of care and reduce the risk of delayed discharge ■ Aids patient recovery ■ Professional roles and responsibilities within the discharge planning process will be made clear and explicit, avoids duplication and improves efficiency ■ To ensure that the GP is able to resume medical responsibility following discharge ■ Discharge will be well planned and co-ordinated. This will ensure patient safety and maintain a consistently high standard of continuity of care ■ Allows time for community nurses to assess the patient on the ward ■ Allows time for care packages to be agreed and set up ■ Community staff can receive training and updates for specialist treatment and care ■ Enables home adaptations to be completed ■ To ensure that equipment is supplied and set up, e.g. variable height bed and manual handling equipment prior to discharge ■ To ensure that the patient is supported at home from day of discharge ■ Reduces the risk of delayed/failed discharge and hospital readmission ■ Promotes/supports patient-centred care and ownership of the process ■ Aids patient recovery

Table 4.1 (*Continued*)

Aims of discharge planning	Principles of good practice	Rationale
To promote effective communication and transfer of information by multi-agency partnership working	■ All professionals involved should maintain accurate up to date shared documentation ■ Joint, locally agreed, health, social services and hospital discharge policy, checklists, trigger forms and guidelines for use by all staff for guidance ■ Where necessary a case conference should be arranged for guidance on how to organise a case conference see Procedure guideline 4.1 ■ Ward staff should have access to up-to-date resource files or the intranet with details of how to refer on to district nurses, social services and voluntary organisations	■ Continuity of care and patient safety is maintained from one care setting to another ■ To improve the quality and standard of information that is passed to and between each discipline ■ This will standardise practice across boundaries and improve the patient journey ■ To discuss particular difficulties or concerns ■ To improve access to primary care services and ensure referrals are made to correct staff
To ensure patient agreement to the discharge plan	■ The patient, and with their consent, their family/significant other/s should be involved throughout discharge planning. This should include acknowledgment of the patients spiritual, cultural and religious beliefs ■ Information regarding care options/choices should be discussed and made available to the patient in an appropriate written format whenever possible ■ Patient/carer should be asked to sign and be given a copy of their discharge care plan. This should include the contact name and details of all relevant community services involved in their care package ■ In the event of the patient declining recommended community services. The patient's GP should be informed and relevant community services contact details and information regarding how to access them should be given to the patient	■ Allows specific concerns/anxieties to be raised, acknowledged and addressed prior to finalising the discharge plan ■ Helps to physically and psychologically prepare the patient and their family for discharge ■ Enables discussion and clarification of roles, expectations and, where appropriate, the degree of informal carer involvement ■ Supports and maintains patient-centred care and independence ■ To enhance concordance with treatment/drug regimen ■ Enables a carer's assessment to be carried out and where appropriate interventions to be put in place to provide more support. ■ To increase patient and carer understanding of the care options/choices available to them ■ Written information may aid decision making, prompt further discussion and act as a source of reference ■ To ensure that agreement and consent has been obtained ■ To reduce the risk of inappropriate readmission to hospital. ■ To aid patient safety ■ To reduce the risk of failed discharge and hospital readmission ■ To ensure accurate recording of the discharge process

Sources: McHale (1997); Biddington (2000); Department of Health (2000a, 2001a, 2003a); Shepherd (2001).

Community Care Delayed Discharge Act 2003

The Community Care Delayed Discharge Act (DH 2003b) introduced a system of reimbursement to the NHS for delayed hospital discharges. This is in relation to social services departments failing to carry out prompt assessment of a patient's needs and provide appropriate services, which results in delayed discharge from an acute care setting (Glasby 2003).

The main components of the act are as follows.

- Hospitals are required to notify local authority social services departments of patients who are likely to require social care on discharge.
- Social services departments having a set timescale to complete a community care assessment and provide a social care package.
- Where timescales are not met and social care services are not in place, then the local authority will be required to reimburse the acute trust.

Intermediate care

Intermediate care is one of the major initiatives for services in the NHS Plan and has also been included in the National Service Framework (NSF) for older people (DH 2000a; Thomas & MacMahon 2001).

The primary focus of the intermediate care team is to provide integrated nursing and social care and rehabilitation either in the patient's home or via the provision of step-down beds for an agreed period of time. This may be following hospital discharge or during the acute phase of an illness where hospital avoidance maybe possible. The main aim of the team is to improve the health and wellbeing of older adults and improve the quality of service they receive (DH 2002).

Continuing care/long-term care

Continuing care can be provided in a NHS hospital, the patient's own home or in a registered care home. Nursing intervention may be over an extended period of time or during the terminal stages of an illness (DH 2001c).

Care homes

Since October 2001 all adults over the age of 18 who have required all or some of their care needs met through nursing interventions have been entitled to free nursing care through a Registered Nursing Care Contribution (RNCC) assessment (Angove 2002). The comprehensive assessment is carried out by a registered general nurse, usually employed by the local primary care trust (PCT), using an RNCC tool to determine which level of the registered nursing care payment the patient meets (Angove 2002).

In the event that a patient's nursing needs fall above the top-level payment, the patient should be assessed using the NHS continuing care process. From April 2003 this was extended to include patients who had previously been non self-funding (DH 2005c).

From October 2007 the RNCC has been referred to as Funded Nursing Care (FNC) and a single band was implemented where before there were three levels of contribution (DH 2007a).

Informal carers

The informal caring role is often unexpected and may be a stressful life event that can have a significant impact on both the patient and the carer. For example:

- financial security may be lost if the carer is unable to work
- social isolation
- changes to their lifestyle
- a change of role, responsibilities and expectations of one another
- adaptations to their home/current living arrangements
- the carer's own health may be compromised
- the patient and carer's personal relationship may be affected.

(Carers UK, 2002)

To minimise these risks and ensure the safety of both patient and carer, the carer must be given time to decide if they are willing/able to share the responsibilities of the role (DH 2000c). Also, as decisions may be altered by experience or information it is important that the carer is given a full and clear explanation of what will be involved. This should include:

- what elements of care they will be expected to provide
- the care that will be provided by community nursing staff
- what will be provided by social services
- where appropriate, the provision of respite care
- their right to an individual assessment of their needs (DH 1995).

It may also be beneficial for the community nurse to establish a professional partnership with the patient and their carer prior to discharge, as this will enable the nurse to act as advocate and ensure that the carer is:

- involved
- informed
- offered choices
- emotionally and psychologically supported
- valued as a partner in the caring role.

With a growing older adult population and evidence to suggest that 17.5 million adults in the UK are living with a long-term condition (DH 2005b), it is reasonable to assume that the current expectations and often-ascribed role placed on informal carers may no longer be an option. Consequently, to meet local and national targets and initiatives, community nurses are at the forefront of community care and play a leading role in its provision (Vincent 1998; DH 2005a).

Risk management

Effective risk management ensures that the possibility of adverse incidents occurring to patients and staff are reduced to a minimum. This can be achieved through the following.

- Systematic assessment.
- The implementation of evidence-based care, action plans and their continuous review.
- Adaptation of plans and procedures to meet the requirements of all individual situations.
- Appropriate delegation and recognition of individual/team competency.
- Adherence to local risk management policy and strategies.

(NMC 2008)

Risk management strategies should be guided and supported by clear and explicit local clinical governance frameworks and healthcare standards to ensure that all community staff have a shared understanding and work in partnership to achieve the following.

- Quality assurance, e.g. measuring the quality and appropriateness of referrals to the district nursing service.
- Auditing practice, e.g. auditing delayed, failed or problematic discharges.
- Risk management assessments, e.g. assessing patients requiring equipment in the home.

- Setting and monitoring standards, e.g. developing procedures and guidelines for the administration of intravenous drug therapy in the community.
- Evidence-based best practice, e.g. the management of long-term conditions.

(Zeh 2002)

Environmental assessment

For those patients that live alone or have complex needs, it may be necessary to carry out a joint home assessment with the patient and occupational therapist prior to discharge to establish the following.

- Actual/potential risks to the patient, e.g. lack of space to accommodate equipment or allow the patient to mobilise safely with mobility aids.
- If home adaptations are necessary, e.g. stair rail, bath/kitchen aids.
- If a personal assistance call system, entry phone or digital key-box is necessary.
- If there are any actual/potential risks to community staff that may compromise their safety when carrying out prescribed care, e.g. manual handling procedures and infection control, and risks to their personal safety.

Any identified risk to either the patient or community staff must be addressed prior to discharge and the commencement of services should be in accordance with local risk management strategies and policies.

Cot sides

Where possible, the use of cot sides should be avoided and only considered after all other alternatives have been explored, for example changing the position of the patient's bed (MDA 2001; Geoff 2002; MHRA 2006). They should never be used as an aid to help patients to change their position while in bed, or prior to a comprehensive risk assessment being carried out. See Box 4.2 for an exemplar checklist that can be used in conjunction with local risk management strategies. Assessment should include assessment of the patient's:

- cognitive ability
- physical ability
- mobility
- sensory state.

(Gallinagh *et al.* 2001)

Box 4.2 Example of a community nursing cot side checklist

[To be used in conjunction with local risk assessment/guidelines for the use of cot sides]	
Does the patient have a known history of falling out of bed?	Yes/No
Have the patient's basic care needs been met prior to them sleeping?	Yes/No
Has a risk assessment been undertaken?	Yes/No
Is the patient confused?	Yes/No
Is confusion an ongoing problem?	Yes/No
If the patient is confused has a reason been identified?	Yes/No
If replied yes to the above question will treatment reduce the confusion?	Yes/No
Does the patient become disorientated at night	Yes/No
Does the patient sleep in a room on their own?	Yes/No
Has a nursing history from carers, patient and community colleagues been collated?	Yes/No
Is the patient known to be restless at night?	Yes/No
Does the patient live alone?	Yes/No
Has an occupational therapist/environmental assessment been undertaken?	Yes/No
Has the multidisciplinary team assessed/discussed the safe use of cot sides?	Yes/No
Have the risk factors/rationale for cot sides been discussed with the patient/carer?	Yes/No
Does the patient agree to the use of cot sides?	Yes/No
Have alternatives to cot sides been considered/discussed?	Yes/No
Does the patient have reduced sensation in the limbs?	Yes/No
Does the patient have the physical/cognitive ability to remove limbs if they become entrapped between the bars of the cot side?	Yes/No
Is the patient independently mobile?	Yes/No
Does the use of a pressure relief mattress with cot sides increase the patient's risk of falls or entrapment?	Yes/No
Has the use of an inter room listening device to improve patient safety been discussed with the carer?	Yes/No
Does the patient have the physical ability to climb over the cot sides or out of the end of the bed?	Yes/No
If cot sides are required could the bed be placed against a wall with a cot side on the side facing into the room only?	Yes/No

Training

Effective, safe and efficient discharge planning should be viewed as an important element in the care of all patients. Therefore it is essential that all professionals involved recognise that episodes of patient care are not isolated events and that their duty of care, in terms of accountability and responsibility, extends beyond the environment in which they work (NMC 2008).

The provision of ongoing joint training in discharge planning for community, social services and hospital staff should be considered a priority to improve knowledge understanding and communication of individual professional roles and enhance partnership working (Carers UK 2002).

Conclusion

This chapter clearly demonstrates the complex nature of discharge planning and the increasingly important and vital contribution made by both patients and community nurses to the process.

To ensure that patient choice and independence are at the centre of discharge planning and clinical practice it is essential that community nurses, hospital staff, social services and other community care providers recognise that integrated working is fundamental to its success.

Useful contacts	
Age UK Astral House 1268 London Road London SW16 4ER Carers UK 20 Great Dover Street London SE1 4LX Tel: 020 7378 4999	Department of Health Richmond House 79 Whitehall London SW16 2NS Tel: 020 7210 9177 (Public Office) Disabled Living Foundation 380–384 Harrow Road London W9 2HU Tel: 0845 130 9177

Procedure guideline 4.1 **Guideline for organising a case conference**

Nursing action	Rationale
1 Set clear aims and objectives for having the case conference and identify the chairperson and minute taker	To maintain focus and direction To ensure participants are aware of their individual roles To ensure that the main issues are clarified and prioritised To ensure that documentation is accurate and complies with local and NMC guidelines
2 Invite all appropriate community, multidisciplinary team members and hospital staff, the patient and carer/s or patient advocate	To facilitate the meeting in achieving its objective To enhance collaboration and integrated working partnerships and coordination of services
3 Ensure that all of those invited are given adequate notice of the planned date and time	To ensure that all relevant individuals are able to attend so that decisions can be made and agreed
4 If the patient is unable to attend, the chairperson, where appropriate, should meet with them prior to the meeting so that their views can be noted	To ensure that the patient's views are presented, acknowledged and responded to
5 Book venue	To ensure that the meeting can be held in a comfortable private environment in order to maintain patient confidentiality
6 Where necessary and with the patient's consent the chairperson should organise for an approved independent interpreter to be present	To enable all participants to be fully involved in the meeting To ensure accuracy of information, especially if medical terms are used. It may also be stressful for a carer or friend to accept responsibility for this role and compromise their understanding/participation
7 Provide basic refreshments and a brief explanation of available facilities and where these are located	To enable participants to feel welcome
8 Start and end meeting on time	To facilitate good time management To reduce stress and anxiety to patient/carer To aid focus on objectives

(Continued)

*Procedure guideline 4.1 **Guideline for organising a case conference** (cont'd)*

Nursing action	Rationale
9 Allow patient and carer the freedom to choose where they sit	To help them feel comfortable and relaxed To ensure patient/carer are able to receive support from each other
10 The chairperson should welcome those present and those present should briefly introduce themselves and give an overview of their contribution to the current patient care plan	All of those in attendance will have a clear understanding of people's roles
11 The chair person chairperson should make those present aware that time will be made available to ask questions and ensure that paper and pens are available for personal note taking	To ensure questions are answered The provision of paper and pens will enable individuals to make a note of questions they may want to ask This may reduce patient/carer anxiety To allow participants to clarify their understanding of points discussed
12 The chairperson should verbally summarise the main points at the end of the conference. This should include identifying specific action points and those responsible for ensuring these are completed/ followed up	To make individual participant's responsibilities explicit clarify the responsibilities of participants To give an opportunity to clarify specific points To enhance the development of future plans
13 Chairperson should ensure that the patient/carer are all right and answer any further questions they may have	This may help to reduce any anxiety or concerns that they may have
14 The carer should be given the contact details of the patients named ward and community nurse to contact if they have any further questions	To promote continuity of care and good communication To reduce the patient/carer's anxiety
15 If the patient has been unable to attend they should be given a summary of what has been discussed/ provisionally agreed upon after the meeting	To ensure that the patient is aware of the discharge plan To promote patient-centred care and participation in decision making To obtain patient consent and promote concordance Written documentation may prompt further discussion and reduce fears or anxiety (NMC 2009)

Problem solving table 4.1

Problem	Action
Patient is not registered with a GP	Patient should be advised to register with a GP
	Advise on how to obtain a local GP list from the primary care trust (PCT) or community/hospital Patient Assisted Liaison Service [PALS]
Patient unable to find a GP who will accept them on their list	Advise on how to contact the local PCT who will advise and may assign the patient to a GP practice
Patient does not have a GP and chooses not to register with one but requires district nursing input	Explain and discuss with the patient/carer the risks of not being registered with a GP and encourage them to register as soon as possible
	If the patient declines, liaise with the discharging hospital about the current consultant continuing to accept medical responsibility for the patient and to provide prescriptions for any necessary medication/ treatment
	If appropriate, liaise with the discharging hospital about the possibility of the patient returning to the ward/ assessment unit as an outpatient for follow-up care
	Where appropriate, explore the possibility of the patient attending the local walk-in centre for follow-up care
The patient will require subcutaneous/ intravenous fluids or medication at home	Ensure that the medical team has contacted the GP to ascertain that they will accept medical responsibility once the patient is discharged
	If necessary, liaise with ward staff about updates/training for team members
	Ensure that there is appropriate team cover at weekends, bank holidays and out of hours, and that those team members on duty are competent to carry out the procedure. Alternatively, liaise with colleagues in other teams to negotiate cover
	Intravenous fluids/medication are not generally available on FP10; consult Trust policy/guidelines or the Trust pharmacy team for guidance and advice
The patient lives alone and will be unable to answer the front door	Explore the possibility of a family member or neighbour holding the key and meeting the community nurse on agreed visit days and times to enable access
	Where appropriate, consider the installation of an entry phone or a digital key lock/box
	To aid safety the patient should be discouraged from attaching the key to the inside of the letter box or placing it, for example, underneath a flowerpot
The patient will be unable to obtain prescribed medication/treatment from the chemist	The community nurse should liaise with the community pharmacist about home delivery
The patient/carer may experience difficulties with administration of oral tablet medication	Community nurse should monitor and review medication post discharge. Where necessary, they should liaise with the GP and community pharmacist about the weekly provision of, e.g. dispensed blister pack or suitable alternative
The patient has been discharged home without necessary supplies of, e.g. wound care treatment; urethral/suprapubic catheter equipment	Community nursing base should maintain an appropriate emergency stock of supplies, for example: ■ sterile dressings ■ bandages and tapes

81

References and further reading

Adcock L (2000) Assessing the needs of carers. *Journal of Community Nursing* **14**(3): 4–8.

Age Concern (2002) FS/37/02/10/01.

Angove E (2002) Changes in funding nursing care homes in England. *The Communicator*, RCN Liaison & Discharge Planning Association, pp. 4–5.

Atwal A (2002) Nurses perceptions of discharge planning in acute health care: a case study in one teaching hospital. *Journal of Advanced Nursing* **39**(5): 450–8.

Audit Commission (1999) *First Assessment: a review of district nursing services in England and Wales*. Audit Commission, London, pp. 41–71.

Biddington W (2000) Reviewing discharge planning processes and promoting good practice. *Journal of Community Nursing* **14**(5): 4–6.

Bull MJ, Roberts J (2001) Components of a proper discharge for elders. *Journal of Advanced Nursing* **35**(4): 571–81.

Carers UK (2002) *Hospital Discharge Practice Briefings*. Carers UK, England.

London Borough of Croydon, Croydon PCT (2002) *Continuing Care: NHS and Local Councils Responsibility*. London Borough of Croydon & Croydon PCT, Surrey.

Department of Health (1995) *The Carers [Recognition and Services] Act*. DH, London.

Department of Health (2000a) *The NHS Plan: a plan for investment, a plan for reform*. DH, London.

Department of Health (2000b) *Care Homes for Older People, National Minimum Standards. Care Standards Act*. DH, London.

Department of Health (2000c) *No Secrets: Guidance on Developing and Implementing Multi-Agency Policies and Procedures to Protect Vulnerable Adults from Abuse*. DH, London.

Department of Health (2001a) *NHS Funded Nursing Care – Practice Guide and Workbook*. DH, London.

Department of Health (2001b) *The National Service Framework for Older People*. DH, London.

Department of Health (2001c) *Continuing Care: NHS and Local Councils' Responsibilities*. HSC 2001/015: LAC.

Department of Health (2002) *NSF For Older People – Intermediate Care: Moving Forward*. DH, London.

Department of Health (2003a) *Discharge from Hospital: Pathway, Process and Practice*. London.

Department of Health (2003b) *The Community Care (Delayed Discharges) Act*. DH, London.

Department of Health (2004a) *The NHS Improvement Plan*. DH, London.

Department of Health (2004b) *Achieving Timely 'Simple' Discharge From Hospital. A Toolkit for the Multi-disciplinary Team*. DH, London.

Department of Health (2005a) *Commissioning a Patient Led NHS*. DH, London.

Department of Health (2005b) *Supporting People With Long Term Conditions, Liberating the Talents of Nurses Who Care for People With Long Term Conditions*. DH, London.

Department of Health (2005c) *Ensuring that all recipients of high band NHS-funded nursing care have been correctly considered against eligibility criteria for fully funded NHS continuing care*. DH, London.

Department of Health (2006) *NHS Continuing Health Care: action following the Grogan judgement*. DH, London.

Department of Health (2006a) *Modernising Nursing Careers, Setting the Direction*. DH, London.

Department of Health (2006b) *Our Health, Our Care, Our Say*. DH, London.

Department of Health (2006c) *Practice Based Commissioning*. DH, London.

Department of Health (2007) *The National Framework for NHS Continuing Healthcare and NHS – Funded Nursing Care*. DH, London, pp. 8, 35 (document revised July 2009).

Dougherty L & Lister S (2011) Assessment, discharge and end of life care. In: Dougherty L & Lister S (eds) *The Royal Marsden Hospital Manual of Clinical Nursing Procedures (8e)*, pp. 22–78. Wiley Blackwell, Oxford.

Eaves A, Scanlon L (2003) Equipment choices – using practice guidelines. *Journal of Community Nursing* **17**(9): 34–8.

Gallinagh R, Slevin E, McCormack B [2001] Side rails as physical restraints: the need for appropriate assessment. *Nursing Older People* **13**(7): 22–7.

Geoff A (2000) Ensuring the safe use of cotsides in patient's settings. *Professional Nurse* **15**(4): 278–9.

Glasby J (2003) Delayed reaction. *Community Care* **10–16 July**: 38–9.

Hancock S (2003) Intermediate care and older people. *Nursing Standard* **17**(48): 45–51.

Hill M, Macgregor G (2001) Health's forgotten partners? How carers are supported through hospital discharge. *Carers Health Matters*. Carers UK, London. Available from British Library Document Supply Centre, DSC:m02/11005.

Holzhausen E (2001) *You Can Take Him Home Now: carer's experience of hospital discharge*, pp. 1–8. Carers UK, London.

Holzhausen E, Pearlman V (2000) *Caring on the Breadline: the financial implications of caring*, pp. 1–4. Carers National Association, London.

McHale C (1997) Essential guide to principles of discharge planning. *Nursing Times* **93**: 52–3.

MDA (2001) *Bed Side Rails [cotsides]: Risk of Entrapment and Asphyxiation*. Hazard Notice. Medical Device Agency HN [10], London.

Medicines and Healthcare products Regulatory Agency (2006) Device bulletin DB2006 (06). Safe use of bed rails. MHRA, London.

Nazarko L (2002) Delayed discharges the legal implications. *Nursing Management* **9**(1): 22–3.

Nursing & Midwifery Council (2008) *The Code: Standards for conduct, performance and ethics for nurses and midwives*. NMC, London.

Nursing & Midwifery Council (2009) *Guidelines for Records and Record Keeping*. NMC, London.

Richardson J (1998) Detection of elder abuse. *Journal of Community Nursing* **8**(12).

Rudd C, Smith J (2002) Discharge planning. *Nursing Standard* **17**(5): 33–7.

Salter M (2001) Planning for a smooth discharge. *Nursing Times* **34**(23 Aug): 32–4.

Salter M (2002) Homeward bound – reflection of a complex discharge. *Journal of Community Nursing* **16**(4).

Savage P (1998) Care in the community. *Journal of Community Nursing* **12**(1): 4–6.

Shepherd E (2001) When it's time to go home. *Nursing Times* **97**(34): 22–3.

Thomas S, Macmahon D (2001) Intermediate care. *Journal of Community Nursing* **15**(6): 12–20.

Vafeas C (2002) Referral criteria. *Nursing Standard* **14**(45): 39–41.

Vincent V (1998) Responding to the needs of carers. *Journal of Community Nursing* **12**(9): 4–8.

Wade S, Lees L (2002) The who, why, what of intermediate care. *Journal of Community Nursing* **16**(10): 6–10.

Zeh P (2002) Clinical governance and the district nurse. *Journal of Community Nursing* **16**(4): 4–11.

5

Ear irrigation

This chapter is adapted and updated from 'Ear Syringing' of *The Royal Marsden Hospital Manual of Clinical Nursing Procedures*, Fifth Edition. Edited by Jane Mallett and Lisa Dougherty.

© 2000 The Royal Marsden Hospital. Blackwell Publishing Ltd.

Definition

Ear irrigation is the process of flushing the external auditory canal of the ear with water to remove ear wax (cerumen), or a foreign object that has impaired hearing (Krapp & Cengage 2002).

Background evidence

Anatomy of the ear

The ear can be divided into three parts: the external, middle and inner ear. Irrigation is directed only at the external ear. The pinna or auricle, the external auditory meatus and the tympanic membrane (ear drum) make up the external ear (Figure 5.1).

The first third of the external auditory canal is formed of fibrocartilage; the inner two-thirds are bony (Figure 5.1).

The *pinna* (or auricle) is the prominent, visible part of the external ear which sits over temporal bone of the skull. It consists of cartilage covered by perichondrium and skin. The *external auditory meatus* is an S-shaped canal that leads down from the pinna to the tympanic membrane. It is lined with epithelium continuous with that on the tympanic membrane. The meatus is 2.4–2.5 cm long in the adult with the outer third made of cartilage and the inner two-thirds made of bone (Corbridge 1998). Hair and sebaceous glands cover the cartilaginous part (the hair becomes more prominent in males after middle age). Cerumen is produced in this area by modified sweat glands or apocrine glands

known as ceremonious glands. The tympanic membrane (ear drum) (Figure 5.2) forms the inner end of the external auditory canal. It is normally shiny and described as transparent, opaque or pearly grey/pink. As part of the normal ageing process the ear drum becomes whiter and duller (Webber-Jones 1992). Some structures of the middle ear are faintly visible through the normal tympanic membrane.

Routine cleaning of the ear

In normal circumstances ear hygiene can be maintained by washing the pinna and external auditory meatus with a tissue or alcohol free wipe. Patients should be advised not to insert anything into the ear further than the part that can be seen from the outside (Beare & Myers 1998). Cotton buds, match sticks and hairpins can damage the wall of the canal, cause wax to become impacted, increase the likelihood of otitis externa or perforate the tympanic membrane (Webber-Jones 1992).

Purpose of ear irrigation

Foreign bodies

Foreign bodies are sometimes inserted into the external canal and may become lodged. Alternatively, insects or debris may be blown into the ear (Beare & Myers 1998). If the foreign body is composed of vegetable matter, irrigation and the use of liquids (e.g. olive oil) are contraindicated because vegetable matter (e.g. peas, beans) is absorbent and swells up on contact with the liquid. Once swollen, the foreign body becomes more firmly lodged and therefore more difficult to remove (Beare & Myers 1998).

Insects may be removed by instilling olive oil into the ear. The insect is usually killed and floats to the entrance of the auditory canal where it can be retrieved with a Tilley's or other grasping forceps. Foreign bodies should

District Nursing Manual of Clinical Procedures, First Edition. Edited by Liz O'Brien.
© 2012 Blackwell Publishing Ltd. Published 2012 by Blackwell Publishing Ltd.

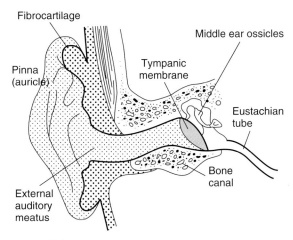

Figure 5.1 External auditory canal. The external one-third is formed of fibrocartilage; the inner two-thirds are bony (Mallett & Dougherty 2000).

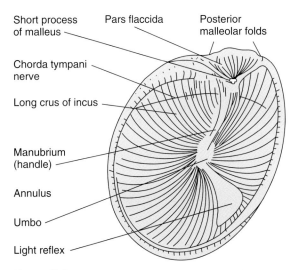

Figure 5.2 Right tympanic membrane (Mallett & Dougherty 2000).

only be removed by specialised medical staff. Referral to an ENT department must be made if:

- the attempt is unsuccessful
- there is suspected trauma to the ear drum
- there is a risk of damaging the eardrum during removal.

(Harkin 2000)

To extract a solid foreign body a hook or Jobson horn probe is passed beyond the foreign body and gently pulled out. Attempting this procedure without the necessary training and skills may result in:

- the foreign body being forced into the bony portion of the canal
- the skin in the canal being damaged
- the eardrum being perforated.

(Corbridge 1998)

Impaction of cerumen

Cerumen is continuously produced by ceruminous glands located in the subcutaneous layer, deep in the sebaceous glands (Lewis 2008). The secretions mix with keratin debris produced by the migration of epithelial cells in the external meatus. Cerumen protects and waterproofs the meatal skin and is slightly acidic, thereby providing antibacterial and antifungal properties (Rodgers 2003). It is gradually moved towards the entrance of the auditory canal by the action of muscles used in chewing and talking, and by surface migration. It is thought by some that their ears should be routinely cleared of ear wax; this is not always the case, and leads to the public misconception that contributes considerably to the increase in ear irrigation (Lewis 2008).

If cerumen production is excessive, or if an obstruction prevents it moving towards the entrance to the auditory canal, the canal may become blocked with wax which hardens over time. People with large amounts of hair in their ears, wear hearing aids, work in dusty or dirty atmospheres or have narrow ear canals are more likely to experience build-up of ear wax. This can usually be resolved by the weekly instillation of one or two drops of olive oil (Beare & Myers 1998; Harkin 2008).

The most common method of cerumen removal is through ear irrigation using warm water. This removes the cerumen occluding the tympanic membrane, therefore restoring hearing (Lewis 2008).

Preparation of the patient prior to irrigation

Examining the outer ear

The external auditory meatus (ear canal) and tympanic membrane must be examined with an otoscope by a qualified practitioner in good light before the decision to irrigate the ear can be made. The otoscope has an ear piece (speculum), illumination to visualise the eardrum and magnification for accurate assessment. Examination should take place with both nurse and patient

85

seated (Harkin 2005). The *Guidance Document in Ear Care* produced by the Action on ENT steering board (Action on ENT 2002) has recently been updated by the Primary Ear Care Trainers (2007). This document gives full step-by-step instructions on ear examination and information that should be followed for safe and effective practice.

A full history must be obtained from the patient of any relevant problems, particularly any:

- previous perforations
- infections
- deafness
- surgery.

It is also important that the community nurse allows the patient to describe their symptoms in detail. In circumstances where the patient is unable to communicate or remember, a full history should be obtained from their medical records, close family members or carers, and an examination done for evidence of surgery, infection or perforations (Kaufman 1998).

If pressure or movement of the pinna is painful, the patient may have an infection of the outer ear (otitis externa). Otitis externa is also associated with redness, scaling and itching, swelling, watery discharge and crusting of the external ear (Phipps 1993). Pain, hearing loss, tinnitus and otorrhoea (ear discharge) may indicate an infection of the middle ear, known as otitis media (Corbridge 1998). If an infection of the outer or middle ear is suspected, the community nurse must seek advice from the patient's GP before carrying out the procedure.

Blockage of the ear with impacted cerumen may cause a feeling of:

- pressure
- fullness
- muffled hearing
- whistling
- squeaking
- crackling noises
- discomfort (rarely pain).

Otoscopic examination using an appropriately sized speculum is carried out by first pulling the pinna upwards and backwards, which stretches the cartilaginous part of the external meatus (Figure 5.3). If infection is present, this procedure will cause pain. The otoscope is held like a pen in the dominant hand while the pinna is gently pulled up and back by the non-dominant hand; to ensure stability the small finger should be rested on the patient's head (Figure 5.4). The external auditory canal can be inspected as the speculum is carefully inserted into the ear. The walls of the

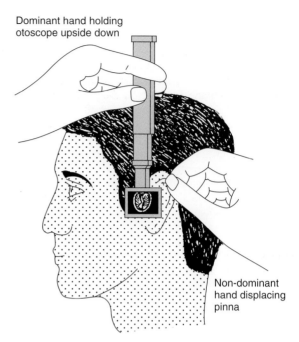

Dominant hand holding otoscope upside down

Non-dominant hand displacing pinna

Figure 5.3 Technique for otoscopic examination (Mallet & Dougherty 2000).

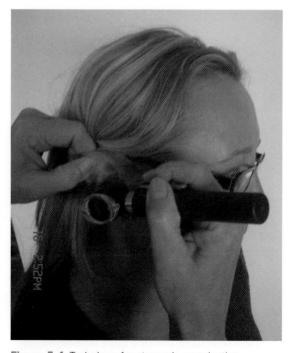

Figure 5.4 Technique for otoscopic examination.

canal are very sensitive and fragile; rough contact with the end of the speculum is painful, and should be avoided (Webber-Jones 1992).

The appearance of the tympanic membrane should be assessed (Figure 5.2). In normal circumstances the tympanic membrane is intact (without perforation). The long and short processes of the malleus (a small bone in the middle ear) are visible through the membrane as white markings, and the umbo, where the malleus is connected with the tympanic membrane, appears as a white spot.

All areas of the tympanic membrane should be observed; light from the otoscope is reflected off the light reflex on the normal tympanic membrane. If the light is reflected in an uneven way, the light reflex is said to be diffuse, and is abnormal. Other parts visible are the handle of malleus (visible at 10 o'clock in the left ear and 2 o'clock in the right), the pars flaccida, pars tensa and the anterior recess (Kaufman 1998).

Changes in the colour of the tympanic membrane (normally shiny, translucent and pearly grey/pink) or the shape (normally slightly concave) may indicate an infection of the middle ear. Otitis media may make the tympanic membrane red, dull or retracted; a bulging tympanic membrane indicates the presence of infection/exudate in the middle ear (Corbridge 1998).

The normal surface of the tympanic membrane is smooth and unmarked, although appearance can vary, and the ability to differentiate this is learnt by practice and experience (Kaufman 1998). Scarring is usually caused by previous infections and/or perforations. It is essential that the community nurse always records what was observed in both ears.

Irrigation is contraindicated if the patient has a history of the following:

- Previous complication with irrigation.
- Previous perforation of the tympanic membrane or surgery, e.g. mastoid, as irrigation could result in unsterile water in the middle ear or mastoid cavity (Cook 1998).
- Recent middle ear infection (previous six weeks), e.g. otitis media, as the tympanic membrane may be under pressure from mucus or pus and irrigation would cause pain as well as the risk of perforation (Cook 1998).
- Pain or tenderness of the pinna.
- The patient has a cleft palate (repaired or not).
- Precautions include tinnitus, healed perforation and dizziness.

Microsuction is used for patients with chronic ear disease, e.g. chronic otitis externa or media, and is performed by a doctor, nurse or audiologist trained in the use of microscope and suction, usually based at an ENT department. For this procedure the ear is examined using a speculum and a light microscope. An aural sucker is then used to identify and remove debris (Primary Care Trainers 2007).

Any abnormality identified in the external ear should be brought to the attention of the patient's GP and advice on further action sought.

Preparation of the external auditory meatus for irrigation

Unless otherwise prescribed, olive oil is the product commonly used prior to irrigation as patients can develop meatal irritation to cerumenolytic ear drops. (Action on ENT 2002). The oil should be at body temperature and instilled with a dropper when the patient is lying with the ear facing upwards. The top of the ear is pulled up to allow the oil to pass down the straightened ear canal (Harkin 2005). The dropper should be placed over the ear canal until one to two drops are instilled, and the tragus of the ear should be massaged, allowing the drops to descend into the canal. The patient should then remain in this position for approximately 5 minutes (Harkin 2005).

Cotton wool is not advised for use as a plug as this will absorb the oil; excess should be wiped with a tissue. The procedure is then repeated on the other side if required. Preparation is usually twice daily for 5–7 days prior to irrigation (Harkin 2005).

Risk management

When irrigation is undertaken in the community, the community nurse must adhere to relevant locally agreed guidelines and policy. The patient's home is not always an ideal location to use as the clinical setting and safety precautions should be taken when using equipment, and if necessary a risk assessment should be completed. Both nurse and patient should be seated comfortably beside a solid surface, e.g. worktop, and as close as possible to a safe electrical socket. If this is not practical, the nurse should create a safe surface next to the patient's chair/bed and use the battery to power the irrigator. It is important to, as far as is practically possible, ensure a good light source.

Because of the danger associated with the pressure created in a metal manual ear irrigation syringe and the difficulty with cleaning, this equipment should no longer be used (Coopey 2001). Electronic jet irrigators allow safe irrigation, for example the Propulse 111; this is both mains and battery operated and has an isolation transformer for electrical safety. The irrigator has minimum/maximum pressure control, and irrigation should be commenced on the minimum setting (Harkin 2005). To maintain both patient and nurse safety it is essential that the manufacturer's instructions are followed and adhered to at all times.

Training

Irrigation of the ear should only be undertaken by a trained nurse/practitioner (Harkin 2005). Appropriate certified training should be undertaken, which will enable the practitioner to work safely, competently and within the current NMC Code (NMC 2008).

The *Guidance Document in Ear Care* (Action on ENT 2002) is regularly updated, and the latest version, Primary Ear Care Trainers (2007), can be downloaded from www.earcarecentre.com. The document has been endorsed by the Royal College of General Practitioners, the Royal College of Nursing, the Primary Ear Care Centre and the Medicines and Healthcare Products Regulatory Agency.

Conclusion

Through patient and/or carer education, and anticipatory preventative treatment, patients will develop an understanding of how to prevent minor ear problems, recognising the first signs of recurrence, and will therefore seek treatment sooner (Rodgers 2003).

Procedure guideline 5.1 **Guideline for ear irrigation**

Equipment

Waterproof cape
Towel (if available)
Otoscope and disposable single-use speculum
Electronic jet irrigator
Head mirror and light or headlight
Jobson Home probe
Lotion thermometer
Cotton wool and tissues
Tap water (at body temperature)
Noots trough or receiver
Disposable single-use apron and gloves

Procedure

Nursing action	Rationale
1 Where appropriate facilities are available wash and dry your hands thoroughly or alternatively cleanse with 70% alcohol-based hand rub (in accordance with local policy)	To reduce the risk of cross-infection
2 If the patient is known to the service review nursing documentation and current care plan	To update knowledge of patient and maintain patient safety
3 If the patient is unknown to the service a full comprehensive assessment must be carried out prior to undertaking the procedure	To identify potential contra-indications and/or cautions To determine if a second nurse is required to assist with the procedure To maintain patient safety

Procedure guideline 5.1 **Guideline for ear irrigation** *(cont'd)*

Nursing action	Rationale
4 Verbally, and where possible visually, explain and discuss the procedure with the patient. Written consent should be obtained from the patient and documented prior to carrying out the procedure	To ensure the patient understands the procedure, assessing their capacity in making a decision to consent (Mental Capacity Act 2005)
	To ensure that the patient can make an informed choice (NMC 2008), to give valid written consent.
	To aid the identification of potential contra-indications and/or cautions
	To maintain patient safety
	Patient information reduces anxiety
	To gain co-operation and consent
5 Prepare the environment; where necessary obtain patient consent to move furniture	To allow freedom of movement when carrying out the procedure
	To maintain patient privacy
6 Assemble all necessary equipment on a clean surface	To prevent disruption to the procedure
7 Assist the patient into the appropriate position, ensuring a good light source	To enhance the visibility of the ear
8 Where appropriate facilities are available wash and dry your hands thoroughly or alternatively cleanse with 70% alcohol-based hand rub (in accordance with local policy)	To reduce the risk of cross-infection
9 Examine both ears, using the otoscope, and inspect the external auditory canal	To detect the presence of abnormalities, e.g. scars, skin defects, discharge, bulging or colour changes of the tympanic membrane. Any signs of infection should be referred to the GP, as treatment may be required (Action on ENT 2007)
	To assess if the ear/s are appropriate for irrigation (Action on ENT 2007).
	To maintain patient safety
10 Place the waterproof protective cape and/or towel around the patient's shoulders	To protect patient clothing
11 Fill the irrigator reservoir with warm water (body temperature) using the lotion thermometer to confirm the temperature (Action on ENT 2007)	Water that is too hot or cold is uncomfortable, may damage tissue, and can cause nausea, vomiting and dizziness by triggering the vestibular reflex (Action on ENT 2007)
12 Set the irrigator pressure to minimum (Action on ENT 2007).	Minimum pressure is required to commence procedure (Action on ENT 2007)
13 Where appropriate facilities are available wash and dry your hands thoroughly or alternatively cleanse with 70% alcohol-based hand rub (in accordance with local policy)	To reduce the risk of cross-infection
14 Apply apron and gloves	To prevent the risk of cross infection

(Continued)

Procedure guideline 5.1 **Guideline for ear irrigation** *(cont'd)*

Nursing action	Rationale
15 Ask the patient, carer or second nurse to hold the Noots trough or receiver in place at the bottom of the ear lobe of the relevant ear	To collect irrigated fluid and debris To protect patient clothing and flooring from irrigation fluid
16 Ensure the irrigator tip is clicked into place, turn on machine and run through to dispel any cold water within the system and check temperature again (Action on ENT 2007)	To ensure tip is secure and ensure water is at body temperature
17 Gentle pull the pinna upwards and backwards using the non dominant hand (Figure 5.4)	To stretch the cartilaginous part of the external meatus To straighten the ear canal and to hold ear steady
18 Position the irrigator tip jet towards the posterior wall of the external auditory canal	To ensure the correct position in preparation for the procedure
19 Inform the patient that you are about to start the procedure	To confirm that the patient continues to consent to the procedure being undertaken To ensure that the patient is relaxed and aware the examination is about to begin To gain patient cooperation To prepare patient and encourage feedback
20 Advise the patient to indicate if they experience any dizziness or pain during the procedure (Action on ENT 2007)	In order to recognise patient discomfort and/or complications and stop the procedure To maintain patient safety To enable the patient to withdraw consent for the procedure
21 Using the foot control, direct the flow of water towards the upper outer wall of the canal (11 o'clock in right ear and 1 o'clock in the left ear) (Action on ENT 2007)	To direct flow behind the wax plug to wash it out
22 If wax proves difficult to remove, increase the pressure slowly. A maximum of two reservoirs are advised in one procedure (Action on ENT 2007)	Too long a period of irrigation can cause trauma to the canal
23 Inspect the canal intermittently throughout the procedure and examine the contents of the receiver for wax and debris during the procedure (Action on ENT 2007)	To assess the condition of the canal To reduce the risk of trauma To ascertain the position of the wax To maintain patient safety
24 Visually examine the contents of the Noots trough/ receiver during the procedure (Action on ENT 2007)	To evaluate the effectiveness of the irrigation procedure
25 If no wax is removed within the first 5 minutes of the procedure, irrigate the second ear then return to the first ear if appropriate	The wax may soften or dislodge during this period of time
26 Once completed, dry the canal with a Jobson Horne probe and cotton wool	This will reduce the risk of infection from excess water (Action on ENT 2007)

Procedure guideline 5.1 Guideline for ear irrigation (cont'd)

Nursing action	Rationale
27 Remove the waterproof protective cape and/or towel from around the patient's shoulders	To promote patient comfort
28 Dispose of all used single-use equipment in accordance with locally agreed infection prevention and control policy	To reduce the risk of cross-infection
29 Discard unused water from the irrigator reservoir and refer to the irrigator manual for guidelines on correct cleaning and disinfectant of the irrigator, back at base	To reduce the risk of cross-infection
30 Remove and dispose of apron in accordance with locally agreed infection prevention and control policy	To reduce the risk of cross-infection
31 Where appropriate facilities are available wash and dry your hands thoroughly or alternatively cleanse with 70% alcohol-based hand rub (in accordance with local policy)	To reduce the risk of cross-infection
32 Replace any moved items of furniture to their original position	To maintain a safe environment for the patient by restoring any furniture moved to its usual place
33 Verbally discuss the outcome of the procedure with the patient giving further advice as indicated. Where possible this should be supported with written information and follow-up visits if appropriate	Advice and education regarding regular oiling of ears, can prevent build up of wax (Stubbs 2000). The ear is susceptible to infection post irrigation; the patient should be made aware of any signs of infection To reinforce verbal information and support patients understanding
34 Document the outcome of the procedure on the community nurse record of visits, this must include: ■ consent ■ findings on examination of both ears ■ the condition of the canal ■ if the tympanic membrane is visible ■ the light reflex ■ pars tensa, pars flaccida, the handle of malleus and the anterior recess ■ result of procedure ■ any further nursing intervention undertaken and the outcome ■ any follow-up action/s to be taken by the community nurse, e.g. follow-up visits, liaison/ referral to the patient's GP (Neno 2006)	If these are visible, it can be recorded as a normal tympanic membrane (Lewis 2008) To maintain patient safety To ensure continuity of care To ensure accurate and contemporaneous records are kept Documentation should provide clear evidence of care planned, decisions made and care delivered (NMC 2009)
35 If wax is difficult to remove, repeat the irrigation following a further 5 days instillation of olive oil. If this continues to be a problem, referral to the ENT department or practitioner for microsuction, would be appropriate	To soften wax for further irrigation. Microsuction by trained practitioners can be undertaken for wax, debris or foreign bodies in patients where irrigation is not appropriate (Action on ENT 2007)

91

References and further reading

Action on ENT (2002) Guidance Document in Ear Care. Available from: www.earcaretrainers.com/protocol (last accessed 1 October 2011).

Beare PJ, Myers JL (1998) *Principles and Practice of Adult Health Nursing* (3e). Mosby, St Louis, pp. 1160–84.

Brunner LS, Suddarth DS (1989) *The Lippincott Manual of Medico-Surgical Nursing* (2e). Harper and Row, London, pp. 867–83.

Cook R (1998) Ear syringing. *Nursing Standard* 16(13): 56–61.

Coopey S (2001) Ear syringing – a case for clinical governance. *Journal of Community Nursing* 15(1): 20–2

Corbridge RJ (1998) Essential ENT Practice. A Clinical Text. Edward Arnold, London, pp. 90–120, 156–62.

Harkin H (2000) Evidence based ear care. *Primary Health Care* **10**(8): 26–30

Harkin H (2005) A nurse led care clinic – sharing knowledge and improving patient care. *British Journal of Nursing* **14**(5): 250–4.

Harkin H (2008) Guidance document in ear care. www.earcarecentre.com/protocols (last accessed 1 October 2011).

Kaufman G (1998) Ear problems: care and prevention. *Practice Nurse* 15(6): 338–42.

Krapp K, Cengage G (eds) (2002) Ear irrigation. In: *Encyclopedia of Nursing and Allied Health*. enotes 2006; www.enotes/nursing encyclopedia/ear irrigation (accessed 15 May 2009).

Lewis H (2008) Ear irrigation: minimising the risks. *Nursing in Practice* **42**: 44–7.

Lewis–Cullinan C, Janken J (1990) Effect on cerumen removal on the hearing ability of geriatric patients. *Journal of Advanced Nursing* 15: 595–600.

Mallett J & Dougherty L (2000) Ear syringing. In: The Royal Marsden Hospital Manual of Clinical Procedures *(5e)*. Blackwell Science, Oxford.

Mental Capacity Act (2005) Code of Practice. The Stationery Office, London.

Neno R (2006) Holistic ear care: cerumen removal techniques. *Journal of Community Nursing* **20**(9): 26–31

Nursing and Midwifery Council (2008) The Code: Standards of Conduct, Performance and Ethics for Nurses and Midwives. NMC, London.

Nursing and Midwifery Council (2009) Records and Record Keeping. NMC, London.

Phipps.W J. (1993) The patient with ear problems. Medico – Surgical nursing. A nursing process approach. 3rd ed; St Louis: Mosby: 1327 – 51.

Primary Care Trainers (2007) *Guidance Document in Ear Care.* Available at www.earcarecentre.com (accessed on 21 June 2008).

Rodgers R (2003) Primary ear care treatments. *Practice Nurse* **25**(9): 69–73.

Stubbs G (2000) Ear syringing and aural care. *Nursing Times* **96**(43): 35–7.

Webber-Jones J (1992) Doomed to deafness? *American Journal of Nursing* **Nov**: 37–9.

6

Infection prevention and control

Glossary

Antibiotic – medication taken to kill or inhibit the growth of micro-organisms.

Antibiotic policy – written guidelines that recommend antibiotics and their dosage for treating and preventing specific infections.

Antimicrobial agent – substances that kills or inhibits the growth of micro-organisms.

Aseptic non-touch technique (ANTT) – refers to practices/procedures that reduce the risk of infection by decreasing the risk that micro-organisms will enter the body during procedures such as wound dressings and injections. Used for simpler and less invasive procedures such as administration of intravenous drugs where only the part of the equipment not in contact with a susceptible site that has to be kept sterile is handled.

Aseptic surgical technique – refers to practices/procedures that reduce the risk of infection by decreasing the risk that micro-organisms will enter the body during invasive procedures such as the insertion of a central venous catheter.

Audit – organise review of current practices and comparison with core-determined standards. Action is then taken to rectify any deficiencies that have been identified in current practice. The review is repeated to see if the pre-determined standards have been met.

Bactericide – chemical that can kill vegetative bacteria (cannot destroy spores).

Benchtop steriliser – machine designed to achieve sterilisation, which requires no permanent connection or installation (Medical Devices Agency 2002).

Blood-borne viruses – viruses that survive in the blood, i.e. HIV, Hepatitis B, C, D, E, F and G.

Carrier – a person who has potentially pathogenic organisms on their body or in their body fluids that are not causing an infection but can cause cross-infection and infection in others.

Cleaning – removal of dirt and some micro-organisms, essential prerequisite to sterilisation and disinfection.

Clinical governance – a framework through which NHS organisations are accountable for continuously improving the quality of their services and safeguarding high standards of care by creating environments in which excellence in clinical care will flourish.

Commensal – an organism, usually harmless, that lives on the body or in body fluids without causing infection but could cause infection in an immunocompromised person.

Communicable disease – a disease that can be transmitted to others.

Community – related to populations or services outside the hospital.

Contact – a person who has been exposed to infection.

Contamination – to make dirty.

Cross-infection – the transfer of infection from one person to another.

Decontamination – general term to cover cleaning, disinfection and sterilisation to remove micro-organisms.

Disinfection – a process to kill or remove micro-organisms, but not usually bacterial spores.

Epidemic – a high incidence of an endemic infection, or a high instance of infection where this infection is not generally found.

Healthcare-associated infection (HCAI) – an infection that was neither present nor incubating at the time of the patient's admission to hospital.

(Continued)

District Nursing Manual of Clinical Procedures, First Edition. Edited by Liz O'Brien.
© 2012 Blackwell Publishing Ltd. Published 2012 by Blackwell Publishing Ltd.

Immune compromised – a person whose natural immunity is impaired either through disease, age or treatment that makes them susceptible to infection.

Immune suppressed – immune response is impaired or prevented from working effectively due to radiotherapy or drug therapy, i.e. cytotoxic drugs, steroids.

Immunisation/vaccination – the use of a vaccine in a protective effect to prevent the person acquiring a particular disease.

Infection – invasion and multiplication of harmful micro-organisms in body tissue.

Medical device – any instrument, appliance, material or other article intended by the manufacturer to be used for a patient or client for the purpose of diagnosis, prevention, monitoring, treatment or alleviation of disease or injury to include control of conception (Medical Devices Agency 2000).

Micro-organism – an organism, including bacteria, fungi, protozoa, viruses and some algae, which can cause infection in susceptible persons.

Needlestick injury/inoculation accident – percutaneous injury where a sharp breaks the skin.

Prophylaxis – medication given to prevent infection. This may be before an operation or when someone has been exposed to infection (needlestick injury) or is vulnerable to infection (HIV-positive person).

Sensitivities – the susceptibility of micro-organisms to antibiotics or disinfectants.

Single use medical device – a device that is intended to be used on an individual patient during a single procedure and then discarded. Not to be reprocessed and used on another patient (NHS Estates 2003).

Spores – dormant micro-organisms that can germinate and cause infection when conditions are suitable. These conditions generally include moisture and warmth.

Sterile – free from viable micro-organisms.

Sterilisation – process that destroys or removes all living micro-organisms including bacterial spores and viruses.

Transmission – the means by which a micro-organism can be spread, and in some cases cause infection.

Introduction

Infection control has been defined as 'measures/actions taken to reduce the incidence of, prevent the spread of, or reduce the complications from any health problems which behave as if it were caused by a transmissible agent'. Infection control in the community is defined as 'the infection control service provided outside acute and major hospitals to those in a care setting' (Public Health Laboratory Service 2002a: 6).

In this era of shorter hospital stays (Pellowe *et al.* 2003) and more surgical procedures being undertaken by general practitioners (GP), the need for effective infection control in the community is essential.

The information contained in this chapter is applicable and appropriate for a variety of settings in primary healthcare including:

- people's own homes
- nursing homes
- residential homes
- schools
- nurseries
- dental practices
- GP surgeries.

Infection control encompasses the whole National Health Service (NHS) healthcare system (National Audit Office 2000) and includes:

- universal precautions
- advice on decontamination
- disinfection

- education and training
- policy
- standards for practice
- surveillance and audit development
- the management of outbreaks of infection
- advice on the use of antibiotics
- immunisation.

The principles of infection control must be firmly grounded in everyday practice. There is a need to continually assess and update these principles to keep pace with new ideas and challenges that are facing the community now, as well as those that are being planned for the future.

Background evidence

The findings of reports by Taylor *et al.* (2001) and the National Audit Commission (1999) suggest that 24% of referrals to the district nursing service come from hospital-based staff. Therefore it is reasonable to assume that if the level of healthcare-associated infection (HCAI) is 1 in 9 for all inpatients, the number of discharged patients who will have had or still have a HCAI is going to be high.

From the 1960s to the 1970s the use of antibiotics and vaccinations had reduced the threat of death from infectious disease in the developed world. This was not the case in the developing world, where tuberculosis, malaria, HIV and AIDS have caused more than

13 000 000 deaths a year, particularly among those on low incomes and children under the age of five years (DH 2002).

A change in epidemiological variables (Box 6.1) and social behaviour (Table 6.1) has meant that the risks of

infectious complications in the developed world have increased. The changes in social behaviour are also thought to be closely linked to outbreaks of infection in the community, for example:

- whooping cough (Jenkinson 2006).
- measles (Stone *et al.* 2007).
- *Salmonella* outbreaks (Calvert *et al.* 2007).
- *Legionella* (Foster *et al.* 2006).
- *Escherichia coli* 0157 (Payne *et al.* 2003).
- multiresistant tuberculosis (Padayatchi & Friedland 2007).
- hepatitis (Meara *et al.* 2007).

More recently new infectious diseases have had a major impact on the community. These include:

- Creutzfeldt–Jakob disease (vCJD): this has already infected an unknown number of people. Predictions of future cases of vCJD remain uncertain. This uncertainty has increased since the identification of cases infected by blood transfusions (Clarke & Ghani 2005)
- multiresistant micro-organisms such as multiresistant *Streptococcus pneumoniae*, the major cause of

---

Box 6.1 Changes in epidemiological variables

- An increasing population of frail older adults (Ward 2001)
- Advances in medical, surgical and cancer treatments and the management of long-term conditions means that patients are living longer. This has resulted in many more people living and receiving nursing care in their local community (Griffiths *et al.* 2007)
- The emergence of antibiotic resistant micro-organisms (Croft *et al.* 2007)
- Reluctance in the population to receive vaccinations (Hobson-West 2007)
- The emergence of new infectious diseases (Smith-Bathgate 2005)

Table 6.1 Changes in social behaviour

Changes in social behaviour	Consequences of changes in social behaviour
International travel: not only to destinations where disease patterns differ, but also the nature of travel causing overcrowding leading to close contact with strangers (DH 2002)	Malaria Meningitis Influenza Ebola virus
Drug misuse (Magura *et al.* 2000)	HIV Hepatitis B Hepatitis C
Change in eating habits, for example cook chilled foods and takeaways (Gillespie *et al.* 2003)	*Escherichia coli* 0157 *Salmonella* *Shigella* *Campylobacter* Varient Creutzfeldt-Jakab disease (vCJD)
Sexual activity, including multiple sexual partners and unprotected sex (McGarrigle *et al.* 2002)	HIV Hepatitis B Hepatitis C Venereal diseases
Changes in work environments, for example increased air conditioning (Sanchez *et al.* 2001)	*Legionella pneumophila*
Increased social activities, for example leisure activities such as fresh water and sea sports (Ward *et al.* 2002)	Hepatitis A Cryptosporidium
Terrorism threats (Bradberry *et al.* 2003).	Smallpox Anthrax Ricin

community acquired pneumonia, and meticillin resistant *Staphylococcus aureus* (MRSA), an important cause of wound infections and bacteraemia (Croft *et al.* 2007).

Healthcare-associated infection (HCAI)

It is estimated that 9% of patients acquire an infection during their admission to hospital (Table 6.2), and approximately 5000 of these patients will die as a direct result of HCA1 (National Audit Office 2000, 2004). With each infection increasing lengths of hospital stay, on average 2.5 times longer per individual patient, the total cost of HCAl to the NHS is suggested to be in the region of £1 billion each year. With the emphasis on the provision of care closer to home, it is envisaged that treatment and care costs for HCA1 will shift from acute to primary and community care services (Plowman *et al.* 1999).

The number of infections diagnosed following discharge from hospital is unknown. However, it is estimated that as many as 48–70% of surgical wound infections are diagnosed following discharge from hospital (Stockley *et al.* 2001; Taylor *et al.* 2001). Furthermore, a separate study of 1449 patients that were followed up in the community found that during the post-discharge phase 19.1% of those who returned their questionnaires reported that while they did not have a HCA1 during their in patient stay, they did report symptoms and were prescribed treatment that met the criteria for a urinary, chest and/or surgical wound infection once at home (Plowman *et al.* 1999).

The National Audit Office (2000) recommends that post-discharge surveillance should take place, either as part of the Nosocomial Infection National Surveillance Scheme (NINSS 2002) or as part of the trust's own surveillance.

Table 6.2 HAI and percentages

Type of infection	Percentage
Urinary tract infection	23.2%
Lower respiratory tract infection	22.9%
Surgical wounds	10.7%
Skin	9.6%
Blood	6.2%
Others	27.4%

(Taylor et al. 2001)

Infections cause increased problems for the patient and their families and can include:

- delayed recovery
- longer hospitalisation
- readmission to hospital
- permanent disability
- increased costs for items such as prescriptions
- loss of earnings
- disruption of family routine
- fear
- pain
- offensive wound discharge and odour, which may lead to social isolation
- antibiotics, which can be toxic
- risk of death
- death.

Not all infections are preventable and some patients, who may be very old or young and those with less efficient or immature immune systems, are particularly susceptible to infection (National Audit Office 2004).

A working group from the Public Health Medicines Environmental Group (PHMEG) (1996) have compiled a list of risk factors for acquiring an infection when at home.

- Extremes of age (i.e. premature babies and frail older people).
- Congenital abnormalities (causing structural/functional deficiencies).
- Previous serious illness.
- Prolonged or intense exposure to a source of infection (living in the same house as someone with untreated tuberculosis for example).
- Malnutrition or obesity.
- Poor personal hygiene, incontinence, general debility.
- Immune suppression by therapy or disease (i.e. cancer, cystic fibrosis, steroid therapy for arthritis).
- Recent antibiotic therapy (reducing normal bacterial colonisation and allowing more virulent or resistant organisms to replace them).
- Breaks in skin (traumatic, chronic ulceration, pressure sores).
- Vascular or urinary catheterisation.
- Smoking, pre-existing lung disease.
- Metabolic disorders (i.e. diabetes).
- Implanted prosthetic material.
- Malignant disease.

(PHMEG 1996)

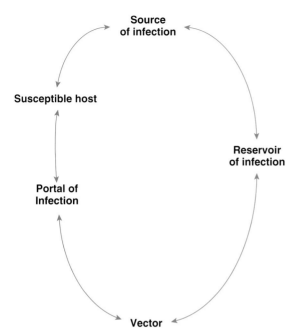

Figure 6.1 Epidemiology of infection. (Adapted from Lawrence & May 2003).

Box 6.2 Portal of entry for micro-organisms

Direct route – unwashed hands (MRSA, *Salmonella*)
Indirect route – contaminated crockery (*Salmonella*), toilets (Vancomycin-resistant enteroccoci [VRE])
Airborne – coughing/sneezing (influenza, tuberculosis), bedmaking (MRSA), building work (aspergillus)
Blood borne – needlestick injuries (HIV, hepatitis B and hepatitis C)
Ingestion –food (*Salmonella*, *Shigella*, *Campylobacter*), water (Cryptosporidium)
Sexually – gonorrhoea, syphilis, HIV, hepatitis

Portal of entry is where micro-organisms are able to enter the body of a susceptible individual (Box 6.2).

A susceptible host is where the patient has reduced resistance to infection, making them more susceptible to acquiring an infection. For example:

- infants
- patients with uncontrolled diabetes
- patients with leukaemia
- patients with severe burns
- patients with poor nutrition
- patients on immunosuppressive therapies (Ayliffe *et al.* 2000).

The epidemiology of infection

Although many micro-organisms can cause an infection, generally only certain micro-organisms, referred to as pathogenic organisms, do cause infection. The term 'chain of infection' has been developed to imply a chain of events that need to occur before an infection can develop. Infection control implies breaking the chain of infection so that infections do not occur (Figure 6.1).

The chain of infection includes several links. These are as follows.

A source of infection where potentially pathogenic micro-organisms are living and in many cases multiplying. Sources of infection include contaminated food, the environment, wounds, the nose or bowel of colonised people or animals.

A reservoir is where micro-organisms can survive and in some cases multiply. Reservoirs of infection include food, carriers of infection, contaminated sink plugs, cracked/damage kitchen surfaces, poorly maintained or malfunctioning equipment, for example refrigerators.

Vector/vehicle for the spread of infection. The most common cause for the spread of infection is unwashed hands.

Infection prevention and control in the community

Infection prevention and control includes all measures and actions that are taken to reduce the incidence of, prevent the spread of, or reduce the complications of infections. The role of infection control includes providing advice on decontamination, disinfection, universal precautions, education and training, audit, policy development, management of outbreaks of infection, advice on the use of antibiotics and immunisation. Loveday *et al.* (2002) state that the practitioners undertaking these tasks are central in the delivery of infection control in the community.

A study commissioned by the Department of Health in December 2000, reported by Loveday *et al.* (2002), reviewed infection control arrangements in the community and found that this was an underdeveloped area. While all districts had an infection control infrastructure that supported the infection control services, problems did occur. These included poor administration support, insufficient financial and other resources, and high workload. This study recommends that there should be a consistent infection control service, with written standards for infection control and appropriately trained staff (Loveday *et al.* 2002).

This study also reviewed infection control staffing levels (Loveday *et al.* 2002). It was found that there were:

- 1.07 whole time equivalent (WTE) consultants in community disease control
- some districts had additional medical support, which meant that there was a total of 1.2 WTE per 500 000 of the population.
- 1.74 WTE infection control in the community (ICIC) nurses per 500 000 of the population.
- 8% of districts had no ICIC nurse
- 41 different variations of the titles for ICIC nurses. These job titles and general responsibilities are all linked in their aim to provide infection control help and advice with the objective of preventing infection, but if infections do occur, to ensure appropriate treatment and care is provided, while preventing the spread of the infection. The role of a nurse involved with infection control is generally defined by the setting within which they work and the type of client population they are responsible for.

Loveday *et al.* (2002) found that the seven key activities of ICIC were:

- providing advice and information
- guidelines development
- outbreak management
- contact tracing
- surveillance
- audit
- meetings.

While the ICIC nurses were found to work closely with public health nurses (PHN) and communicable disease control nurses (CDCN), there were differences in their roles. For example the PHNs took the lead in health protection, including health assessment, health improvement and health promotion, while the CDCNs work with consultants in communicable disease control (CCDC) in the management and control of communicable diseases (Farrow *et al.* 1999).

Link infection control nurses are identified members of staff working in a particular area who are not substitutes for infection control nurses but can be trained by the infection control nurse to give infection control advice, increase awareness of infection control issues and assist in the early detection of infection control outbreaks. In some cases they can be

trained to collect surveillance data for the infection control team. Link nurses must have sufficient clinical experience and standing to have authority with managers and colleagues within their own area, in order to be able to encourage compliance with infection control policies and procedures (National Audit Office 2004).

The DH study undertaken in December 2000 (Loveday *et al.* 2002) found that of the 90 health authorities surveyed, 34% had written standards for the infection control in the community service; 88% had antimicrobial prescribing policy/guidance and a CCDC/microbiologist had been involved in their development. Samples of relevant standards for infection control in the community include the following.

- Appropriate and accessible written infection control policies and procedures. Evidence of review and update.
- Written statement defining the infection control doctor and nurse's roles and responsibilities in the community.
- Designated members of staff who act as infection control link nurses.
- Records kept of suspected and confirmed cases of infection.
- Written policy for outbreak of infection control measures.
- Written procedures for training in infection control, including induction and mandatory training.
- Written statement on universal control precautions, evidence of competence in use of universal control precautions.
- Written policy and evidence of competent handwashing techniques.
- Written policy and evidence of competence on safe handling, labelling and transportation of specimens; waste disposal; handling and disposing of sharps; safe handling of laundry.
- Written policy for safe handling and disposal of all types of clinical/domestic waste.
- Written policy and evidence of competence on sharps and needlestick injuries.
- Written policy and procedures and evidence of competence on the safe use of reusable equipment.
- Written polices and procedures and evidence of competence in tasks such as:
  - intravenous therapy
  - urinary catheterisation
  - enteral feeding
  - parenteral feeding
  - wound care
  - administration of medicines.

- Written policies and procedures and evidence of competence for specific infections such as:
  - meticillin resistant *Staphylococcus aureus* (MRSA)
  - *Clostridium difficile*
  - tuberculosis
  - scabies
  - gastroenteritis
  - HIV and AIDS.

Standards

Standards underpin any quality initiative (Calman 1992). In 1993 the Department of Health issued standards in infection control suggesting that these standards could be used as a point of reference to deliver a high quality infection control service (DH 1993). More recently the Department of Health (2004b) consultative document introduced key standards for the quality of care delivered throughout England. Two categories of standard were developed:

- core standards related to enabling overall quality of healthcare to all patients
- developmental standards designed to enable overall quality of healthcare to rise as additional resources being invested in the NHS take effect.

The need to have national standards for infection control in the community has been suggested by the regional directors of public health in a study of infection control in the community (PHLS 2002a). They recommend five main types of standards (*see* Box 6.3).

Outbreak of infection in the community

Outbreaks of infection can occur and may vary in extent and severity, ranging from a few cases of urinary infection to a major outbreak of food poisoning. Each primary care trust (PCT) should have an outbreak committee, policy, procedure and plan to deal with outbreaks of infection. A core of relevant persons including the CCDC, nurses, GPs and regional managers would make up the outbreak committee, and the committee could request other relevant persons with particular expertise for a current outbreak for their help and advice. For example, in the case of water-borne infections this could be the local water supply representative. The outbreak committee is responsible for agreeing an outbreak policy, procedure and plan. Once an outbreak of infection is identified the outbreak committee would

---

Box 6.3 Quality initiative standards

Standard 1

ICIC nurses should be competent for this role and maintain their competence through appropriate professional development

Standard 2

There should be sufficient staffing resources devoted to infection control to enable the functions to be carried out satisfactorily and in accordance with national standards

Standard 3

There should be sufficient support for the infection control team

Standard 4

Primary care trusts must have robust arrangements to fulfil their infection control functions

Standard 5

There should be formally agreed infection control guidance for community healthcare settings and other establishments that have particular infection control needs

(PHLS 2002a)

take all necessary steps to investigate the source and cause of the outbreak, co-ordinate control measures and prepare a report (DH 1995a).

Health clearance for healthcare workers

All healthcare workers must be well and fit to undertake the work that they do. Occupational health clearance is essential and is required in the pre- and post-appointment checks for all new persons working in the NHS in England (HSC 2002/2008). New DH guidance now requires certain healthcare workers to be checked for:

- tuberculosis disease/immunity
- hepatitis B, with post-immunisation testing of response
- hepatitis C and HIV.

This is to ensure that staff, including, for example, all medical, surgical, dental, midwifery, paramedics and ambulance workers, are free of TB and are provided with appropriate vaccinations. Extra checks are required for all new healthcare workers who go on to perform exposure-prone procedures (EPP). These checks will need to be made to ensure they are free from hepatitis B, hepatitis C and HIV (DH 2007a).

Universal/Standard precautions

The use of universal precautions safeguards the health-care worker from all risks that may occur while at work (ICNA 2003a), as well as helping to prevent the spread of infection, and assists in the containment of known infections. A questionnaire survey of community nurses found that universal precautions were not always followed, mainly because care was often provided in less than ideal home conditions (Bennett & Mansell 2004). Strategies are required for improving compliance, especially related to sharps management (Cutter & Gammon 2007) to ensure compliance with NICE guidelines is achieved (NICE 2002).

The key premise of universal precautions is that all patients should be assumed to be a risk and the same precautions should be applied routinely to all patients (Stein *et al*. 2003). This universal approach protects the health of the staff and ensures that all patients' dignity and respect is maintained (Lymer *et al*. 2003).

Universal precautions protect healthcare workers from pathogens, potentially toxic chemicals and drugs spread by:

- infected blood (i.e. HIV, hepatitis)
- infected body fluids (i.e. HIV, hepatitis)
- airborne particles (i.e. tuberculosis)
- contaminated specimens (i.e. HIV, hepatitis)
- blood and body fluids contaminated with toxic drugs (i.e. incontinence following administration of cytotoxic drugs), radioactivity (incontinence following nuclear medicine investigation that involved administration of diagnostic doses of a radionuclide)
- spilt potentially toxic chemicals and drugs.

(Hart 2008)

Protection is obtained by:

- handwashing
- wearing gloves
- wearing plastic aprons/barrier gowns
- wearing face masks
- wearing goggles
- wearing armlets and over shoes
- safe handling and disposal of sharps and contaminated waste

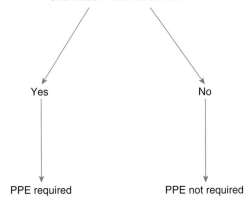

Figure 6.2 Risk assessment and use of PPE.

- safe handling of specimens
- safe handling of spillages.

(Pratt *et al*. 2007)

The use of protective clothing is known as personal protective equipment (PPE) and refers to single-use items that are worn for one patient and then disposed of in a clinical waste bag (Figure 6.2).

PPE is designed to cover and protect the health care worker from every eventuality (Principles table 6.1). A risk assessment must be undertaken for every procedure to establish four key risks and to ensure that the most suitable PPE is utilised (Pratt *et al*. 2007). All risk assessment must include:

- the risk of transmission of micro-organisms to the patient
- the risk of contamination of healthcare workers by the patient's blood and body fluids, secretions and excretions
- selection and utilisation of the most suitable PPE
- evaluation of the PPE in use to ensure it is providing the necessary protection to the user.

Risk assessment ensures that the decision to use or wear PPE is based on a specific clinical procedure, the patient's general condition and takes into consideration current health and safety legislation (Pratt *et al*. 2007). In general, the following factors should be considered for all of those people providing direct care to a patient.

- Risk of fluid splashes/aerosol in eye – goggles to be worn.

- Risk of fluid splashes/aerosol to nose and mouth – mask to be worn.
- Known airborne infection, i.e. meningococcus meningitis/ tuberculosis – mask to be worn.
- Risk of handling blood or body fluids (known or expected) – gloves to be worn.
- Contact with non-intact skin and mucous membranes – gloves to be worn.
- When handling contaminated instruments/equipment – gloves to be worn.
- Risk of contamination to uniform/clothing – plastic apron to be worn. It is unlikely that fuller cover is required in the community, but if it is required a barrier gown must be worn.

Mask

A facemask must be worn where there is a risk of blood, body fluids, secretions or excretions splashing the face. Respiratory protective equipment, for example a particulate filter mask, must be worn correctly and used when caring for patients with respiratory infections transmitted by airborne particles (Pratt *et al.* 2007). In the event of pandemic influenza, particulate filter masks will be worn when in close contact with a patient with pandemic influenza (DH 2005).

NB All community nurses should be issued with a facemask with one-way valves; this must be used for cardiopulmonary resuscitation of all persons suffering a cardiorespiratory arrest and receiving cardiopulmonary resuscitation (Idris & Gabrielli 2002).

Goggles

Goggles are worn to prevent the eyes from becoming contaminated with aerosolised blood and body fluids. A study to estimate the frequency with which goggles become contaminated with blood during care in the home setting found that contamination occurred in 2% of all procedures (Beltrami *et al.* 2000).

Uniforms for nurses

Traditionally, a nurse's uniform has been representative of professional status, power, infection control, identity, modesty, symbolism. and health and safety (Pearson *et al.* 2001). However, it has been questioned whether uniforms should be worn in all settings, and a differentiation should be drawn between uniform and protective clothing (Richardson 1999).

It is important that personal protective clothing is worn in the community to protect the community nurse's uniform, because micro-organisms can be spread to other home care patients by nurses unknowingly carrying the micro-organisms to another home care patient's home (Friedman 1999). Micro-organisms can survive on fabrics for long periods of time. One study found that micro-organisms could survive on fabric for more than 60 days (Neely 2000).

In the community, laundry and changing facilities are not always available. This means nurses wear their uniforms home and launder them in domestic washing machines to reduce the risk of cross-infection. The uniform should be removed as soon as the community nurse gets home and machine washed following the manufacturer's instructions. Care should be taken to ensure that the washing machine is not overfilled as this could inhibit removal of micro-organisms from the used uniform. A clean uniform should be worn each day.

Handwashing

Healthcare workers' unwashed hands are considered to be the major vehicle for the transmission of micro-organisms between patients, which means that correct handwashing is considered to be one of the most important infection control practices to ensure hands are clean and free from contamination (Pratt *et al.* 2007). An audit of community healthcare workers' handwashing practices found that there was a need to pay greater attention to hand hygiene (Gould *et al.* 2000). Correct handwashing should be undertaken by all community staff providing care to a patient and by the patient themselves when, for example, they have been to the toilet prior to handling or eating food or may be involved in their own care.

The aim of handwashing is twofold.

1 To remove transient micro-organisms on the skin surface (routine handwashing).
2 To remove resident micro-organism on the skin surface prior to aseptic/surgical techniques.

Routine handwashing
Routine handwashing is aimed at removing dirt, organic matter and transient micro-organisms, making the hands socially clean, and in most instances liquid soap and water is adequate (NICE 2003). Preparations containing antimicrobial handwashing agents are more effective in removing resident micro-organisms and should be used for all surgical hand washes (Pratt *et al.* 2007). A risk assessment must be completed by community nurses in order to establish the method of handwashing that should be undertaken for each patient (Carroll 2001a).

Principles table 6.1 Use of personal protective equipment

Action	Rationale
1 Gloves	
1.1 Gloves must be available when contact with patients is likely to occur (Carroll 2001b)	Gloves are more likely to be used appropriately if they are readily available
1.2 Gloves must comply with European Community (CE) standards (NICE 2003)	To ensure they are of a suitable quality and standard for their intended use
1.3 Powdered gloves must not to be used (NICE 2003)	Powder is associated with drying of hands, adhesions, latex allergy and contamination of the environment and equipment with powder
1.4 Polythene gloves must not to be used (NICE 2003)	Polythene gloves can easily become damaged during use
1.5 Alternatives to natural rubber latex gloves must be available. Alternatives include vinyl and Nitrile (Korniewicz et al. 2002)	While latex gloves offer increased dexterity, vinyl gloves made to CE standards and used appropriately provide the same protection as latex gloves (Hampton 2002). Some hospitals have changed to nitrile gloves (Brown et al. 2003); these must be checked to ensure that they do not contain latex (Crippa et al. 2003).
1.6 Clean-boxed gloves must be worn to protect hands from contamination with blood, body fluids, secretions and excretions	Clean-boxed gloves are sufficient and more economical to use when providing a barrier to hands and reduce the risk of hand contamination from micro-organisms, toxic drugs and chemicals (Rossoff et al. 1993)
1.7 Sterile gloves must be worn when there is a need to prevent the risk of transmission of micro-organisms to patients during aseptic surgical techniques	Sterile gloves are indicated for aseptic surgical procedures, for example during wound care, when sterile gloves may replace forceps when cleaning wounds (St Clair & Larrabee 2002)
1.8 Gloves must be used as a single-use item and must be changed after each patient (NICE 2003)	To prevent cross-infection
1.9 Gloves must not be washed	Washing of gloves can reduce the integrity of the glove material and therefore reduce the protection (Hampton 2002)
1.10 Gloves must be changed as soon as they become damaged	To prevent contamination of the hands
1.11 Used gloves contaminated with blood, body fluids, secretions, excretions or chemicals must be disposed of as clinical waste (NICE 2003)	To prevent cross-infection
1.12 Gloves must be worn for all cleaning tasks (Lawrence & May 2003)	To protect hands from the area being cleaned and the chemicals being used
1.13 Gloves must fit correctly	Poorly fitting gloves that are too large can interfere with dexterity and performance, exposing the wearer to potential risk. Gloves that are too small can become damaged and cause friction, which may cause skin irritations (Powell et al. 1994)
1.14 Gloves should not be worn for too long	Wearing gloves for long periods of time causes excessive sweating, which creates an ideal environment for micro-organism growth and skin damage (Kownatzki 2003)

Principles table 6.1 *Use of personal protective equipment* (cont'd)

Action	Rationale
2 Gowns	
2.1 Fluid-repellent gowns must be worn when there is a risk of extensive splashing from blood, body fluids, secretions, excreta, chemicals or toxic substances (NICE 2003)	Gowns provide increased cover and more protection than a plastic apron (Seto *et al.* 2003)
2.2 Gowns are single-use items	Gowns can easily become contaminated and may contaminate the wearer or the next patient if used more than once (Zachary *et al.* 2001)
2.3 Disposable gowns (Lankester *et al.* 2002) contaminated with blood, body fluids, secretions, excretions or chemicals must be disposed of as clinical waste (NICE 2003)	To prevent cross-infection
2.4 Reusable fabric gowns must be processed at a hospital laundry	Reusable gowns must be properly decontaminated before reuse
3 Plastic aprons	
3.1 Disposable plastic aprons are cheap, easy to put on and generally provide good cover to the wearer's clothing and should be worn when contamination to clothing is suspected (Pratt *et al.* 2007).	To prevent contamination of clothing that could result in cross-infection to other persons exposed to the contamination, i.e. other patients, family and friends
3.2 Plastic aprons are single-use items and must be changed after each patient care (NICE 2003)	To prevent cross-infection
3.3 Used plastic aprons must be disposed of as clinical waste (NICE 2003)	Plastic aprons maybe contaminated
4 Filter facemask	
4.1 Filter facemasks must be worn when there is a risk of aerosol blood, body fluids, secretions, excretions and splashing into the face (NICE 2003)	To prevent contamination of the face
4.2 Filter facemasks must be worn when in close contact with a person with an infectious respiratory disease, e.g. untreated pulmonary tuberculosis, Influenza, meningococcus meningitis	To reduce the risk of cross infection
4.3 The specifications for facemasks must be established to ensure the correct filtration is being used	Micro-organism and chemical droplets for example vary in size and the filtration of the mask must be suitable for its intended use (Lipp 2003)
4.4 Masks are single-use items and once used must be disposed of as clinical waste	Reusing masks can lead to cross infection as micro-organisms can be transferred to the clean side of the mask during storage
5 Armlets	
5.1 While rarely required, they should be kept in case of gross spillage or contamination from toxic chemicals, blood, body fluids, secretions or excretions	To prevent contamination of arms
5.2 Armlets are single-use items and should be disposed of as clinical waste after use	Used armlets may be contaminated and therefore must be disposed of as clinical waste
6 Goggles/Safety spectacles/Eye protection	
6.1 Eye protection must be worn when there is a risk of contamination to the eyes from toxic chemicals, blood, body fluids, secretions or excretions (NICE 2003)	To prevent contamination to the eyes, during certain minor procedures such as wound irrigation and when manually cleaning instruments
6.2 Goggles are not single use items.	Goggles/safety spectacles can be easily washed with hot soapy water and dried with a paper towel after use

Reusable handwashing equipment in patients' homes must not be used by community nurses; these include bars of soap, nail brushes and reusable towels, as they can become readily contaminated with micro-organisms and are therefore a potential source of cross-infection (Malik *et al.* 2003).

It is essential that the nurse's skin integrity be maintained following repeated handwashing. Skin damage is generally related to the preparation being used and poor technique, and can lead to changes in microbial flora to those with increased pathogenicity (Larson *et al.* 1998). Sore skin is also a predisposing factor for why nurses reduce the number of times they clean their hands. Alcohol-based hand rubs are better tolerated than the traditional soap and running water hand wash (Winnefeld *et al.* 2000).

Handwashing is not only for healthcare workers, as hands of healthy persons in the community can be colonised with pathogenic organisms, therefore if providing care for a sick relative or friend in the community it is essential that carers also undertake handwashing before and after providing care (Larson *et al.* 2003).

There is no set frequency for handwashing, but times that hands must be washed include:

- before starting and when finishing work
- whenever hands become soiled
- before and after every patient contact
- between different care activities for the same patient
- after handling equipment used by patients
- after handling specimens, waste and used linen
- after removing gloves
- before preparing, handling or eating food
- after going to the toilet
- after coughing and blowing one's nose.

Aseptic/surgical handwashing
Aseptic/surgical handwashing is required prior to invasive procedures to remove both transient and resident micro-organisms. Aqueous antiseptic or alcoholic solutions are required.

Interventions to improve handwashing/cleansing
These include the following.

- Promotion of effective hand hygiene practice through in-service education programmes (ICNA 2003b). Programmes should actively involve staff rather than the use of posters or leaflet information.
- As handwashing cannot be carried out successfully if facilities are inadequate (Cochrane 2003), there should be provision of suitable handwashing/

cleansing solutions. Alcohol-based products provide an effective means of cleansing hands (Kampf 2003).
- Risk assessment approach to ensure adequate decontamination of hands is achieved in patient's homes where optimum facilities are often not available (Carroll 2001a).
- Provision of suitable handwashing facilities, for example in community nursing bases and clinics.
- Contributing to the National Patient Safety Agency (NPSA) Cleanyourhands campaign to sustain year-on-year improvement in compliance with hand hygiene (Storr 2005).
- Involvement of the patients by asking patients to remind staff of the need to undertake handwashing (Pearson & Duncanson 2006) has been seen to increase soap usage in hospital by 34% (McGuckin *et al.* 1999).
- Audit and feedback to staff (Pratt *et al.* 2007). One observation audit of community nurses' handwashing practices found that inadequate handwashing facilities in some patient's homes compromised nurses' ability to perform good handwashing (Gould *et al.* 2000). This supports the use of alcoholic hand rub in the community setting.

Washing of gloved hands
Disposable gloves are single-use items and should not be cleansed and reused for the same or a second patient (Pratt *et al.* 2007).

Safe handling and disposal of sharps

The safe handling and disposal of used sharps is essential to prevent sharps accidents. The risk of transmission of blood-borne pathogens following a single percutaneous exposure has been estimated as:

- hepatitis B virus 33.3% (1 in 3)
- hepatitis C virus 3.3% (1 in 30)
- human immunodeficientcy virus (HIV) (0.31% 1 in 319).

(Pratt *et al.* 2007).

This is higher than the risk of seroconversion after a mucocutaneous exposure to HIV-infected blood, which is estimated to be about 0.03% (1 in 3000) (Public Health Laboratory Service (PHLS) AIDS & STD Centre 1999).

Most of the information connected to percutaneous injuries is related to inpatient care, but studies of HIV post-exposure prophylaxis does include community workers (Braitstein *et al.* 2002), which indicates that accidents are occurring in the community.

All accidents must be reported to an occupational service. A survey in 2002 to assess occupational health requirements in the community highlighted the need for a core occupational health service for all community staff (Harrison & Harrison 2002). In one such service that has been set up in London, they found that uptake was poor, but those who had used the service found it helpful (Grime 2005). Any incident or accident that involves a patient who is known to be infected with HIV, hepatitis B, hepatitis or CJD has to be reported to the Health and Safety Executive, which will fully investigate each incident (HSE 1985). There is also a system for surveillance of healthcare workers who occupationally acquire HIV infection. This includes reporting occupational exposure to the Communicable Disease Surveillance Centre (DH 1997).

Healthcare workers infected with HIV, hepatitis B or hepatitis C must adopt safe universal precautions at all times to protect patients from the risk of transmission of blood-borne pathogens (DH 1999).

Practices to prevent sharps accidents include the following.

■ Used needles must not be resheathed as resheathing predisposes to accidents when the sheath is missed.
■ Used needles must not be disconnected by hand from the syringe, but disposed of as a single unit.
■ Needles must not be bent or broken prior to use or disposal as bending or breaking needles can cause splashing with blood or drugs and sharp accidents.
■ Sharps must not be passed directly from hand to hand and handling should be kept to a minimum. The more times sharps are handled the more likely an accident will occur.
■ Used sharps, whether produced by a healthcare worker or by self-caring persons with diabetes for example, must be disposed of in a sharps container that complies with UN3291 and BS7320 standards and it must be correctly fitted together. Properly used sharps disposal bins can prevent accidents.
■ Sharp containers used in the community must also be of the type approved within the carriage of Dangerous Goods Regulations (Lawrence & May 2003). Care must be taken during the movement of used sharps bins, which are being transported from the home for incineration. This may be a patient taking the container back to the hospital that supplied it, or a community nurse carrying sharps containers in their bags and cars.
■ Under the COSHH regulations (HSC 2002) the employer is responsible for ensuring all risks related to clinical waste, which includes sharps, are properly controlled. Policies appropriate for each area where clinical waste/sharps are produced must be available (HSC 2002). Clinical waste and used sharps must be disposed of safely (DH 2006a).
■ Sharps disposal bins must not be overfilled. When filled to the mark indicating that they are full, containers must be sealed shut, labelled with the date, clinic/place of origin and the initials of the person sealing shut the container, before being placed in a secure area for collection. Most accidents occur during the disposal of used needles, so sharps must be disposed of as soon as possible. Accidents are less likely to occur if sharps are disposed of quickly by the person who has most control of the sharps.
■ Whenever possible take sharps disposal bins to the point of use. Speedy disposal of used sharps reduces the risk of accidents.
■ When working in difficult circumstances arrange a joint visit with a colleague.
■ Consider the use of needlestick prevention devices, for example needle-less systems and syringes and needles with a protective shield (Pratt *et al.* 2007).
■ Risk management dictates that every effort must be made to provide suitable equipment, which will reduce the risk of percutaneous injuries as far as practically possible.

The use of needlestick-prevention devices is being advocated and newly designed devices are now much more freely available. It is essential that these devices are evaluated, and when introduced into patient areas, a full programme of education and training should be provided for staff, as it has been suggested that an increase in accidents may occur:

■ when staff are resistant to new devices.
■ when staff are confused by the complexity of some devices
■ through improper use and poor training.

(Pratt *et al.* 2007).

If a percutaneous injury or contamination of mucous membranes or non-intact skin does occur, immediate action must be taken (Principles table 6.2).

Blood and body fluids spillage

Blood and body fluids containing blood must be handled with caution to prevent contamination occurring. All spillages must be dealt with as soon as possible. Commercially available spillage packs that contain bleach solutions should be used when dealing with large

Principles table 6.2 Actions to be taken following a sharps incident involving blood or body fluids

Action to be taken	Rationale
1 Encourage puncture site or cut to bleed and wash with copious amounts of water	To reduce the number of micro organisms on the wound/skin
2 Wash puncture site or cut with copious soap and running water without scrubbing	To reduce the number of micro-organisms on the wound/skin
3 Cover area with a water-proof plaster.	To prevent an open wound from becoming contaminated with other micro-organisms
4 Complete an incident/accident form. Inform manager and occupational health	To ensure a record is made of incident. The manager must review the incident to establish whether practices need to be changed in view of the accident. Occupational health will ensure policy has been followed and all necessary care is given
5 Arrange for a blood specimen to be obtained from the patient and self as soon as possible	To test the patient's blood for hepatitis B, hepatitis C and HIV. If positive, then prophylactic treatment and care can be provided for the injured healthcare worker (DH 2006b)

amounts of blood. Full protective clothing must be worn and the instructions closely followed, as bleach is covered by strict COSHH regulations (HSC 2002) due to its toxic nature and the toxic reaction that can occur, particularly if mixed with body fluids such as urine (Ayliffe *et al.* 2000).

In the community, locally agreed policies and guidelines should be followed to prevent further contamination of the environment. In most cases of spillage in the community, it is more appropriate to wear disposable gloves and a plastic apron, to use disposable cloths to clear up the spillage and then to clean the area with hot soapy water (Lawrence & May 2003).

Foodborne illnesses

Each year it is estimated that as many as 5.5 million people in the UK may suffer from foodborne illnesses; this is 1 in 10 people. Outbreaks of foodborne illnesses among patients in healthcare institutions, for example hospitals and residential care facilities, are much more likely to be prolonged and associated with significantly higher death rates (Lopman *et al.* 2003). Children are also particularly susceptible to foodborne illnesses, as they tend to have close contact with other children and put their fingers and other potentially contaminated items in their mouths, as well as not always understanding the importance of hygiene (Cleary *et al.* 2003).

Micro-organisms can be hard to detect as they often do not affect the taste, appearance or smell of food. These micro-organisms multiply slowly below 5°C and rapidly between temperatures of 5 and 63°C, and can generally be killed by temperatures of 70°C (Ayliffe *et al.* 2000). Fortunately, most bacteria multiply very slowly and proper cooking and chilling of food can reduce the risk of food poisoning, although it is not possible to completely eliminate the risk.

The Food Safety (General Food Hygiene) Regulations 1995 apply to all food other than food cooked at home. The Food Safety (Temperature Control) Regulations 1995 (DH 1995a) include the temperatures at which particular types of food should be stored before consumption. The local authority health department has a responsibility and legal powers to ensure food and water will not harm health (Ayliffe *et al.* 2000). In the community, this includes meals on wheels when food must be delivered hot and the client encouraged to eat the food while it is hot. Pre-cooked frozen meals have to be delivered frozen and stored in a freezer in the client's home until they are ready to reheat the meal. Examples of micro-organisms implicated in food poisoning include the following.

Viruses
Small round structure viruses
Small round structure viruses (SRSVs) (Lachlan *et al.* 2002; Meakins *et al.* 2003) are the main cause of hospital

and community outbreaks of gastroenteritis, particularly during the winter months. SRSVs can be spread by faecal/oral route, aerosols during vomiting, and food and water. SRSV infection is associated with relatively mild symptoms, in particular nausea and projectile vomiting. It is short in duration and the infected person rarely seeks medical advice. The incubation period is 15–48 hours without a prodormal (early manifestation of symptoms) period (Chadwick *et al.* 2000).

Bacteria

Commonly *Salmonella*, *Shigella*, *Campylobacter* and *Escherichia coli* (Adak *et al. 2002*; O'Donnell *et al. 2002*).

Salmonella

There are several species of *Salmonella* that cause human disease. Some, such as *Salmonella typhi*, cause enteric fever, while others such as *Salmonella enteritidis* and *typhmurium* cause food poisoning. *Salmonella* is found in the intestines of humans and animals and is particularly linked to foods containing raw eggs and inadequate cooking of food such as chicken (Wilson 2002).

Shigella

Shigella species are the cause of bacillary dysentery, the most common being *Shigella sonnei*. Infection is characterised by bloody, mucopurulent stools, often associated with poor standards of hygiene (Long *et al.* 2002).

Campylobacter

Campylobacter species are commonly found in the gastrointestinal tract of wild and domesticated animals and are a major cause of bacterial gastroenteritis causing symptoms of infection that includes fever, headache, myalgia, malaise and diarrhoea that can vary from loose stools to bloody diarrhoea (Tam *et al.* 2003). Contact with animals, eating chicken and drinking bottled water has been implicated in infection (Evans 2003).

Escherichia coli *0157*

A common cause of foodborne infection, associated with haemorrhagic colitis. Contact with animals and eating contaminated meat and milk products are associated with infection (O'Brien *et al.* 2001; Gillespie *et al.* 2003).

Fungal
Cryptosporidium

Cryptosporidium causes profuse watery diarrhoea. It is generally due to contamination of food and water by infected farm and domestic animals (Department of the Environment and Health 1990; Fournier *et al.* 2002). Person-to-person spread can occur (Glaberman *et al.* 2002).

Aspergillus

Kitchens can be heavily contaminated with a variety of moulds that can cause infection (Loudon *et al.* 1996).

The following advice on food hygiene should be adopted at all times.

- All staff preparing food for others must have documented training in personal and catering hygiene.
- All staff who handle food require food hygiene training relevant for the task that is being undertaken. In the community this may include staff who buy food and deliver food to patients in their own homes and those who prepare a snack or beverage for patients in their own home, for example home care staff and community nurses.
- Staff who deliver hot meals and frozen foods to patients in their own homes must understand the importance of food being properly transported, delivered in a good condition and at the right temperature.
- Carers should avoid preparing food if they are ill, especially with vomiting and/or diarrhoea.
- Older people, people with existing illnesses, babies, young children and pregnant women are particularly susceptible to food illness and should only eat eggs cooked until both yolk and white are solid and should not eat raw or partially cooked fish and shellfish, pâté or soft cheeses.
- Hands must be washed and dried thoroughly before handling and eating food.
- Every area and item in the kitchen must be clean and in working order.
- Cooked and uncooked food must be kept separate during purchase, storage and preparation.
- No food lasts forever however well it is stored. Most pre-packed foods carry either a 'use by' or 'best before' date. Check them carefully and look out for advice on how long food can be kept or once packaging has been opened.
- Even if food is within these dates don't eat it if it looks, tastes or smells off.
- Food must not be cooked too far in advance, and once cooked must be covered and served piping hot (above 63°C). Prepared cold food must be kept in the fridge until it is time to eat.
- Refrigerators and freezers must be kept clean, defrosted and in good working order. Temperatures

should be maintained at less than 8°C for refrigerators and −18°C for freezers.

- Keep pets away from food dishes and worktops (Ministry of Agriculture, Fisheries and Food 1994).

The prevention of the spread of food-related infections relies on the implementation of measures that will prevent the transmission of infection to others. *See* Procedure guideline 6.4: Guideline for the prevention and care of food-related infections.

Waterborne infections

Legionella

Legionella pneumophilia can cause a potentially severe respiratory infection. The organism multiplies readily in temperatures between 20 and 45°C. Colonisation of water systems is common and can cause outbreaks of infection. Vulnerable persons, particularly older people and those with existing respiratory conditions, are especially susceptible to infection (HSE 2004).

Health and Safety Executive (2004) guidelines are available on the prevention of legionella and must be adopted for all healthcare facilities in the community. Sterile water must be used for all procedures such as nebulised drug administration. Equipment such as benchtop sterilisers which require distilled water, must be emptied after use and stored dry. Contents of part-used containers of sterile water should be discarded as their microbiological purity will be compromised once opened (MDA 2002).

Cryptosporidium

Cryptospridium is a major cause of diarrhoea infection and can cause serious infection in immune-compromised persons, while in a healthy person a self-limiting illness occurs. Cryptosporidium is widely distributed in the community, commonly infecting livestock, which can lead to contamination of the water supply (Department of the Environment and Health 1990). Infection in humans is generally caused by eating or drinking contaminated food or drink, or from direct contact with farm animals (Robinson & Pugh 2002). All unexplained diarrhoea should be fully investigated and specimens of stool sent to the microbiology laboratory for culture and sensitivity testing. Prevention relies on efficient cleaning, filtration and disinfection procedures at the water supply site (Fournier *et al.* 2002).

Antibiotic-resistant micro-organisms

Micro-organisms resistant to antibiotics emerged soon after the introduction of antibiotics in the 1940s, and have led to infections that are now difficult to treat (Bhattacharyya & Bradley 2006). Treatment required is often expensive and can be toxic. While some very effective new antibiotics have become available, resistance to these has already been seen (Croft *et al.* 2007).

The most common antibiotic-resistant micro-organism is *meticillin-resistant Staphylococcus Aureus* (MRSA), which can cause serious disease (Coia *et al.* 2006).

Other resistant micro-organisms that have a major impact on the provision of community care are *Streptococcus pneumoniae*, which is a major cause of pneumonia, meningitis and bacteraemia; *Mycobacterium tuberculosis*; and viral infections, such as cytomegalovirus, which are a common cause of serious infection in persons with immune suppression, such as with HIV.

Many resistant micro-organisms such as vancomycin-resistant enterococci (VRE), multi-drug-resistant coliforms, *Pseudomonas* and *Klebsiella* are often carried harmlessly in a person's bowel or sputum, or they may colonise slow healing wounds such as leg ulcers and cause infection (Tacconelli 2006).

Meticillin-resistant Staphylococcus aureus (MRSA)

Staphylococcus aureus is a gram-positive micro-organism. It is a common commensal organism that can be found in warm moist areas of the body, particularly the nose.

Staphylococcus aureus produces and secretes a range of toxins and enzymes, which make it a major pathogenic micro-organism (Jacobsson *et al.* 2007). It is a very common cause of skin and wound infections but can also cause serious infections such as septicaemia, pneumonia, toxic shock syndrome, scalded skin syndrome, osteomyelitis and food poisoning.

MRSA is increasing as new strains of resistance are emerging, but they remain rare.

- **Vancomycin-intermediate *Staphylococcus aureus* (VISA)** – micro-organisms that are not fully susceptible to vancomycin (low-level resistance)
- **Vancomycin-resistant *Staphylococcus aureus* (VRSA)** – vancomycin would not be effective for treating VRSA infection (higher levels of resistance).
- **Glycopeptide intermediate *Staphylococcus aureus* (GISA)**, which refers to *Staphylococcus aureus* that are resistant to glycopeptide antimicrobial agents, including vancomycin.

It has been suggested that VRSA and GISA are the same (Coia *et al.* 2006).

Fortunately, the majority of people with MRSA carry it harmlessly in their nose, and do not develop any infection. Even those with MRSA in their wounds who do not have clinical signs and symptoms of infection can, with good wound care, have normal healing (Mendelson *et al.* 2003). However, while 47% of surgical site infections were due to *Staphylococcus*, of these 82% were *Staphylococcus aureus* and 62% of these were MRSA-positive (Nosocomial Infection National Surveillance Service NINSS 2002). Serious infection with MRSA is associated with death (Coia *et al.* 2006). Therefore every effort must be made to prevent a patient acquiring MRSA, and if they do, good infection control practice must be used to prevent further spread.

The epidemiology of MRSA is changing, with reports of MRSA spreading in the community (Patel 2007). There are a large number of people living in the community who are either infected or colonised with MRSA, most of whom acquired MRSA during a hospital admission (Wyllie *et al.* 2005). Generally these people do not present a risk to the community and should continue their normal lives without restrictions (Coia *et al.* 2006). The exception to this would be if they were in contact with immune-suppressed persons who may be at risk of significant infection if they do acquire MRSA. In such cases a risk assessment would need to be undertaken (*see* Table 6.3).

Table 6.3 Risk assessment for MRSA colonisation or infection

Site of MRSA colonisation or infection	Risk assessment	Risk management controls
Nose	No risk	Careful handwashing and safe disposal of any used tissues down the toilet
Throat		
1 No cough	1 No risk	1 Nil
2 Cough	2 Low risk	2 Sit away from immunosuppressed persons. Explain the importance of the patient covering mouth with hand when coughing, careful handwashing and safe disposal of tissues
Sputum		
1 Minimal sputum mainly on waking	1 Low risk	1 Explain the importance of the patient covering mouth with hand when coughing as well as careful handwashing and safe disposal of tissues
2 Productive cough, copious sputum	2 High risk	2 Sit away from immunosuppressed person. Provide covered container for sputum, which must be emptied and washed regularly. Explain the importance of the patient covering mouth with hand when coughing as well as careful handwashing and safe disposal of tissues
Faeces		
1 Continent	1 No risk	1 Nil
2 Incontinent	2 Medium risk	2 Provide supervision and incontinence aids, to reduce the risk. Incontinence aids to be disposed of as clinical waste
Urine		
1 Continent	1 No risk	1 Nil
2 Incontinent	2 Medium risk	2 Provide supervision and incontinence aids to reduce the risk of contamination of the environment and carers. Incontinence aids to be disposed of as clinical waste
Wound		
1 Healed or covered with dressing	1 No risk	1 Nil
2 Wound covered with dressing but dressing insufficient to prevent strike through or leakage	2 Medium risk	2 Reassess wound to establish correct dressing and if necessary increase frequency of wound dressings to reduce the risk of contamination of the environment. Used dressings must be disposed of as clinical waste.

(Ayliffe *et al.* 2000; ICNA/Pharmacia 2002)

MRSA is principally transmitted by unwashed hands, but can also spread by the airborne route from contaminated skin squames carried in dust particles. The single most effective method of preventing and controlling the spread of MRSA is by effective decontamination of hands before and after every patient contact (Coia *et al.* 2006).

Vancomycin-resistant enterococci (VRE)

A sub-therapeutic dose of a growth promoter containing a glycopeptide antibiotic drug called avoparcin that is fed to food-producing animals is thought to be the cause of human colonisation with VRE (McDonald *et al.* 1997).

VRE can be spread by the hands of carers, contaminated patient care equipment or environmental surfaces (Morbidity and Mortality Weekly Report [MMWR] 1995). Contamination leads to colonisation of the patient's gastrointestinal tract, which can lead to endogenous infection in vulnerable patients particularly those undergoing intra-abdominal surgery.

VRE is not as intrinsically virulent as other organisms, with many infections resolving without antimicrobial therapy. VRE has the ability to survive temperatures up to 65°C for 20 minutes and 71°C for 3 minutes and can withstand disinfectants such as chlorine. This means if the environment or equipment such as bedpans and commodes become contaminated, VRE will survive in the environment for long periods of time (Bradley & Fraise 1996).

Streptococcus pneumoniae

There are more than 80 serotypes of *Streptococcus pneumoniae*, some of which are pathogenic to humans, and are the major cause of community-acquired pneumonia, meningitis, sinusitis and otitis media (DH 2006b). Most people who develop *Streptococcus pneumoniae* infection have risk factors that predispose them to infection, with more than 80% of those admitted to hospital having more than one other diagnosis (Melegaro *et al.* 2006). *Streptococcus pneumoniae* colonises the nasopharynx of healthy persons, providing a reservoir of infection for susceptible persons. Person-to-person spread by airborne droplets can easily occur, particularly in crowded areas (DH 2006b). Advice on the control of the spread of *Streptococcus pneumoniae* infection can be sort from the community infection control specialist nurses.

Care of patients with *Streptoccus pneumoniae* chest infection would be the same as those for patients with MRSA colonisation of sputum. See Principle table 6.1 for the risk assessment of MRSA colonisation or infection.

Tuberculosis (TB)

Tuberculosis is a major health problem, with more than 3 million deaths a year worldwide, and only 15% of people infected with TB receiving treatment. This makes TB the second leading cause of death from communicable diseases (DH 2002).

Tuberculosis affects the most vulnerable; this includes children, older people, homeless people, immigrants and the immunocompromised. In the UK, the number of reported TB cases continues to rise: from 6323 in 2000 to 8113 in 2005, with around 350 people dying every year in England from TB (Health Protection Agency Press Statement 2007).

London has a particular TB problem, with 42% of the total number of cases in the UK from London (Health Protection Agency Press Statement 2007). This is mainly because its population is made up of many different ethnic groups, coupled with a high rate of HIV-related tuberculosis. Cross-infection does occur, which can lead to major outbreaks of TB. The Royal College of Physicians (2006) has produced guidelines for the clinical diagnosis and management of tuberculosis and measures for its prevention and control. The Department of Health (2004c) has produced an action plan to stop TB in England. The National Institute for Health and Clinical Excellence (2006b) has produced advice on implementing guidelines related to TB.

Symptoms of TB include fever, night sweats and a productive cough. In advanced cases symptoms may include haemoptysis, weight loss and anorexia. The diagnosis of TB normally relies on Mantoux testing (DH 2006b) and the microscopic identification of acid-fast bacilli found in:

- sputum
- urine
- cerebrospinal fluid for central nervous system disease
- biopsy specimens from tissue such as lymph nodes.

Those with 'smear positive' results should be considered for interferon-gamma immunological testing if available (NICE 2006a). In some cases patients may be 'smear negative', but culturing of the specimen provides a positive diagnosis termed 'culture positive'. In such cases the patient is not considered to be infectious (DH 1998) (Table 6.4).

Control of tuberculosis is dependent on:

- BCG immunisation prevention programme (DH 2006b)
- identifying people with TB
- rapid identification and management of outbreaks
- effective treatment

110

Table 6.4 Tuberculosis infectivity

Microbiological report	Infectious status
Smear positive (this result can be available on the day the specimen arrives at the microbiology laboratory)	Infectious
Smear negative	Not infectious
Smear positive – culture positive (full result will take longer, although modern PCR tests have reduced this time) (Marais & Pai 2007)	Infectious
Smear negative – culture positive	Not infectious
Smear negative – culture negative	Not infectious as specimen is negative. If the patient continues to have signs and symptoms of TB, patient should provide further sputum or urine samples

(NICE 2006b)

- tracing and examining infected persons' close contacts
- treating contacts at the earliest opportunity to prevent them from developing overt disease in the future
- monitoring trends to identify where resources and care is required
- raising awareness of tuberculosis, particularly among healthcare workers, so that infection is recognised early
- provision of adequate resources
- patient-centred care, particularly supervised treatment in the community, to ensure people with TB comply with treatment programmes
- recognising the link between HIV infection and TB
- maintaining effective screening and identification among new entrants to the country
- promoting research into better drugs, diagnosis and vaccines
- contributing to international efforts towards a worldwide control of TB to ensure that people in developing countries have assess to diagnosis, treatment and care (DH 2002).

The treatment of TB involves a combination of drugs that contribute to the rapid reduction in the number of viable bacteria while limiting the risk of ineffective treatment if the patient is infected with drug-resistant bacteria. Treatment normally involves combination therapy of four drugs for two months, then three drugs for two months, followed by two drugs for seven months (NICE 2006b). The increase in multi-drug-resistant TB (MDR-TB) seen in the UK is of major concern and is thought to occur following:

- prior drug treatment
- poor compliance leading to treatment failure
- contact with known case of MDR-TB
- birth in a foreign country, particularly in high incidence countries
- HIV infection
- residence in London (NICE 2006a).

All patients with TB should have a risk assessment for drug resistance and for HIV. Those with no risk will not need to be admitted to hospital for diagnosis and treatment. The admission and discharge to and from hospital for those with a risk would need to be discussed with the infection control team at the hospital and the local TB service and consultant in communicable diseases (NICE 2006a).

Human immunodeficiency virus (HIV)

HIV is the cause of the acquired immune deficiency syndrome (AIDS). It is principally transmitted by risk behaviours such as sharing needles and syringes, and unsafe sexual behaviour such as unprotected sexual intercourse, both anal and vaginal, with a person infected with HIV. Spread is less common from mother to child because antiretroviral drugs can be taken during pregnancy to protect the unborn child. Spread by blood and tissue is rare because careful screening of donors is now undertaken (Public Health Laboratory Service 2002b).

Following infection, the natural history of HIV is of an initial flu-like illness that often goes unnoticed, followed by an incubation period. By the late 1990s the median incubation period where there are no signs and symptoms of the disease had improved from 10 years to 21–23 years (Artzrouni 2004). Once the virus becomes active it causes a variety of infections and malignancies. AIDS occurs when the immune system is so weakened by HIV that severe, sometimes life-threatening, infections such as *Pneumocystis carinii* pneumonia, tuberculosis or cytomegalovirus infection and certain AIDS-defining cancers such as cerebral lymphomas and Kaposi's sarcoma occur (Hart 2008).

Combination therapy with antiviral drugs, plus the use of prophylactic antibiotics to prevent infections such as herpes and cytomegalovirus, has meant that persons with HIV can live very successfully in the community, receiving treatment, support and care from HIV specialist and community nurses (Rogers *et al.* 2000). Community HIV specialist nurses and genitourinary medicine departments tend to take the lead in the clinical care of patients with HIV and AIDS (Petchey *et al.* 2000).

Nursing care for patients with HIV is very similar to that for all patients. The concept of no safe patient, only safe technique is applicable for contact and care with all patients (DePaola & Carpenter 2002; Stein *et al.* 2003).

The exceptions to this are as follows.

- All specimens being sent for processing should have a biohazard label attached to the specimen container and request card.
- Needlestick injury or contamination of mucous membranes or damaged skin accident must be fully reported and investigated immediately to establish the need for prophylactic therapy with anti-HIV antiviral drugs for the injured healthcare worker.
- If a person with HIV dies, embalming is not recommended because of the risk of infection to the embalmer. Therefore the funeral director should be made aware of the risk from bloodborne viruses but does not need to know which virus is involved.
- Relatives and friends of the deceased may wish to view the body, either in the home or in the funeral directors chapel of rest. Viewing and superficial contact such as touching and kissing need not be discouraged.

Infestation

With the exception of scabies, human infestation ranging from lice and mites to worms, do not cause a serious health problem and can be easily treated in the community. Scabies (Sarcoptes scabiei var hominis) can be diagnosed from clinical signs of intense itch, especially at night, skin rashes often starting on the hands and in a few cases burrows may be visible where female mites form burrows to lay their eggs. Signs and symptoms may be relatively mild in early cases, unless the infected person is immune suppressed, very young or an older person, when extensive crusted skin lesions may be present. Transmission is by skin-to-skin contact. Evidence of infection often takes 2–6 weeks to appear (Burgess 2003).

Immunisation/Vaccination

The Department of Health, Welsh and Northern Ireland office produces guidance on the immunisation against infectious disease (DH 2006b). This book, often referred to as the 'Green Book', provides advice on all vaccines and immunoglobulins as well as a wealth of information on procedures, adverse reactions and vaccine damage. There are also phone numbers for expert advice on professional matters, vaccine supplies, pharmaceutical and nursing matters. Travel advice is also included, although detailed country-to-country risks and recommendations are now included in the new companion volume *Health Information for Overseas Travel* (DH 2006b).

The aims and objectives of vaccination programmes are to reduce the number of susceptible persons as much as practically possible, to reduce death from preventable illnesses and to prevent epidemics of infection (Crowcroft *et al.* 2002). Vaccination programmes reduce the instances of infection and also reduce healthcare costs (Carabin *et al.* 2002). Patients' compliance with vaccine initiatives vary. One study found that the decision whether to accept or refuse a vaccine was often influenced by trust of modern medicines, perceived risk of the infection that the vaccine is to prevent and prior experience of vaccination (Telford & Rogers 2003).

Community nurses make an important contribution in the prevention of infection by promoting immunisation programmes. This includes the following.

- Encouraging compliance with programmes.
- Identifying economic, environmental and social factors that may reduce the likelihood of immunisation programmes being taken up and completed.
- Identifying those groups most in need of immunisation, for example:
  - pneumococcal vaccine to protect all those aged two years or older in whom infection is likely to be more common and serious, for example those people with long-term heart, lung or liver disease, diabetes mellitus and HIV
  - selective influenza vaccine for those people with a long-term condition, older adults and those living in private or care homes where rapid spread is likely to occur following initial infection.
- Monitoring vaccination programmes. For example this could include surveys of correct vaccine storage and transplantation to patients' homes and clinics (Finn & Crook 1999) or vaccine uptake (Arthur *et al.* 2002).
- Being involved with educational initiatives to encourage compliance with immunisation programmes (Bellaby 2003).
- Keeping up to date, to ensure new vaccines are offered to the appropriate persons.

All persons should be encouraged to receive the relevant vaccines, and should be provided with the benefits and risks involved in a suitable language in order to obtain consent to the proposed vaccine programme. It is essential that a person's fitness and suitability to receive the vaccine is established. If fitness and suitability cannot be established immunisation should be deferred and specialist advice obtained (DH 2006b).

A GP may delegate responsibility for vaccination to a community nurse providing that certain local, national, legal and professional conditions are met. These include the following.

- The nurse is willing to be professionally accountable for this task.
- The nurse has received appropriate training and updates and is competent in all aspects of vaccination. This should include knowledge of the contraindications to specific vaccines and potential side effects.
- Training has been received in basic life support and in the recognition and treatment of anaphylaxis. While anaphylactic reactions to vaccines are rare, they cannot be predicted and can be fatal. Adrenaline and an appropriate one-way valve facemask must always be immediately available whenever vaccinations are given (DH 2006b).
- Community nurses should only carry out vaccinations if agreed protocols are in place and written instructions have been received from the relevant GP or under a patient group direction.

Last offices

While most bodies are not infectious, community nurses may be required to undertake last offices for a person who is known to be infected with a disease such as HIV, hepatitis, tuberculosis, *Salmonella* or vCJD, for example. Precautions used prior to death are still relevant for those handling blood and body fluids after death (National End of Life Care Programme 2011).

Specimen collection

Specimens collected in the community must be delivered in a safe manner to the relevant laboratory as soon as possible, as this ensures that accurate results are obtained.

Inaccurate results can occur for a number of reasons.

- Delays in specimens arriving in the microbiology department can cause micro-organisms to multiply or die. If a delay is anticipated the specimen should be kept cool, but must not be stored in a refrigerator used for food or drugs.
- If during specimen collection contamination of the specimen with the patient's own normal flora occurs.

During transportation to the laboratory, these organisms may multiply and provide false results.

- Multiplication of some micro-organisms in the sample may flourish more readily than weaker organisms and a false result will be obtained.
- Specimens should be obtained prior to the patient being prescribed antibiotics; this is to prevent the antibiotics distorting the patient's normal flora by selective pressure of the antibiotics where some commensal and pathogenic bacteria can survive in the presence of antibiotic (ICNA/Pharmacia 2002).

Laboratory specimen containers

Approved specimen containers must always be used to ensure the container is suitable for the purpose it is intended and will not break or leak. Advice can be sort from the microbiology laboratory that will be dealing with the specimen. The container must be placed in a double sealable bag, one bag for the specimen and the second for the fully and correctly completed specimen request card. This is to ensure that if the container leaks or is damaged or the outside has become contaminated during collection of the specimen, the transport bag will prevent contamination of the environment or the persons handling the specimen. If the patient is known to have an infectious disease such as hepatitis B or C, or HIV, the transport bag, the specimen request card and the container must be labelled with a risk of infection biohazard label (HSAC 2003). The specimen must then be placed in a lockable, washable box that is strong enough to withstand transportation and constructed to prevent loss of contents if the specimen becomes damaged. Warning labels must be attached to the box stating 'Diagnostic specimens, not to be opened' and a contact number in case it is found unattended (HSAC 2003)

The request card accompanying the specimen should contain all necessary details:

- name
- age
- type of specimen (including site of swab or whether the urine was a mid-stream or catheter specimen, for example)
- diagnosis
- suspected infection
- current antibiotic therapy
- doctor requesting the sample
- details of the person taking the sample
- to whom the results are to be sent
- date and time of specimen collection.

All samples, including specimens for laboratories other than the microbiology laboratory, must be transported in a safe manner to prevent loss and damage of the sample that may result in contamination of the environment or the persons handling the specimen (HSAC 2003). If sent by post, the specimen must be packed in an approved container which contains enough absorbent material to absorb the entire contents of the specimen if the container becomes damaged. The outer package must be correctly addressed with the sender and the laboratory name and address and marked 'Pathological specimens, fragile with care'. Specimens that may contain biological agents in hazard group 2 (a biological agent that can cause human disease) or hazard group 3 (a biological agent that can cause severe human disease) require special arrangements, which are included in the current Royal Mail packaging specification for carriage of pathological specimens through the post and is available from Royal Mail Business and Consumer Markets, Room 120, Royal London House, 22 Finsbury Square, London EC2A INL.

Healthcare waste disposal in the community

'Waste legislation has been adapted and improved over the past 25 years to ensure waste is collected, managed, transported, stored, recovered and disposed without harm to human health or the environment' (Waste Strategy 2000: 6).

All waste generated in the community during nursing and medical interventions, whether undertaken by community nurses, care staff, the patient or the patient's family, has to be segregated, contained and disposed of in a safe manner. Compliance with national and local recommendations is essential to reduce the risk of accidents and contamination of the environment (DH 2006a).

All community nurses should make themselves familiar with local procedures related to waste disposal. In general waste generated in the community can be divided into:

- hazardous waste (infectious waste)
- non-hazardous waste (domestic waste)
- offensive/hygiene waste (DH 2006a).

To determine its classification, all healthcare waste must be assessed by the producer at the time of production for medicinal, chemical and infectious properties (DH 2006a)

Hazardous waste
- Waste that poses known or potential risk of infection, regardless of the level of infection posed.
- Medicinal waste.

Medicinal waste
This includes all unused drugs in all forms including tablets, capsules, liquids and cartridges, in containers

such as vials, glass bottles and plastic bottles. Medicinal waste is further divided into:

- cytotoxic and cytostatic medicines, which is classed as hazardous waste and must be disposed of by incineration. This includes all toxic, carcinogenic, toxic for reproduction and mutagenic waste
- pharmaceutically active but not cytotoxic and cytostatic medicines
- not pharmaceutically active and possessing no hazardous properties (e.g. saline bags).

To establish the category of medicinal waste refer to the product material safety sheets (COSHH sheets, HSC 2002) (DoH 2006a).

Domestic waste
This includes all types of waste generated in the home, with the exception of that contaminated with blood, body fluids and drugs.

The method of storage and collection for domestic waste does vary between and within localities and can include reusable bins and polythene bags. At a minimum, domestic waste should be disposed of in robust black plastic bags that are not overfilled, and are tied securely shut and placed in a suitable container to await collection by the routine council collection service. Domestic waste is generally disposed of by landfill disposal (DH 2006a).

Offensive/Hygiene waste
The term offensive/hygiene waste describes waste that is non-infectious and does not require special treatment or disposal but which may cause offence to those coming into contact with it. Examples are incontinence pads, sanitary waste and nappies (DH 2006a).

All clinical waste generated in the community has to be handled with care. If an accident does occur during transportation and incineration it is much more difficult to provide informed first aid and follow-up care. This is because it is often difficult to discover exactly where the waste came from and the patient involved.

The transportation and disposal of clinical waste is included in the following.

- The Health and Safety at Work Act 1974.
- Control of Substances Hazardous to Health Regulations (COSHH, HSC 2002).
- Environmental Protection Act (Duty of Care) Regulations (1991).
- *Safe Working and the Prevention of Infection in Clinical Laboratories and Similar Facilities* (Health Service Advisory Committee 2003).

- Carriage of Dangerous goods by Road Regulations (1996) SI 1996/2095.
- *Environment and Sustainability*. Health Technical Memorandum 07-01: Safe management of health-care waste (DH 2006a).

Control of Substances Hazardous to Health (COSHH)

COSHH provides a risk assessment and management framework for controlling the risks from hazardous substances including, for example, chemicals used for infection control purposes and biological agents such as micro-organisms. The objective of COSHH is to protect all those persons involved in a particular activity from risk by eliminating or controlling risk (HSC 2002).

This framework requires all employers to assess the risk from hazardous substances to employees, patients and visitors who may be affected by the hazard. This involves a full assessment of the potential risk from the agent being assessed and the control strategies needed to ensure that any risk is as low as practically possible. Emphasis is placed on providing information, instruction and training. Health surveillance may be included for agents such as chemicals that could potentially cause asthma (HSC 2002).

Principles for cleaning, decontamination and sterilisation

Cleaning, decontamination and sterilisation is a combination of processes to ensure that reusable medical devices are safe to use for other patients. This process also makes reusable items safe to be handled by staff (Table 6.5). Failure of these processes can lead to cross-infection. Inadequate processing may be the result of poor technique, lack of equipment and resources, and poorly trained and unsupervised staff (NHS Estates 2003).

The Department of Health and the National Health Service Estates recommend that reusable medical devices should be reprocessed in a central processing unit. The reprocessing of medical devices in the clinical area should be the exception rather than the norm (NHS Estates 2000).

There are three main methods of decontamination.

Cleaning/Decontamination

Micro-organisms need warmth, moisture and nutrition to survive and multiply on used equipment and in the environment. If these conditions are removed most bacteria will not survive and multiply, although some will remain dormant until more suitable conditions are provided. Cleaning/decontamination removes dust and organic matter and can be achieved by using detergent/warm water and drying carefully. Failure to decontaminate equipment or the environment can result in cross-infection, which puts patients, carers, community staff and the family at risk. Caution must be taken when substituting liquid soap and hot water for alcoholic wipes (70% isopropyl alcohol solution), as a study has demonstrated that cleaning with alcoholic wipes can leave a scanty growth of micro-organisms (O'Malley & Lok 2003).

Disinfection

Disinfection refers to any process used to reduce the number of micro-organisms; however, many of these processes cannot effectively remove spores. Cleaning of equipment prior to sterilisation is an essential pre-requisite to ensure effective disinfection has occurred. The use of disinfectant is no substitute for thorough cleaning.

Sterilisation

Sterilisation refers to the complete removal of all organic matter and micro-organisms, including bacteria, fungus, viruses and spores. Cleaning of equipment prior to sterilisation is an essential pre-requisite to ensure effective sterilisation will occur.

It is essential that the cleaning process does not result in equipment failure, which could interrupt or compromise the patient's treatment. All staff must read the manufacturer's instructions before using equipment that is unfamiliar to them as equipment can vary. Most manufacturers provide clear instructions and a customer service helpline. An example of such a device is electronic ear irrigation equipment that requires cleaning of the reservoir and tubing with chlorine solutions after use.

Cleaning of the environment

Routine domestic cleaning in the home setting is important to prevent cross-infection to those living in the home and to the community carers providing care. Particular attention should be paid to the toilet and kitchen. In general when the home environment becomes contaminated with urine, faeces and vomit, it needs to be cleaned using disposable gloves (plastic apron for large spillage) and disposable paper towels and the area should then be washed with hot soapy water. It is unlikely that large amounts of blood that will require a spillage kit will be present. A risk assessment needs to be completed if a patient in their own home has a medical condition that

115

Table 6.5 Example of cleaning recommendations

Equipment	Non-infected patient, wearing gloves and plastic apron	Infected patient, wearing gloves and plastic apron, plus other personal protective equipment as directed in the COSHH assessment for the disinfectant being used
Single-use item	Never clean and reuse	
Baths/showers	Cream cleaner after each use	Chlorine-based non-abrasive cleaner
Hospital beds	Wash with hand hot water and detergent and dry	Detergent and hot water, dry wipe over with a 1000 ppm chlorine-releasing agent (bleach/Milton) (check manufacturer's instructions)
Crockery/cutlery	Ideally machine wash at 80°C. If machine not available, wash in hot soapy water, rinse in clean hot water, leave to dry	Machine wash at 80°C. If machine not available, wash in hot soapy water, rinse in clean hot water, leave to dry
Bedding	Machine wash and dry 65°C for 10 min or 71°C for 3 min, taking care not to overfill washing machine	As for non-infected patient
Flooring	Vacuum, wash with hand-hot water and detergent	Vacuum, wash with hand-hot water and detergent. If contamination has occurred wipe over with a 1000 ppm chlorine-releasing agent (bleach/Milton) after initial cleaning
Carpets	Vacuum, wash with hand-hot water and detergents	Vacuum, wash with hand-hot water and detergent. If contamination has occurred that cannot be removed by washing. A 1000 ppm chlorine-releasing agent (bleach/Milton) will damage the carpet, therefore steam cleaning is the only effective means of decontamination
	Wash with hand-hot water and detergent	Wash with hand-hot water and detergent. If contamination has occurred wipe over with a 1000 ppm chlorine-releasing agent (bleach/Milton) after initial cleaning
Commode	Wash with hand-hot water and detergent	Wash with hand-hot water and detergent. If contamination has occurred wipe over with a 1000 ppm chlorine-releasing agent (bleach/Milton) after initial cleaning
Bedpans/urinals/bowls	Machine wash before use by another patient. In person's home empty into toilet, wash with detergent and water, being careful not to contaminate environment	Machine wash before being used by another patient. In person's home, empty into toilet, wash with detergent and water, being careful not to contaminate environment
Pressure-relieving mattresses	Wash with hand-hot water and detergent	Check manufacturer's instructions. Generally wash with detergent and hand-hot water, followed by wiping with alcohol 70% or 1000 ppm of a chlorine-releasing agent (bleach /Milton)
Urine bag holders, etc.	Wash with hand-hot water and detergent	Wash with detergent and hand hot water, followed by wiping with alcohol 70% or 1000 ppm of a chlorine-releasing agent (bleach/Milton)
Pumps, i.e. nutritional feeding pumps	Damp wipe with detergent and hand-hot water	Check manufacturer's instructions. Generally damp wipe with detergent and hand-hot water, followed by wiping with alcohol 70% or 1000 ppm of a chlorine-releasing agent (bleach/Milton)
Digital thermometers	A disposable probe cover to be used for each recording	A disposable probe cover to be used for each recording. Consider the use of single-use clinical thermometers
Blood pressure monitoring machines	Damp wipe machine. Only cuffs that can be wiped over with detergent and hand-hot water or disposable cuffs are to be used	Damp wipe machine. Wipe cuff over with detergent and hand-hot water and alcohol 70% or 1000 ppm of a chlorine-releasing agent (bleach/Milton)

Table 6.5 (*Continued*)

Equipment	Non-infected patient, wearing gloves and plastic apron	Infected patient, wearing gloves and plastic apron, plus other personal protective equipment as directed in the COSHH assessment for the disinfectant being used
Stethoscope	Damp wipe with detergent and hand-hot water	Damp wipe with detergent and hand-hot water; consider the use of disposable stethoscope diaphragm cover
Doppler	Damp wipe with detergent and hand-hot water	Check manufacturer's instructions. Generally damp wipe with detergent and hand-hot water, followed by wiping with alcohol 70% or 1000 ppm of a chlorine-releasing agent (bleach/Milton)
Blood glucose monitoring machines	Check manufacturer's instructions	Check manufacturer's instructions
Ear irrigation equipment	Check manufacturer's instructions	Check manufacturer's instructions
Nebulisers	Discard all single-use attachments. Reusable sections damp wipe with detergent and hand-hot water dry carefully	Check manufacturer's instructions. Discard all single use attachments, damp wipe with detergent and hand hot water, followed by wiping with alcohol 70% or 1000 ppm of a chlorine-releasing agent (bleach/Milton)

may suggest bleeding is likely to occur, in such cases a spillage kit maybe required (DH 2006c).

Healthcare facilities

Healthcare facilities in the community such as GP practices, health centres and walk-in clinics are governed by the same strict regulations as hospitals. The National Health Service Estates (2002) has produced extensive guidance on the principles that must be considered when designing and planning healthcare premises. This includes new builds as well as changes to existing buildings. The emphasis is on designers, architects, engineers, planners and managers working in collaboration with infection control personnel to provide facilities in which infection control measures need to have been anticipated and provided for. Good standards can only be achieved by all those involved understanding the infection control risks that will be present during the construction of the facilities and when the facility is in use. This is to ensure that all buildings are fit for their purpose and safe from a health, safety and infection control perspective. Important considerations include:

- adequate handwashing facilities
- quality finishes in all areas to ensure that all surfaces and equipment can be easily cleaned and are wear resistant
- adequate ventilation to ensure airborne contamination can be removed
- clean water to prevent infections such as cryptosporidium and legionella

- adequate storage to protect equipment from contamination
- laundry facilities; this may be separate storage of clean and dirty linen that is washed elsewhere, or provision of washers and dryers that comply with laundry regulations (Department of Health 1987; NHS Estates 1995)
- all healthcare establishments must comply with the food safety requirements (Food Safety Act 1990).

Home care environment facilities

Patients being cared for in the community will have home, social and cultural conditions that will vary. It is important that all patients requiring care in their own homes have basic amenities to ensure that cleanliness and a basic diet are achievable. Social Services have a responsibility to ensure that basic hygienic amenities are available and this should be part of the discharge planning process that is undertaken before a patient is discharged home (NHSE 2001).

Discharge planning

Discharge planning of the hospitalised patient must take into consideration any infection that the patient might have which may cause a potential risk following discharge into the community. Communication is an essential component to ensure effective infection control assessments can be undertaken prior to the patient being discharged into the community so that any requirements can be organised (Dellasega & Fisher 2001).

Discharge planning includes assessment of:

- the patient (Rowe *et al.* 2000).
- their family and/or carers (Heaton *et al.* 1999).

Discharge planning should provide:

- information for the patient and carers (Worth *et al.* 2000)
- support for informal carers and primary health teams (Simon 2001) to ensure that the discharge of infected patients from hospital is problem-free.

Risk assessment

The importance of minimising the risks of infection is laid out in the Health and Safety at Work Act (1974), the Management of Health and Safety at Work Regulations (1994), the Control of Substances Hazardous to Health (COSHH) Regulations (Health and Safety Commission 2002) and the Provision and Use of Work Equipment Regulations (PUWER 1998). One survey with a response rate of 85% to assess general practitioners' knowledge and compliance with risk assessment found that fewer than 1 in 10 GPs had completed the required risk assessments (Kennedy *et al.* 2002).

Health and Safety at Work Act (1974)

Health and Safety at Work Act (1974) requires the employer to provide, as far as reasonably possible, a safe environment for employees, patients and visitors. Importantly, it requires all employees to take reasonable precautions to ensure their own and others' safety. One survey with a response rate of 85% to assess GPs' knowledge and compliance with health and safety and occupational health guidance found that although they were aware of legislation, compliance was poor (Kennedy *et al.* 2002).

Management of Health and Safety at Work Regulations (1994)

Management of Health and Safety at Work Regulations (1994) require all employers to assess the risk to their employees' health and to put in place control measures to ensure staffs are protected from risk. In relation to infection control this would be protection from infection hazards through the provision of safe working systems. These include the following:

1 Use of standard/universal precautions.
2 Systems for reporting incidents and accidents that occur at work.
3 Provision of care following an incident or accident at work.

4 Provision of facilities to facilitate infection control practices, in particular for handwashing.
5 Systems for the management of used medical devices.
6 Arrangements for the disposal of waste.
7 Arrangements for the laundering of used linen.

Control of Substances Hazardous to Health (COSHH) Regulations (2002)

COSHH provides specific guidance related to the protection against hazardous substances, which include micro-organisms and chemicals.

Provision and Use of Work Equipment Regulations (PUWER) (1998)

PUWER requires the employer to ensure that equipment used during work activities is suitable for the intended use and is safe to use. All equipment must have documented maintenance checks to ensure it is maintained in a safe condition and must be inspected periodically to ensure that it remains safe. The users of the equipment must have received information, instruction and training to ensure they can operate the equipment confidently and safely.

Reporting of Injuries, Diseases and Dangerous Occurrences Regulations (RIDDOR) (1995)

RIDDOR requires employers to report any infection attributed to work.

The Carriage of Dangerous Goods (Classification, Packaging and Labelling) Regulations (1996)

The Carriage of Dangerous Goods (Classification, Packaging and Labelling) Regulations (1996) is involved in the carriage of potentially dangerous goods by road or rail and includes specimens and waste (*see* Specimen collection and waste disposal).

Safe management of healthcare waste. Health Technical Memorandum 07-01 (DH 2006a)

This is a best practice guide to the management of healthcare waste, and refers to any waste produced by, and as a consequence of, healthcare activities. It replaces the Health Service Advisory Committee (1999) Safe disposal of clinical waste. The guidance includes storage, carriage, treatment and disposal of waste (DoH 2006a).

Clinical governance

Clinical governance applies to all health authorities, primary care trusts and to NHS trusts, providing the framework for maintenance and where necessary the improvement in the standards of patient care, while safeguarding high standards of care. Clinical governance creates an environment in which excellence in clinical care develops and flourishes, so that incidents, crises and serious failures in standards of care will no longer occur. Included within clinical governance is the means to identify and provide services that are both clinically and cost-effective, as well as the institution and maintenance of systems to ensure clinical quality (NHSE 1999b).

Evidence-based practice is one aspect of improvement in quality care (Gould 2002). An important part of evidence-based practice involves orientation and update education programmes and the proper use of standards, guidelines and audit.

The NHSE (1999b) states that for clinical governance to be successful all health authorities must demonstrate:

- that education, research and the sharing of good practice is valued and expected
- that all managers and staff have a commitment to quality care and this is supported by clearly identified local human and financial resources
- a tradition of active working with patients, users, carers and the public
- multidisciplinary team working at all levels
- use of information to plan and assess progress.

Clinical governance requires good information to assess the quality and performance of services. This can be achieved by:

- undertaking baseline assessments to identify scope for improvement
- monitoring progress to ensure planned improvements have resulted in the desired change
- establishing leadership and accountability arrangements
- benchmarking (essence of care) between local services to identify scope for improvement and for sharing good practice
- providing information to the public
- monitoring to obtain early warning of serious service failures. This also includes learning from complaints and adverse incidents.

Clinical governance includes ensuring that the infection control service is monitored, to ensure the provision of high-quality care, with the benefit of clinical risk management in the infection control setting being emphasised (Masterton & Teare 2001).

Guidelines

Guidelines provide statements of good practice based on systematic review of research and other evidence.

These can be adapted to local need so they are relevant and appropriate to assist practitioners and managers to achieve sound clinical governance (Department of Health 2001). National guidelines are available for:

- standard infection control principles
- care of patients with long-term urinary catheters
- care during enteral feeding
- care of patients with central venous catheters.

These guidelines can be used as standard principles by all healthcare workers (NICE 2003).

Audit

Clinical governance includes monitoring standards to assess whether clinical effectiveness is achieved and if not where improvements can be made. It is the duty of all those providing healthcare to put and keep in place arrangements for monitoring and improving the quality of healthcare. Audit provides the means to achieve this (DH 2004a).

Audit is essential in monitoring infection control procedures, by seeking to improve the quality and outcome of patient care through structured peer review, whereby staff examine their practices and results against agreed standards/policies and modify their practices where the data indicate that improvements can be made.

Examples of infection control audits that could be undertaken by community nurses:

- waste disposal to ensure guidelines are followed, particularly disposal of clinical waste and sharps disposal bins as community policies do vary (Lawrence & May 2003: 97)
- safe handling of sharps (ICNA in partnership with PORTEX 2003)
- laundry arrangements
- handwashing (Pratt *et al.* 2007)
- access to appropriate equipment (NICE 2003)
- community staff infection control training (NICE 2003)
- patients' and, where appropriate, carers' information and training to carry out infection control measures (NICE 2003)
- disinfection and decontamination of equipment and medical devices used by community nurses (NHS Estates 2003).

Infection control audit checklists/tools have been developed (Millward *et al.* 1993). The Department of Health's 2007 *Saving Lives: reducing infection, delivering clean and safe care*, provides high impact interventions guidelines on appropriate care that needs to be achieved to

119

prevent infections. Included in these interventions are tools to identify if appropriate care has been achieved and where improvements can be made (DH 2007b). These can be adapted for use in most healthcare settings. All community nurses should be involved in audit initiatives to ensure evidence-based practice is in everyday use.

indication of the complexities involved in the effort to prevent infection. This information provides advice on how to safeguard patients, their families and friends, and staff from the risk from infections. This knowledge will improve the understanding of infection control in the community setting and provide the trigger to allow community nurses to develop and use this knowledge to ensure patients can be cared for safely in the community.

Conclusion

This chapter has provided evidence on the importance of infection control in the community and some

Procedure guideline 6.1 **Guideline for routine handwashing**

When hands are free from dirt and organic matter, a decontaminating alcoholic hand rub can be used (NICE 2003). If gloves are worn to keep hands clean during nursing procedures, alcoholic hand rub can replace routine handwashing, once the intial routine handwashing has been undertaken at the beginning of a shift (ICNA 1997). However, alcoholic hand rub must be used once the gloves have been removed (NICE 2003).

Nursing action	Rationale
1 Besides normal handwashing following a visit to the toilet for example, hands must be washed when arriving and leaving work and before all meal and beverage breaks	To prevent cross-infection to yourself and those persons with whom you are in contact
2 Nails should be short and clean. False nails and nail varnish must not be used (ICNA 1997)	To ensure thorough handwashing can be undertaken. False nails can encourage the growth of micro-organisms (Porteous 2002)
3 Remove wrist watches, jewellery and roll up/remove long-sleeved clothing	To enable thorough handwashing – long sleeves and jewellery can inhibit handwashing
4 Wet hands under warm running water and apply liquid soap into cupped hands	To ensure hands are being cleaned in clean running water during the whole procedure. Soap is more effective in removing dirt when mixed with warm water
5 Rub hands together vigorously to cover all parts of the hands thoroughly for 10–15 seconds, paying particular attention to tips of fingers, the thumb and areas between the fingers (ICNA 1997)	To ensure that all areas of the hands are thoroughly cleansed
6 Rinse hands thoroughly under warm running water	To ensure all dirt and soap residue is removed To ensure hands are clean and free from the risk of developing sore hands from the soap residue
7 Dry hands thoroughly with disposable paper towel (ICNA 1997)	To ensure hands are dried thoroughly as bacteria can thrive on warm moist hands. The skin of hands that are not dried thoroughly can become sore, which predisposes to colonisation with micro-organisms
8 Emollient hand creams should be applied regularly (NICE 2003)	To protect skin from the drying effects of regular handwashing

Procedure guideline 6.2 **Guideline for aseptic/surgical handwashing**

Nursing action	Rationale
1 Nails should be short and clean. False nails and nail varnish must not to be used	To ensure thorough handwashing can be undertaken. False nails can encourage the growth of micro-organisms (Porteous 2002)
2 Remove wrist watches, jewellery and roll up/remove long-sleeved clothing	To ensure thorough handwashing – long sleeves and jewellery may inhibit handwashing
3 Wet hands under warm running water and apply liquid aqueous antiseptic solution into cupped hands	To ensure hands are being cleaned in clean running water during the whole procedure. Aqueous antiseptic solution is more effective than soap in removing dirt, dead skin squames and bacteria when mixed with warm water
4 Rub hands together vigorously to cover all parts of the hands thoroughly for 10–15 seconds, paying particular attention to tips of fingers, the thumb and areas between the fingers	To ensure that all areas of the hands are thoroughly cleansed
5 Rinse hands thoroughly under warm running water	To ensure all dirt and soap residue is removed

To ensure hands are clean and free from the risk of developing sore hands from the soap residue |
| 6 Dry hands thoroughly with disposable paper towel. If undertaking a surgical procedure a sterile towel should be used | To ensure hands are dried thoroughly as bacteria can thrive on warm moist hands. The skin of hands that are not dried thoroughly can become sore, which predisposes to colonisation with micro-organisms

A sterile towel ensures contamination does not occur from the socially clean but unsterile paper towels (Griffith *et al.* 2003) |
| 7 If hands have already been cleaned with a surgical handwash immediately prior to the current procedure and did not become contaminated during the previous procedure, an alcoholic hand rub may be used instead of undertaking steps 1 to 5 above. The alcoholic solution should be rubbed on to the whole surface of the hands. Alcoholic hand rubs contain an emollient hand cream | Alcoholic hand rub/gel is a quick and convenient means of cleansing clean hands. All areas of the hands must be covered to ensure all areas have been cleansed. Emollient hand cream prevents the hands becoming dry and sore |
| 8 Emollient hand creams should be applied regularly (ICNA 1997; NICE 2003) | To protect skin from the drying effects of regular handwashing |

121

Procedure guideline 6.3 **Guideline for cleansing of clean hands with alcoholic hand rub**

Nursing action	Rationale
1 Where possible when arriving and leaving each patient's home hands should be washed using the routine handwashing guidelines above to ensure hands are free from dirt and organic material (NICE 2003)	To ensure hands are clean
2 When hands are free from dirt and organic matter a decontaminating alcoholic hand rub can be used (NICE 2003)	Alcohol cannot penetrate dirt and organic matter
3 If gloves are worn to keep hands clean, during nursing procedures alcoholic hand rub can replace routine handwashing, once the initial routine handwashing has been undertaken at the beginning of a shift (ICNA 1997)	While wearing gloves when handling blood and body fluids will prevent hands becoming dirty, hands must still be cleansed before and after every patient contact
4 Alcoholic hand rub must be used once the gloves have been removed (NICE 2003)	Hands must be cleansed before and after patient contact; the wearing of gloves does not replace handwashing, as wearing gloves does not completely prevent contamination of the hands (Tenorio *et al.* 2001)
5 Nails should be short and clean. False nails and nail varnish must not to be used (NICE 2003)	To ensure thorough handcleansing can be undertaken. False nails can encourage the growth of micro-organisms (Porteous 2002)
6 Remove wrist watches, jewellery and roll up/remove long-sleeved clothing	Long sleeves and jewellery inhibits thorough handwashing
7 Apply the alcoholic hand rub on to the hands following the manufacturer's instructions. Hands must be rubbed together vigorously until the hand rub has evaporated and the hands are dry. All areas of the hands must be included, particularly the tips of the fingers, the thumbs and the areas between the fingers	To ensure cleansing of hands. Alcoholic hand rub/gel is a quick and convenient means of cleansing clean hands, particularly when liquid soap, running water and paper towels are not readily available (Cochrane 2003). All areas of the hands must be covered to ensure all areas have been cleansed

The tips of the fingers, the thumb and the areas between the fingers are often missed when applying alcoholic hand rub (ICNA 1997) |
| 8 Individual containers of hand rub are now available which can be kept in community nurses pockets (Hugonnet *et al.* 2002) | To ensure hand rub is available at all times; this is particularly important in the community where some homes may have inadequate handwashing facilities |
| 9 Emollient hand creams should be applied regularly (ICNA 1997; NICE 2003) | To protect skin from the drying effects of regular handwashing |

Procedure guideline 6.4 **Guideline for the prevention and care of food-related infections**

Action	Rationale
1 Food infections are notifiable under Section 10 of the Public Health Control of Disease Act (1984). The environmental health officer will review all reports to quickly establish whether an outbreak of infection is occurring	Earlier recognition of an outbreak of infection can enable effective management to start early to prevent the further spread of infection
2 Segregation of infected person; this may include sleeping in a separate bed from their partner and if the home has two toilets keeping one for the infected person	To reduce the risk of cross-infection
3 Careful handwashing by those in contact with the infected person. Nurses and other home care staff such as chiropodist and physiotherapist to use alcoholic hand rub. Family members to use separate soap and towels	To reduce the risk of cross-infection
4 Careful handwashing by the infected person	Unwashed hands are one of the main routes of cross-contamination
5 Infected persons should not prepare food for others until signs and symptoms of infection have resolved for 48 hours	Infected person could contaminate the food or the kitchen environment, leading to cross-infection
6 Careful cleaning of the environment, especially if contamination has occurred, is generally sufficient. However, during household outbreaks of infection a disinfectant should be used (Kagan *et al.* 2002)	To reduce the risk of cross-infection as micro-organisms can survive in the environment for some time. Home environments, particularly kitchens and bathrooms, serve as a reservoir for infection
7 Infected person not to share personal items such as towels and toothbrushes	To reduce the risk of cross-infection
8 Community nurses and others to wear a plastic apron and gloves to prevent spreading infection to other households	To prevent contamination of uniform and clothing, which could be a source of infection to other patients, nurses and the healthcare worker and their families

Procedure guideline 6.5 **Guideline for care of a patient diagnosed with MRSA**

Nursing action	Rationale
1 Where appropriate facilities are available wash and thoroughly dry hands. Alternatively cleanse hands with anti bactericidal alcoholic hand rub **NB** Handwashing/cleansing should be performed on entering and prior to leaving the patient's home, and at appropriate times during all nursing procedures	To maintain patient and practitioner safety. Contaminated hands are the main route for the spread of infection

(Continued)

Procedure guideline 6.5 **Guideline for care of a patient diagnosed with MRSA** *(cont'd)*

Nursing action	Rationale
2 Explain how MRSA will affect the patient, their family and friends, and all restrictions and precautions that will be necessary. The explanation should include reiteration of the importance for strict hand washing/cleansing techniques. All explanations given should be supported by written information in the appropriate language and/or format	Patients may become distressed when told they have MRSA and this could affect their ability to retain any information given To enable the patient to ask questions To allay any fears or concerns the patient may have To promote and aid concordance with treatment and restrictions that may be required
3 Appropriate standard precautions should be fully utilised when carrying out all nursing procedures	To prevent cross-infection/contamination To maintain patient, practitioner and others safety
4 Provide education and practical instruction on correct handwashing/cleansing techniques. This is particularly relevant where the patient is performing their own wound dressing changes or intermittent self-catheterisation (ISC), for example	To ensure patients understand that if they are colonised with MRSA they can contaminate other areas, if their hands become contaminated with MRSA Alcohol-based hand rub is an effective method of cleansing hands and may be a more convenient and acceptable alternative for the patient
5 Where appropriate offer advice on the importance for the home environment to be kept clean	To ensure that patients understand that MRSA can survive in the environment for long periods of time, providing a reservoir of infection
6 All healthcare equipment used in the home, e.g. hoist, commode, nebuliser, syringe driver/pump, should be cleaned after use **NB** The transportation of equipment to and from a patient's home in the community nurse's car is not recommended	To prevent cross-contamination as MRSA can survive for long periods of time in or on contaminated equipment Cleaning with soap and water will remove dust and body fluids and the MRSA
7 Where possible and practicable, single-use medical devices, e.g. forceps, scissors, should be used **NB** Single use medical devices are not designed to be cleaned and reuse and may be damaged or ineffectively cleaned	Guidelines related to decontaminating of reusable equipment must always be followed to prevent cross-infection A central sterile service department (SSD) may not be available to community nursing staff. Reusable medical devices such as dressing forceps must go back to the sterile service department for reprocessing
8 Waste disposal – segregation or restriction of a person with MRSA is not required in the community if the above actions are undertaken and if obvious sources of infection are contained. See Table 6.3 for the risk assessment of MRSA colonisation or infection	MRSA is unlikely to cause infection to healthy persons in the community, as long as the infected person seeks advise when wanting to visit, for example, a premature baby or a relative or friend receiving cancer therapy
9 Advice can be sought from the infection control nurse in the community or hospital	The infection control nurse can assist with risk assessment and care planning to ensure good care is provided with only the necessary restrictions to the patient and their families
10 If there appears to be evidence of MRSA cross-infection the infection control nurses advice should be sought	Cross-infection must be fully investigated so the cause can be isolated in order to prevent further cross-infection

References and further reading

Adak GK, Long SM, O'Brien SJ (2002) Trends in indigenous food-borne disease and deaths, England and Wales 1992–2000. *Gut* **51**(6): 831–41.

Arthur AJ, Matthews RJ, Jagger C et al. (2002) Improving uptake of influenza vaccination among older people: a randomised controlled trial. *British Journal of General Practice* **52**(482): 717–22.

Artzrouni M (2004) Back-calculation and projection of the HIV/AIDS epidemic a homosexual/bisexual men in three European countries: evaluation past projection and updates allowing for treatment effects. *European Journal of Epidemiology* **19**(2): 171–9.

Ayliffe GAJ, Fraise AP, Geddes AM et al. (2000) *Control of Hospital Infections. A Practical Handbook* (4e). Arnold, London.

Baumann MA, Rath B, Fischer JH, Iffland R (2000) The permeability of dental procedure and examination gloves by an alcohol based disinfectant. *Dental Materials* **16**(2): 139–44.

Bellaby P (2003) Communication and miscommunication of risk: understanding UK parents' attitudes to combined MMR vaccination. *British Medical Journal* **327**: 725–8.

Beltrami EM, McArthur MA, Mc Geer A et al. (2000) The nature and frequency of blood contact among home health care workers. *Infection Control and Hospital Epidemiology* **21**(12): 765–70.

Bennett G, Mansell I (2004) Universal precautions: a survey of community nurses experience and practice. *Journal of Clinical Nursing* **13**(4): 413–21.

Bhattacharyya M, Bradley H (2006) Management of a difficult-to heal chronic wound infected with meticillin-resistant staphylococcus aureus in a patient with psoriasis following a complex knee surgery. *International Journal of Low Extremity Wounds* **5**(2): 105–8.

Bradberry SM, Dickers KJ, Rice P et al. (2003) Ricin poisoning. *Toxicology Review* **22**(1): 65–70.

Bradley CR, Fraise AP (1996) Heat and chemical resistance of enterococci. *Journal of Hospital Infection* **34**(3): 191–6.

Braitstein P, Chan K, Beardsell A et al. (2002) Prescribing practices in a population-based HIV postexposure prophylaxis program. *AIDS* **16**(7): 1067–70.

Brown RH, Hamilton RG, McAllister MA et al. (2003) How health care organizations can establish and conduct a program for the latex-safe environment. *Joint Commission Journal on Quality and Patient Safety* **29**(3): 113–23.

Burgess IF (2003) Understanding scabies. *Nursing Times* (Suppl.) **99**(7): 44–5.

Calman R (1992) Quality: a view from the centre. *Quality in Health Care* **1**: S28–33.

Calvert N, Murphy L, Smith A et al. (2007) A hotel-based outbreak of salmonella enterica subsp. Enterica serovar Enterititis (Salmonella Enteritidis) in the United Kingdom 2006. *Eurosurveillance* **12**(3):222.

Campbell S, O'Malley C, Watson D et al. (2000) The image of the children's nurse. A study of the qualities required by families of children's nurses uniform. *Journal of Clinical Nursing* **9**(1): 71–82.

Carabin H, Edmunds WJ, Kou U et al. (2002) The average cost of measles cases and adverse events following vaccination in industrial countries. *BMC Public Health* **19**(2): 11.

Carroll A (2001a) Handwashing for health care workers in domestic settings. *British Journal of Community Nursing* **6**(5): 217–23.

Carroll A (2001b) Use of gloves in the community: why, when, which and how? *British Journal of Community Nursing* **6**(9): 459–66.

Chadwick PR, Beards G, Brown D et al. (2000) Management of hospital outbreak of gastro-enteritis due to small round structured viruses. *Journal of Hospital Infection* **45**(1): 1–10.

Clarke P, Ghani AC (2005) Projections of the future course of the primary vCJD epidemic in the UK: Inclusion of subclinical infection and the possibility of wider genetic susceptibility. *Journal of Royal Society Interface* **2**(2): 19–31.

Cleary V, Slaughter R, Heathcock R (2003) An infection control programme in primary schools and the wider public health impact. *British Journal of Infection Control* **4**(5): 11–16.

Cochrane J (2003) Infection control audit of hand hygiene facilities. *Nursing Standard* **17**(18): 33–8.

Coia JE, Duckworth GJ, Edwards DI et al. (2006) Guidelines for the control and prevention of meticillin resistant *Staphylococcus aureus* (MRSA) in healthcare facilities. *Journal of Hospital Infection* **63**(Suppl. 1): S1–S44.

Crippa M, Belleri L, Mistrell OG et al. (2003) Prevention of latex allergy among health care workers: evaluation of the extractable latex protein content in different types of medical gloves. *American Journal of Industrial Medicine* **44**(1): 24–31.

Croft AC, D'Antoni AV, Terzulli SL (2007) Update on the antibacterial resistance crisis. *Medical Science Monitor* **13**(6): 103–18

Crouch D (2003) Thinking the unthinkable. *Nursing Times* **99**(113): 22–7.

Crowcroft NS, Andrews N, Rooney C et al. (2002) Deaths from pertussis is underestimated in England. *Archives of Disease in Childhood* **86**(5): 336–8.

Curran E, Ahmed S (2000) Do health care workers need to wear masks when caring for patients with tuberculosis. *Communicable Disease and Public Health* **3**(4):240–3.

Cutter J, Gammon J (2007) Review of standard precautions and sharp management in the community. *British Journal of Community Nursing* **12**(2): 54–60.

Davies E, Linklater KM, Jack RH et al. (2006) How is place of death from cancer changing and what affects it? Analysis of cancer registration and service data. *British Journal of Cancer* **95**(5): 593–600.

Dellasega CA, Fisher KM (2001) Posthospital home care for frail older adults in rural locations. *Community Health Nursing* **18**(4): 247–60.

DePaola LG, Carpenter WM (2002) Bloodborne pathogens: current concepts. *Compendium on Continuing Education in Dentistry* **23**(3): 207–14.

Department of Health (1984) *The Public Health (Control of Disease) Act*. HMSO, London.

Department of Health (1987) *Hospital Laundry Arrangements for Used and Infected Linen*. HC(87)30. HMSO, London.

Department of Health (1989) *Chilled and Frozen. Guidelines on Cook-Chill and Cook-Frozen Catering Systems*. HMSO, London.

125

Department of Health (1991) *Hospital Mattress Assemblies, Care and Cleaning.* DH, London.

Department of Health (1993) *Standards in Infection Control in Hospitals.* HMSO, London.

Department of Health (1995a) *Hospital Infection Control.* DH, London.

Department of Health (1995b) *The Food Safety (General Food Hygiene) Regulations 1995.* HMSO, London.

Department of Health (1997) *Guidelines for the Post Exposure Prophylaxis for Health Care Workers Occupationally Exposed to HIV.* PL/CO(97). The Stationery Office, London.

Department of Health (1998) *The Prevention and Control of Tuberculosis in the United Kingdom.* HSC 1998/196. The Stationery Office, London.

Department of Health (1999) *AIDS/HIV Infected Health Care Workers: guidance on the management of infected health care worker and patient notification.* UK Health Department, London.

Department of Health (2001) *Shifting the Power, Securing Delivery.* HMSO, London.

Department of Health (2002) *Getting Ahead of the Curve. A strategy for combating infectious diseases (including other aspects of health protection). A report by the Chief Medical Officer for England.* HMSO, London.

Department of Health (2004a) *Primary Care Contracting.* HMSO, London.

Department of Health (2004b) *Standards for Better Health.* HMSO, London.

DoH (2004c) *Stopping Tuberculosis in England. An action plan from the Chief Medical Officer.* HMSO, London.

Department of Health (2005) *Explaining Pandemic Flu: a guide from the Chief Medical Officer.* DH, London.

Department of Health (2006a) *Environment and Sustainability.* Health Technical Memorandum 07-01: Safe management of healthcare waste. HMSO, London.

Department of Health (2006b) *Immunisation Against Infectious Disease.* HMSO, London.

Department of Health (2006c) *Infection Control: guidance for care homes.* DH, London.

Department of Health (2007a) *Health Clearance for Tuberculosis, Hepatitis B, Hepatitis C, and HIV. New Healthcare Workers.* DH, London.

Department of Health (2007b) *Saving Lives: reducing infection, delivering clean and safe care.* DH, London.

Department of Health NHS Executive (1995a) *Food Safety (Temperature Control) Regulations.* HMSO, London.

Department of Health NHS Executive (1995b) *Food Safety (General Food Hygiene) Regulations.* HMSO, London.

Department of Health NHS Executive (1996) *Management of Food Hygiene and Food Service in the National Health Service.* Department of Health, London.

Department of the Environment and Health (1990) *Report of the Group of Experts on Cryptosporodium in Water Supplies.* HMSO, London.

Dougherty L, Lister S (2011) *The Royal Marsden Hospital Manual of Clinical Nursing Procedures* (8e). Wiley-Blackwell, Oxford.

Evans MR (2003) Hazards of healthy living: bottles water and salad vegetables as risk factors for campylobacter infection. *Emerging Infectious Diseases* **9**(10): 1219–25.

Farrow SC, Zeuner D, Hall C (1999) Improving infection control in general practice. *Journal of the Royal Society of Health* **119**(1): 17–22.

Finn L, Crook S (1999) A district survey of vaccine cold chain protection in general practitioners' surgeries. *Communicable Disease and Public Health* **2**(1): 47–9.

Food Safety Act (1990) HMSO, London.

Foster K, Gorton R, Waller J (2006) Outbreak of legionellois associated with spa pool. *UK Eurosurveillance* **11**(9): E060921.2.

Fournier S, Dubrou S, Liguory O *et al.* (2002) Detection of Microsporidia, Cryptosporidia and Giardia in swimming pools: a one-year prospective study. *FEMS Immunology and Medical Microbiology* **33**(3): 209–13.

Friedman MM (1999) Preventing and controlling the transmission of antibiotic-resistant microorganisms in the home setting. *Caring* **18**(11): 6–11.

Gillespie IA, O'Brien SJ, Adak GK *et al.* (2003) Point source outbreaks of Campylobacter jejuni infection – are they more common than we think and what might cause them ? *Epidemiology and Infection* **130**(3): 367–75.

Glaberman S, Moore JE, Lowery CJ *et al.* (2002) Three drinking water associated cryptosporidiosis outbreaks, Northern Ireland. *Emerging Infectious Diseases* **8**(6): 631–633.

Gould D (2002) Health-related infection and hand hygiene part 1. *Nursing Times Plus* **98**(38): 48–51.

Gould D, Gammon J, Donnelly M *et al.* (2000) Improving hand hygiene in community health care settings: the impact of research and clinical collaboration. *Journal of Clinical Nursing* **9**(1): 95–102.

Griffith CJ, Malik R, Cooper RA *et al.* (2003) Environmental surface cleanliness and the potential for contamination during handwashing. *American Journal of Infection Control* **31**(2): 93–6.

Griffiths J, Ewing G, Rogers M *et al.* (2007) Supporting cancer patients with palliative care needs: district nurses' role perceptions. *Cancer Nursing* **30**(2): 156–62.

Grime P (2005) Evaluation of an occupational health service for general practitioners and their staff in a primary care trust. *Occupational Medicine (Lond)* **55**(6): 494–7.

Hampton S (2002) Nurses' inappropriate use of gloves in caring for patients. *British Journal of Nursing* **12**(17): 1024–7.

Harrison J, Harrison CE (2002) Developing a model for occupational health provision in primary care. *International Journal of Occupational Medicine and Environmental Health* **15**(2): 185–92.

Hart S (2008) Infection control in intravenous therapy. In: Dougherty L, Lamb J (eds) *Intravenous Therapy in Nursing Practice* (2e), chapter 5. Wiley Blackwell, Oxford.

Health and Safety at Work Act (1974) The Stationery Office, London. ISBN 0 11 141439 X.

Health and Safety Commission (2002) *Control of Substances Hazardous to Health Regulations (COSHH).* The Stationery Office, London. ISBN 0 11 042919 2.

Health and Safety Executive (2004) *Controlling Legionella in Nursing and Residential Care Homes.* HSE Books, Suffolk.

Health Protection Agency Press Statement (2007) Cases of tuberculosis continue to rise during 2006.

Health Service Circular (HSC) (2002) Pre and post appointment checks for all persons working in the NHS in England. London, Department of Health 2002/008.

Health Services Advisory Committee (1991) *Safety in Health Service Laboratories. The labelling, transport and reception of specimens.* HMSO, London.

Health Services Advisory Committee (2003) *Safe Working and the Prevention of Infection in Clinical Laboratories and Similar Facilities.* HMSO, London.

Health Service Executive (1985) *The Reporting of Injuries, Diseases and Dangerous Occurrences Regulations (1985) RIDDOR.* HSE, London.

Heaton J, Arksey H, Sloper P (1999) Carers' experience of hospital discharge and continuing care in the community. *Health and Social Care in the Community* **7**(2): 91–9.

Hobson-West P (2007) 'Trusting blindly can be the biggest risk of all': organised resistance to childhood vaccination in the UK. *Social Health and Illness* **29**(2): 198–215.

Hugonnet S, Peregar TV, Pittet D (2002) Alcohol-based handrub improves compliance with hand hygiene in intensive care units. *Archives of Internal Medicine* **162**(9): 1037–43.

Idris AH, Gabrielli A (2002) Advances in airway management. *Emergency Medicine Clinics of North America* **20**(4): 843–57.

Infection Control Nurses Association (1997) *Guidelines for Hand Hygiene.* Fitwise, Edinburgh.

Infection Control Nurses Association in partnership with Pharmacia (2002) *Antibiotic Resistance Theory and Practice.* Fitwise, Edinburgh.

Infection Control Nurses Association in partnership with Portex (2003a) *Reducing Sharps Injury. Prevention and Risk Management.* Fitwise, Edinburgh.

Infection Control Nurses Association (2003b) Infection control prevention of HCAI in primary and community care. *British Journal of Infection Control* **5**(5): 10–11.

Jacobsson G, Dashti S, Wahlberg T, Anderson R (2007) The epidemiology of the risk factors for invasive *Staphylococcus aureus* infection in Western Sweden. *Scandinavian Journal of Infectious Diseases* **39**(1): 6–13.

Jenkinson D (2006) Whooping cough is quite common and can be diagnosed clinically. *British Medical Journal* **333**(7563): 352.

Kagan LJ, Aiello AE, Larson E (2002) The role of the home environment in the transmission of infectious diseases. *Journal of Community Health* **27**(4): 247–67.

Kampf G (2003) State-of-the-art hand hygiene in community medicine. *International Journal of Hygiene and Environmental Health* **206**(6): 465–72.

Kennedy I, Williams S, Reynolds A et al. (2002) GPs' compliance with health and safety legislation and their occupational health needs in one London health authority. *British Journal of General Practice* **52**(482): 741–2.

Kocent H, Corke C, Alajeel A, Graves S (2002) Washing of gloved hands in antiseptic solution prior to central venous line insertion reduces contamination. *Anaesthetic Intensive Care* **30**(3): 338–40.

Korniewicz DM, El-Masri M, Broyles JM et al. (2002) Performance of latex and non-latex medical examination gloves during simulated use. *American Journal of Infection Control* **30**(2): 133–8.

Kownatzki E (2003) Hand hygiene and skin health. *Journal of Hospital Infection* **55**(4): 239–45.

Lachlan M, Licence K, Oates K et al. (2002) Practical lessons from the management of an outbreak of small round structures virus (Norwalk-like virus) gastroenteritis. *Communicable Disease and Public Health* **5**(1): 43–7.

Lankester BJ, Bartlett GE, Garneti N et al. (2002) Direct measurement of bacterial penetration through surgical gowns: a new method. *Journal of Hospital Infection* **50**(4): 281–5.

Larson EL, Hughes CA, Pyrek JD et al. (1998) Changes in bacterial flora associated with skin damage on hands of health care personnel. *American Journal of Infection Control* **26**(5): 513–21.

Larson EL, Gomez-Duarte C, Lee LV et al. (2003) Microbial flora of hands of homemakers. *American Journal of Infection Control* **31**(2): 72–9.

Lawrence J, May D (2003) *Infection Control in the Community.* Churchill Livingstone, Edinburgh.

Lipp A (2003) The effectiveness of surgical face masks: what the literature shows. *Nursing Times* **99**(39): 22–4.

Long SM, Adak GK, O'Brien SJ, Gillespie IA (2002) General outbreaks of infectious intestinal disease linked with salad vegetables and fruit, England and Wales 1992–2000. *Communicable Disease and Public Health* **5**(2): 101–5.

Lopman BA, Adak GK, Reacher MH, Brown DW (2003) Two epidemiologic patterns of norovirus outbreaks: surveillance in England and Wales, 1992–2000. *Emerging Infectious Diseases* **9**(1): 71–7.

Loudon KW, Coke AP, Burnie JP et al. (1996) Kitchens as a source of *Aspergillus niger* infection. *Journal of Hospital Infection* **32**(3): 191–8.

Loveday HP, Harper PF, Mulhall A et al. (2002) Informing the future 1. A review of the nursing roles and responsibilities in community infection control. *British Journal of Infection Control* **3**(6): 20–4.

Lymer UB, Richt B, Isaksson B (2003) Health care workers' action strategies in situations that involve risk of blood exposure. *Journal of Clinical Nursing* **12**(5): 660–7.

Magura S, Nwakeze PC, Rosenblum A, Joseph H (2000) Substance misuse and related infectious diseases in a soup kitchen. *Substance Use and Misuse* **35**(4): 551–83.

Malik R, Cooper RA et al. (2003) Environmental surface cleanliness and the potential for contamination during handwashing. *American Journal of Infection Control* **31**(2): 93–6.

Management of Health and Safety at Work Regulations (1994) The Stationery Office, London. ISBN 0 11 0856252 2

Marais BJ, Pai M (2007) Recent advances in the diagnosis of childhood tuberculosis. *Archives of Disease in Childhood* **92**(5): 446–452.

Masterton RG, Teare EL (2001) Clinical governance and infection control in the United Kingdom. *Journal of Hospital Infection* **47**(1): 25–31.

McDonald LC, Kuehnert MJ, Tenover FC, Jarvis WR (1997) Vancomycin-resistant enterococci outside the health care setting: prevalence sources, and public health implications. *Emerging Infectious Diseases* **3**(3): 1–10.

McGarrigle CA, Fenton KA, Gill ON et al. (2002) Behavioural surveillance: the value of national co ordination. *Sexually Transmitted Infections* **78**: 398–405.

McGuckin M, Waterman R, Porten L et al. (1999) Patient education model for increasing handwashing compliance. *American Journal of Infection Control* 27(4): 309–14.

Meakins SM, Adak GK, Lopman BA, O'Brien SJ (2003) General outbreaks of infectious intestinal disease (IID) in hospitals, England and Wales 1992–2000. *Journal of Hospital Infection* 53(1): 1–5.

Meara MO, Barry J, Mullen L (2007) Epidemiology of hepatitis C infection. ERHA/HSE Eastern region. *Irish Medical Journal* 100(2): 365–6.

Medical Devices Agency (2000) *Equipped to Care. The Safe Use of Medical Devices in the 21st Century*. DH, London.

Medical Devices Agency (2002) *Benchtop Steam Sterilizers – Guidance on Purchase, Operation and Maintenance*. MDA DB 2002(06). DH, London.

Melegaro A, Edmunds WJ, Pebody R et al. (2006) The current burden of pneumococcal disease in England and Wales. *Journal of Infection* 52(1): 37–48.

Mendelson G, Yearmack Y, Granot E et al. (2003) *Staphylococcus aureus* carrier state among elderly residents of a long term care facility. *Journal of American Medical Directors Association* 4(3): 125–7.

Millward S, Barnett J, Thomlinson D (1993) A clinical infection control audit programme: evaluation of the audit tool used by infection control nurses to monitor standards and assess effective staff training. *Journal of Hospital Infection* 24(3): 219–32.

Ministry of Agriculture, Fisheries and Food (1994) *Food Safety*. Food Safety Directorate, Ministry of Agriculture, Fisheries and Food, London.

Morbidity and Mortality Weekly Report (MMWR) (1995) Recommendations for preventing the spread of vancomycin resistance. Recommendations of the hospital infection control practice advisory committee (HICPAC). 44 (RR-12) 1–13.

National Audit Commission (1999) *First Assessment. A review of district nursing in England and Wales*. National Audit Commission, London.

National Audit Office (2000) *The Management of Hospital Acquired Infection in Acute NHS Trusts in England*. HMSO, London.

National Audit Office (2004) *Improving Patients' Care by Reducing the Risk of Hospital Acquired Infection: a progress report*. The Parliamentary Bookshop, London.

National End of Life Care Programme (2011) *Guidance for Staff Responsible for Care After Death (Last Offices)*. NHS National End of Life Care Programme, London.

NHS Estates (1995) *Hospital Laundry Arrangements for Used and Infected Linen*. HSG(95)18. HMSO, London.

NHS Estates (2001) *A Protocol for the Local Decontamination of Surgical Instruments*. Department of Health, London.

NHS Estates (2002) *Infection Control in the Built Environment*. Department of Health, London

NHS Estates (2003) *A Guide to the Decontamination of Reusable Surgical Instruments*. Department of Health, London.

National Health Service Executive (1999a) *Controls Assurance in Infection Control. Decontamination of Medical Devices*. HSC 1999/179. Department of Health, London.

National Health Service Executive (1999b) *Clinical Governance: Quality in the New NHS*. HSC1999/065. Department of Health, London.

National Health Service Executive (2000) *Decontamination of Medical Devices*. HSC 2000/032. Department of Health, London.

National Health Service Executive (2001) *Your Guide to the National Health Service*. HMSO, London.

National Institute for Clinical Excellence (2002) *Clinical Guideline on Community Infection Control*. NICE, London.

National Institute for Clinical Excellence (2003) *Infection Control Prevention and Healthcare-associated Infection in Primary and Community Care*. NICE, London.

National Institute for Clinical Excellence (2006a) *Tuberculosis. Clinical Diagnosis and Management of Tuberculosis and Measures for its Prevention and Control*. NICE, London.

National Institute for Clinical Excellence (2006b) *Implementation Advice. Suggested Actions for Implementing the NICE Clinical Guideline on Tuberculosis*. NICE, London.

Neely AN (2000) A survey of gram-negative bacteria survival on hospital fabrics and plastics. *Journal of Burn Care and Rehabilitation* 21(6): 523–7.

Nosocomial Infection National Surveillance Service (2002) *Surveillance of Surgical Site Infection*. Public Health Laboratory Service, London.

O'Brien SJ, Murdoch PS, Ruley AH et al. (2001) A foodborne outbreak of Vero cytotoxin-producing *Escherichia coli* 0157: H-phage type 8 in hospitals. *Journal of Hospital Infection* 49(3): 167–72.

O'Donnell JM, Thornton L, McNamara EB et al. (2002) Outbreak of Vero cytotoxin-producing *Escherichia coli* 0157 in a child day care facility. *Communicable Disease and Public Health* 5(1): 54–8.

O'Malley A, Lok S (2003) Cross-infection in hospitals: an audit of stethoscope use. *Clinical Governance Bulletin* 4(1): 9–10.

Padayatchi N, Friedland G (2007) Managing multiple and extensively drug-resistant tuberculosis and HIV. *Expert Opinion in Pharmacotherapy* 8(8): 1035–7.

Patel S (2007) Managing MRSA in hospital and in the community. *Nursing Times* 103(10): 48–9.

Payne CJ, Petrovic M, Poberts RJ et al. (2003) Vero cytotoxin producing *Escherichia coli* 0157 gastroenteritis in farm visitors, North Wales. *Emerging Infectious Diseases* 9(5): 526–30.

Pearson A, Baker H, Walsh K, Fitzgerald M (2001) Contemporary nurses uniforms history and traditions. *Journal of Nursing Management* 9(3): 147–52.

Pearson L, Duncanson V (2006) Involving patients in staff hand hygiene. *Nursing Times* 102(24): 46–7.

Pellowe CM, Pratt RJ, Harper P et al. (2003) Infection control: prevention of healthcare-associated infection in primary and community care. *British Journal of Infection Control* (Suppl) 4(6): 1–100.

Petchey R, Farnsworth B, Williams J (2000) The last resort would be to go to the GP. Understanding the perceptions and use of general practitioners service among people with HIV/AIDS. *Social Care and Medicine* 50(2): 233–45.

Plowman R, Graves N, Griffin M et al. (1999) The Social-Economic Burden of Hospital Acquired Infection. Executive Summary. Public Health Laboratory Service, London

Porteous J (2002) Artificial nails… very real risks. Canadian Operating Room Nursing Journal 20(3): 16–17, 20–1.

Powell BJ, Winkley GP, Brown JO, Etersque S (1994) Evaluating the fit of ambidextrous and fitted gloves: implications for hand discomfort. Journal of the American Dental Association 125(9): 1235–42.

Pratt RJ, Pellowe CM, Wilson JA et al. (2007) Epic 2: National evidence-based guidelines for preventing healthcare-associated infections in NHS hospitals in England. Journal of Hospital Infection 65(Suppl. 1): S1–S59.

Provision and Use of Work Equipment Regulations (PUWER) (1998) The Stationery Office, London.

Public Health Laboratory Service AIDS & STD Centre (1999) Occupational Transmission of HIV. PHLS, London.

Public Health Laboratory Service (2002a) Infection Control in the Community Study. PHLS, London.

Public Health Laboratory Service (2002b) HIV and AIDS in the UK in 2001. An update: November 2002. PHLS, London.

Public Health Medicines Environmental Group (1996) Guidelines on the Control of Infection in Residential and Nursing Homes. Department of Health, London.

Reporting of Injuries, Diseases and Dangerous Occurrences Regulations (RIDDOR) (1995) ISBN 01 1053 7523. The Stationery Office, London.

Richardson M (1999). The symbolism and myth surrounding nurses' uniform. British Journal of Nursing 8(3): 169–75.

Robinson RA, Pugh RN (2002) Dogs, zoonoses and immunosuppression. Journal of the Royal Society of Health 122(2): 95–8.

Rogers PA, Sinka KJ, Molesworth AM et al. (2000) Survival after diagnosis of AIDS among adults resident in the United Kingdom in the era of multiple therapies. Communicable Disease and Public Health 3(3): 188–94.

Rossoff LJ, Lam S, Hilton E et al. (1993) Is the use of boxed gloves in an intensive care unit safe? American Journal of Medicine 94(6): 602–7.

Rowe WS, Yaffe MJ, Pepler C et al. (2000). Variables impacting on patients perceptions of discharge from short-stay hospitalisation or same day surgery. Health Soc Care Community 8(6): 362–71.

Royal College of Nursing (1992) Standards of Care Project. Royal College of Nursing, London.

Royal College of Physicians (2006) Tuberculosis. Clinical Diagnosis and Management of Tuberculosis, and Measures for its Prevention and Control. Royal College of Physicians, London.

Sanchez JL, Polyak CS, Kolavic SA (2001) Investigation of a cluster of Legionella pneumophila infection among staff at a federal research facility. Military Medicine 166(9): 753–8.

Seto WH, Tsang D, Yung RW et al. (2003) Effectiveness of precautions against droplet and contact in prevention of nosocomial transmission of severe acute respiratory syndrome (SARS). Lancet 361(368): 1519–20.

Simon C (2001) Informal carers and the primary care team. British Journal of General Practice 51(472): 920–3.

Smith-Bathgate B (2005) Creutzfeldt-Jakob disease: diagnosis and nursing care. Nursing Times 101(20): 52–3.

St Clair K, Larrabee JH (2002) Clean versus sterile gloves: which to use for postoperative dressing changes? Outcomes Management 6(1): 17–21.

Stein AD, Makarawo TP, Ahmad MFR (2003) A survey of doctors' and nurses' knowledge, attitudes and compliance with infection control guidelines in Birmingham teaching hospitals. Journal of Hospital Infection 54(1): 68–73.

Stockley JM, Allen RM, Thomlinson DF et al. (2001) A district general hospitals method of post-operative infection surveillance including post-discharge follow up developed over a five year period. Journal of Hospital Infection 49(1): 48–54.

Stone L, Olinky R, Huppert A (2007) Seasonal dynamics of recurrent epidemics. Nature 446(7135): 533–6.

Storr J (2005) The effectiveness of the national cleanyourhands campaign. Nursing Times 101(8): 50–1.

Tacconelli E (2006) New strategies to identify patients harbouring antibiotic resistant bacteria at hospital admissions. Clinical Microbiology and Infection 12(2): 102–9.

Tam CC, O'Brien SJ, Adak GK et al. (2003) Campylobacter coli – an important foodborne pathogen. Journal of Infection 47(1): 28–32.

Taylor K, Plowman R, Roberts J (2001) The Challenge of Hospital Acquired Infection. National Audit Office. HMSO, London.

Telford R, Rogers A (2003) What influences elderly peoples' decisions about whether to accept the influenza vaccination? A qualitative study. Health Education Research 18(6): 743–53.

Tenorio AR, Badri SM, Sahgal NB et al. (2001) Effectiveness of gloves in the prevention of hand carriage of vancomycin-resistant enterococcus species by health care workers after patient care. Clinical Infectious Diseases 32(5): 826–9.

The Carriage of Dangerous Goods (Classification, Packaging and Labelling) Regulations (1996) ISBN 01 1043 6695. The Stationery Office, London.

The Carriage of Dangerous Goods by Road Regulations (1996) SL 1996/2095. ISBN 0 11 062926 4. The Stationery Office, London.

Thielemann P (2000) Educational needs of home caregivers of terminally ill patients: literature review. American Journal of Hospital Palliative Care 17(4): 253–7.

Wagenvoort JH, Sluijsmans W, Penders RJ (2000) Better environmental survival of outbreaks. Sporadic MRSA isolates. Journal of Hospital Infection 45(3): 231–4.

Ward D (2001) Infection control policies in nursing homes. Nursing Standard 15(46): 40–4.

Ward PI, Deplazes P, Regli W et al. (2002) Detection of eight Cryptosporidium genotypes in surface and waste water in Europe. Parasitology 124(Pt 4): 359–68.

Waste Strategy (2000) Waste Strategy 2000 for England and Wales. Part 1 & 2. Department for Environment, Food and Rural Affairs, London.

Wendt C, Wiesenthal B, Dietz E, Ruden H (1998) Survival of vancomycin-resistant and vancomycin-susceptible enterococcu on dry surfaces. Journal of Clinical Microbiology 36(12): 3734–6.

129

Wilson A, Wynn A, Parker H (2002a) Patient and care satisfaction with 'hospital at home': quantitative and qualitative results from a randomised controlled trial. *British Journal of General Practice* **52**(474): 9–13.

Wilson IG (2002) Salmonella and campylobacter contamination of raw retail chickens from different producers: a five year survey. *Epidemiology and Infection* **129**(3): 635–45.

Winnefeld M, Richard MA, Drancourt M, Grob JJ (2000) Skin tolerance and effectiveness of two hand decontamination procedures in everyday hospital use. *British Journal of Dermatology* **143**(3): 546–50.

Worth A, Tierney AJ, Watson NT (2000) Discharge from hospital: should more responsibility for meeting patients' and carers' information needs now be shouldered in the community. *Health and Social Care in the Community* **8**(6): 398–405.

Wyllie DH, Peto TE, Crook D (2005) MRSA bacteraemia in patients on arrival in hospital: a cohort study in Oxfordshire 1997–2003. *British Medical Journal* **331**(7523): 992–7.

Zachary KC, Bayne PS, Morrison VJ *et al.* (2001) Contamination of gowns, gloves and stethoscopes with vancomycin-resistant enterococci. *Infect Control Hosp Epidemiol* **22**(9): 560–4.

7

Intravenous therapy and central vascular access devices

Definition of vascular access device (VAD) and central vascular access device (CVAD)

The administration of any IV therapy treatment, regardless of the setting, requires a vascular access device (VAD). A VAD is defined by Dougherty & Watson (2011) as 'a device that is inserted into either a vein or an artery, via the peripheral or central vessels, to provide vascular access for either diagnostic (blood sampling, central venous pressure reading) or therapeutic purposes (administration of medications, fluids and/or blood products)'. A central vascular access device (CVAD) is a catheter inserted into a centrally located vein with the tip residing in the superior vena cava (Goodwin & Carlson 1993; RCN 2010).

Background evidence

Intravenous (IV) therapy is routine practice in hospital in the UK and the requirement for IV therapy is frequently a reason for admission to hospital. It is a natural and necessary development for some IV therapies to take place outside the hospital inpatient setting, particularly in the context of increasing demand for acute hospital beds and lengthening waiting lists (Kayley 2008; O'Hanlon *et al.* 2008). Patients now have a greater influence on the choice and location of treatment, and in many circumstances prefer the comfort and familiarity of their own home environment (Kayley 2008).

Community IV therapy itself is not a new concept. It has been a well-established practice for some years for a very small number of chronic conditions that require long-term IV therapy such as parenteral nutrition, factor VIII and IX for haemophilia, immunoglobulin therapy and IV antibiotics for cystic fibrosis (Kayley

2008) (Table 7.1). These programmes have evolved because it is impractical both socially and economically for them to be carried out in hospital or on an outpatient basis (Kayley *et al.* 1996). Over the past 5 years there has been a general increase in the range and complexity of IV treatments administered in the community (Table 7.2). Also recent developments in technology, and drugs with pharmacokinetic profiling, such as some antimicrobials that allow once- or twice-daily dosing, has enabled community IV therapy to be a more realistic and viable option (Kayley *et al.* 1996). The main growth areas over the past 5 years have been IV antimicrobial therapy for acute and chronic infections (Kayley 2000) and ambulatory chemotherapy (Daniels 1996; Dougherty *et al.* 1998; Aston 2000).

Patients receiving community IV therapy need a reliable VAD, which could either be peripherally or centrally placed, that meets the patient's clinical needs and is acceptable to them (Gabriel 1996; Kayley 2000). The type of VAD and location of vein used to administer the IV therapy is dependent on:

- the pH and osmolarity of the drug
- the nature and duration of the treatment
- the patient's lifestyle
- who is administering the treatment
- how it is administered in the community.

Peripheral cannula are used for some short-term community IV therapies; however, in many primary care trusts peripheral IV therapy is not part of the core community nursing service provided. If a patient is discharged home with a peripheral cannula it can be problematic to find someone in the community to take on responsibility for resiting the cannula. The patient may have to return to hospital each time the cannula needs resiting, which in some situations could be daily

District Nursing Manual of Clinical Procedures, First Edition. Edited by Liz O'Brien.
© 2012 Blackwell Publishing Ltd. Published 2012 by Blackwell Publishing Ltd.

Table 7.1 Established community IV therapies

Conditions	Treatment	Started
Haemophlia A & B	Factor VIII & IX	1971
Intestinal failure	Parenteral nutrition	late 1970s
Primary antibody deficiency	Immunoglobulin	mid-1980s
Cystic fibrosis	Antibiotics	mid-1980s

(Kayley 2008)

Table 7.2 More recent community IV therapies

Condition	Treatment
Acute or chronic infection	Antibiotics
Cytomegalovirus	Antivirals
Serious fungal infection	Antifungals
Haematological disorders	Blood products/platelets
Cancer	Chemotherapy
Nausea/vomiting	Anti-emetic
Acute/chronic pain	Analgesia
Gaucher's disease	Ceredase
Dehydration	Intravenous fluid
Hyperemesis	Intravenous fluid

(Kayley 2008)

(Kayley 2008). While a peripheral cannula may be suitable for some specific situations there is a growing acceptance that peripherally inserted central catheters (PICCs) or midline catheters are more appropriate for community IV therapy (Hamilton 2000; Kayley 2008).

This chapter will explore the range of CVADs most commonly seen in the community (Table 7.3), their indication for use and the particular issues that need considering in relation to their management in the community. It will also provide guidance on how to prepare and administer IV medications using a bolus or infusion method. In the context of this chapter community IV therapy is considered to be any IV treatment administered at home, in general practitioner (GP) surgeries, community hospitals and care homes.

Referrals

Nurses working in the community will be asked to accept patients for community IV therapy, and therefore need to be aware of the different types of CVAD and the advantages and disadvantages of each one (Table 7.4). It is also important to know of any particular aspects related to the care and management of the CVAD, as well as understanding any possible complications that could develop, and how those complications might be recognised.

When a referral is made there are a number of questions related to the CVAD that need to be answered by the referring unit, before the patient is accepted for community IV therapy.

- What type of CVAD does the patient have?
- Is the CVAD suitable for the prescribed IV therapy?
- When was the CVAD placed/inserted?
- If centrally placed, where is the tip positioned?
- What is the external measurement of the CVAD?
- What are the complications of this type of CVAD?
- What are the signs and symptoms of these complications?
- Who should be contacted if any problems occur and what are their contact details?
- Does the patient/family/carer understand about the treatment and the CVAD, how to recognise and deal with any complications, and who to contact throughout the day or night?
- Is there a planned date for the CVAD to be removed?
- Who will remove the CVAD and where?

(Kayley & Finlay 2003)

Education and training

Community nurses are ideally placed to provide IV therapy as well as support to patients and carers in the community. While community nurses may have many of the skills required, they do need access to a community-based theoretical IV training programme, supervised practice and ongoing support (Kayley 2008).

As IV therapy is still not routine practice in many areas, community nurses may only encounter it on an infrequent basis, which makes it difficult for them to maintain their practical skills and have the confidence to use them (Kayley 2008). Community nurses may also come across a range of different IV therapies and vascular access devices and therefore require the specific knowledge and practical skills to enable them to cope with each situation.

Therefore it must be recognised that community nurses need to keep updating their practical skills and theoretical knowledge. This may be achieved by visiting the hospital unit when a patient is referred, although time and distance constraints may make this difficult. Some areas of the UK now have specialist community IV nurses and part of their role is to provide practical training and ongoing support for community nurses within the home environment.

Table 7.3 CVADs most commonly seen in the community*

Catheter	Material	Site of insertion	No of lumens	Dwell time	General indications
Open ended peripherally inserted central catheter (PICC)	Silicone or polyurethane	Antecubital fossa Upper arm	Single, double or triple lumen	Optimal dwell time is unknown (INS 2011). Recommended 4 weeks (or less) to 6 months (Todd 1998)	Blood sampling. All types of IV therapy whose duration is more than several days
Valved PICC	Silicone	Antecubital fossa Upper arm	Single, double or triple lumen	Optimal dwell time is unknown (INS 2006). Recommended 4 weeks (or less) to 6 months (Todd 1998)	Blood sampling. All types of IV therapy whose duration is more than several days
Open-ended tunnelled catheter	Silicone or polyurethane	Chest wall	Single, double or triple lumen	Months to several years if no complications occur (Gabriel 2008)	Blood sampling. All types of IV therapy where long term venous access is required
Valved tunnelled catheter	Silicone	Chest wall	Single, double or triple lumen	Months to several years if no complications occur (Gabriel 2008)	Blood sampling. All types of IV therapy where long term venous access is required
Open-ended implantable port	Silicone catheter with stainless steel, titanium or plastic port	Chest wall or antecubital fossa	Single or double port	Months to several years if no complications occur (Gabriel 2008)	Blood sampling. All types of IV therapy where long term venous access is required
Valved implantable port	Silicone catheter with titanium port	Chest wall or antecubital fossa	Single or double port	Months to several years if no complications occur (Gabriel 2008)	Blood sampling. All types of IV therapy where long term venous access is required

*Vascular access devices may vary between different manufacturers. The above table is a general guide only, and not an exhaustive list. It is important to seek specific guidance related to the care and management from individual manufacturers.

The Royal College of Nursing (2008) states:

Standard
The nurse inserting devices and/or providing infusion therapy shall be competent in all clinical aspects of infusion therapy and have validated competency in clinical judgement and practice in accordance with the Nursing & Midwifery Council's (NMC) *Code*: that is, they will maintain their knowledge and skills (Scales 1996; Hyde 2008; NMC 2008).

Practice criteria
Nurses undertaking the administration of infusion therapy and care and management of vascular access devices will have undergone theoretical and practical training in the following aspects (Hyde 2002; NPSA 2003; MDA 2003; NICE 2003).

- Legal, professional and ethical issues
- Anatomy and physiology
- Fluid balance and blood administration
- Mathematical calculations
- Pharmacology and pharmaceutics related to reconstitution and administration
- Local and systemic complications
- Infection control issues
- Use of equipment, including infusion equipment
- Drug administration

133

Table 7.4 Advantages and disadvantages of CVADs*

CVAD	Advantages	Disadvantages
Open-ended PICC	No discomfort with use	Can be dislodged/pulled out
	Easy to conceal under clothing	Not recommended for swimming
	No scar once removed	Need to avoid heavy lifting and excessive use of arm
	Suitable for needle-phobic patients	Difficult for self-administration without an extension set
	Easy to remove	Dressing required at the entry site for the whole time the catheter remains in situ
Valved PICC	As above	As above
	Only requires flushing with sodium chloride 0.9% to maintain patency (Weinstein 2007; Perucca 2010)	
Open-ended tunnelled catheter	Dacron cuff anchors catheter in place	Altered body image
	No discomfort with use	Can get caught in clothing and bedding
	Easily accessible	Vulnerable to activities that may catch or pull catheter
	Can be used for blood sampling	External clamps (if required) are bulky
	Suitable for needle-phobic patients	May require minor surgical procedure to remove
		Discomfort with car seat belts
		Requires very secure waterproof protection for swimming
Valved tunnelled catheter	As above	As above
	Only requires flushing with sodium chloride 0.9% to maintain patency (Weinstein 2007; Perucca 2010)	
Open-ended implantable port	Concealed under skin – only small, raised area visible	Each use requires a needle puncture (unless non-coring needle with extension tubing left in situ)
	Requires only monthly flush, when not in use, to maintain patency (Weinstein 2007; Perucca 2010)	More difficult to access, particularly self-access for the patient
	No restrictions on physical activities	Skin can become sore with frequent accessing
	Suitable for bathing, showering and swimming	Not suitable for needle-phobic patients
	No dressing required	Requires a surgical procedure to remove
Valved implantable port	As above	As above

(Kayley 2008)
*Vascular access devices vary between different manufacturers. The above table is a general guide only, and not an exhaustive or inclusive list.

- Risk management/health and safety
- Care and management of vascular access devices
- Infusion therapy in specialist areas covered separately (paediatrics, oncology, parenteral nutrition, transfusion therapy).

All staff have a professional obligation to maintain their knowledge and skills (NMC 2008a,b). It is also the responsibility of the organisation to support and provide staff with training and education (RCN 2010: 7).

Quality of life issues

It is very important that the chosen CVAD meets the clinical needs of the individual patient and matches their lifestyle. Patients will be expected to 'live' with their CVAD and in some instances they will assume responsibility for its care and management (Gabriel 2008). It is essential therefore that patients are involved in the decision-making process (Dougherty & Watson

2011) and understand any restrictions the CVAD may have on normal daily activities such as bathing, swimming and other sporting activities (Gabriel 2000).

Community nurses can play an important role in providing support, advice and information for patients with a CVAD in relation to:

- activities of daily living especially bathing and showering
- sporting activities
- sexual activity
- exemption from wearing a seat belt in a car
- altered body image
- preventing external catheters getting caught in clothing.

Peripherally inserted central catheters (PICCs)

Definition

A peripherally inserted central catheter (PICC) is inserted in the region of the antecubital fossa or the upper arm and advanced into the superior vena cava (SVC) (NAVAN 1998). A PICC is placed by cannulation of the basilic, cephalic or median cubital vein in the patient's arm (Gabriel 2003; INS 2011) and the gauge size can range from 3 Fr to 7 Fr. A valved PICC may have the valve located in the tip of the catheter or in the hub (Dougherty & Watson 2011) (Figure 7.1).

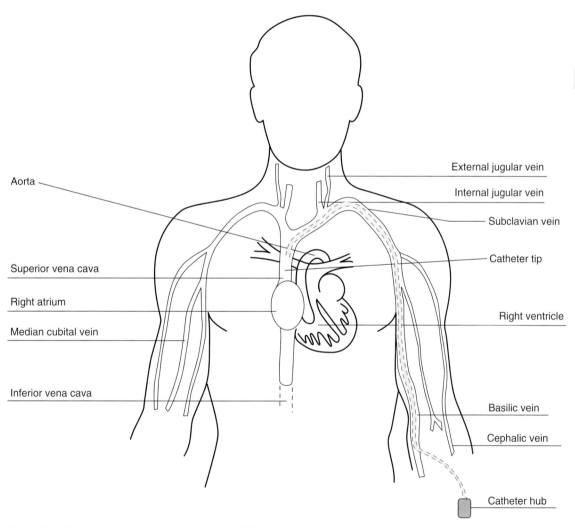

Figure 7.1 Peripherally inserted central catheter (PICC).

Indications for placement of a PICC

- Intermediate to long term IV therapy.
- Administration of hyperosmolar/irritant solutions, parenteral nutrition or chemotherapy (Philpot & Griffiths 2003; Dougherty & Watson 2011).
- Lack of peripheral venous access.
- The requirement for blood sampling and/or regular venous access (Kayley & Finlay 2003).
- Patient preference.
- Patients with needle phobia who wish to avoid multiple cannulations (Dougherty & Watson 2011).

Contraindications to placement of a PICC

- Inability to locate suitable antecubital fossa veins, although with the use of ultrasound this is not always a contraindication (Dougherty & Watson 2011).
- Anatomical distortions from surgery, burns or trauma, for example lymphoedema or scarring from mastectomy surgery (Todd 1998), which may prevent the tip of the catheter being advanced to the correct position (Dougherty & Watson 2011).
- Patient is unable to lie supine for the insertion procedure (Macrae 1998).
- Patient wants to go swimming during treatment period (Todd 1998).
- Patient confused and therefore may be likely to remove PICC or has a history of non- compliance with vascular access devices (Philpot & Griffiths 2003).

Location/placement

An accurate and detailed patient assessment should be carried out prior to PICC placement (Hamilton 2000). It should include:

- the condition of the patient's veins (Philpott & Griffiths 2003)
- the patient's clinical condition (Gabriel 2003)
- the patient's lifestyle (Gabriel 2003)
- the patient's preference of CVAD (Gabriel 2003).

In many hospitals PICCs are commonly placed by nursing staff who have been trained in this procedure, and they can be inserted at the bedside using a strict aseptic technique. The basilic vein is preferred as, anatomically, it is the largest of the three veins and the straightest route for catheter advancement to the SVC (Sansivero 1998; Dougherty & Watson 2011). The distal tip of the catheter should be located in the lower third of the SVC, close to the junction of the SVC and the right atrium (NAVAN 1998; Vesely 2003). The catheter tip location must be confirmed by a chest X-ray or fluoroscopy, and documented clearly by a medical practitioner in the patient's medical notes prior to the initiation of IV therapy (Wise *et al.* 2001; Gabriel 2008). If a patient is being discharged into the community with a PICC then the community nurses should have written documentation of the exact catheter tip location and the measurement of the external portion of the PICC. However, it is advisable that the community nurse also measures and documents the external portion of the PICC once the patient is discharged. If the length of the external portion of the PICC then changes, the original measurement can be used as the guide.

Care and management

Dressing
Following PICC insertion, the dressing should be changed after 24 h, as there may be some bleeding from the exit site (Todd 1998; Ryder 2001; LSC 2002; RCN 2010). The dressing technique should be performed aseptically using 2% chlorhexidine with alcohol 70% or aqueous solution for cleaning the site (Maki *et al.* 1991; DH 2007; Pratt *et al.* 2007). Sutures should not routinely be used for stabilisation of PICCs due to their potential for contributing to the risk of infection (CDC 2002; RCN 2010). Products that can be used to stabilise the catheter include:

- sterile tapes
- transparent semi-permeable membrane (TSM)
- catheter securement devices, e.g. StatLock
- sterile surgical strips.

(Hanchett 1999; Gabriel 2001; INS 2011; RCN 2010)

The frequency of dressing change after the first 24 h depends on the type of dressing used. Ideally a gauze dressing should be replaced by a TSM dressing as soon as possible, and should be replaced every 7 days or sooner if they are no longer intact or moisture collects under the dressing (Todd 1998; NICE 2003; DH 2007; Pratt *et al.* 2007; Gabriel 2008). However, if a gauze dressing is used then it should be maintained with an occlusive material (INS 2011; Gabriel 2008), and changed routinely every 24–48 hours, and immediately if the integrity of the dressing is compromised (NICE 2003).

Maintaining patency
Flushing of the catheter is essential to ensure and maintain patency, and prevent the mixing and precipitation of incompatible drugs and/or infusates (RCN 2010). The frequency of flushing and the solution used is often

Table 7.5 Guidelines for maintaining CVAD patency*

CVAD	Flushing solution	Volume of flushing solution	Frequency	Rationale
Open-ended PICC	Heparinised sodium chloride solution (Kelly 1992; Dougherty & Watson 2011; RCN 2010)	5 ml (10 iu heparin in 1 ml solution of sodium chloride, 5 ml = 50 iu)	Weekly	To maintain patency if the CVAD is not in regular or continuous use
Valved PICC	Sodium chloride 0.9% (Weinstein 2007; Perucca 2010)	10 ml	Weekly	To maintain patency if the CVAD is not in regular or continuous use
Open ended tunnelled catheter	Heparinised sodium chloride solution (Kelly 1992; Dougherty & Watson 2011; RCN 2010)	5 ml (10 iu heparin in 1 ml solution of sodium chloride, 5 ml = 50 iu)	Weekly	To maintain patency if the CVAD is not in regular or continuous use
Valved tunnelled catheter	Sodium chloride 0.9% (Weinstein 2007; Perucca 2010)	10 ml	Weekly	To maintain patency if the CVAD is not in regular or continuous use
Open ended implantable port	Heparinised sodium chloride, usually 100 iu per ml (Weinstein 2007; Perucca 2010)	5 ml (100 iu per ml of heparinised sodium chloride solution, 5 ml = 500 iu)	Monthly	To maintain patency if the CVAD is not in regular or continuous use
Valved implantable port	Heparinised sodium chloride, usually 100 iu per ml (Dougherty & Watson 2011)	5 ml	Monthly	To maintain patency if the CVAD is not in regular or continuous use
All CVADs	Sodium chloride 0.9% (INS 2011; NICE 2003)	10 ml	Before and after blood sampling	To check for patency prior to blood sampling and to prevent the CVAD occluding with blood after sampling
All CVADs	Sodium chloride 0.9% (NICE 2003; INS 2011)	10 ml	Before and after the administration of drugs or infusion	To ensure that no drug is left within the lumen of the CVAD and to prevent precipitation of incompatible drugs and/ or infusates (RCN 2010)
Double or triple lumen CVADs	See above (depending on type of CVAD)	See above for volume depending on type of CVAD. Each separate lumen of CVAD must be flushed with this amount	Weekly or monthly (depending on type of CVAD)	To maintain patency of the lumens of the CVAD if not in regular or continuous use

*Vascular access devices may vary between different manufacturers. The above table offers general guidelines and it is important to seek specific guidance related to the care and management from individual manufacturers and the referring hospital unit.

137

dictated by individual units and hospitals; however, this should also depend on catheter size and the manufacturer's recommendations (Todd 1998; Dougherty & Watson 2011) (Table 7.5).

The concentration of heparin should be the lowest that will maintain patency (RCN 2010). In valved catheters there should be no reflux of blood into the catheter when the valve is closed, therefore heparinised sodium chloride solution is not routinely required to maintain patency (Todd 1998; Philpot & Griffiths 2003). Goodwin and Carlson (1993) recommended a turbulent flush using a push/pause flushing technique to reduce the risk of fibrin and platelets becoming adhered to the catheter wall, which may cause an occlusion. A positive pressure should be maintained within the lumen(s) of the catheter to prevent reflux of blood (INS 2011). This should be achieved by using the correct technique (*see* Procedure guideline 7.4) or by using a specially designed 'positive pressure or positive displacement cap' on the end of the catheter (Berger 2000; Lenhart 2000; Mayo 2001a).

Removal

The removal of a PICC can be done in the hospital setting or the patient's home, providing the community nurse has received specific practical instruction and supervision on the procedure. PICCs can be easily removed by applying gentle traction to the device once the dressings and any securement devices have been removed (Gabriel 2008). The practitioner should apply gentle traction at the skin exit site, regrasping the catheter near the skin every few centimetres (Philpot & Griffiths 2003; Drewett 2009). Regrasping the catheter near the skin allows for better control and a more even force along the length of the catheter (Drewett 2009).

Any resistance felt during the removal procedure may be caused by venospasm, vasoconstriction or phlebitis (Wall & Kierstead 1995). If this occurs, the arm, and particularly the upper arm, should be wrapped in a warm compress for 20 minutes as the heat will encourage vasodilation, and therefore aid the removal of the PICC (Gabriel 2008; Drewett 2009; Dougherty & Watson 2011). An alternative is to apply slight tension to the catheter and use a piece of adhesive tape to secure it to the patient's forearm (Gabriel 2008; Drewett 2009). This should be left in situ for approximately 30 minutes to allow the venous spasm to subside before attempting to remove the catheter (Wall & Kierstead 1995; Drewett 2009). Pressure should not be applied to the exit site or vein as the catheter is removed as this encourages the catheter to touch the vein wall and can cause venous spasm (Drewett 2009). The PICC should never be pulled or stretched against resistance as the catheter may break (Wall & Kierstead 1995; Philpot & Griffiths 2003).

If a PICC is being removed outside the hospital setting by a community nurse and resistance is felt during the removal procedure, then advice should be sought from the referring hospital unit or community IV specialist nurse (if appropriate). If the community nurse is in any doubt about the procedure or the advice offered, then the patient should be referred back to the hospital for removal of the PICC.

Skin-tunnelled cuffed catheters

Definition

A skin-tunnelled central catheter is inserted into the central venous system via the subclavian or internal jugular vein with the distal tip located in the lower third of the SVC or right atrium (Wise *et al.* 2001; Vesely 2003; Gabriel 2008). The catheter lies in a subcutaneous tunnel and usually exits on the chest wall. Skin-tunnelled central catheters are available in single, double or triple lumen configurations with a variety of sizes referred to as a French e.g. 10 Fr, and they can be open-ended or valved. A valved tunnelled catheter may have the valve located in the tip of the catheter or in the hub (Dougherty & Watson 2011). (Figure 7.2)

Indications for placement of a skin-tunnelled cuffed catheter

- All types of IV therapy when long-term venous access is required (Kayley & Finlay 2003).
- Blood sampling.
- Patient preference.

Contraindications to placement of a skin-tunnelled cuffed catheter

There are a number of co-morbid conditions that impede conventional placement, for example:

- cutaneous lesions in proximity to the VAD exit site
- previous surgical interventions
- SVC syndrome
- irradiation to the chest
- fractured clavicle
- malignancy at the base of the neck
- morbid obesity.

(Sansivero 1998; Dougherty & Watson 2011)

Location/placement

The placement of skin-tunnelled central catheters is generally considered a medical procedure in many hospitals and is usually performed in the operating theatre or anaesthetic room (Benton & Marsden 2002). However, there are a growing number of clinical nurse specialists in the UK who are now successfully performing this procedure at the bedside (Hamilton *et al.* 1995; Gabriel 2003). A skin-tunnelled central catheter can be placed either under general anaesthetic or under sedation and using local anaesthetic (Gabriel 2008).

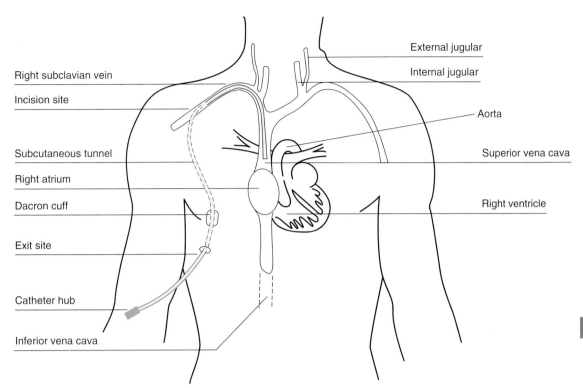

Right subclavian vein

Incision site

Subcutaneous tunnel

Right atrium

Dacron cuff

Exit site

Catheter hub

Inferior vena cava

External jugular

Internal jugular

Aorta

Superior vena cava

Right ventricle

Figure 7.2 Skin tunnelled cuffed catheter.

Access to the central venous circulation can be achieved either by a cut-down technique or by direct puncture (percutaneous approach) using a guidewire and Seldinger approach (Sansivero 1998; Gabriel 2008). Image guidance in the form of ultrasound or fluoroscopy is becoming more common practice for the insertion of CVADs to assess the patency and availability of target vessels, and to reduce complications (Sansivero 1998; Anstett & Royer 2003).

Central catheters specifically designed for tunnelling have a small Dacron cuff, which is situated around the catheter approximately 30 cm from the external hub (Kayley 1997; Dougherty & Watson 2011). When the catheter is inserted the Dacron cuff is positioned in the subcutaneous tunnel, and after 2–3 weeks tissue granulates around the cuff, which helps to stabilise the catheter and reinforces the barrier to potential infection (Gabriel 2008; Dougherty & Watson 2011). Post insertion, the catheter is secured with a suture at the exit site, this suture should not be removed for 21 days, allowing the Dacron cuff time to fibrose (INS 2011; Dougherty & Watson 2011).

The exit site suture is often encrusted with dried blood from the insertion procedure and may be very close to the exit site. This can make the removal procedure quite difficult and there could be a risk of nicking the catheter with the suture removal blade during the procedure. Therefore if community nurses are asked to carry out this procedure without any practical support or prior experience, it may be advisable to refer the patient back to hospital for the removal of the exit site suture.

If a patient is being discharged into the community with a skin-tunnelled cuffed catheter then the community nurses should have written documentation of the exact catheter tip location and the measurement of the external portion of the catheter. However, it is advisable that the community nurse also measure and document the external portion of the catheter once the patient is discharged. If the length of the external portion of the catheter then changes then the original measurement can be used as the guide.

Care and management

Dressing

Following insertion of a skin-tunnelled central catheter, the dressing should be changed after 24 h, as there may be some bleeding from the exit site (Ryder 2001; LSC 2002; RCN 2010). The dressing technique should be performed aseptically using 2% chlorhexidine with alcohol 70% or aqueous solution for cleaning the site (Maki *et al.* 1991; DH 2007; Pratt *et al.* 2007).

The frequency of dressing change after the first 24 hours depends on the type of dressing used. Ideally a gauze dressing should be replaced by a TSM dressing as soon as possible, and should be replaced every 7 days or sooner if they are no longer intact or moisture collects under the dressing (Todd 1998; NICE 2003; DH 2007; Pratt *et al.* 2007; Gabriel 2008). However, if a gauze dressing is used then it should be maintained with an occlusive material (INS 2011; Gabriel 2008), and changed routinely every 24–48 hours, and immediately if the integrity of the dressing is compromised (NICE 2003). Once the exit site sutures have been removed after 21 days, a dressing is not usually required unless the patient requests one (Kayley 1997; Dougherty & Watson 2011). The skin closure sutures at the entry/incision site can be removed after 7 days (Kayley 1997; Dougherty & Watson 2011).

Maintaining patency
Flushing of the catheter is essential to ensure and maintain patency, and prevent the mixing and precipitation of incompatible drugs and/or infusates (RCN 2010). The frequency of flushing and the solution used is often dictated by individual units and hospitals; however, this should also depend on catheter size and the manufacturer's recommendations (Dougherty & Watson 2011) (Table 7.5).

Goodwin and Carlson (1993) recommended a turbulent flush using a push/pause flushing technique to reduce the risk of fibrin and platelets becoming adhered to the catheter wall thus causing an occlusion. A positive pressure should be maintained within the lumen of the catheter to prevent reflux of blood (INS 2011). This should be achieved by using the correct technique (see Procedure guideline 7.4) or by using a specially designed 'positive pressure or positive displacement cap' on the end of the catheter (Berger 2000; Lenhart 2000; Mayo 2001).

Removal
There are a number of complications that can occur during or after the removal of skin-tunnelled central catheters (Drewett 2009) and therefore this procedure should only be undertaken in hospital by authorised and appropriately trained nurses or doctors (Drewett 2009; Dougherty & Watson 2011).

Skin-tunnelled central catheters can either be removed by using gentle traction or surgical excision to release the Dacron cuff (Drewett 2009; Dougherty & Watson 2011). An aseptic technique should be used throughout either procedure (Dougherty & Watson 2011). Following either removal method a sterile dressing should be applied to the exit site and incision site, and covered with an occlusive dressing (Drewett 2009). The dressings should be left in place for 24–48 hours (Drewett 2009; Dougherty & Watson 2011), then the incision site should be redressed until the sutures are removed.

Implantable ports

Definition

An implantable port consists of a subcutaneous injection port attached to a silicone catheter. The reservoir of the port has a self-sealing, thick silicone septum and this is accessed through the skin using a non-coring needle (Huber needle). It is a totally implanted CVAD, which is designed for long-term use (Dougherty & Watson 2011), and is available as a single or double port and can be open-ended or valved (Gabriel 2008) (Figure 7.3).

Indications for placement of an implantable port

- All types of IV therapy when long-term venous access is required, especially intermittent therapies (Kayley & Finlay 2003).
- Blood sampling.
- Patient preference.

Contraindications to placement of an implantable port

- Patients who are needle phobic (Dougherty & Watson 2011).

There are a number of co-morbid conditions that impede conventional placement, for example:

- cutaneous lesions in proximity to the CVAD exit site
- previous surgical interventions
- SVC syndrome
- irradiation to the chest
- fractured clavicle
- malignancy at the base of the neck
- morbid obesity.

(Sansivero 1998; Dougherty & Watson 2011)

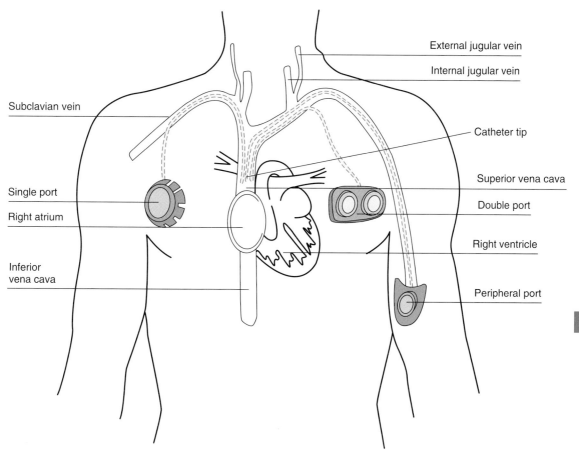

Figure 7.3 Implantable ports.

Location/placement

Implantable ports are placed surgically (Viale 2003) and inserted either on the chest wall or in the antecubital area (Gabriel 2008; Dougherty & Watson 2011). A subcutaneous pocket is created under the patient's skin, and the portal body is placed in this pocket, often positioned over a bony prominence to provide stability for the device (Viale 2003; Gabriel 2008; Dougherty & Watson 2011). The portal body is then sutured to the underlying muscle to keep the device in the appropriate anatomical position (Gabriel 2008; Dougherty & Watson 2011). The silicone catheter is then threaded through the vessel until the tip terminates in the SVC/right atrial junction (Wise *et al.* 2001; Gabriel 2008). The most appropriate veins for implantable device cannulation include the basilic (Sansivero 1998), internal jugular and subclavian (Hamilton 2000; Dougherty & Watson 2011).

Care and management

Accessing an implantable port

It is important to seek specific training and instruction on how to access a port because there is a risk of extravastion of drugs/infusate if the needle is wrongly placed (Viale 2003; Gabriel 2008; Dougherty & Watson 2011). Accessing a port can be painful for the patient, as the needle has to pass through the skin before reaching the silicone membrane of the portal body (Dougherty & Watson 2011). This can be overcome with the use of a prescribed topical local anaesthetic cream (Dougherty & Watson 2011).

Implantable ports are accessed by palpating the portal body through the patient's skin and using a non-coring needle, such as a Huber point needle, to puncture the portal body's silicone membrane (Gabriel 2008). Is it essential to use a non-coring needle for accessing the port as it prevents the risk of 'coring' and

141

damaging the silicone membrane. Once the port has been accessed the Huber needle should be supported by gauze and covered with a transparent dressing to prevent needle dislodgement (Dougherty & Watson 2011).

Huber point needles are available in a variety of lengths and gauge sizes, and can be straight or angled (Gabriel 2008). They are also available with a small length of extension tubing attached to the needle and these can be left in situ once the port has been accessed, and then changed every 7 days (Springhouse 2002).

When removing the Huber needle it is important to hold the port firmly down using your thumb and first finger, the needle can then be pulled out using the other hand. There are a number of different types of Huber needles available incorporating safety systems that prevent the risk of needle stick injury, and these should always be used (NICE 2003; Gabriel et al 2004; NHS Employers 2007).

Site care

Once the Huber needle is removed and the port is not in use the site does not require a dressing. The port site should be checked regularly for signs of erythema, swelling, tenderness, warmth or purulent discharge, as this could indicate the presence of an infection (Viale 2003; Dougherty & Watson 2011). If the skin over the portal body becomes inflamed, accessing the port is not recommended as it is possible to seed the bloodstream with infectious material from the device (Wickham et al. 1992).

Maintaining patency

Flushing of the implantable port is essential to ensure and maintain patency, and prevent the mixing and precipitation of incompatible drugs and/or infusates (RCN 2010). The frequency of flushing and the solution used is often dictated by individual units and hospitals; however, it will also depend on the type of port and the manufacturer's recommendations (Dougherty & Watson 2011) (Table 7.5).

Removal

The removal of an implantable port is usually performed in a theatre setting (Dougherty & Watson 2011). An incision is made close to the portal body to enable it to be removed from the subcutaneous pocket (Dougherty & Watson 2011). Skin closure sutures may be used to close the incision site and these can be removed after 7–10 days. The dressings should be left in place for 24–48 hours (Drewett 2009; Dougherty & Watson 2011), then the incision site redressed until the sutures are removed.

Administration of medications and/or infusions

The RCN Standards for infusion therapy (RCN 2010: 32) state that 'the nurse should aspirate the catheter and check for blood return to confirm patency prior to the administration of medications and/or solutions'.

As well as confirming the patency of the CVAD, obtaining an adequate blood return signifies that the catheter tip is positioned within a large blood vessel (Masoorli 2003). However, obtaining only a 'flash' of blood or 'pink-tinged sodium chloride' is not an indication that the catheter is functioning properly within the vein (Masoorli 2003). Determining that the catheter tip is positioned within a large blood vessel and that the CVAD is functioning properly will minimise the risk of extravasation injury to the patient (Masoorli 2003). Therefore checking for blood return is essential if vesicant drugs are to be administered (Masoorli 2003).

While checking for blood return prior to the administration of medication and/or infusions is best practice (INS 2006; RCN 2010), there are a number of other equally important issues that should also be taken into account.

- The exact tip position of the catheter should be known and documented. This means that if a patient is discharged from hospital with a CVAD, then the information about the tip location should be passed on, in writing, by the referring hospital to the community nurses. It is not acceptable for the tip location to be described as 'in a good place, safe to use'.
- Whether the hospital has ever been able to get a blood return from the catheter.
- Information about the CVAD, including possible complications and the signs and symptoms of these.

A thorough patient assessment should be carried out each time the community nurse visits to administer any IV medication and/or infusion. This should include:

- asking the patient if they have any pain, discomfort, swelling in the area of the CVAD or if they are experiencing any new/different symptoms
- asking the patient if they have pulled or caught the catheter
- measuring the length of the external portion of the catheter at each visit to ensure it remains the same, and recording the measurement
- checking the exit site and surrounding area to ensure there is no visible swelling, exudate, redness or signs of infection.

All the relevant information at each patient assessment should be clearly documented even if nothing abnormal is detected. If the community nurse is concerned about any aspect of the assessment then advice should be sought from the referring hospital unit or community IV specialist nurse (if appropriate).

As well as the patient assessment it is important to know about the prescribed medication/infusion that is to be administered (NMC 2008b).

- What is the pH and osmolarity of the drug?
- Is the drug a vesicant or hyperosmolar solution?
- How it should be given, i.e. via a centrally placed catheter?
- Should the medication be given as an infusion or slow bolus?
- What are the possible side effects of the medication?
- Are there any contraindications?
- Are there any possible interactions with other medications?

Flushing with 0.9% sodium chloride (5–10 ml) using a 10 ml syringe should be performed before and after the administration of any medication and/or infusion (INS 2011; RCN 2010).

This is often referred to as the **SASH** method:

Sodium chloride 0.9%
Antibiotic (or other medication)
Sodium chloride
Heparinised sodium chloride (if used).

(Kayley 1997)

It is also important to check that the patient does not experience any pain or discomfort when the first sodium chloride 0.9% flush is being administered. If this should occur the community nurse should stop immediately and advice should be sought from the referring hospital unit or community IV specialist nurse (if appropriate). See Procedure guideline 7.1.

CVAD insertion complications

There are a number of complications that could occur during the insertion procedure or in the first few days following insertion (Gabriel 2008) (Table 7.6). If any of these should occur they should be diagnosed and treated before patients are discharged into the community. However, if a patient had a CVAD inserted in day care, for example, then it is possible that some insertion complications could manifest themselves once the patient is home. It is therefore important that any nurse caring for patients with a CVAD is aware and informed of all possible complications.

Complications of CVADs

There are a number of complications that can occur days, weeks or months after insertion. Potential complications are numerous, but infection and thrombotic events represent the most significant (Ryder 2001). It is therefore essential that community nurses understand the possible complications and can recognise the signs and symptoms. The incidence of some complications occurring can be reduced or prevented by good technique and care of the CVAD (Tables 7.7 and 7.8).

CVAD-related infection

Infection is the most significant risk of vascular access devices (Ryder 2001), and a large body of clinical evidence points to skin flora as the source of infection (Hadaway 1998; Jackson 2001). Micro-organisms migrate from the skin down the catheter tract and colonise the catheter tip (Hadaway 1998). It is also thought that the catheter hub is a source of microorganisms, especially for long-term catheters (Hadaway 1998). Infection rates from catheters inserted via the antecubital fossa are lower than those for catheters inserted via the chest and trunk area as there are fewer colony-forming units (CFUs) of skin flora on the arm than the chest (Todd 1998).

Most data on catheter-related infections are derived from hospitalised patients, and very few studies have attempted to collect data from patients with vascular access devices in the community (Hadaway 1998; Jackson 2001). However, patients in the community are thought to be at lower risk of developing catheter-related infections, as the home environment is less likely to contain the resistant strains of bacteria found in the hospital environment (Jackson 2001).

Catheter-related infections can be potentially very serious and therefore it is important to make every effort to prevent them, not just diagnose and treat (Hadaway 1998). If any patient with a CVAD becomes unwell or develops an unexplained pyrexia then a catheter-related infection should be considered as the most likely diagnosis.

Management of CVAD-related infection
- If a catheter-related infection is suspected the community nurses should contact the referring hospital immediately and refer the patient back for review and assessment.

143

Table 7.6 Insertion complications

Complication	Detail	Clinical features	CVAD
Pneumothorax	A pneumothorax occurs if the chest wall is damaged allowing air to enter the space between the pleural lining and the lung (Gabriel 2008). Interpleural pressure is then equal to atmospheric pressure and the surface tension and recoil of elastic fibres cause the lung to collapse (Tortora & Grabowski 2000)	Pain on inspiration and expiration, dyspnoea	Valved and open-ended tunnelled catheters. Valved and open-ended implantable ports
Haemothorax	Haemothorax can occur as a result of a puncturing the subclavian vein or artery during insertion of the CVAD (Gabriel 2008) and blood then leaks into the pleural cavity	Dyspnoea, tachycardia, hypotension	Valved and open-ended tunnelled catheters. Valved and open-ended implantable ports
Arterial puncture	Arterial puncture during the insertion of the CVAD (Gabriel 2008)	Pulsating or spurting of bright red blood into the cannula or introducer	Valved and open-ended tunnelled catheters, implantable ports, PICCs
Catheter malposition	A CVAD may be malpositioned as a result of the insertion procedure	Coughing, ear/neck pain on the side of the insertion, patient may be able to hear the fluid/drug administration in the ear on the side of the insertion palpitations, arrhythmias, difficulty or inability aspirating blood, backflow of blood into the catheter. However the patient may be asymptomatic	Valved and open-ended tunnelled catheters, implantable ports, PICCs
Air embolus	Air embolus occurs as a result of air entering the venous circulation and travelling to the pulmonary vein (Gabriel 2008; Drewett 2009). It is a potentially preventable complication of CVAD insertion and can be minimised by placing the patient in the Trendelenburg position on insertion and removal of cvc (Gabriel 2008; Drewett 2009)	Dyspnoea, cyanosis, hypotension, tachycardia, weak pulse, confusion, reduced conscious level, cardiac arrest (Drewett 2009)	Valved and open-ended tunnelled catheters, implantable ports Open-ended PICCs
Nerve damage	Nerve damage can occur if the ulna or median nerves are damaged during PICC placement (Gabriel 2008). The radial cords of the brachial plexus can be damaged during subclavian placement of CVADs (Richardson & Bruso 1993)	Tingling, loss of movement down part or all of the affected arm	Valved and open-ended tunnelled catheters, implantable ports, PICCs
Atrial fibrillation, cardiac arrhythmias	These can occur if the tip of the catheter extends beyond the superior vena cava (Gabriel 2008; Vesely 2003)	Weak irregular pulse Patient may feel heart beating forcefully Reduced conscious level	Valved and open-ended tunnelled catheters, implantable ports, PICCs

Table 7.7 Signs and symptoms of CVAD-related infection

Site of the CVAD-related infection	Signs and symptoms
Exit site infection	Tenderness, induration, exudate or erythema within 2 cm of the skin at the exit site
Skin tunnel infection	Tenderness, induration and erythema in the tissue overlying the catheter tunnel and <2 cm from exit site
Pocket infection	Erythema over the reservoir of an implantable port, or purulent exudate in the subcutaneous pocket
Colonised within the catheter	Positive blood culture growth from catheter blood cultures in the absence of accompanying clinical symptoms
Catheter-related bloodstream infection	Positive blood culture from catheter blood cultures and peripheral blood cultures (same organism). Patient has signs and symptoms of a blood stream infection (pyrexia, rigors, hypotension, sore throat, feeling unwell) and no other apparent source of infection
Infusate-related bloodstream infection	Isolation of the same organism from infusate and from peripheral blood cultures, and no other identifiable source of infection

(Pearson 1996)

Table 7.8 CVAD problems/complications, possible causes and suggested action

Problem/complication	Possible cause	Suggested action for community nurses
Inability to administer medication, flush catheter and/or aspirate blood	Position of clamp Venous thrombosis Drug precipitate Catheter tip position Pinch-off syndrome Intraluminal clotting	Check clamp, if this does not resolve problem refer patient back to hospital unit for review/assessment
Inability to aspirate blood but ability to administer medication, flush catheter	Fibrin sheath	Take blood sample peripherally Contact referring unit and ask for review/assessment of patient's catheter at their next hospital appointment
Difficulty administering medication, flushing catheter and/or aspirating blood	Position of clamp Venous thrombosis Catheter tip position Pinch-off syndrome	Check clamp, if this does not resolve problem refer patient back to hospital unit for review/assessment
Redness and/or exudate at exit site of CVAD	Exit site infection	Check whether patient is pyrexial. Clean exit with chlorhexidine with alcohol 70% or aqueous solution and apply new dressing. Ask GP to visit and contact referring unit for advice
Redness at exit site of skin-tunnelled cuffed catheter spreading along and around subcutaneous tunnel area, with/without exudate at exit site	Exit site and tunnel infection	Check whether patient is pyrexial. Clean exit with chlorhexidine with alcohol 70% or aqueous solution and apply new dressing. Refer patient back to hospital unit for review/assessment
Patient unwell and/or has any of the following signs and symptoms: pyrexia, rigors, tachycardia, hypotension, sore throat, aching, headache, nausea, diarrhoea	Catheter infection Bacteraemia Septicaemia	Refer patient back to hospital unit **immediately** for review/assessment. If patient very unwell dial 999 and ask for an ambulance

(*Continued*)

Table 7.8 *(Continued)*

Problem/complication	Possible cause	Suggested action for community nurses
Signs of redness, warmth, swelling, pain, induration and a hard, palpable venous cord in the upper arm above PICC, occurring within first 7 days following PICC insertion	Mechanical phlebitis	Ask GP to visit and contact referring unit for advice Monitor daily Apply heat to affected area 4 times per day Elevate affected arm and advise only gentle movement Use of prescribed non-steroidal anti-inflammatory drugs
Purulent discharge from exit site and above signs and symptoms but occurring more than 7 days after insertion of PICC. Patient may be unwell and pyrexial	Infective phlebitis	Check whether patient is pyrexial. Refer patient back to hospital unit immediately for review/ assessment
Fluid leaking from the catheter or exit site on administration of flush/ drugs/infusion	Damaged, split or ruptured catheter	The damage/split part of the catheter may be external and therefore visible or the catheter may be damaged/split internally. Clamp catheter (if possible) above damaged portion using non-toothed forceps or by manually pinching the catheter. Refer the patient back to hospital immediately for review and possible catheter repair
Fluid or blood leaking from injection cap	Damage to injection cap possibly caused by use of a needle	Do not use. Remove injection cap (as per guideline) and replace with a new sterile injection cap
Length of external portion of PICC is longer than original measurement	PICC may not have been secured properly. PICC may have been pulled or caught in clothing	Re-dress PICC as per guideline. Contact referring unit for advice explaining by how much (cm) the PICC has come out. Do not use CVAD until advice has been sought
PICC has come out completely	PICC may not have been secured properly. PICC may have been pulled or caught in clothing	If PICC has just come out apply pressure to exit site. Clean exit site with chlorhexidine with alcohol 70% or aqueous solution and apply a sterile dressing (as per guideline). Contact referring unit to inform then that PICC has come out
Dacron cuff visible at exit site of skin-tunnelled cuffed catheter	Catheter may not have been secured properly. Exit site sutures may have been removed too soon or catheter may have been pulled or caught in clothing	Check original measurement. Redress catheter as per guidelines ensuring it is well secured and supported. Contact referring unit for advice explaining by how much catheter has come out (if appropriate). Patient may need to return to hospital for repeat chest X-ray and re-suturing at exit site
Skin-tunnelled cuffed catheter has come out completely	Catheter may not have been secured properly. Exit site sutures may have been removed too soon or catheter may have been pulled or caught in clothing	If catheter has just come out apply pressure to exit site and incision site for 5 min. Clean exit with chlorhexidine with alcohol 70% or aqueous solution and apply a sterile occlusive dressing to exit site (as per guideline). Contact referring unit to inform them that skin-tunnelled catheter has come out. Patient may need to be reviewed in hospital
Blood visible in the external portion of PICC	Blood has back tracked down PICC – cause may not be known/obvious	Flush PICC (as per guideline) using push pause technique. Ensure all blood is cleared from PICC

- Catheter blood cultures and peripheral blood cultures (Gabriel 2008).
- Swabs for microbiological culture and sensitivity (Gabriel 2008).
- Treatment of the infection with antimicrobials.
- Possible catheter removal.

The management of a catheter-related infection and the possible decision to remove the CVAD would be carried out in hospital and may depend on a number of issues, for example:

- the device
- the site of the infection
- the specific microbiology
- how ill the patient is
- whether the CVAD is required for long-term or short-term use.

(Hadaway 1998; Gabriel 2008)

Prevention of CVAD-related infection
- Thorough handwashing should be performed before and after any CVAD-related procedure, and before putting on and after removing gloves (RCN 2010).
- The use of alcohol hand rub as an additional hand cleansing agent (DH 2001; NICE 2003).
- The injection port or catheter hub should be cleaned and left to air dry using an alcoholic solution of 2% chlorhexidine before and after it has been used to access the system (NICE 2003; DH 2007; Pratt *et al.* 2007).
- An aseptic technique must be used for catheter site care and for accessing the system (NICE 2003) (Box 7.1).
- Following handwashing and the use of alcohol hand rub, clean gloves and a non-touch technique, or sterile gloves, should be used when changing the exit site dressing (NICE 2003).

Box 7.1 NICE (2003) clinical guidelines on catheter site care

Preferably, a sterile transparent, semi-permeable polyurethane dressing should be used to cover the catheter site

If a patient has profuse perspiration, or if the insertion site is bleeding or oozing, a sterile gauze dressing is preferable to a transparent, semi-permeable dressing

Gauze dressings should be changed when they become damp, loosened or soiled, and the need for a gauze dressing should be assessed daily. A gauze dressing should be replaced by a transparent dressing as soon as possible

Dressings used on tunnelled or implanted CVC sites should be replaced every 7 days until the insertion site has healed, unless there is an indication to change them sooner

An alcoholic chlorhexidine gluconate solution should be used to clean the catheter site during dressing changes, and allowed to air dry. An aqueous solution of chlorhexidine gluconate should be used if the manufacturer's recommendations prohibit the use of alcohol with the product

Healthcare personnel should ensure that catheter-site care is compatible with catheter materials (tubing, hubs, injection ports, luer connectors and extensions) and carefully check compatibility with the manufacturer's recommendations

Transparent dressings should be changed every 7 days, or sooner if they are no longer intact or moisture collects under the dressing

Individual sachets of antiseptic solution or individual packages of antiseptic-impregnated swabs or wipes should be used to disinfect the dressing site

---

Phlebitis

The basic definition of phlebitis is inflammation of the vein, and it is associated with three causes:

- mechanical
- infective
- chemical.

(Hadaway 1998)

Mechanical phlebitis
This is usually caused by:

- trauma to the venous intima during insertion or too large a device being placed in an individual with small veins (Todd 1998; Philpott & Griffiths 2003; Gabriel 2008)
- repeated movement of the device within the vessel (Jackson 1998).

This type of phlebitis is more obvious in patients with PICCs and peripheral implantable ports (Gabriel 2008). It is more likely to occur in the first 7 days following insertion of the CVAD (Goodwin & Carlson 1993; Gabriel 2008). The risk of developing mechanical phlebitis is higher in women, as the internal diameter of their veins is smaller than men's (Goodwin & Carlson 1993).

147

Signs and symptoms of mechanical phlebitis

- Pain, redness, warmth, swelling, induration and a hard, palpable venous cord in the upper arm above the PICC/implantable port insertion site (Todd 1998).

Management of mechanical phlebitis

- If mechanical phlebitis is suspected the community nurse should contact the referring hospital and ask them to see the patient to review and assess.
- If the patient is not admitted to hospital, the community nurse should ask the GP to visit.
- The community nurse should observe the affected area at every visit and document all relevant information.
- Application of heat compresses to the affected area at least four times per day (Todd 1998).
- Elevation of the affected arm and only gentle movement should be encouraged (Todd 1998; Philpott & Griffiths 2003).
- The use of prescribed non-steroidal anti-inflammatory drugs (Todd 1998).

Prevention of mechanical phlebitis

- Placement of the smallest appropriate device for the patient and the therapy (Todd 1998).
- Stabilisation of the CVAD using an appropriate securement device/dressing (RCN 2010).

Infective phlebitis

If phlebitis presents more than 7 days post insertion of the CVAD, or a suspected mechanical phlebitis is not resolved with heat treatment, then infection could be the cause (Richardson & Bruso 1993).

For signs and symptoms, treatment and prevention, *see* CVAD-related infection section.

Chemical phlebitis

This occurs as a result of drugs/infusates with extremes of pH and osmolarity, which damage the endothelium of the vessel wall (Philpott & Griffiths 2003) and predispose the vessel to thrombus formation (Ryder 1993). It would be unusual to see this type of phlebitis in patients with a CVAD because the tip of the catheter terminates in a large blood vessel and therefore any drugs/infusates are quickly diluted by the volume of circulating blood (Gabriel 2008).

Catheter occlusion

Occlusion is the most common non-infectious complication (Kryzwda 1999; Wise *et al.* 2001) and can be divided into mechanical, thrombotic (either intra-

luminal or extraluminal) and non-thrombotic causes (Gabriel 2008).

Non-thrombotic

This could be due to precipitation formation resulting from inadequate flushing between incompatible medications or lipids and can be resolved by use of specific agents (Dougherty 2006).

Thrombotic

There are two types of thrombotic occlusion – persistent withdrawal occlusion (PWO) caused by fibrin sheath, and total occlusion. This can be intraluminal when a clot forms within the lumen as a result of insufficient or incorrect flushing of the device or an administration set being turned off accidently and left for a prolonged period (Dougherty 2006), or due to fibrin in the form of a sheath or sleeve.

Fibrin sheath **(also referred to as a fibrin sleeve)**

It is thought that a fibrin sheath can develop within seconds of insertion and all catheters are at risk of developing a fibrin sheath (Ryder 1999; Mayo 2001b). If the fibrin sheath accumulates around the distal tip of the catheter forming a fibrin tail, it can affect catheter function by acting as a 'one-way' valve, allowing drugs/fluids to be infused, but preventing withdrawal of blood (Wise *et al.* 2001; Dougherty 2006). The fibrin sheath can completely encase the catheter from the tip to the entry site, causing a retrograde flow of drug/fluid along the catheter track resulting in extravastion of drugs/fluids into the surrounding tissue (Wickham *et al.* 1992)

Signs and symptoms of fibrin sheath

- Inability or difficulty aspirating blood from the catheter but flushing, drug administration or infusion can be performed without any difficulty (Krzywda 1999; Wise *et al.* 2001). This is referred to as persistent withdrawal occlusion (PWO) (Mayo 2001b).
- Leaking of drug/fluid from entry site indicating retrograde flow between the fibrin sheath and the catheter (Hadaway 1998).
- Tenderness, pain and oedema on the ipsilateral side of the catheter (Hadaway 1998).

Management

- The community nurse should contact the referring hospital and refer the patient back for review and assessment.
- Early recognition of signs and symptoms and assessment of catheter function.

- A thorough assessment of any signs and symptoms experienced by the patient (Hadaway 1998; Wise *et al.* 2001).
- Venogram or venous flow study, in hospital, to confirm or exclude the presence of a fibrin sheath (Gabriel 2008).
- The use of thrombolytic agents, in hospital, such as urokinase or tissue plasminogen activator (TPA), either as a bolus or infusion (Hadaway 1998; Wise *et al.* 2001).
- Possible catheter removal in hospital.

Prevention
- Regular assessment of the patient and catheter function (Wise *et al.* 2001).
- The use of prescribed prophylactic anticoagulation (Hadaway 1998).

Thrombosis

Venous thrombi are composed of fibrin and erythrocytes interwoven with platelets and leucocytes (Hadaway 1998). Virchow's triad was described in the 19th century and still forms the basis for current theory on thrombus formation. The three components are:

- vessel wall damage
- blood flow changes
- alteration in the chemical composition of blood.

(Hadaway 1998; Krzywda 1999)

Signs and symptoms of thrombosis
- Pain or discomfort and oedema in the chest, neck, jaw, ear or extremity (Krzywda 1999; Wise *et al.* 2001).
- Engorged peripheral veins in the chest wall, neck or extremity (Hadaway 1999; Krzywda 1999).
- Catheter occlusion (Krzywda 1999).
- Difficulty swallowing (Hadaway 1998).
- Difficulty turning head (Hadaway 1998).
- Paresthesia and/or numbness in hand and fingers on catheter side (Krzywda 1999).
- Cyanotic/discoloured arm on catheter side (Wise *et al.* 2001).

Management
- The community nurse should contact the referring hospital and refer the patient back for review/assessment.
- Early recognition of signs and symptoms and assessment of catheter function.
- A thorough assessment of any signs and symptoms experienced by the patient (Hadaway 1998; Wise *et al.* 2001).

- Venogram or venous flow study, in hospital, to confirm or exclude the presence of thrombosis (Wise *et al.* 2001; Gabriel 2008).
- Treatment with prescribed anticoagulation therapy (Wise *et al.* 2001).
- The use of thrombolytic agents, in hospital, such as urokinase or tissue plasminogen activator (TPA), either as a bolus or infusion (Hadaway 1998; Wise *et al.* 2001).
- Possible catheter removal in hospital (Dougherty 2006).

Prevention
- Educate the patient about the signs and symptoms of thrombosis and when to report them (Wise *et al.* 2001).
- Regular assessment of the patient and catheter function (Wise *et al.* 2001).
- The use of prescribed anticoagulation therapy (Hadaway 1998).

Clamps on skin-tunnelled cuffed catheters

Non-valved skin-tunnelled cuffed catheters have a clamp on each lumen, which is situated on a reinforced portion of the catheter near to the hub. Repeated clamping of the catheter in the same place can cause the two internal sides of the catheter to stick together.

Signs of catheter occlusion caused by the clamp
Inability or difficulty administering IV medication/flushing the catheter and/or aspirating blood.

Management
Release clamp and then slide the clamp off the reinforced portion of catheter. Using your finger and thumb hold the reinforced portion of catheter where clamp has been positioned and rub firmly – this will release the two sides of the catheter. Slide the clamp back on to the reinforced portion of catheter but in a different position.

Prevention
Change position of the clamp weekly, always ensuring it remains on the reinforced portion of the catheter; rub that portion of the catheter firmly to ensure that the two sides are not sticking.

Pinch-off syndrome

Pinch-off syndrome is a well documented but often unrecognised problem with tunnelled catheters and implanted ports, and most common when subclavian venepuncture is used (Andris & Krzywda 1997; Krzywda 1999). It occurs when the catheter is compressed between the clavicle and the first rib causing occlusion related to postural changes (Krzywda 1999). The clavicle and first rib form a narrow triangle as they join the sternum, and when venepuncture is made close to the small triangle or medially, the catheter may pass under the clavicle before it enters the subclavian vein (Hadaway 1998). If left unresolved it can cause partial or complete catheter fracture (Hadaway 1998).

Signs and symptoms
- Resistance to flushing, infusion or aspiration (Dougherty 2006).
- If the patient rolls their shoulder or raises their arm on the ipsilateral side and there is immediate resolution of the problem, then this is a definite indicator of pinch-off syndrome (Hadaway 1998).
- There may be points on the external catheter that 'balloon out' during flushing.

Management
- The community nurse should contact the referring hospital and refer the patient back for review/ assessment.
- Early recognition of the problem and confirmation by observing the catheter narrowing under fluoroscopy or chest X-ray, in hospital (Andris & Krzywda 1997; Hadaway 1998).
- Catheter removal and subsequent catheter replacement, in hospital (Krzywda 1999).

Prevention
This is related to the insertion of the catheter and may involve the following techniques.

- Venepuncture in the axillary vein at or lateral to the midclavicular line (Krzywda 1999).
- Avoiding subclavian venepuncture medial to the middle of the clavicle.
- Using other approaches, such as internal or external jugular puncture, and tunnelling over the clavicle (Hadaway 1998).
- Using a PICC as an alternative CVAD.

Catheter damage/split/rupture

This may be caused by:

- excessive syringe pressure
- poor catheter care
- accidental puncture of the catheter
- pinch-off syndrome

- repeated twisting of the catheter if not securely anchored to the patient's skin
- damage caused by scissors or toothed forceps.

(Todd 1998; Philpott & Griffiths 2003; Gabriel 2008)

Signs and symptoms
- Fluid leaking from the catheter or exit site on administration of flush/drugs/infusion (Todd 1998).
- The damage/split may be obvious.

Management
- The community nurse should clamp the catheter above the damaged portion (if possible) with non-toothed forceps or by manually pinching the catheter.
- The referring hospital should be contacted and the patient referred back immediately for re-assessment and catheter repair.

Prevention
- Never use syringes smaller than 10 ml due to the higher pressure generated with smaller syringes (Hadaway 1998; Gabriel 2008).
- Never use toothed forceps to clamp a catheter.
- Avoid the use of scissors near a catheter.
- Stabilisation of the CVAD using an appropriate securement device/dressing (RCN 2010).

Air embolus

Air embolus occurs as a result of air entering the venous circulation (Drewett 2009). The air, which may be bolus of air or a collection of small air bubbles, enters the vein and travels to the right atrium of the heart and proceeds to the ventricle and pulmonary arterioles, thus blocking the pulmonary blood flow (Gabriel 2008; Scales 2008) (Figure 7.4).

Air may enter the venous circulation:

- during catheter insertion
- as a result of a damaged catheter
- during drug/infusion administration
- during catheter hub manipulation
- upon catheter removal.

(Scales 2008)

Signs and symptoms
- Dyspnoea
- Cyanosis
- Hypotension

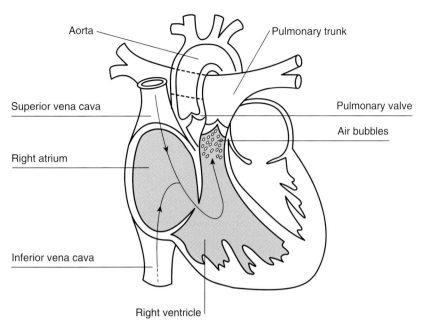

Figure 7.4 Air embolism.

- Tachycardia
- Weak pulse
- Confusion
- Reduced conscious level
- Cardiac arrest

(Drewett 2009)

Management
- Dial 999 immediately and request an ambulance. State that the patient may have an air embolus and that they have a central venous catheter in place (Kayley 1997).
- Occlude air entry point (if possible).

- Where possible, place patient on to left side in a modified Trendelenburg position (left lateral with head down), to prevent air entering the pulmonary artery (Lamb & Dougherty 2008).

Prevention
- Always clamp the catheter when removing or changing the injection cap (Kayley 1997).
- Maintain a closed-catheter system (Richardson & Bruso 1993).
- If the catheter is damaged or ruptures, then clamp (using non-toothed forceps or by manually pinching the catheter) immediately above the damaged portion (Kayley 1997).

Procedure guideline 7.1 **Guideline for administering a bolus intravenous injection**

Equipment

Intravenous (IV) medication vial(s) (plus drug package insert)
Prescribed diluent for reconstitution, for example water for Injection
Sodium chloride 0.9% for Injection, 10 ml ampoule × 2
Heparinised saline (10 units per ml) – 5 ml (50 units) if required
10 ml syringes × 3 or 4
23 g needles × 3 or 4

(Continued)

Procedure guideline 7.1 **Guideline for administering a bolus intravenous injection** *(cont'd)*

Dressing pack with sterile towel, gloves and non-linting gauze swabs
70% alcohol swabs
2% chlorhexidine in 70% alcohol wipe
Single-use disposable plastic apron
Gloves (sterile) if not in dressing pack (1–2 pairs)
Sharps bin
Alcohol hand-cleansing gel
Disposable tape measure (one per patient for course of treatment)
Tray (if available)
Clean hand towel or paper kitchen towel
Community drug chart
Anaphylaxis equipment

Nursing action	Rationale
1 Explain and discuss procedure and medication treatment plan with the patient	To ensure that patient understands the procedure and gives their verbal consent to proceed
2 Identify a suitable place/room in the patient's home to carry out the procedure	To ensure patient is comfortable and privacy is maintained
3 Check IV medication drug, dose and route are prescribed on Community Drug Chart for this patient (drug details transferred from hospital discharge drug sheet and signed by the general practitioner) Read the drug package insert to check about dosage, reconstitution and administration details	To ensure that the correct medication and dose is being given to the correct patient, at the correct time via the correct route
4 Check allergy history is recorded on Community Drug Chart Ask patient about any known allergies, type of reaction and document these even if no known allergies	To avoid allergic reaction to medication
5 Put on plastic apron	To reduce the risk of cross-infection and minimise risk of infection
6 Wash hands using (bactericidal) soap and water, dry with paper towels and apply alcohol hand gel	To reduce the risk of cross-infection and minimise risk of infection
7 Ensure patient is comfortable and VAD is accessible	To gain access to VAD
8 Check insertion site and observe for any complications, for example: ■ redness ■ swelling ■ exudate ■ pain ■ discomfort Discuss any discomfort with the patient and document the findings	To ensure complications are managed promptly, and ensure that the patient is comfortable during the drug administration procedure
9 If patient has a PICC in situ then using the disposable tape measure, take and record measurement of PICC from entry/exit point of catheter to tip (far end) of needleless injection cap	To compare measurement with previous recording in order to ensure catheter remains in place; to ensure prompt action is taken if catheter has become displaced

Procedure guideline 7.1 **Guideline for administering a bolus intravenous injection** *(cont'd)*

Nursing action	Rationale
10 Wash hands using soap and water, dry with paper towels, apply alcohol hand gel	To reduce the risk of cross-infection and minimise risk of infection
11 Identify a suitable clean surface to place dressing pack and equipment	To minimise the risk of introducing infection
12 Create a clean area for drug preparation, assemble the equipment required for the procedure and place beside the tray/preparation area	To ensure safe preparation of IV medication and minimise risk of infection To ensure all equipment is sterile and in date **NB** Sometimes more appropriate to prepare medication in different room to the patient, maximises concentration
13 Check all packaging is intact and check expiry dates	To ensure all equipment is sterile and in date
14 Check the expiry date of the medication, diluent, sodium chloride 0.9% flushes and heparinised saline if required	To ensure all equipment is sterile and in date
15 Wipe tray (if available) or surface (if appropriate) with an alcohol wipe, allow to dry (30 seconds)	To ensure safe preparation of IV medication and minimise the risk of introducing infection
16 Apply alcohol hand gel to both hands	Hands may have become contaminated during preparation of tray and equipment/supplies
17 Open the outer cover of the sterile dressing pack and slide the inner pack on to the tray/surface. Open the sterile field using the corners of the paper only	To create a sterile area for procedure To reduce the risk of contamination of sterile working area
18 Remove clinical waste bag and position between patient and sterile working area	To reduce the risk of contamination by enabling clinical waste to be placed straight into clinical waste bag and not passed over sterile field
19 Place sharps bin between patient and sterile dressing area	To enable sharps to be placed straight into sharps bin after use
20 Prepare equipment: open packages of needles, syringes, alcohol wipes, gauze swabs (if used) and sterile gloves (if not in dressing pack) on the sterile field. Use a non-touch technique, ensuring all key parts remain covered with their protective caps	To ensure all equipment and medication is assembled and ready for medication preparation
21 Clean hands using alcohol hand gel and put on sterile gloves	To reduce risk of infection and protect nurse preparing medication from exposure to the drug
22 Draw up the appropriate prescribed diluent into 10 ml syringe (or larger) using a 23 g needle	To ensure correct diluent used to reconstitute medication
23 If using a vial then remove the plastic cap from the vial and clean the rubber stopper with an alcohol swab	To ensure the top of the vial is decontaminated. The plastic cap does not provide sterility only prevents damage to the rubber stopper

(Continued)

Procedure guideline 7.1 **Guideline for administering a bolus intravenous injection** *(cont'd)*

Nursing action	Rationale
24 Inject the diluent into the vial slowly and mix with the contents checking there is no precipitation	To ensure the reconstitution procedure is completed as per drug manufacturer's instructions and is ready for further dilution process
25 Draw up 2 × sodium chloride 0.9% 10 ml flushes into 10 ml syringes using 23 g needles Draw up heparinised saline 5 ml into 10 ml syringe using 23 g needle (if required)	To ensure that catheter patency is checked prior to dose administration and the catheter is flushed following administration of medication
26 If equipment prepared in a different room to the patient, take the tray and sharps bin, and place beside patient on suitable clean and firm surface	To ensure medication and equipment is ready for administration process
27 Continue procedure with the same pair of gloves, unless clearly contaminated, for example equipment is carried from one room to another. In this situation remove gloves and apply another pair of sterile gloves	To minimise risk of infection
28 Place sterile towel under catheter, wipe end of needleless injection cap firmly with 2% chlorhexidine in alcohol swab. Lay catheter on sterile field while allowing it to dry (30 seconds)	To minimise risk of infection
29 Remove needle from first sodium chloride 0.9% syringe and discard the needle into the sharps bin	Needle not required for connection to needleless injection cap
30 Attach the sodium chloride syringe to the needleless injection cap **either** by screwing on (Luer Lok) **or** by pushing the tip of the syringe firmly on to the needleless injection cap (Luer slip) and twisting a ¼ turn until firmly in place	To establish secure connection between injection cap and syringe
31 Using a push-pause method (approximately 1 ml at a time) inject the contents of the sodium chloride 0.9% syringe. Discard into the sharps bin	To ensure that the VAD is patent and to create turbulence in the catheter in order to flush thoroughly
32 Wipe end of needleless injection cap firmly with 2% chlorhexidine in alcohol wipe. Allow to dry (30 seconds)	To minimise risk of infection
33 Attach the medication syringe to the needleless injection cap **either** by screwing on (Luer Lok) **or** by pushing the tip of the syringe firmly on to the needleless injection cap (Luer slip) and twisting a ¼ turn until firmly in place	To establish secure connection between injection cap and syringe
34 Administer the medication slowly at the correct rate as per manufacturer's instructions. It may be easier to give 0.5 ml, wait 30 seconds, give 0.5 ml, wait 30 seconds and repeat until all medication administered	To ensure medication infusion is administered at correct rate
35 Wipe end of needleless injection cap firmly with 2% chlorhexidine alcohol wipe. Allow to dry (30 seconds)	To minimise risk of contamination of needless injection cap To ensure correct completion of disinfection process

Procedure guideline 7.1 **Guideline for administering a bolus intravenous injection** *(cont'd)*

Nursing action	Rationale
36 Remove needle from second sodium chloride 0.9% syringe and discard the needle into the sharps bin	Needle not required for connection to needleless injection cap
37 Attach the sodium chloride syringe to the needleless injection cap **either** by screwing on (Luer Lok) **or** by pushing the tip of the syringe firmly on to the needleless injection cap (Luer slip) and twisting a ¼ turn until firmly in place	To establish secure connection between injection cap and syringe
38 Inject the first 2 ml of sodium chloride 0.9% at the same rate as the medication, then using a push-pause method (approximately 1 ml at a time) inject the contents of the sodium chloride 0.9% syringe. Discard into the sharps bin	To ensure the remaining medication in the VAD is flushed at the correct rate To create turbulence in the catheter in order to flush thoroughly

If using heparinised saline then proceed with next steps

Nursing action	Rationale
39 Wipe end of needleless injection cap firmly with 2% chlorhexidine alcohol wipe. Allow to dry (30 seconds)	To minimise risk of contamination of needless injection cap To ensure correct completion of disinfection process
40 Remove needle from heparinised saline syringe and discard the needle into the sharps bin	Needle not required for connection to needleless injection cap
41 Attach the heparinised saline syringe to the needleless injection cap **either** by screwing on (Luer Lok) **or** by pushing the tip of the syringe firmly on to the needleless injection cap (Luer slip) and twisting a ¼ turn until firmly in place	To establish secure connection between injection cap and syringe
42 Using a push-pause method (approximately 1 ml at a time) inject the contents of the heparinised saline syringe	To create turbulence in the catheter in order to flush thoroughly and reduce risk of occlusion
43 Maintain pressure on the plunger as the syringe is disconnected from the cap then clamp catheter and discard syringe into the sharps bin	To maintain positive pressure and prevent back flow of blood into the catheter and possible clot formation
44 Remove gloves and apron and discard into clinical waste bag together with used dressing pack	To prevent contamination and reduce the risk of cross-infection
45 Wash hands with (bactericidal) soap and water. Dry well on clean towel or paper kitchen towel	To reduce the risk of cross-infection
46 Apply alcohol-based hand rub to both hands	To reduce the risk of cross-infection
47 Dispose of clinical waste	To prevent contamination and reduce the risk of cross-infection
48 Discuss procedure with patient, manage any questions or concerns and make plan for next home visit	To offer the patient an opportunity to discuss and express queries or concerns about IV treatment and the venous access device
49 Document actions, observations, decisions and rationale	To ensure adequate records and provide continuity of care for the patient

Procedure guideline 7.2 **Guideline for administering an intravenous infusion**

Equipment

Intravenous (IV) medication vial(s) (plus drug package insert)
Prescribed diluent for reconstitution, for example water for Injection
Sodium chloride 0.9% for Injection 10 ml ampoule × 2
Sodium chloride 0.9% infusion solution (volume dependent on medication requirements)
IV solution administration set
White sticky-backed label × 1
Heparinised saline (10 units per ml) – 5 ml (50 units) if required
10 ml syringes × 3 or 4
23 g needles × 3 or 4
Dressing pack with sterile towel, gloves and non-linting gauze swabs
70% alcohol swabs
2% chlorhexidine in 70% alcohol wipe
Single-use disposable plastic apron
Gloves (sterile) if not in dressing pack (1–2 pairs)
Sharps bin
Alcohol hand-cleansing gel
Disposable tape measure (one per patient for course of treatment)
Tray (if available)
Drip stand
Clean hand towel or paper kitchen towel
Community drug chart
Anaphylaxis equipment

Nursing action	Rationale
1 Explain and discuss procedure and medication treatment plan with the patient	To ensure that patient understands the procedure and gives their verbal consent to proceed
2 Identify a suitable place/room in the patient's home to carry out the procedure	To ensure patient is comfortable and privacy is maintained
3 Check IV medication drug, dose and route are prescribed on Community Drug Chart for this patient (drug details transferred from hospital discharge drug sheet and signed by the general practitioner) Read the drug package insert to check about dosage, reconstitution and administration details	To ensure that the correct medication and dose is being given to the correct patient, at the correct time via the correct route
4 Write drug, dose, date, patient's name on white sticky label and sign (add time the infusion commences)	To ensure label is ready and all information will be available on infusion bag if required
5 Check allergy history is recorded on Community Drug Chart Ask patient about any known allergies, type of reaction and document these even if no known allergies	To avoid allergic reaction to medication
6 Put on plastic apron	To reduce the risk of cross-infection and minimise risk of infection
7 Wash hands using (bactericidal) soap and water, dry with paper towels and apply alcohol hand gel	To reduce the risk of cross-infection and minimise risk of infection

Procedure guideline 7.2 **Guideline for administering an intravenous infusion** *(cont'd)*

Nursing action	Rationale
8 Ensure patient is comfortable and VAD is accessible	To gain access to VAD
9 Check insertion site and observe for any complications, for example: ■ redness ■ swelling ■ exudate ■ pain ■ discomfort Discuss any discomfort with the patient and document the findings	To ensure complications are managed promptly, and ensure that the patient is comfortable during the drug administration procedure
10 If patient has a PICC in situ then using the disposable tape measure, take and record measurement of PICC from entry/exit point of catheter to tip (far end) of needleless injection cap	To compare measurement with previous recording in order to ensure catheter remains in place; to ensure prompt action is taken if catheter has become displaced
11 Wash hands using soap and water, dry with paper towels, apply alcohol hand gel	To reduce the risk of cross-infection and minimise risk of infection
12 Identify a suitable clean surface to place dressing pack and equipment	To minimise the risk of introducing infection
13 Create a clean area for drug preparation, assemble the equipment required for the procedure and place beside the tray/preparation area	To ensure safe preparation of IV medication and minimise risk of infection To ensure all equipment is sterile and in date **NB** Sometimes more appropriate to prepare medication in different room to the patient, maximises concentration
14 Check all packaging is intact and check expiry dates	To ensure all equipment is sterile and in date
15 Check the expiry date of the: medication, diluent, sodium chloride 0.9% flushes and heparinised saline if required	To ensure all equipment is sterile and in date
16 Wipe tray (if available) or surface (if appropriate) with an alcohol wipe, allow to dry (30 seconds)	To ensure safe preparation of IV medication and minimise the risk of introducing infection
17 Apply alcohol hand gel to both hands	Hands may have become contaminated during preparation of tray and equipment/supplies
18 Open the outer cover of the sterile dressing pack and slide the inner pack on to the tray/surface. Open the sterile field using the corners of the paper only	To create a sterile area for procedure To reduce the risk of contamination of sterile working area
19 Remove clinical waste bag and position between patient and sterile working area	To reduce the risk of contamination by enabling clinical waste to be placed straight into clinical waste bag and not passed over sterile field
20 Place sharps bin between patient and sterile dressing area	To enable sharps to be placed straight into sharps bin after use

(Continued)

Nursing action	Rationale
21 Prepare equipment: open packages of needles, syringes, alcohol wipes, gauze swabs (if used) and sterile gloves (if not in dressing pack) on the sterile field Use a non-touch technique, ensuring all key parts remain covered with their protective caps	To ensure all equipment and medication is assembled and ready for medication preparation
22 Clean hands using alcohol hand gel and put on sterile gloves	To reduce risk of infection and protect nurse preparing medication from exposure to the drug
23 Draw up the appropriate prescribed diluent into 10 ml syringe (or larger) using a 23 g needle	To ensure correct diluent used to reconstitute medication
24 If using a vial then remove the plastic cap from the vial and clean the rubber stopper with an alcohol swab	To ensure the top of the vial is decontaminated. The plastic cap does not provide sterility only prevents damage to the rubber stopper
25 Inject the diluent into the vial slowly and mix with the contents checking there is no precipitation	To ensure the reconstitution procedure is completed as per drug manufacturer's instructions and is ready for further dilution process
26 Clean access port on the IV infusion bag with alcohol wipe and allow to dry (30 seconds)	To minimise infection risk
27 Keep the infusion bag flat and insert needle of reconstituted medication syringe into the access port of the IV infusion bag and inject medication into bag. Remove needle and syringe and discard into sharps bin	To reduce risk of pushing needle through side of access port and puncturing the bag
28 Gently invert the bag	To ensure the dilution and mixing procedure is completed safely as per manufacturer's instructions
29 Remove IV administration set from packaging and turn roller clamp on set to off position	To prevent the solution leaking from end of set when priming it
30 Remove protective covering from spike end of the set and push it firmly into access site of infusion bag	To ensure IV drug solution is ready for infusion process and infection risk minimised
31 Release roller clamp slowly to prime administrator's set and then turn it off when solution reaches end of set	To remove air from the set and fill with solution
32 Hang bag on drip stand	To prepare for attachment
33 Put the prepared white sticky label on to the infusion bag	To ensure all relevant information is available on infusion bag if required
34 Draw up 2 × sodium chloride 0.9% 10 ml flushes into 10 ml syringes using 23 g needles Draw up heparinised saline 5 ml into 10 ml syringe using 23 g needle (if required)	To ensure that catheter patency is checked prior to dose administration and the catheter is flushed following administration of medication
35 If equipment prepared in a different room to the patient, take the tray and sharps bin, and place beside patient on suitable clean and firm surface	To ensure medication and equipment is ready for administration process

Procedure guideline 7.2 **Guideline for administering an intravenous infusion** *(cont'd)*

Nursing action	Rationale
36 Continue procedure with the same pair of gloves, unless clearly contaminated, for example equipment is carried from one room to another. In this situation remove gloves and apply another pair of sterile gloves	To minimise risk of infection
37 Place sterile towel under catheter, wipe end of needleless injection cap firmly with 2% chlorhexidine in alcohol swab. Lay catheter on sterile field while allowing it to dry (30 seconds)	To minimise risk of infection
38 Remove needle from first sodium chloride 0.9% syringe and discard the needle into the sharps bin	Needle not required for connection to needleless injection cap
39 Attach the sodium chloride syringe to the needleless injection cap **either** by screwing on (Luer Lok) **or** by pushing the tip of the syringe firmly on to the needleless injection cap (Luer slip) and twisting a ¼ turn until firmly in place	To establish secure connection between injection cap and syringe
40 Using a push-pause method (approximately 1 ml at a time) inject the contents of the sodium chloride 0.9% syringe. Discard into the sharps bin	To ensure that the VAD is patent and to create turbulence in the catheter in order to flush thoroughly
41 Wipe end of needleless injection cap firmly with 2% chlorhexidine in alcohol wipe. Allow to dry (30 seconds)	To minimise risk of infection
42 Remove protective cap from end of administration set and screw set on to needleless injection cap	To attach the infusion to the catheter
43 Release roller ball clamp slowly on administration set slowly until fluid is seen dripping in the chamber. Set to correct drip rate (see Box 7.2 for drip rate calculation)	To ensure infusion is administered at correct rate
44 When infusion completed, turn roller clamp to off position, disconnect administration set and discard into sharps bin	To disconnect set and dispose of waste correctly
45 Wipe end of needleless injection cap firmly with 2% chlorhexidine alcohol wipe. Allow to dry (30 seconds)	To minimise risk of contamination of needless injection cap To ensure correct completion of disinfection process
46 Remove needle from second sodium chloride 0.9% syringe and discard the needle into the sharps bin	Needle not required for connection to needleless injection cap
47 Attach the sodium chloride syringe to the needleless injection cap **either** by screwing on (Luer Lok) **or** by pushing the tip of the syringe firmly on to the needleless injection cap (Luer slip) and twisting a ¼ turn until firmly in place	To establish secure connection between injection cap and syringe
48 Inject the first 2 ml of sodium chloride 0.9% at the same rate as the medication then using a push-pause method (approximately 1 ml at a time) inject the contents of the sodium chloride 0.9% syringe. Discard into the sharps bin	To ensure the remaining medication in the VAD is flushed at the correct rate To create turbulence in the catheter in order to flush thoroughly

159

(Continued)

Procedure guideline 7.2 **Guideline for administering an intravenous infusion** *(cont'd)*

Nursing action	Rationale
If using heparinised saline then proceed with next steps	
49 Wipe end of needleless injection cap firmly with 2% chlorhexidine alcohol wipe. Allow to dry (30 seconds)	To minimise risk of contamination of needless injection cap To ensure correct completion of disinfection process
50 Remove needle from heparinised saline syringe and discard the needle into the sharps bin	Needle not required for connection to needleless injection cap
51 Attach the heparinised saline syringe to the needleless injection cap **either** by screwing on (Luer Lok) **or** by pushing the tip of the syringe firmly on to the needleless injection cap (Luer slip) and twisting a ¼ turn until firmly in place	To establish secure connection between injection cap and syringe
52 Using a push-pause method (approximately 1 ml at a time) inject the contents of the heparinised saline syringe	To create turbulence in the catheter in order to flush thoroughly and reduce risk of occlusion
53 Maintain pressure on the plunger as the syringe is disconnected from the cap then clamp catheter and discard syringe into the sharps bin	To maintain positive pressure and prevent back flow of blood into the catheter and possible clot formation
54 Remove gloves and apron and discard into clinical waste bag together with used dressing pack	To prevent contamination and reduce the risk of cross-infection
55 Wash hands with (bactericidal) soap and water. Dry well on clean towel or paper kitchen towel	To reduce the risk of cross-infection
56 Apply alcohol-based hand rub to both hands	To reduce the risk of cross-infection
57 Dispose of clinical waste	To prevent contamination and reduce the risk of cross-infection
58 Discuss procedure with patient, manage any questions or concerns and make plan for next home visit	To offer the patient an opportunity to discuss and express queries or concerns about IV treatment and the venous access device
59 Document actions, observations, decisions and rationale	To ensure adequate records and provide continuity of care for the patient

---

Box 7.2 Drip rate calculation

$$\frac{\text{Volume required}}{\text{Duration (hours)}} \times \frac{\text{Set value (drops/ml)}}{\text{minutes (60)}} = \text{drops per minute}$$

Example

$$\frac{1000\,\text{ml}}{8\,\text{h}} \times \frac{20}{60} = 42 \text{ drops per minute}$$

Procedure guideline 7.3 **Guideline for changing the needleless injection cap on a PICC or skin-tunnelled cuffed central catheter**

The frequency of the needless injection cap change should be in accordance with the manufacturers instructions.

Equipment

Sterile needleless injection cap
Sterile dressing pack containing non-linting gauze
Chlorhexidine 2% with alcohol 70% or aqueous solution
Alcohol-based hand rub
Sterile gloves
Apron
Clean hand towel or paper towels

Nursing action	Rationale
1 Explain and discuss the procedure with the patient	To ensure that the patient understands the procedure and gives their valid consent
2 Identify a suitable place/room in the patient's home to carry out the cap change	To ensure patient is comfortable and privacy is maintained
3 Identify a suitable clean surface to place dressing pack and equipment	To minimise the risk of introducing infection
4 Assemble equipment and inspect all packaging to ensure it is intact and not damaged	To ensure all equipment is sterile and in date
5 Assist the patient into a comfortable position with CVAD and needleless injection cap exposed and easily accessible	To enable injection cap change procedure to be carried out
6 Put on apron	To reduce the risk of cross-infection
7 Wash hands with (bactericidal) soap and water. Dry well on clean towel or paper towels	To reduce the risk of cross-infection
8 Apply alcohol-based hand rub to both hands	To reduce the risk of cross-infection
9 Open the outer cover of the sterile dressing pack and slide the inner pack on to the clean surface. Open the sterile field using the corners of the paper only	To create a sterile area for procedure To reduce risk of contamination of sterile working area
10 Remove clinical waste bag and position between patient and sterile working area	To reduce the risk of contamination by enabling clinical waste to be placed straight into bag and not passed over sterile field
11 Open 2% chlorhexidine-impregnated swab then open the packaging of the injection cap and remove any protective coverings. Place on the sterile field	To ensure all equipment is accessible and to prevent interruptions to the procedure
12 Apply alcohol-based hand rub to both hands	Hands may have become contaminated by handling the outer packs
13 Put on sterile gloves	To reduce the risk of cross-infection

(Continued)

Procedure guideline 7.3 Guideline for changing the needleless injection cap on a PICC or skin-tunnelled cuffed central catheter (cont'd)

Nursing action	Rationale
14 Place a sterile towel under the cap end of the CVAD	To ensure that cap end of CVAD does not touch a non-sterile area during the procedure
15 Ensure CVAD is clamped (if appropriate)	To prevent blood loss or any risk of air entry
16 Unscrew needleless injection cap from CVAD (anti-clockwise). Discard in clinical waste bag	
17 Using 2% chlorhexidine-impregnated swab, clean around the screw thread of the CVAD, taking care not to touch the end of CVAD with gloves. Allow the area to air dry before applying new needleless injection cap	To ensure the screw thread area of the CVAD is clean before applying new needleless injection cap To ensure completion of disinfection process
18 Take new needleless injection cap from sterile field, taking care not to touch the end of the cap which is to be screwed directly on to the CVAD. Screw (clockwise) onto end of CVAD	To prevent contamination of end of cap and therefore reduce risk of introducing infection into CVAD
19 Remove gloves and apron and dispose into clinical waste bag together with used dressing pack	To reduce the risk of cross-infection
20 Wash hands with (bactericidal) soap and water. Dry well on clean towel or paper towels	To reduce the risk of cross-infection
21 Apply alcohol-based hand rub to both hands	To reduce the risk of cross-infection
22 Dispose of clinical waste	To prevent contamination and reduce risk of cross-infection
23 Document actions, observations, decisions and rationale	To ensure adequate records and provide continuity of care for the patient

162

Procedure guideline 7.4 **Guideline for maintaining patency of a PICC or skin-tunnelled cuffed catheter**

Equipment

Sterile dressing pack containing non-linting gauze
Sodium chloride 0.9% – 10 ml
Heparinised sodium chloride (10 iu per ml) – 5 ml (50 units) (may not be required for valved catheters)
10 ml syringes × 2
23 g needles × 2
2% chlorhexidine with alcohol 70% or aqueous solution
Sharps bin
Alcohol-based hand rub
Sterile gloves
Apron
Clean hand towel or paper towels

Procedure guideline 7.4 **Guideline for maintaining patency of a PICC or skin-tunnelled cuffed catheter** *(cont'd)*

Nursing action	Rationale
1 Explain and discuss the procedure with the patient	To ensure that the patient understands the procedure and gives their valid consent
2 Identify a suitable place/room in the patient's home to carry out the flushing procedure	To ensure patient is comfortable and privacy is maintained
3 Identify a suitable clean surface to place dressing pack and equipment	To minimise the risk of introducing infection
4 Assemble and inspect all packaging to ensure it is intact and not damaged	To ensure all equipment is sterile and in date
5 Assist the patient into a comfortable position with CVAD and needleless injection cap exposed and easily accessible	To enable the flushing of CVAD procedure to be carried out
6 Put on apron	To reduce the risk of cross-infection
7 Wash hands with (bactericidal) soap and water. Dry well on clean towel or paper towels	To reduce the risk of cross-infection
8 Apply alcohol-based hand rub to both hands	To reduce the risk of cross-infection
9 Open the outer cover of the sterile dressing pack and slide the inner pack on to the clean surface. Open the sterile field using the corners of the paper only	To create a sterile area for procedure To reduce risk of contamination of sterile working area
10 Remove clinical waste bag and position between patient and sterile working area	To reduce the risk of contamination by enabling clinical waste to be placed straight into bag and not passed over sterile field
11 Place sharps bin between patient and sterile dressing area	To enable sharps to be placed straight into sharps bin after use
12 Open 2% chlorhexidine-impregnated swab	To ensure all equipment is accessible and to prevent interruptions to the procedure
13 Draw up 10 ml sodium chloride in to a 10 ml syringe using a 23 g needle, place on sterile field	To ensure sodium chloride flush is then ready for use once needed
14 Draw up 5 ml heparinised sodium chloride (if required) into a 10 ml syringe using a 23 g needle, place on sterile field	To ensure heparinised sodium chloride flush is then ready for use once needed
15 Apply alcohol-based hand rub to both hands	Hands may have become contaminated during drawing up of flush solutions
16 Put on sterile gloves	To protect the nurse from any contact with the patients blood and prevent cross-infection
17 Place a sterile towel under the cap end of the CVAD	To ensure that cap end does not touch a non-sterile area during the procedure
18 Using 2% chlorhexidine-impregnated swab, clean the end of the needleless injection cap and allow to air dry	To minimize the risk of contamination of the needleless infection cap To ensure completion of disinfection process

163

(Continued)

Procedure guideline 7.4 **Guideline for maintaining patency of a PICC or skin-tunnelled cuffed catheter** *(cont'd)*

Nursing action	Rationale
19 Remove needle from sodium chloride 0.9% syringe and discard into the sharps bin	Needle not required for connection to needleless cap and to prevent any risk of needlestick injury
20 Attach the syringe to the needleless injection cap **either** by screwing on (Luer Lok) **or** by pushing the tip of the syringe firmly on to the needleless injection cap (Luer slip) and twisting a ¼ turn until firmly in place	To establish secure connection between cap and syringe
21 Release the catheter clamp	To allow administration of flush solution
22 Using a push-pause method (approximately 1 ml at a time) inject the contents of the sodium chloride 0.9% syringe	To create turbulence in the catheter in order to flush thoroughly and reduce risk of occlusion
23 Remove syringe and dispose into the sharps bin	To reduce risk of cross-infection
24 Using 2% chlorhexidine-impregnated swab, clean the end of the needleless injection cap and allow to air dry	To minimize the risk of contamination of the needleless infection cap To ensure completion of disinfection process
25 Remove needle from heparinised sodium chloride syringe (if required) and discard into the sharps bin	Needle not required for connection to needleless bung and to prevent any risk of needlestick injury
26 Attach the syringe to the needleless injection cap **either** by screwing on (if syringe is Luer Lok) **or** by pushing the tip of the syringe firmly on to the needleless injection cap (if syringe is Luer slip) and twisting a ¼ turn until firmly in place	To establish secure connection between cap and syringe
27 Using a push-pause method (approximately 1 ml at a time) inject the contents of the heparinised sodium chloride syringe	To create turbulence in the catheter in order to flush thoroughly and reduce risk of occlusion
28 Maintain pressure on the plunger as the syringe is disconnected from the cap	To maintain positive pressure and prevent back flow of blood into the catheter and possible clot formation
29 Clamp the catheter (if appropriate)	As a safety measure to prevent entry of air in case the cap is removed
30 Remove syringe and dispose into the sharps bin	To reduce risk of cross-infection
31 Remove gloves and apron and dispose into clinical waste bag	To reduce risk of cross-infection
32 Wash hands with (bactericidal) soap and water. Dry well on clean towel or paper towels	To reduce the risk of cross-infection
33 Apply alcohol-based hand rub to both hands.	To reduce the risk of cross-infection
34 Dispose of clinical waste	To prevent contamination and reduce risk of cross-infection
35 Document actions, observations, decisions and rationale	To ensure adequate records and provide continuity of care for the patient

Procedure guideline 7.5 **Guideline for dressing change – peripherally inserted central catheter (PICC)**

Equipment

Sterile dressing pack containing non-linting gauze
Anti-microbial skin cleansing solution – 2% chlorhexidine with alcohol 70% or aqueous solution
Transparent semi-permeable membrane (TSM) dressing
Sterile tapes (steristrips) or manufactured catheter securement device
Micropore tape
Tubigrip or tubigauze
Pair of clean gloves (for removing old dressing)
Alcohol-based hand rub
Sterile gloves
Apron
Clean hand towel or paper towels

Nursing action	Rationale
1 Explain and discuss the aseptic dressing procedure with the patient	To ensure that the patient understands the procedure and gives their valid consent
2 Identify a suitable place/room in the patient's home to carry out the dressing change	To ensure patient is comfortable and privacy is maintained
3 Identify a suitable clean surface to place dressing pack and equipment	To minimise the risk of introducing infection
4 Assemble and inspect all packaging to ensure it is intact and not damaged	To ensure all equipment is sterile and in date
5 Assist the patient into a comfortable position with arm with PICC in situ supported straight on a pillow	To enable dressing procedure to be carried out
6 Put on apron	To reduce the risk of cross-infection
7 Wash hands with (bactericidal) soap and water. Dry well on clean towel or paper towels	To reduce the risk of cross-infection
8 Apply alcohol-based hand rub to both hands	To reduce the risk of cross-infection
9 Open the outer cover of the sterile dressing pack and slide the inner pack on to the surface. Open the sterile field using the corners of the paper only	To create a sterile area for procedure To reduce risk of contamination of sterile working area
10 Remove clinical waste bag and position between patient and sterile working area	To reduce the risk of contamination by enabling clinical waste to be placed straight into bag and not passed over sterile field
11 Open 2% chlorhexidine-impregnated swab and open the other sterile packs and tip their contents gently onto the sterile field	To ensure all equipment is accessible and to prevent interruptions to the procedure To reduce the risk of contamination of contents
12 Apply alcohol-based hand rub to both hands	Hands may have become contaminated by handling the outer packs

(Continued)

Procedure guideline 7.5 **Guideline for dressing change – peripherally inserted central catheter (PICC)** *(cont'd)*

Nursing action	Rationale
13 Using tape secure the lower part of the PICC (hub end) to the skin	To prevent the PICC from hanging loose and pulling the catheter out at the entry site
14 Loosen the old dressing on all sides	So that the dressing can be lifted off easily
15 Apply alcohol-based hand rub to both hands	Hands may have become contaminated by handling the dressing
16 Put on clean gloves	To protect the nurse from any contact with the patients blood and soiled dressing
17 Using gloved hands remove the old dressing, steristrips (if used) and securement device (if used) carefully from around the exit site, taking care not to pull on or dislodge the PICC as the dressing is removed. Discard into clinical waste bag	To prevent contamination and reduce risk of cross-infection
18 Remove gloves and discard in clinical waste bag	Gloves have been contaminated by the old dressing
19 Apply alcohol-based hand rub to both hands	To reduce the risk of cross-infection
20 Put on sterile gloves	To reduce the risk of cross-infection
21 Inspect exit site of PICC for any redness, swelling or exudate	To check for any sign of infection
22 Take a piece of sterile gauze and use it to hold the PICC firmly in place whilst the exit site is cleaned. Position the gauze approximately 5 cm from the entry site	To prevent movement of PICC at exit site during cleaning procedure
23 Using 2% chlorhexidine swab, clean the entry site with friction. Allow the area to air dry before applying the new dressing	To ensure completion of disinfection process and prevent skin reaction in response to the application of TSM dressing to moist skin
24 **Either** apply a new sterile tape 0.5 cm away from entry site across PICC and the other 2–3 sterile tapes at 0.5 cm intervals. **And/or** apply new catheter securement device	To secure PICC at exit site
25 Apply TSM dressing to cover exit site	To secure PICC, protect exit site and enable visual inspection of site
26 Remove tape securing the lower part of the PICC	No longer required
27 Place a small gauze dressing on the patient's arm where the hub of the PICC will lie and secure this in place	To prevent a pressure area from the hub resting on the patient's arm
28 Cover the remaining lower part of the PICC with a TSM dressing or adhesive tape	To ensure full length of PICC is secure
29 Apply either a piece of tubigrip or tubigauze to cover the external length of the PICC	For patient comfort and help prevent PICC/hub getting caught in clothing

Procedure guideline 7.5 Guideline for dressing change – peripherally inserted central catheter (PICC) (cont'd)

Nursing action	Rationale
30 Remove gloves and apron and dispose into clinical waste bag together with used dressing pack	To reduce risk of cross- infection
31 Wash hands with (bactericidal) soap and water. Dry well on clean towel or paper towels	To reduce the risk of cross-infection
32 Apply alcohol-based hand rub to both hands	To reduce the risk of cross-infection
33 Dispose of clinical waste	To prevent contamination and reduce risk of cross-infection
34 Document actions, observations, decisions and rationale	To ensure adequate records and provide continuity of care for the patient

Procedure guideline 7.6 **Guideline for dressing change – skin-tunnelled cuffed central catheter**

Equipment

Sterile dressing pack containing non-linting gauze
Anti-microbial skin cleansing solution – 2% chlorhexidine with alcohol 70% or aqueous solution
Transparent semi-permeable membrane (TSM) dressing
Pair of clean gloves (for removing old dressing)
Alcohol-based hand rub
Sterile gloves
Apron
Clean hand towel or paper towels

Nursing action	Rationale
1 Explain and discuss the aseptic dressing procedure with the patient	To ensure that the patient understands the procedure and gives thei valid consent
2 Identify a suitable place/room in the patient's home to carry out the dressing change	To ensure patient is comfortable and privacy is maintained
3 Identify a suitable clean surface to place dressing pack and equipment	To minimise the risk of introducing infection
4 Assemble and inspect all packaging to ensure it is intact and not damaged	To ensure all equipment is sterile and in date
5 Assist the patient into a comfortable position with dressing site exposed	To enable dressing procedure to be carried out
6 Put on apron	To reduce the risk of cross-infection
7 Wash hands with (bactericidal) soap and water. Dry well on clean towel or paper towels	To reduce the risk of cross-infection

(Continued)

Procedure guideline 7.6 **Guideline for dressing change – skin-tunnelled cuffed central catheter** *(cont'd)*

Nursing action	Rationale
8 Apply alcohol-based hand rub to both hands	To reduce the risk of cross-infection
9 Open the outer cover of the sterile dressing pack and slide the inner pack on to the surface. Open the sterile field using the corners of the paper only	To create a sterile area for procedure To reduce risk of contamination of sterile working area
10 Remove clinical waste bag and position between patient and sterile working area	To reduce the risk of contamination by enabling clinical waste to be placed straight into bag and not passed over sterile field
11 Open 2% chlorhexidine-impregnated swab. Open the other sterile packs and tip their contents gently onto the sterile field	To ensure all equipment is accessible and to prevent interruptions to the procedure To reduce the risk of contamination of contents
12 Apply alcohol-based hand rub to both hands	Hands may have become contaminated by handling the outer packs
13 Loosen the old dressing on all sides	So that the dressing can be lifted off easily
14 Apply alcohol-based hand rub to both hands	Hands may have become contaminated by handling the dressing
15 Put on clean gloves	To protect the nurse from any contact with the patients blood and soiled dressing
16 Using gloved hands remove the old dressing carefully from around the exit site, taking care not to pull on the catheter as the dressing is removed. Discard into clinical waste bag	To prevent contamination and reduce risk of cross-infection
17 Remove gloves and discard in clinical waste bag	Gloves have been contaminated by the old dressing
18 Apply alcohol-based hand rub to bath hands	To reduce the risk of cross-infection
19 Put on sterile gloves	To reduce the risk of cross-infection
20 Inspect exit site of catheter for any redness, swelling or exudate	To check for any sign of infection
21 Using 2% chlorhexidine swab, clean the site with friction. Allow the area to air dry before applying the new dressing	To ensure completion of disinfection process and prevent skin reaction in response to the application of TSM dressing to moist skin
22 Apply TSM dressing to cover exit site	To protect exit site and enable visual inspection of site
23 Remove gloves and apron and dispose into clinical waste bag together with used dressing pack	To reduce risk of cross-infection
24 Wash hands with (bactericidal) soap and water. Dry well on clean towel or paper towels	To reduce the risk of cross-infection
25 Apply alcohol-based hand rub to both hands	To reduce the risk of cross-infection
26 Dispose of clinical waste	To prevent contamination and reduce risk of cross-infection
27 Document actions, observations, decisions and rationale	To ensure adequate records and provide continuity of care for the patient

Procedure guideline 7.7 **Guideline for obtaining blood samples from a PICC or skin-tunnelled cuffed central catheter**

There is no requirement to routinely withdraw blood and discard it prior to flushing a CVAD except prior to blood sampling (RCN 2010). If blood cultures are required then a blood sample must be withdrawn without flushing the CVAD first, and this blood sample is then used for culture. If a multi-lumen catheter is in situ then the largest diameter lumen should be used for blood taking.

Syringe sampling using blood transfer device

Equipment

Sterile dressing pack
Sodium chloride 0.9% – 10 ml × 2 ampoules
Heparinised saline (10 units per ml) – 5 ml (50 units) (may not be required for valved catheters)
10 ml syringes × 3
23 g needles × 3
Syringe for blood samples (10 ml or larger)
Appropriate vacuumed blood sample bottles
Blood transfer device
Completed blood test request form
2% chlorhexidine with alcohol 70% or aqueous solution
Sharps bin
Alcohol-based hand rub
Clean hand towel or paper towels
Sterile gloves
Apron

Nursing action	Rationale
1 Explain and discuss the procedure with the patient	To ensure that the patient understands the procedure and gives their valid consent
2 Identify a suitable place/room in the patient's home to carry out the blood sampling procedure	To ensure patient is comfortable and privacy is maintained
3 Identify a suitable clean surface to place dressing pack and equipment	To minimise the risk of introducing infection
4 Assemble and inspect all packaging to ensure it is intact and not damaged	To ensure all equipment is sterile and in date
5 Assist the patient into a comfortable position with CVAD and needleless injection cap exposed and easily accessible	To enable blood sampling procedure to be carried out
6 Put on apron	To reduce the risk of cross-infection
7 Wash hands with (bactericidal) soap and water. Dry well on clean towel or paper towels	To reduce the risk of cross-infection
8 Apply alcohol-based hand rub to both hands	To reduce the risk of cross-infection
9 Open the outer cover of the sterile dressing pack and slide the inner pack on to the surface. Open the sterile field using the corners of the paper only	To create a sterile area for procedure To reduce risk of contamination of sterile working area

(Continued)

Procedure guideline 7.7 **Guideline for obtaining blood samples from a PICC or skin-tunnelled cuffed central catheter** (cont'd)

Nursing action	Rationale
10 Remove clinical waste bag and position between patient and sterile working area	To reduce the risk of contamination by enabling clinical waste to be placed straight into bag and not passed over sterile field
11 Place sharps bin between patient and sterile dressing area	To enable sharps to be placed straight into sharps bin after use
12 Open 2% chlorhexidine-impregnated swab	To ensure all equipment is accessible and to prevent interruptions to the procedure
13 Draw up 2 × 10 ml sodium chloride into 10 ml syringes using 23 g needles, place on sterile field	Sodium chloride flushes are then ready for use once needed
14 Draw up 5 ml heparinised sodium chloride (if required) into a 10 ml syringe using a 23 g needle, place on sterile field	Heparinised saline flush is then ready for use once needed
15 Apply alcohol-based hand rub to both hands	Hands may have become contaminated during drawing up of flush solutions
16 Put on sterile gloves	To protect the nurse from any contact with the patients blood and prevent cross infection
17 Place a sterile towel under the cap end of the CVAD	To ensure that cap end does not touch a non-sterile area during the procedure
18 Using 2% chlorhexidine swab, clean the end of the needleless injection cap and allow to air dry	To minimize the risk of contamination of the needleless infection cap
	To ensure completion of disinfection process
19 Remove needle from first sodium chloride 0.9% syringe and discard the needle into the sharps bin	Needle not required for connection to needleless bung
20 Attach the sodium chloride syringe to the needleless injection cap **either** by screwing on (Luer Lok) **or** by pushing the tip of the syringe firmly on to the needleless injection cap (Luer slip) and twisting a ¼ turn until firmly in place	To establish secure connection between cap and syringe
21 Release the clamp (if appropriate)	To allow administration of flush solution
22 Using a push-pause method (approximately 1 ml at a time) inject the contents of the sodium chloride 0.9% syringe	To create turbulence in the catheter in order to flush thoroughly and reduce risk of occlusion
23 Do not remove the syringe, use it to withdraw approximately 5 ml blood	To check for blood return prior to taking samples and for discard as a mixture of blood and sodium chloride
24 Clamp the catheter (if appropriate)	To maintain patient safety
25 Remove syringe and discard into the sharps bin	For safe disposal of discard blood sample and to reduce the risk of cross infection

Procedure guideline 7.7 **Guideline for obtaining blood samples from a PICC or skin-tunnelled cuffed central catheter** *(cont'd)*

Nursing action	Rationale
26 Using 2% chlorhexidine swab, clean the end of the needleless injection cap and allow to air dry	To minimize the risk of contamination of the needleless infection cap To ensure completion of disinfection process
27 Attach the empty syringe to the needleless injection cap **either** by screwing on (if syringe is Luer Lok) **or** by pushing the tip of the syringe firmly on to the needleless injection cap (if syringe is Luer slip) and twisting a ¼ turn until firmly in place	To establish secure connection between cap and syringe
28 Release the clamp (if appropriate)	To allow blood to be withdrawn
29 Gently withdraw required amount of blood	To obtain the sample
30 Clamp the catheter (if appropriate)	To maintain patient safety
31 Remove syringe and attach to blood transfer device	For safe transfer of blood to sample bottles
32 Attach required vacuumed blood sample bottles for requested specimens	For safe transfer of blood to sample bottles
33 Dispose of syringe and blood transfer device into the sharps bin	To reduce the risk of cross-infection
34 Using 2% chlorhexidine swab, clean the end of the needleless injection cap and allow to air dry	To minimise the risk of contamination of the needleless infection cap To ensure completion of disinfection process
35 Remove needle from second sodium chloride 0.9% syringe and discard the needle into the sharps bin	Needle not required for connection to needleless cap
36 Attach the sodium chloride syringe to the needleless injection cap **either** by screwing on (Luer Lok) **or** by pushing the tip of the syringe firmly on to the needleless injection cap (Luer slip) and twisting a ¼ turn until firmly in place	To establish secure connection between cap and syringe
37 Release the clamp (if appropriate)	To allow administration of flush solution
38 Using a push-pause method (approximately 1 ml at a time) inject the contents of the sodium chloride 0.9% syringe	To create turbulence in the catheter in order to flush thoroughly and ensuring that all traces of blood are cleared from the catheter
39 Clamp the catheter (if appropriate)	To maintain patient safety
40 Remove syringe and discard into the sharps bin	To reduce risk of cross-infection
41 Using 2% chlorhexidine swab, clean the end of the needleless injection cap and allow to air dry	To minimize the risk of contamination of the needleless infection cap To ensure completion of disinfection process

171

(Continued)

Procedure guideline 7.7 **Guideline for obtaining blood samples from a PICC or skin-tunnelled cuffed central catheter** *(cont'd)*

Nursing action	Rationale
42 If required – remove needle from heparinised sodium chloride syringe and discard the needle into the sharps bin	Needle not required for connection to needleless bung
43 Attach the heparinised sodium chloride syringe to the needleless injection cap **either** by screwing on (Luer Lok) **or** by pushing the tip of the syringe firmly on to the needleless injection cap (Luer slip) and twisting a ¼ turn until firmly in place	To establish secure connection between cap and syringe
44 Release the clamp (if appropriate)	To allow administration of flush solution
45 Using a push-pause method (approximately 1 ml at a time) inject the contents of the heparinised sodium chloride syringe	To create turbulence in the catheter in order to flush thoroughly and reduce risk of occlusion
46 Maintain pressure on the plunger as the syringe is disconnected from the cap	To maintain positive pressure and prevent back flow of blood into the catheter and possible clot formation
47 Clamp the catheter (if appropriate)	Catheter should remain clamped once procedure completed
48 Remove syringe and discard into sharps bin	To reduce risk of cross-infection
49 Label blood sample bottles with patient's name, date of birth and other relevant information, and send to laboratory with the appropriate forms	To ensure correct documentation for laboratory so blood tests can be carried out and results returned to correct patient's notes
50 Remove gloves and apron and discard into clinical waste bag together with used dressing pack	To prevent contamination and reduce the risk of cross-infection
51 Wash hands with (bactericidal) soap and water. Dry well on clean towel or paper towels	To reduce the risk of cross-infection
52 Apply alcohol-based hand rub to both hands	To reduce the risk of cross-infection
53 Dispose of clinical waste	To prevent contamination and reduce the risk of cross-infection
54 Document actions, observations, decisions and rationale	To ensure adequate records and provide continuity of care for the patient

Blood sampling can be carried out using a vacuum holder and adaptor. Instead of discarding a syringe of blood, attach the vacuum holder to the needle-less injection cap, then attach a sample bottle and once filled discard. The other samples can then be taken directly from the catheter using the vacuum system.

Procedure guideline 7.8 **Guideline for de-accessing the needle from an implanted port**

Patients who are receiving intravenous therapy via an implanted port (e.g. infusional chemotherapy) may go home with a port needle in situ, which will require removal once therapy is completed. This guidance provides the community nurse with the necessary steps in how to remove the needle (de-access) from the port.

Equipment

Plastic apron
Sterile gloves
Dressing pack
2% chlorhexidine in 70% alcohol
10 ml syringe containing 0.9% sodium chloride × 1
10 ml containing 500 iu heparin in 5 ml in 0.9% sodium chloride × 1
Plaster
Sharps bin

Nursing action	Rationale
1 Explain and discuss the procedure with the patient	To ensure that the patient understands the procedure and gives their valid consent
2 Identify a suitable place/room in the patient's home to carry out the procedure	To ensure patient is comfortable and privacy is maintained
3 Identify a suitable clean surface to place dressing pack and equipment	To minimise the risk of introducing infection
4 Assemble and inspect all packaging to ensure it is intact and not damaged	To ensure all equipment is sterile and in date
5 Assist the patient into a comfortable position with port needle and extension set easily accessible	To enable the removal of needle to be carried out
6 Put on apron	To reduce the risk of cross-infection
7 Wash hands with (bactericidal) soap and water. Dry well on clean towel or paper towels	To reduce the risk of cross-infection
8 Apply alcohol-based hand rub to both hands	To reduce the risk of cross-infection
9 Open the outer cover of the sterile dressing pack and slide the inner pack on to the clean surface. Open the sterile field using the corners of the paper only	To create a sterile area for procedure To reduce risk of contamination of sterile working area
10 Remove clinical waste bag and position between patient and sterile working area	To reduce the risk of contamination by enabling clinical waste to be placed straight into bag and not passed over sterile field
11 Place sharps bin between patient and sterile dressing area	To enable sharps to be placed straight into sharps bin after use
12 Open 2% chlorhexidine-impregnated swab	To ensure all equipment is accessible and to prevent interruptions to the procedure

173

(Continued)

Procedure guideline 7.8 **Guideline for de-accessing the needle from an implanted port** *(cont'd)*

Nursing action	Rationale
13 Put on sterile gloves	To protect the nurse from any contact with the patients blood and prevent cross-infection
14 Place a sterile towel under the cap end of the port extension set	To ensure that cap end does not touch a non-sterile area during the procedure
15 Using 2% chlorhexidine-impregnated swab, clean the end of the needleless injection cap and allow to air dry	To minimize the risk of contamination of the needleless infection cap To ensure completion of disinfection process
16 Attach the syringe of 0.9% sodium chloride to the needleless injection cap **either** by screwing on (if syringe is Luer Lok) **or** by pushing the tip of the syringe firmly on to the needleless injection cap (if syringe is Luer slip) and twisting a ¼ turn until firmly in place	To establish secure connection between cap and syringe
17 Using a push-pause method (approximately 1 ml at a time) inject the contents of the sodium chloride syringe. Remove and discard	To create turbulence in the catheter in order to flush thoroughly and reduce risk of occlusion
18 Repeat this process with heparinised saline syringe	
19 Maintain pressure on the plunger as the syringe is disconnected from the cap and clamp the catheter	To maintain positive pressure and prevent back flow of blood into the catheter and possible clot formation
20 Dispose of syringe into the sharps bin	To reduce risk of cross-infection
21 Press down on either side of the portal body of the port with two fingers (one on each side of port)	To support port while removing the needle
22 Withdraw the needle using steady traction and discard needle immediately into a sharps bin	To remove the needle and prevent needlestick injury
23 Apply pressure with a gauze swab over the puncture wound and apply a plaster if necessary	To prevent oozing at the site
24 Document removal date and time in patients notes	To ensure adequate records and to enable continued care of the patient

References and further reading

Andris DA, Krzywda EA (1997) Catheter pinch-off syndrome: recognition and management. *Journal of Intravenous Nursing* **20**(5): 233–7.

Anstett M, Royer TI (2003) The impact of ultrasound on PICC placement. *Journal of the Association for Vascular Access* **8**(3): 24–8.

Aston V (2000) Community management of peripherally inserted central catheters. *British Journal of Community Nursing* **5**(7): 318, 320–5.

Benton S, Marsden C (2002) Training nurses to place tunnelled central venous catheters. *Professional Nurse* **17**(9): 531–5.

Berger L (2000) The effects of positive pressure devices on catheter occlusions. *Journal of Vascular Access Devices* **5**(4): 31–3.

Communicable Disease Council (CDC) (2002) Guidelines for the prevention of intravascular catheter-related infections. *Morbidity and Mortality Weekly Report* **51**(RR 10): S35–S63.

Daniels LE (1996) Innovations in cancer care in the community; home therapy. *British Journal Community Health Nurse* **1**(3): 163–8.

Dougherty L (2006) *Central Venous Access Devices*. Essential Skills series Blackwell Publishing, Oxford.

Dougherty L, Watson J (2011) Vascular access devices: insertion and management. In: Dougherty L, Lister S (eds) *Royal Marsden Manual of Clinical Nursing Procedures* (8e). Blackwell Publishing, Oxford.

Dougherty L, Viner C, Young J (1998) Establishing ambulatory chemotherapy at home. *Professional Nurse* **13**(6): 356–8.

Drewett SR (2009) Removal of central venous access devices. In: Hamilton H, Bodenham A (eds) *Central Venous Catheters*, pp. 238–48. Wiley-Blackwell, Chichester.

Gabriel J (1996) Care and management of peripherally inserted central catheters. *Surgical Nurse* **5**(10): 594–6.

Gabriel J (2000) What patients think of a PICC. *Journal of Vascular Access Devices* **5**(4): 26–9.

Gabriel J (2001) PICC securement: minimising potential complications. *Nursing Standard* **15**(43): 42–4.

Gabriel J (2003) Improved levels of patient care in the United Kingdom as nurses gain experience with PICCs. *Journal of Vascular Access Devices* **8**(2): 18–20.

Gabriel J (2008) Long-term central venous access. In: Dougherty L, Lamb J (eds) *Intravenous Therapy in Nursing Practice* (2e). Blackwell Publishing, Oxford.

Gabriel J, Dailly S, Kayley J (2004) Needlestick and sharps injuries: avoiding the risk in clinical practice. *Professional Nurse* **20**(1): 25–8.

Goodwin ML, Carlson I (1993) The peripherally inserted central catheter: a retrospective look at three years of insertions. *Journal of Intravenous Nursing* **16**(2): 22–6.

Hadaway LC (1998) Major thrombotic and nonthrombotic complications. *Journal of Intravenous Nursing* **21**(5S): S143–S160.

Hamilton HC (2000) Selecting the correct IV device: nursing assessment. *British Journal of Nursing* **9**(15): 968–78.

Hamilton HC, O'Byrne M, Nickolai L (1995) Central lines inserted by clinical nurse specialists. *Nursing Times* **91**(17): 38–9.

Hanchett M (1999) Science of IV securement. *Journal of Vascular Access Devices* **4**(3): 30–5.

Hyde L (2008) Legal and professional aspects of intravenous therapy. In: Dougherty L, Lamb J (eds) *Intravenous Therapy in Nursing Practice* (2e). Blackwell Publishing, Oxford.

Intravenous Nursing Society (INS) (2011) *Standards for Infusion Therapy*. USA, INS and Becton Dickinson (BD).

Jackson A (1998) A battle in vein: intravenous cannulation. *Nursing Times* **94**(4): 68–9.

Jackson D (2001) Infection control principles and practices in the care and management of vascular access devices in the alternate care setting. *Journal of Intravenous Nursing* **24**(3S): S28–S34.

Kayley J (1997) Skin-tunnelled cuffed catheters. *Community Nurse* **3**(5): 21–2.

Kayley J (2000) Home IV antibiotic therapy. *Primary Health Care* **10**(6): 25–30.

Kayley J (2008) Intravenous therapy in the community. In: Dougherty L, Lamb J (eds) *Intravenous Therapy in Nursing Practice* (2e). Blackwell Publishing, Oxford.

Kayley J, Finlay T (2003) Vascular access devices used for patients in the community. *Community Practitioner* **76**(6): 228–31.

Kayley J, Berendt AR, Snelling MJM *et al.* (1996) Safe intravenous antibiotic therapy at home: experience of a UK based programme. *Journal of Antimicrobial Chemotherapy* **37**(5): 1023–9.

Kelly C (1992) A change in flushing protocols of central venous catheters. *Oncology Nursing Forum* **19**(4): 599–605.

Krzywda EA (1999) Predisposing factors, prevention, and management of central venous catheter occlusion. *Journal of Intravenous Nursing* **22**(6S): S11–S17.

Lamb J, Dougherty L (2008) Local and systemic complications of intravenous therapy. In: Dougherty L, Lamb J (eds) *Intravenous Therapy in Nursing Practice* (2e). Blackwell Publishing, Oxford.

Lenhart C (2000) Prevention vs treatment of vascular access devices occlusions. *Journal of Vascular Access Devices* **5**(4): 34–5.

London Standing Conference (LSC) (2002) *Standards of Care of External Central Venous Catheters in Adults*. London Standing Conference, London.

Macrae K (1998) Hand held dopplers in central catheter insertion. *Professional Nurse* **14**(2): 99–102.

Maki DG, Ringer M, Alvarado CJ (1991) Prospective randomised trial of povidone-iodine alcohol and clhorhexidine for prevention of infection associated with central venous and arterial catheters. *Lancet* **338**: 339–43.

Masoorli S (2003) Extravasation Injuries associated with the use of central venous access devices. *Journal of Vascular Access Devices* **8**(1): 21–3.

Mayo DJ (2001a) Reflux in vascular access devices – a manageable problem. *Journal of Vascular Access Devices* **6**(4): 39–40.

Mayo DJ (2001b) Catheter-related thrombosis. *Journal of Intravenous Nursing* **24**(35): 13–22.

Medical Devices Agency (MDA now Medicines and Healthcare products Regulatory Agency MHRA) (2003) *Infusion System Device Bulletin*. London, MDA.

NAVAN (1998) Clinical position statement: tip location and peripherally inserted catheters. *Journal of Vascular Access Devices* **3**(2): 8–10.

NHS Employers (2007) *The Management of Health, Safety and Welfare Issues for NHS Staff*. NHS Employers, London.

National Institute for Clinical Excellence (NICE) (2003) *Infection Control: prevention of healthcare-associated infection in primary and community care* (clinical guidelines 2). NICE, London.

National Patient Safety Agency (NPSA) (2003) *Risk Analysis of Infusion Devices*. NPSA, London.

Nursing & Midwifery Council (NMC) (2008a) *Standards for Medicines Management*. NMC, London.

Nursing & Midwifery Council (NMC) (2008b) *The Code. Standards of conduct, performance and ethics for nurses and midwives*. NMC, London.

O'Hanlon S, Glenn R, Hasler B (2008) Delivering intravenous therapy in the community setting. *Nursing Standard* **22**(31): 44–8.

Pearson ML (1996) Hospital Infection Control Practices Advisory Committee. Guidelines for prevention of intravascular device related infections. *Infection Control Hospital Epidemiology* **17**(7): 438–73.

Perucca R (2010) Peripheral venous access devices. In: Alexander M, Corrigan A, Gorski L et al. (eds) *Infusion nursing: an*

175

evidence-based approach (3e), pp. 456–79. Saunders Elsevier, St Louis.

Philpott P, Griffiths V (2003) The peripherally inserted central catheter. *Nursing Standard* **17**(44): 39–46.

Pratt RJ, Pellowe CM, Wilson JA *et al.* (2007) epic2: National evidence-based guidelines for preventing healthcare-associated infections in NHS hospitals in England. *Journal of Hospital Infection* **65**(Suppl 1): S1–64.

Richardson D, Bruso P (1993) Vascular access devices – management of common complications. *Journal of Intravenous Nursing* **16**(1): 44–9.

Royal College of Nursing (RCN) (2010) *Standards for Infusion Therapy*. RCN, London.

Ryder M (2001) The Role of biofilm in vascular-related infections. *New Developments in Vascular Diseases* **2**(2): 15–25.

Ryder M (1993) Peripherally inserted central venous catheters. *Nursing Clinics of North America* **28**(4): 937–71.

Ryder M (1999) The future of vascular access: will the benefits be worth the risk? *Nutrition in Clinical Practice* **14**(4): 165–9.

Sansivero GE (1998) Venous anatomy and physiology. *Journal of Intravenous Nursing* **21**(5S): S107–S114.

Scales K (1996) Legal and professional aspects of intravenous therapy. *Nursing Standard* **11**(3): 41–8.

Springhouse Corporation (2002) *Intravenous Therapy Made Incredibly Easy*. Springhouse, Lippincott, Williams & Wilkins, Philadelphi.

Todd J (1998) Peripherally inserted central catheters. *Professional Nurse* **13**(5): 297–302.

Tortora GJ, Grabowski SR (2000) *Principles of Anatomy and Physiology* (9e). Harper Collins College Publishers, New York.

Vesely TM (2003) Central venous catheter tip position: a continuing controversy. *Journal of Vascular Interventional Radiology* **14**: 527–34.

Viale PH (2003) Complications associated with implantable vascular access devices in the patient with cancer. *Journal of Intravenous Nursing* **26**(2): 97–102.

Wall JL, Kierstead VL (1995) Peripherally inserted central catheters. Resistence to removal: a rare complication. *Journal of Intravenous Nursing* **18**(5): 251–62.

Weinstein S (2007) *Plumer's Principles and Practices of Intravenous Therapy* (8e). Lippincott, Philadelphia.

Wickham R, Purl S, Welker D (1992) Long-term central venous catheters: issues for care. *Seminars in Oncology Nursing* **2**(8): 133–47.

Wise M, Richardson D, Lum P (2001) Catheter tip position. A sign of things to come! *Journal of Vascular Access Devices* **6**(6): 18–27.

8

Medicines management

The administration of medicines is a key element of nursing care. Every day some 7000 doses of medication are administered in a typical NHS hospital, with thousands more being self-administered by patients and administered by community nurses in the home environment (Audit Commission 2002).

Background evidence

The main legal framework for the prescribing and administration of medicines includes the following.

- The Medicines Act 1968, which classifies medicines into four categories (Table 8.1).
- The Prescription Only Medicines (Human Use) Order (1997).
- The Misuse of Drugs Act (1971).

Section 58a of the Medicines Act (1968) places a duty on the Secretary of State for Health to place all medicines that represent a danger to patients, if their use is not supervised by an appropriate practitioner on the prescription-only medicine list (POM).

Accountability, responsibility and consent

Nurses administering medications must exercise accountability, professional judgement and apply knowledge and skill (NMC 2010). To achieve this they must know, for example:
the therapeutic uses of all drugs being administered

- the normal dose ranges
- potential side effects
- precautions and contraindications.

(NMC 2010)

Prior to the administration of medication to a patient at each visit the community nurse should do the following.

- Ensure that the aspect of care they are undertaking is not beyond their level of knowledge, skills and competence or outside their area of registration (NMC 2008).
- Correctly identify the patient.
- Through observation and discussion with the patient, their carer or significant other, undertake an assessment of the patient's condition. This should include consideration of changes in presenting symptoms and any over-the-counter (OTC) medication that the patient may be self-administering. This should be recorded in the nursing documentation.
- Exercise their professional responsibility by providing and discussing appropriate information regarding the drug/s to be administered with the patient in order to obtain consent, e.g. why they have been prescribed, potential side effects and contraindications (Cable *et al.* 2003).
- Check, discuss and where necessary update documentation to record all known and potential allergies.
- Read, and where appropriate update the current nursing care plan and relevant documentation.
- Ensure that the administration chart clearly details:
  - the patient's full name
  - the name of the drug/s to be administered
  - the correct dose
  - the correct route of administration
  - the time of administration
  - the duration of treatment.

These details should also be checked against the drug/s to be administered.

District Nursing Manual of Clinical Procedures, First Edition. Edited by Liz O'Brien.
© 2012 Blackwell Publishing Ltd. Published 2012 by Blackwell Publishing Ltd.

Table 8.1 Classification of medicines (NMC 2007)

Prescription-only medicines (POM)	Pharmacy-only medicines (P)	General sales list medicines (GSL)	Controlled drugs (CD)
May only be prescribed or administered by or in accordance with the directions of an appropriate practitioner, e.g. doctor, independent or supplementary prescriber	May be purchased over the counter, without a prescription, from a registered pharmacist or under the supervision of a registered pharmacist	May be purchased from, e.g. supermarkets, without a prescription or pharmacist supervision	Prescription-only medicines that include e.g. opioids and major stimulants. **Please refer to relevant act/s and amendments for specific regulations regarding prescribing, dispensing and safety**

- Discuss any concerns that may arise with the prescriber or qualified district nurse and record this in the nursing documentation.
- Ask the patient and/or carer and check the administration chart and nursing documentation to ensure that the drug/s have not already been administered.
- Check the expiry date of the drug/s to be administered.
- Where relevant, a visual inspection of the drug should be undertaken to check for colour abnormalities or precipitation.

(Figure 8.1) (Audit Commission 2002; NMC 2008, 2010)

Risk management

During the period from January 2005 to June 2006 of all community medication-related incidents reported to the National Patient Safety Agency (NPSA), 52.4% were recorded as having occurred in the patient's home, 36.1% in community pharmacies and 11.5% within general practice (NPSA 2007a). While the data relating to patient's home include care homes, and reporting is thought to be initiated by nursing staff visiting the patient, responsibility for administration is not identified (NPSA, 2007a).

Areas highlighted by NPSA data that community nurses should be aware of include:

- poor communication and documentation
- incomplete or incorrect information supplied on discharge from hospital
- non-recording of patient's allergy status
- wrongly prescribed or dispensed drug, dose, strength or frequency of administration
- availability and access to medicines out of hours, especially controlled drugs

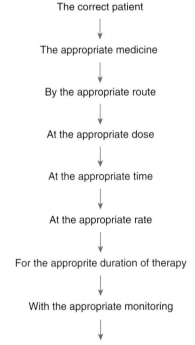

The correct patient
↓
The appropriate medicine
↓
By the appropriate route
↓
At the appropriate dose
↓
At the appropriate time
↓
At the appropriate rate
↓
For the approprite duration of therapy
↓
With the appropriate monitoring
↓
With the appropriate reporting of adverse incidents

Figure 8.1 Medicines administration process (Adapted from Dougherty & Lister 2008).

- the need for the promotion of concordance and safe self-administration by enabling and empowering patient's through education and, where necessary, skills training
- the need for continued training and education in medicines management including injectable medicines.

(NPSA 2007, 2010)

Delegation of administration

Team members within the community setting work without direct clinical supervision, therefore to ensure patient and staff safety, and maintain controls assurance in line with clinical governance requirements, it is essential that the community nurse:

- carries out a full nursing needs assessment and risk assessment of the procedure to be undertaken prior to delegation
- delegates all nursing procedures in accordance with local trust and Nursing & Midwifery Council (NMC) policies, guidelines and standards.

If delegation is to a junior nurse or a healthcare assistant or other non-regulated healthcare staff, e.g. generic support worker, risk management should include periods of planned supervision in practice. This is to assess competency and to ensure that the team member understands and works within the limitations of their knowledge and skills and knows what action to take if changes occur (NMC 2007, 2008).

Storage

All medicines must be stored in accordance with the patient information leaflet supplied with the relevant medication (NMC 2010). Community nurses should ensure that they and the patient are aware of and adhere to the relevant storage conditions for each drug. Any drug that has been stored outside the correct temperature may become inactivated (this includes active ingredients within wound dressings, therefore they should never be stored in the boot of a car).

All drugs should be observed for signs of deterioration prior to administration and any concerns should be discussed with the community pharmacist or relevant drug company. In the patient's home, medicines should be stored away from areas of dampness and away from children and vulnerable adults.

Insulin

Insulin cartridges, vials and pre-filled pens that are in use can be kept out of the refrigerator as long as the room temperature does not exceed 25–28°C for a maximum period of 4 weeks. Products for future use must be stored in a refrigerator away from the internal walls at a temperature of 2–8°C (Trend UK 2010; NPSA 2011a).

Cartridges, vials and pre-filled pens that have been opened must not be used after 28 days (NPSA 2011a).

Vaccines

Recommended storage temperatures will vary according to individual vaccines so the most up-to-date guidelines should be available for staff. If there is any uncertainty manufacturer's guidance should be sought.

If vaccines are being stored at district nurse bases or GP surgeries and require the cold chain procedure the following guidelines should be followed.

- A specialist pharmacy fridge should be used for storage.
- There should be a named clinician to take responsibility for storage, monitoring and regular recording of the vaccine fridge temperature in a designated book.
- General guidance recommends that the fridge should be kept within the range of 2–8°C degrees centigrade, ideally around 4 or 5°C.
- The fridge temperature, including the maximum, minimum and mean temperature, should be read and recorded during each working day. Each entry must be signed and the time of reading recorded. One of the readings should be carried out first thing in the morning before any vaccines have been removed for use.
- The fridge thermometer should be re-set each evening and recorded. This process will enable any variance in temperature to be detected. If, on a number of occasions, the temperature in the evening at the time of re-set is high but the reading in the morning is within normal limits it is essential to (a) confirm that the fridge is not being opened unnecessarily or for long periods during the day and (b) contact the manufacturer for advice.
- The fridge door should not be left open for long periods and the frequency of door opening should be kept to a minimum.
- In summer months when room temperatures may rise above average e.g. 18–20°C, the fridge temperature may rise quickly when the fridge door is opened. During this time the fridge temperature should be closely monitored.
- Vaccines should never be stockpiled and there should be rotation of stock so that the oldest is used first.
- Vaccines should not be packed into the fridge too tightly and should never come into contact with ice.
- Vaccines must be protected from light.

(National Patient Safety Agency [NPSA], 2010)

A nurse responsible for administering medicines that require the cold chain procedure to be carried out when stored must ensure that prior to administration, the drug has been stored at the correct temperature. Where necessary, clarification and advice should be sought from the community or principal pharmacist.

Transportation of medication

If taking vaccines from district nurse bases or GP surgeries to patients' homes or clinics for administration, the minimum amount of vaccine required should be taken out of the fridge and transported in a cool box/bag containing a frozen ice block. It is essential that the ice block does not come into contact with the vaccine packaging as this may remove vital information and make the checking procedure prior to administration impossible, e.g. drug name, expiry date and batch number. It may also affect the storage temperature rendering the vaccine inactive.

Where a patient or carer is unable to collect a prescribed and dispensed medication, including controlled drugs, a community nurse may, if in accordance with local policy, transport the medication directly to the patient (NMC 2010). In the case of receiving controlled drugs from, e.g. a community pharmacist or local hospice, it is advised that the community nurse:

- Presents their identity badge
- ensures that all relevant packaging is sealed and has not been tampered with
- checks the prescription details against the dispensed drug/s and counts medication prior to signing for receipt.

(NMC 2010)

In the patient's home the community nurse should:

- record the name and quantity of all controlled drugs in accordance with local policies when all new supplies are received.

All drugs and dressings that have been prescribed and dispensed to an individual patient becomes their legal property and removal from the patient's home by a community nurse, e.g. for use with another patient, is considered as theft. It also places other patients at risk in terms of cross-infection (NMC 2010).

Transcribing

Where community nurses transcribe medication from discharge letters, faxes or dispensing labels to local patient administration charts, they are accountable for their actions and any errors or omissions in the information transcribed (NMC 2008, 2010).

Changes to medication doses

Where a change in drug dose for a previously prescribed drug is thought to be necessary, but the prescriber is unable to supply a new prescription, the use of information technology, e.g. faxes or email, is advocated. It is essential that this confirms the new dose and the direction to administer. This must be stapled to the existing administration chart and a new prescription should be issued by the prescriber within 24–72 hours (NMC 2010). Authorisation must be received prior to administration (NMC 2010). The above standards of practice should also be followed in circumstances when drugs have not been previously prescribed, for example where a local hospice home care team supplies a crisis box containing drugs for symptom control. However, this should only be in exceptional circumstances and the fax or email must confirm the prescription (NMC 2010). To avoid this situation it is suggested that a prescription, with a range of doses, should be issued with the crisis box; this also enables the community nurse to respond promptly and effectively to the patient's needs.

Incident reporting

To minimise the risk of drug errors all community staff should have access to up-to-date policies and guidelines that reflect NPSA recommendations.

All errors and near misses should be reported through locally agreed risk management systems.

Adverse drug reaction (ADR)

An adverse drug reaction is described as a harmful or unwanted response to a drug or combination of drugs that have been administered under normal conditions of use and can be either minor or life threatening (Prodigy 2004).

In those aged 65 years and over it is suggested that 16% of hospital admissions are due to suspected ADR compared with 4% in younger adults (Beijer & Blaey 2002).

Suspected drug reactions must be treated promptly and appropriately (see section on diagnosis and treatment of anaphylaxis) reported according to local policy and by completing the Yellow Card contained at the back of the *British National Formulary* (BNF) or online at www.yellowcard.gov.uk (NMC 2010).

Disposal

Unused or expired patient drugs must be returned to a community pharmacist for safe disposal. If the patient is unable to do this the community nurse may, if supported by local policy, act as their representative (NMC 2010).

Non-medical prescribing

Prescribing by district nurses and health visitors was first introduced in England in 1998. There are a number of types of prescribing courses now available to all registered nurses. Once the prescribing qualification is registered with the NMC community nurses are able to prescribe in the following ways.

Nurse prescribers formulary for community practitioners
This type of prescribing is included in the community specialist practitioner pathway and enables the district nurse to prescribe from a limited formulary, providing it is within their area of competency (NMC 2008). This can be found in the BNF.

Nurse supplementary prescribing
A supplementary nurse prescriber is able to prescribe any medicine, e.g. licensed, unlicensed and controlled drugs, that has been voluntarily agreed with the patient and an independent prescriber, and has been documented in an individualised clinical management plan (DH 2005).

Nurse independent prescribing
Once trained and registered with the NMC or relevant professional body as an independent prescriber, a nurse or pharmacist working within their level of experience and competency may prescribe any licensed medication. For independent nurse prescribers this includes some controlled drugs for specific medical conditions (DH 2006b; BNF 2010).

Legal requirement for nurse prescribing training

To be legally eligible to become a prescriber a nurse must be a first level registered nurse or registered midwife with active NMC registration.

In addition, applicants for nurse prescribing are required to have:

- the ability to study at level 3 (degree level)
- a minimum of 3 years post-registration clinical nursing experience
- a medical supervisor, for example a general practitioner (GP), to contribute to and supervise the nurse's 12 days learning in practice element of the training
- confirmation from their employer that their post is one in which they: (a) will have the need and opportunity to prescribe; (b) will have access to a prescribing budget; and (c) will have access to continuing professional development opportunities on completion of the course.

(www.dh.gov.uk/nonmedicalprescribing)

Administration

The therapeutic benefit, in terms of expected clinical outcomes of drug administration, can be affected by a number of factors, including the following.

- **The timing of administration** To ensure that blood concentration level of the prescribed drug does not fall below or rise above the therapeutic range, potentially causing loss of disease control or drug toxicity, drugs must be administered in accordance with prescribing/dispensing instructions. This is particularly relevant for drugs with narrow therapeutic ranges, e.g. digoxin, insulin, anti-epileptics and warfarin.
- **Food/meal times** The absorption of some drugs is co-dependent on the level of gastric acidity, for example some drugs are destroyed by high levels of digestive enzymes and must be administered to the patient when they have an empty stomach (Dougherty & Lister 2011). Gastric irritant drugs should be administered with snacks or meals to prevent mucosal damage. Therefore the relationship between administration and ingestion of food must be accurate and consistent to ensure that blood plasma concentration levels remain constant and do not fluctuate (Schmidt & Dalhoff 2002). The incidence of interactions between drugs and food and herbs remains unknown; however, this type of

interaction is becoming increasingly recognised as an avoidable cause of both therapeutic failure and adverse drug reactions (Jordan *et al.* 2003).

- **Concomitant medication** Increased/decreased drug absorption, e.g. the anticoagulant effect of warfarin may be enhanced by the influenza vaccine (BNF 2007). Therapeutic failure can also occur as a result of poly pharmacy and co-administration of some drugs, including OTC medication and complementary therapies such as St Johns wort (Rang & Dale 2007; Bailey 2000; Chan 2002; BNF 2010).
- **Excipients** It is essential to be aware that excipients may differ between brands of the same drug. As a result of this, where a patient is prescribed or dispensed another brand or generic drug, disease control may be lost. For example modified release formulations, anti-epileptic drugs, lithium preparations and antipsychotic medications (Chappell 1993).

The relationship between clinical outcomes, patient safety, reduced risk of adverse reactions and the correct route of drug administration is also extremely important.

Oral tablets/capsules

Unless contraindicated, tablets and capsules should be administered with a full glass of water, where possible the patient should be sitting upright and remain upright for 30 minutes following administration (McKenry & Salerno 1998). Unless otherwise stated, tablets should not be chewed or crushed; similarly, the contents of capsules should not be removed for administration as this may alter the rate of release of the drug, destroy its properties or cause gastric irritation (Downie *et al.* 2000; Jevon *et al.* 2010). In circumstances where a patient experiences difficulty swallowing the prescribed drug the community nurse should seek advice from the community pharmacist and discuss alternative modes of administration with the prescriber (Table 8.2).

Injections

The mode in which the injection should be administered is normally pre-determined by factors relating to patient safety and the type, volume and therapeutic use of the drug being administered.

Injection sites should be systematically rotated to reduce the risk of localised irritation and ensure optimum absorption (Dougherty & Lister 2011). The site of injection, batch number and expiry date of the drug administered should be recorded in the relevant nursing documentation.

Table 8.2 Examples of routes for drug administration

Oral	Injection	Intravenous	Other
Tablet	Subcutaneous	Bolus	Rectal
Capsule	Intramuscular	Intermittent infusion	Vaginal
Liquid	Intradermal		Transdermal
Sub-lingual		Continuous infusion	Intranasal
			Auricular
			Ophthalmic
			Via enteral feeding tubes
			Inhalation
			Topical

Continuous subcutaneous (SC) infusion/fluids

This type of administration is not recommended for emergency rehydration but is suggested as having some beneficial effects in aiding the control of nausea and relieving the distressing symptoms of thirst for those patients receiving end of life care (Cerchietti *et al.* 2000; Dougherty & Lister 2011).

When selecting infusion devices, research evidence suggests that the use of, e.g. a plastic peripheral cannulae as opposed to a steel-winged infusion device, presents fewer complications that may result in the need for frequent resiting of the device (Dawkins *et al.* 2000). This may also enhance patient comfort (*see* Chapter 12).

Selection of the site for cannula placement should take the following into consideration.

- The patient's physical abilities – are they currently able to mobilise independently?
- The patient's mental state – do they have periods of agitation or are they confused?
- The importance of body image to the patient.
- The patient's and, where relevant, their carer's ability to recognise and take appropriate action if problems occur.

If there are no contraindications the recommended sites for cannulae placement are:

- the abdomen
- the anterior chest
- the lateral aspects of the upper arm
- the thigh.

If the patient is receiving drugs for symptom control at the same time as the infusion and is unable to tolerate oral medication or this route is ineffective, a syringe driver or pump is recommended (*see* Chapter 12).

Intravenous (IV) drug administration

With the shift to primary and community care closer to home, IV drug administration should be viewed as an integral part of the community nurse's role (DH 2002, 2005, 2006a, 2007). Nurses who undertake the administration of intravenous therapy should have undergone practical training and education in the following aspects:

- legal, professional and ethical issues
- related anatomy and physiology
- mathematical calculations related to medications
- pharmacology and pharmaceutics related to reconstitution and administration
- local and systemic complications
- infection control issues
- use of equipment, including infusion equipment
- drug administration
- risk management/health and safety
- care and management of vascular access devices.

(Hyde 2008; NPSA 2009; RCN 2010)

When administering drugs via the intravenous route the community nurse must adhere to the strict principles of aseptic technique and universal precautions throughout the procedure to prevent the risk of infection (Pratt *et al.* 2007). Each Trust should ensure that there are policies and procedures related to administration of IV therapy and the care and management of vascular access devices. For further details and guidelines *see* Chapter 7).

Diagnosis and management of anaphylaxis

What is anaphylaxis?

An anaphylactic reaction can vary in severity ranging from a mild response to a severe reaction and sometimes death. It can be triggered by a number of agents but most notably hypersensitivity following re-exposure to an antigen. The principal manifestation of the allergic response usually has a rapid onset.

Reducing the risk

A through patient assessment and comprehensive nursing documentation prior to drug administration will aid continuity of care and enable the community nurse to identify actual and potential problems associated with previous drug therapy (NMC 2002).

Assessment of the potential for anaphylactic reaction can also be enhanced by the community nurse asking key questions such as the following.

- Have you ever been diagnosed or suffered from hay fever, asthma or skin conditions?
- Have you ever reacted to insect bites or stings or any drugs including injections? (If possible ascertain the name of the drug or what the patient was being treated for.)
- Are you allergic to any foods? (Influenza vaccine is contraindicated in those patients with an allergy to eggs because it is grown using chick embryos [BNF 2010].)
- Are you currently taking any prescribed or OTC medication?
- Are you allergic to anything?

If there is any doubt or uncertainty regarding a patient's allergy status or any identified contraindications, the community nurse should, in the interest of patient safety, withhold administration of the prescribed drug, seek further information from the GP and immediately record the rationale for this in the nursing documentation (NMC 2002, 2004, 2007a).

Recognition and treatment of the signs and symptoms of anaphylactic reaction

The clinical signs and symptoms of anaphylaxis very rarely occur in isolation; however, due to other clinical conditions manifesting in a similar manner, diagnosis can sometimes be problematic (Table 8.3).

Anaphylaxis is life threatening, therefore if there is any doubt about the diagnosis the community nurse should explain what is happening to the patient and reassure them and any carers that may be present. Treatment should be commenced immediately and where indicated include the administration of adrenaline (epinephrine). The recommended dose of adrenaline (epinephrine) should be repeated every 5 minutes until the patient shows signs of improvement and further help arrives (Table 8.4).

The recommended route for administration of adrenaline (epinephrine) in adults is by intramuscular (IM) injection in the middle third of the anterolateral thigh. If previous administration of a SC or IM injection is considered to be the cause of the reaction, adrenaline (epinephrine) should not be injected into the same limb as local vaso-constriction may result in poor absorption. If necessary, administration can occur straight through clothing (Resuscitation Council (UK) 2008).

If the patient's condition necessitates, basic life support should be initiated while waiting for emergency

Table 8.3 Signs and symptoms of anaphylaxis and vaso-vagal reaction (Resuscitation Council [UK] 2005)

Signs and symptoms	Vaso-vagal reaction	Anaphylaxis
Dizziness, weakness, collapse	Present	Present
Tachycardia, weak pulse	Present	Present
Pruritus. Possible sneezing, rhinorrhoea, lacrimation, nasal congestion	Absent	Present
Hoarseness. Possible stridor, cough, dyspnoea, tachypnoea, angioedema, e.g. lips, face and tongue	Absent	Present
Possible airway obstruction, cyanosis	Absent	Present
Erythema, flushing, urticaria	Absent	Present
Pallor, pale, clammy	Present	Absent
Hypotension	Present	Present

Table 8.4 Adrenaline (epinephrine) doses for the treatment of anaphylaxis (Resuscitation Council [UK] 2005)

Age	Epinephrine dose, volume of 1:1000 (1 mg/ml)
Less than 6 months	150 µg IM (0.15 ml)
6 months to 6 years	150 µg IM (0.15 l)
6–12 years	300 µg IM (0.3 ml)
Above 12 years	500 µg IM (0.5 ml)
	NB 300 µg should be given if a child is prepubertal or small

Caution

Patients being treated with non-cardioselective beta-blockers may not respond to adrenaline (epinephrine).

Patients being treated with tricyclic antidepressants may require a reduced dose of adrenaline (epinephrine).

British National Formulary (2010)

services to arrive (Figure 8.2) (Resuscitation Council (UK) 2008).

It is recommended that all community nurses administering medication:

- are fully trained and up to date in the treatment of anaphylaxis and basic life support
- are fully aware of relevant Trust policies and procedures
- are able to call for additional help/emergency services, e.g. are provided with a mobile telephone
- carry an in date anaphylaxis pack.

The pack should include:

- adrenaline (epinephrine) 1:1000 and a dosage guide
- appropriate needles and syringes

- all equipment necessary for basic life support to be initiated and maintained until help arrives.

When administering adrenaline (epinephrine) for the emergency treatment of anaphylaxis the recommended route is IM using a 25 mm (25 gauge/orange) needle. For larger adults a 38 mm (21 gauge/green) may be used to ensure muscle penetration (Resuscitation Council (UK) 2008).

NB Although adrenaline (epinephrine) is a prescription-only medicine it is exempt from the Medicines Act (1968) when administered for life-saving purposes.

Post-treatment management

In all cases of anaphylactic reactions there is a potential risk, following initial treatment, that acute symptoms may reoccur and further treatment could be necessary. Therefore all patients must be transferred to hospital by ambulance for observation. The community nurse should discuss the incident and any necessary follow-up care, post hospital discharge, with the patient's GP.

Documentation

The treatment and management of all actual and suspected anaphylactic reactions must be recorded in accordance with local policy and in the nursing documentation, and should include the following.

- All relevant patient history obtained prior to treatment – including documenting the source of the information.
- Date and time of event.
- Trigger factor(s) if known.
- The condition of the patient on initial presentation.
- Any treatment carried out, including drugs that were administered, the route, time and where relevant the site of administration.

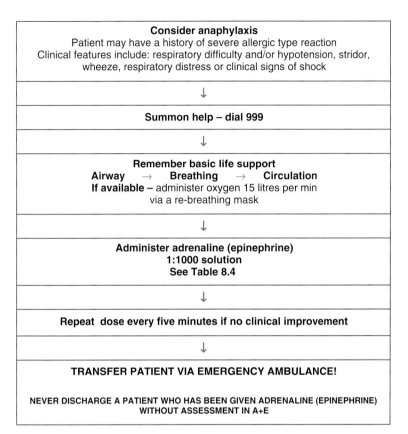

Figure 8.2 Anaphylactic reactions in adults – treatment by the first clinical respondent (Resuscitation Council UK 2008)

- The batch numbers, pack supplier and expiry dates of all drugs administered.
- All observations made during treatment.
- The condition of the patient on transfer to another care provider, e.g. emergency care practitioner, paramedics.
- Full written details (as above) of all drugs administered by the emergency services prior to the patient being transferred to hospital.
- Where the patient was transferred to and the time of transfer.
- Full details of all staff present for all/part of the incident.
- Information supplied to the patient's GP.

All adverse drug reactions should be reported using the Yellow Card system in the current BNF (NMC 2010).

Advice to patients

Patients with a known allergy should be offered information regarding the medic-alert system, and the community nurse should discuss with them the benefit of wearing a medic-alert bracelet/neck chain. Where the causative allergen has not been confirmed the patient should be advised that as far as practically possible, the suspected allergen should be avoided.

Conclusion

Medicines management within the community environment emphasises the importance that administration should not be viewed in isolation of the psychological and emotional benefits to patients. For many patients and their carers successful medicines administration and management by community nurses' extends far beyond expected therapeutic outcomes. For example:

- it facilitates and supports the patient's choice to remain in their own home if they wish
- it enables the patient to remain as independent as possible

- it enables the patient to work in partnership with the community nurse, GP and allied healthcare professionals involved in their care and to have increased involvement in decision making regarding current and future care/treatment needs
- it facilitates and supports planned early discharge from hospital
- it reduces the risk of unplanned hospital admission for those with long-term conditions, especially respiratory conditions, by, for example, the development of integrated multidisciplinary team care management plans that incorporate the provision

and supply of pre-emptory medication for use during periods of exacerbation
- it respects the wishes of patients and their carers in their request to receive end of life care in their own home.

To achieve safe and successful medicines management the community nurse, working in partnership with the patient, GP, primary healthcare team and other colleagues, must exercise accountability and professional judgement, and at all times apply knowledge and skill (NMC 2010).

Procedure guideline 8.1 **Guideline for self-administration of medication**

Equipment

Relevant nursing documentation
Prescribed medication
Aids to support self-medication (where appropriate)

Nursing action	Rationale
1 Obtain a full, current, patient medication history from the GP	To ensure an accurate record of all prescribed medication is available for the first assessment visit
2 Carry out and record a full medication review and evaluation of effectiveness with the patient. Where necessary this should include asking the patient to present all of the medication they are currently taking including OTC and dietary supplements	If there have been frequent changes to the patient's prescription they may still be in possession of a number of unnecessary medications that could potentially be used inappropriately
	To maintain patient safety by enabling the community nurse to advise/arrange for the safe disposal of out-of-date or inappropriate medication
3 Carry out and document a full nursing assessment of the patient's ability to self-medicate, this should include for example the patient's: (a) allergy status (b) willingness and ability to participate in self-care (c) understanding of their drug regimen, e.g. what the medication is for and potential side effects, dosage and time of administration (d) ability to accurately use medication aids and equipment, e.g. oral inhalers/spacer, insulin pens, blister pack (e) mental capacity, e.g. are they confused/forgetful (f) physical ability, e.g. are they able to open the containers (g) preferred language and eyesight, e.g. are they able to read the container labels (h) current presenting symptoms	To maintain patient safety and identify actual and potential problems that may inhibit safe, accurate self administration To assess the need for medication aids or, e.g. alternative containers or labelling that will enable the patient to participate in self-care and improve independence To identify and address any additional learning/teaching needs that the patient may have. To enhance concordance and independence To enable the community nurse to share information regarding the prescribed drug regimen To enable the community nurse to identify where additional support or monitoring is necessary to ensure that the patient receives their prescribed medication To enable the community nurse to evaluate the effectiveness of ongoing treatment To aid the development of an appropriate care plan

Procedure guideline 8.1 **Guideline for self-administration of medication** *(cont'd)*

Nursing action	Rationale
4 Discuss with the patient and document systems that they have in place for obtaining any necessary repeat prescriptions and dispensed medication	To prevent disruption to treatment and where necessary enable the community nurse to negotiate a collection and delivery service with the local community pharmacist
5 Where necessary liaise and discuss the patient's drug regimen with the GP or, in the case of medication dispensed on hospital discharge, the prescribing hospital doctor	To explore and discuss potential changes to the prescribed regimen that would make it less complicated for the patient to self-administer or reduce the number of community nurse visits, e.g. converting Oramorph to morphine sulphate tablets (*see* Chapter 12)

Procedure guideline 8.2 **Guideline for oral drug administration**

Unless otherwise stated, tablets should not be chewed or crushed; similarly the contents of capsules should not be removed for administration as this may alter the rate of release of the drug, destroy its properties or cause gastric irritation (Downie *et al.* 2000; Jevon *et al.* 2010) (For more information see Administration).

Equipment

Record of administration chart and nursing documentation
Prescribed medication

Nursing action	Rationale
1 Where appropriate facilities are available wash hands. Alternatively cleanse hands with antibactericidal alcoholic hand rub and apply disposable apron	To prevent the risk of cross-infection/contamination
2 Read nursing documentation, care plan and administration chart Explain and discuss the prescribed treatment with the patient	To update previous knowledge and maintain patient safety, e.g. last date and time of administration, duration of treatment and allergy status To prevent duplication of treatment and maintain patient safety To enable the patient time to give feedback regarding existing or new symptoms and express any concerns they may have To enable the community nurse to evaluate the effectiveness of ongoing treatment To provide patient education and information regarding the prescribed treatment To obtain patient consent (Mental Capacity Act 2007)
3 Check prescribed drug against administration record	To ensure that the correct patient receives: (a) the correct drug (b) the correct dose and strength (c) at the correct time (d) via the correct route
4 Identify and select all of the medication to be administered and check the expiry date/s	To ensure patient safety and efficacy of treatment

(Continued)

Procedure guideline 8.2 **Guideline for oral drug administration** *(cont'd)*

Nursing action	Rationale
5 Cleanse hands with antibactericidal alcoholic hand rub	To prevent the risk of cross-infection
6 Gently shake the required dose into the container cap or pour the liquid into a measured medicine pot and give to the patient to take with, e.g. a glass of water Pour liquid into a measured medicine pot or spoon Offer assistance where necessary	To ensure that the patient receives the correct medication as prescribed and to minimise the risk of contamination
7 Place sub-lingual tablets under the patient's tongue and buccal tablets between the patient's gum and cheek	To ensure correct administration route and rate of absorption
8 Following administration wash or cleanse hands as in step 1 above, remove and appropriately dispose of apron (*see* Chapter 6)	To prevent the risk of cross-infection and contamination
9 Record relevant information on the drug administration chart and patient records	To avoid potential duplication of treatment and maintain patient safety To ensure continuity of care To ensure accurate and contemporaneous records are kept To reduce the risk of drug errors Documentation should provide clear evidence of care planned

Procedure guideline 8.3 **Guideline for reconstitution/preparation of drugs for injection**

Ampoule – powder

Equipment

Syringes – various sizes
Needles – various sizes
Single use sterile gloves
Alcohol swabs
Sharps bin
Record of administration chart and nursing documentation
Prescribed medication
Dilutent (where appropriate)
Sterile gauze

Nursing action	Rationale
1 Where appropriate facilities are available wash hands. Alternatively cleanse hands with antibactericidal alcoholic hand rub apply disposable apron	To prevent the risk of cross-infection/contamination
2 Check the details of the dispensed drug with the record of administration chart	To ensure patient and staff safety

Procedure guideline 8.3 **Guideline for reconstitution/preparation of drugs for injection** *(cont'd)*

Nursing action	Rationale
3 Prepare a clean area for drug preparation, e.g. table/worktop with a disposable tray	To minimise the risk of infection and prevent cross-contamination
4 Collect and assemble all necessary equipment and visually inspect packaging. Discard any equipment that is damaged, where sterile seals are broken or dates have expired	To maintain patient safety To prevent disruption to the procedure
5 Check expiry dates on all drugs to be administered, including the diluent to be used for reconstitution	To ensure patient safety
6 Gently tap the neck of the drug and diluent ampoules	To dislodge any powder/fluid that may have accumulated
7 Using a sterile gauze swab cover the individual neck of the ampoules, gently apply pressure to snap it open	To prevent injury and the risk of contamination
8 Draw up correct amount of diluent	To ensure that the patient receives the correct dose and strength of drug
9 Slowly inject the diluent into the ampoule containing the drug powder then gently agitate the ampoule	To thoroughly dissolve the powder and maintain safety by preventing the release of the powder into the atmosphere
10 Visually inspect the contents of the ampoule	To identify the presence of particulate matter or glass fragments and precipitation. **If present discard in accordance with health and safety regulations and locally agreed policy and recommence procedure**
11 When the solution is thoroughly dissolved/clear withdraw the prescribed amount	To maintain patient safety
12 Expel air bubbles from the syringe by replacing the needle sheath and tapping gently to dislodge	To ensure that the correct amount of drug has been drawn up and to prevent aerosol formation
13 Discard used needle into sharps bin, remove apron and cleanse hands as in step 1 above	To prevent the risk of cross-contamination and injury to the nurse and others, e.g. carers, children and refuse collectors
Proceed with administration using correct gauge needle	To ensure correct administration route and rate of absorption and reduce the risk of increased patient discomfort

Ampoule – solution For list of equipment see Ampoule – powder

Nursing action	Rationale
1 Where appropriate facilities are available wash hands. Alternatively cleanse hands with antibactericidal alcoholic hand rub and apply disposable apron	To prevent the risk of cross-infection/contamination
2 Visually inspect the solution for particulate matter/cloudiness. **If present discard in accordance with health and safety regulations and locally agreed policy**	To maintain the safety of patient and others safety
3 Check the details of the dispensed drug with the record of administration chart	To ensure patient and staff safety

189

(Continued)

Procedure guideline 8.3 **Guideline for reconstitution/preparation of drugs for injection** *(cont'd)*

Nursing action	Rationale
4 Prepare a clean area for drug preparation, e.g. table/worktop with a disposable tray	To minimise the risk of infection and prevent cross-contamination
5 Collect and assemble all necessary equipment and visually inspect packaging. Discard any equipment that is damaged, where sterile seals are broken or dates have expired	To maintain patient safety To prevent disruption to the procedure
6 Check expiry dates on all drugs to be administered	To ensure patient safety
7 Gently tap the neck of the ampoule	To dislodge any fluid that may have accumulated
8 Using a sterile gauze swab cover the neck of the ampoule, gently apply pressure to snap it open	To prevent injury and the risk of contamination
9 Visually inspect the contents of the ampoule	To identify the presence of glass fragments. **If present discard in accordance with health and safety regulations and locally agreed policy and recommence procedure**
10 Withdraw the prescribed amount	To ensure that the patient receives the correct drug dose
11 Expel air bubbles from the syringe by replacing the needle sheath and tapping gently to dislodge	To ensure that the correct amount of drug has been drawn up and to prevent aerosol formation
12 Discard used needle into sharps bin, remove apron and cleanse hands as in step 1 above. Proceed with administration using correct gauge needle	To prevent the risk of cross contamination and injury to the nurse and others, e.g. carers, children and refuse collectors To ensure correct administration route and rate of absorption and reduce the risk of increased patient discomfort

Single/multi-dose vial – powder For list of equipment see ampoule – powder

Nursing action	Rationale
1 Where appropriate facilities are available wash hands. Alternatively cleanse hands with antibactericidal alcoholic hand rub apply disposable apron	To prevent the risk of cross-infection/contamination
2 Check the details of the dispensed drug with the record of administration chart	To ensure patient and staff safety
3 Prepare a clean area for drug preparation, e.g. table/worktop with a disposable tray	To minimise the risk of infection and prevent cross-contamination
4 Collect and assemble all necessary equipment and visually inspect packaging. Discard any equipment that is damaged, where sterile seals are broken or dates have expired	To maintain patient safety To prevent disruption to the procedure
5 Check expiry dates on all drugs to be administered, including the diluent to be used for reconstitution	To ensure patient safety
6 Clean the rubber cap with an alcohol swab and allow to air dry	To prevent contamination

Procedure guideline 8.3 **Guideline for reconstitution/preparation of drugs for injection** *(cont'd)*

Nursing action	Rationale
7 Vent the vial by inserting a needle through the rubber cap, bevel up at a 45 to 60° angle	To prevent back pressure that may cause separation of the needle from the syringe and minimise the risk of coring
Draw up the correct amount of diluent	To ensure that the patient receives the correct dose and strength of drug
8 Slowly inject the diluent into the vial containing the drug powder	To thoroughly wet the powder
9 Remove the needle and syringe and discard	To enable the vial to be safely agitated
Apply sterile gloves, place a sterile gauze swab over the venting needle and gently agitate the vial	To maintain nurse safety, prevent release of the drug into the atmosphere and ensure that the drug powder is thoroughly dissolved
10 Visually inspect the contents of the vial	To identify the presence of particulate matter and precipitation. **If present discard in accordance with health and safety regulations and locally agreed policy and recommence procedure**
11 Clean the rubber cap with an alcohol swab and allow to air dry	To prevent contamination
12 Withdraw the prescribed amount	To ensure that the patient receives the correct drug dose
13 Expel air bubbles from the syringe by replacing the needle sheath and tapping gently to dislodge	To ensure that the correct amount of drug has been drawn up and to prevent aerosol formation
14 Discard used needle into sharps bin, remove gloves, and cleanse hands as in step 1 above	To prevent the risk of cross-contamination and injury to the nurse and others, e.g. carers, children and refuse collectors
Proceed with administration using correct gauge needle	To ensure correct administration route and rate of absorption and reduce the risk of increased patient discomfort

Procedure guideline 8.4 **Guideline for administration of subcutaneous and intramuscular injections**

Pre-administration procedure

- **Nursing documentation** – The community nurse should update themself on the patient's progress to date and any actual/potential problems that may have arisen during or following previous administration. This will also enable the community nurse to confirm: (a) the patient's care plan; (b) the last date and time of administration; and (c) the duration of the prescribed treatment.
- **Drug/s to be administered** – The community nurse should make a visual inspection of the packaging to ensure it is not damaged, and the drug to check for, e.g. precipitation. The drug should be clearly labelled with: (a) the name and contact details of the dispensing pharmacist; (b) the name of the drug, strength and date dispensed; (c) the patient's name; and (d) the dose, route and frequency of administration and, where relevant, appropriate information regarding the diluent to be used for reconstitution.
- **Drug administration chart/record** – To maintain patient and staff safety the chart should include: (a) the patient's full name and date of birth; (b) all known and potential allergies; (c) the name of the drug/s to be administered; (d) the dose, route and method of administration; (e) the duration of treatment; and (f) a clear record/history of previous administration. The community nurse should check this information against the dispensed drug/s to ensure it is correct; any anomalies must be clarified.

(Continued)

Procedure guideline 8.4 *Guideline for administration of subcutaneous and intramuscular injections* (cont'd)

Equipment

Patient nursing records and drug administration chart/record
Insulin administration chart/record clearly identifying the dose to be administered in units
Drug/s to be administered
Correct diluent (where required)
Syringe/s appropriate to the volume of drug to be administered
21G needle/s for reconstitution and drawing up (where relevant)
Appropriate needle/s, e.g. 21, 23 or 25G, depending on the size of the patient
Insulin syringe marked in units or international units (NPSA 2011a)
Sterile alcohol swabs
Sterile gauze swabs
Protective clothing/equipment according to health and safety regulations, e.g. disposable apron and gloves
    (see Chapter 6)
Sharps bin

Subcutaneous injection

Nursing action	Rationale
1 Where appropriate facilities are available wash hands. Alternatively cleanse hands with antibactericidal alcoholic hand rub	To prevent the risk of cross-infection/contamination
2 Read nursing documentation, care plan and administration chart ■ Explain and discuss the procedure with the patient and establish if they have any known or potential allergies ■ Where new actual or potential allergies are identified this must be recorded in the nursing documentation and administration chart record	To update knowledge of the patient and prevent potential duplication of treatment To enable the patient time to give feedback regarding previous administration and express any concerns they may have To enable the community nurse to evaluate the effectiveness of ongoing treatment To maintain patient safety To provide patient education and information regarding the prescribed treatment To obtain patient consent (Mental Capacity Act 2007)
3 Prepare a clean area for drug preparation, e.g. table/worktop with a disposable tray	To minimise the risk of infection and prevent cross-contamination
4 Collect all necessary equipment and visually inspect packaging. Discard any equipment that is damaged, where sterile seals are broken or dates have expired	To prevent disruption to the procedure To maintain patient safety
5 Check expiry dates on all drugs to be administered and where relevant, diluent to be used for reconstitution	To ensure patient safety
6 Cleanse hands with antibactericidal alcoholic hand rub and apply disposable apron	To prevent the risk of cross-infection
7 Open and assemble all equipment and draw up drug/s to be administered in the correct dose, volume and where appropriate dilution	To prevent disruption to the procedure To maintain patient safety and ensure that the correct dose of medication is administered

Procedure guideline 8.4 **Guideline for administration of subcutaneous and intramuscular injections** *(cont'd)*

Nursing action	Rationale
8 Discuss the potential site/s for administration with the patient, where necessary reiterating the need for site rotation **NB** Thigh and buttocks are the recommended sites for intermediate acting insulin and the abdomen for soluble human insulin (Trend UK 2010)	To enable the patient to be involved in decision making and state preference To ensure maximum drug absorption
9 Assist the patient into a safe appropriate position	To ensure patient safety and comfort and access to the injection site
10 Expose the site of administration, where necessary use a blanket/towel to cover the patient	To enable ease of access to the injection site and maintain patient dignity
11 Cleanse hands with antibactericidal alcoholic hand rub	To prevent the risk of cross-infection
12 Expose the injection site and cleanse the skin with a sterile 70% alcohol swab and allow to air dry	To reduce the amount of pathogens present in the skin flora that may be introduced further into skin layers through needle insertion To prevent the stinging sensation sometimes associated with needle insertion and ensure disinfection of the skin
13 Using the non-dominant hand, form a fold by gently pinching the skin between your thumb and index finger **NB** When administering insulin, formation of a skin fold may not be necessary with 4 mm needles but may be indicated where the patient is slim	To lift tissue away from muscle and ensure that needle insertion is into subcutaneous tissue To prevent the possible risk of intra-muscular administration (Trend, 2011)
14 Insert the needle into the skin fold at a 45° angle quickly in one smooth motion. Release the skin fold and inject the drug slowly When administering insulin, needle insertion should be at a 90° angle when using needles that are 4, 5 or 6 mm in length (Diabetes in the UK 2011)	To ensure correct administration route and rate of absorption and reduce the risk of increased patient discomfort Shorter needles are used on insulin syringes and pens (Trounce & Gould 2000)
15 Withdraw the needle quickly and apply direct pressure to puncture site with sterile gauze	To stem any slight bleeding that may occur and prevent the development of haematoma formation at the injection site
16 Place sharps immediately into sharps bin. **Do not re-sheath needle**	To prevent needlestick injury and the risk of contracting blood-borne infection
17 Assist the patient into a comfortable position and where relevant to dress or adjust clothing	To maintain patient dignity and comfort
18 Dispose of all used equipment in accordance with health and safety regulations and locally agreed policy (*see* Chapter 6)	To prevent the risk of cross-infection and injury to the nurse and others, e.g. carers, children and refuse collectors
19 Remove and appropriately dispose of apron. Where appropriate facilities are available wash hands. Alternatively cleanse hands with antibactericidal alcoholic hand rub	To prevent the risk of cross-infection

(Continued)

Procedure guideline 8.4 **Guideline for administration of subcutaneous and intramuscular injections** *(cont'd)*

Nursing action	Rationale
20 Record relevant information on the drug administration chart and in the patient's records, e.g. the date, time and dose, site of medication administration, batch number and expiry date of drug. Also where relevant the type, amount and expiry date of diluent used and any additional relevant information	To maintain patient safety through the completion of contemporaneous accurate record keeping (NMC, 2005)
	When units are abbreviated as 'U' it could be mistaken as a zero, this could lead to a higher/dangerous dose of insulin being administered (NPSA 2011a)
When transcribing or recording the dose or administration of insulin abbreviations must not be used, i.e. 'U' to indicate the units this must be written in full, i.e. 'Units'	

NB Where single nurse administration is not practised, the community nurse who has prepared the drug should be the administering nurse (NMC 2010)

Intramuscular injection

Nursing action	Rationale
1 Where appropriate facilities are available wash hands. Alternatively cleanse hands with antibactericidal alcoholic hand rub	To prevent the risk of cross-infection/contamination
2 Read nursing documentation, care plan and administration chart	To update knowledge of the patient and prevent potential duplication of treatment
■ Explain and discuss the procedure with the patient and establish if they have any known or potential allergies	To enable the patient time to give feedback regarding previous administration and express any concerns they may have
■ Where new actual or potential allergies are identified this must be recorded in the nursing documentation and administration chart	To enable the community nurse to evaluate the effectiveness of on going treatment
	To maintain patient safety
	To provide patient education and information regarding the prescribed treatment
	To obtain patient consent (Mental Capacity Act 2007)
3 Prepare a clean area for drug preparation, e.g. table/worktop with a disposable tray	To minimise the risk of infection and prevent cross-contamination
4 Collect all necessary equipment and visually inspect packaging. Discard any equipment that is damaged, where sterile seals are broken or dates have expired	To prevent disruption to the procedure
	To maintain patient safety
5 Check expiry dates on all drugs to be administered and where relevant, diluent to be used for reconstitution	To ensure patient safety
6 Cleanse hands with antibactericidal alcoholic hand rub and apply disposable apron	To prevent the risk of cross-infection

Procedure guideline 8.4 **Guideline for administration of subcutaneous and intramuscular injections** *(cont'd)*

Nursing action	Rationale
7 Open and assemble all equipment and draw up drug/s to be administered in the correct dose, volume and where appropriate dilution	To prevent disruption to the procedure To maintain patient safety and ensure that the correct dose of medication is administered
8 Discuss the potential site/s for administration with the patient, where necessary reiterating the need for site rotation	To enable the patient to be involved in decision making and state preference To ensure maximum drug absorption
9 Assist the patient into a safe appropriate position	To ensure patient safety and comfort and access to the injection site
10 Expose the site of administration, where necessary use a blanket/towel to cover the patient	To enable ease of access to the injection site and maintain patient dignity
11 Wash or cleanse hands as in step 1 above	To prevent the risk of infection
12 Expose the injection site and cleanse the skin with a sterile 70% alcohol swab and allow to air dry	To reduce the amount of pathogens present in the skin flora that may be introduced further into skin layers through needle insertion To prevent the stinging sensation sometimes associated with needle insertion and ensure disinfection of the skin
13 Using the non-dominant hand spread the skin at the injection site	To move underlying subcutaneous tissue
14 With one quick motion insert the needle at a 90° angle	To ensure that the needle penetrates through any underlying subcutaneous tissue into the muscle To ensure correct administration route and rate of absorption and reduce the risk of increased patient discomfort
15 Draw back syringe plunger to check for blood aspiration; if blood is not present slowly depress plunger to administer drug. If blood appears, withdraw the needle, replace contaminated equipment and commence procedure again Discuss and explain what has happened to the patient	To maintain patient safety by confirming that the needle is correctly placed and not, for example, in a vein, confirmed by the observation of blood at the needle hub To address any concerns they may have and obtain consent to continue with the procedure
16 Allow the needle to remain in situ for approximately 10 seconds before withdrawing	To prevent drug leakage through puncture site and facilitate dispersion into muscle
17 Withdraw the needle quickly and apply direct pressure to puncture site with sterile gauze	To stem any slight bleeding that may occur and prevent the development of haematoma formation at the injection site
18 Place sharps into sharps bin immediately. **Do not re-sheath needle**	To prevent needlestick injury and the risk of contracting blood-borne infection
19 Assist the patient into a comfortable position and where relevant to dress or adjust clothing	To maintain patient dignity and comfort
20 Dispose of all used equipment in accordance with health and safety regulations and locally agreed policy (*see* Chapter 6)	To prevent the risk of cross-infection and injury to the nurse and others, e.g. carers, children and refuse collectors

195

(Continued)

Procedure guideline 8.4 *Guideline for administration of subcutaneous and intramuscular injections* (cont'd)

Nursing action	Rationale
21 Remove disposable apron, where appropriate facilities are available wash hands. Alternatively cleanse hands with antibactericidal alcoholic hand rub	To prevent the risk of cross-infection
22 Record relevant information on the drug administration chart and also in the patient's records, e.g. the date, time and dose, site of medication administration, batch number and expiry date of drug. Also where relevant the, type, amount and expiry date of diluent used and any additional relevant information	To maintain patient safety through the completion of contemporaneous accurate record keeping (NMC 2005)

NB Where single nurse administration is not practised the community nurse who has prepared the drug should be the administering nurse (NMC 2010)

Procedure guideline 8.5 **Guideline for instillation of eye drops and eye ointment**

Equipment

Record of administration chart and nursing documentation
Prescribed eye drops/ointment
Sterile gauze swabs
0.9% sterile sodium chloride or sterile water
Disposable apron
Sterile gloves (where relevant)

Eye drops

Nursing action	Rationale
1 Where appropriate facilities are available wash hands. Alternatively cleanse hands with antibactericidal alcoholic hand rub and apply disposable apron	To prevent the risk of cross-infection/contamination
2 Read nursing documentation, care plan and administration chart Explain and discuss the procedure with the patient	To update previous knowledge and maintain patient safety, e.g. last date and time of administration, duration of treatment and allergy status To prevent duplication of treatment To enable the patient time to give feedback regarding previous administration and express any concerns they may have To enable the community nurse to evaluate the effectiveness of ongoing treatment To provide patient education and information regarding the prescribed treatment To obtain patient consent (Mental Capacity Act 2007)

*Procedure guideline 8.5 **Guideline for instillation of eye drops and eye ointment** (cont'd)*

Nursing action	Rationale
3 Collect all necessary equipment and visually inspect packaging. Discard any equipment that is damaged, where sterile seals are broken or dates have expired	To maintain patient safety
4 Check expiry date on eye drop bottle and date of first opening recorded by community nursing staff, discard in accordance with manufacturers instructions	To ensure patient safety
5 Cleanse hands with alcohol-based hand rub	To prevent the risk of cross-infection/contamination
6 If the patient has undergone eye surgery or suffered a traumatic eye injury the procedure should be carried out using a strict aseptic technique	Infection may lead to loss of sight/eye
7 Assist the patient into a safe appropriate position, i.e. sitting with head tilted backwards or lying down	To ensure patient safety and comfort and ease of access to the eye To reduce the risk of excess solution running down the patients face
8 If discharge is present the eye area should be first cleansed with the eye closed. Apply single-use gloves and cleanse with a moistened gauze swab, starting from the nose outwards using one motion. Ask the patient to open their eye and look upward to gently cleanse the lower lid and downward to cleanse the upper lid dry thoroughly (see Chapter 11) Using a new swab each time repeat as necessary	To reduce the risk of corneal damage To reduce the risk of cross-infection, e.g. to other eye To prevent the reintroduction of debris back into the eye and reduce the risk of cross infection Debris may inactivate the drug (Watkinson & Seewoodhary 2007)
9 Remove and dispose of gloves and cleanse hands with alcohol-based hand rub	To prevent the risk of cross-infection/contamination
10 Using a slightly moistened gauze swab against the lower lid margin, gently pull down to expose the upper rim of the inferior fornix, ask the patient to look upward and instil the prescribed number of drops	To open the eye and ensure the correct dose and route of administration. To reduce the risk of the patient blinking during instillation of the eye drop
11 Ask the patient to close their eye immediately following instillation and remove excess solution with gauze swab	To facilitate solution absorption and aid patient comfort
12 Assist the patient to readjust their position	Assist the patient to readjust their position
13 Remove and dispose of all used equipment in accordance with health and safety regulations and locally agreed policy (see Chapter 6)	To reduce the risk of cross-infection
14 Remove apron and dispose of it; where appropriate facilities are available wash hands. Alternatively cleanse hands with antibactericidal alcoholic hand rub	To prevent the risk of cross-infection/contamination
15 Record relevant information on the drug administration chart and patient records	To avoid potential duplication of treatment and maintain patient safety

Procedure guideline 8.5 **Guideline for instillation of eye drops and eye ointment** *(cont'd)*

Eye ointment

Nursing action	Rationale
1 Where appropriate facilities are available wash hands. Alternatively cleanse hands with antibactericidal alcoholic hand rub and apply disposable apron	To prevent the risk of cross-infection/contamination
2 Read nursing documentation, care plan and administration chart Explain and discuss the procedure with the patient	To update previous knowledge and maintain patient safety, e.g. last date and time of administration, duration of treatment and allergy status To prevent duplication of treatment To enable the patient time to give feedback regarding previous administration and express any concerns they may have To enable the community nurse to evaluate the effectiveness of on going treatment To provide patient education and information regarding the prescribed treatment To obtain patient consent (Mental Capacity Act 2007)
3 Collect all necessary equipment and visually inspect packaging. Discard any equipment that is damaged, where sterile seals are broken or dates have expired	To maintain patient safety
4 Check expiry date on ointment tube and date of first opening recorded by community nursing staff, discard in accordance with manufacturers instructions	To ensure patient safety
5 Wash or cleanse hands as in step 1 above	To prevent the risk of cross-infection/contamination
6 If the patient has undergone eye surgery or suffered a traumatic eye injury the procedure should be carried out using a strict aseptic technique	Infection may lead to loss of sight/eye
7 Assist the patient into a safe appropriate position, i.e. sitting with head tilted backwards or lying down	To ensure patient safety and comfort and ease of access to the eye To reduce the risk of excess solution running down the patients face
8 If discharge is present the eye area should be first cleansed with the eye closed. Cleanse with a moistened gauze swab starting from the nose outwards using one motion. Ask the patient to open their eye and look upward to gently cleanse the lower lid and downward to cleanse the upper lid dry thoroughly Using a new swab each time repeat as necessary	To reduce the risk of corneal damage To reduce the risk of cross-infection, e.g. to other eye To prevent the reintroduction of debris back into the eye and reduce the risk of cross infection Debris may inactivate the drug (Watkinson & Seewoodhary 2007)
9 Cleanse hands as in step 1 above	To prevent the risk of cross-infection/contamination

Procedure guideline 8.5 **Guideline for instillation of eye drops and eye ointment** *(cont'd)*

Nursing action	Rationale
10 Using a slightly moistened gauze swab against the lower lid margin, gently pull down to expose the upper rim of the inferior fornix, ask the patient to look upwards	To open the eye and reduce the risk of the patient blinking during instillation of the ointment
11 Apply the ointment to the lower eyelid by holding the tube approximately 2 cm above the eye and placing a line of ointment starting from the nose outwards	To prevent the risk of corneal damage and ensure the correct route of administration To reduce the risk of cross-infection
12 Ask the patient to close their eye immediately following instillation, remove excess ointment with gauze swab	To facilitate absorption and aid patient comfort
13 Assist the patient to readjust their position	Assist the patient to readjust their position
14 Remove and dispose of all used equipment in accordance with health and safety regulations and locally agreed policy	To reduce the risk of cross-infection
15 Cleanse hands as in point 1 above remove apron	To prevent the risk of cross-infection/contamination
16 Record relevant information on the drug administration chart and patient records	To avoid potential duplication of treatment and maintain patient safety

199

References and further reading

Audit Commission (2002) *A Spoonful of Sugar – Medicines Management in NHS Hospitals.* Audit Commission, London.

Bailey D (2000) Grapefruit-felodipine interaction: effect of unprocessed fruit and probable active ingredients. *Clinical Pharmacology and Therapeutics* **68**(5): 468–77.

Baird A (2004) Recent developments in prescribing. *Journal of Community Nursing* **18**(3).

Beijer HJ, de Blaey CJ (2002) Hospitalisations caused by adverse drug reactions, a meta-analysis of observational studies. *Pharmacy World and Science* **24**(2): 46–54.

British National Formulary 60 (2010) British Medical Association & Royal Pharmaceutical Society of Great Britain, London.

Cable S, Lumsdaine J, Semple M (2003) Informed consent. *Nursing Standard* **18**(12): 47–55.

Cerchietti L, Navigante A, Sauri, Palazzo F (2000) Hypodermoclysis for control of dehydration in terminal stage cancer. *International Journal of Palliative Nursing* **6**(8): 370–4.

Chadwick C, Forbes A (1996) Pharmaceutical problems for the nutrition team pharmacist. *The Hospital Pharmacist* **3**(6): 139–43.

Chappell B (1993) Implications of switching antiepileptic drugs. *Prescriber* **4**(18): 37–8.

Chan L (2002) Drug-nutrient interaction in clinical nutrition. *Current Opinion in Clinical Nutrition and Metabolic Care* **5**(3): 327–32.

Cox AR, Anton C, McDowell SE *et al.* (2010) Correlates of spontaneous reporting of adverse drug reactions within primary care: the paradox of low prescribers who are high reporters. *British Journal of Clinical Pharmacology* **69**(5): 529–34.

Dawkins L, Britton D, Johnson I *et al.* (2000) A randomised trial of winged vialon cannulae & metal butterfly needles. *International Journal of Palliative Nursing* **6**(3): 110–16.

Department of Health (2000) *An Organisation with a Memory – Report of an Expert Group on Learning from Adverse Events in the NHS.* London, The Stationery Office.

Department of Health (2004) *Extending Independent Nurse Prescribing within the NHS in England – A Guide for implementation* (2e). DH, London.

Department of Health (2005) *Supplementary Prescribing by Nurses and Pharmacists within the NHS in England – A Guide for Implementation.* DH, London.

Department of Health (2006a) *Our Health, Our Care, Our Say.* DH, London.

Department of Health (2006b) *Improving Patients' Access to Medicines; a guide to implementing nurse and pharmacist independent prescribing within the NHS in England.* DH, London.

Department of Health (2002) *Liberating the Talents: helping primary care trusts and nurse deliver the NHS plan.* DH, London.

Department of Health (2005) *Supporting People With Long Term Conditions: liberating the talents of nurses who care for people with long term conditions.* DH, London.

Department of Health (2007) *Implementing Care Closer to Home: convenient quality care for patients.* DH, London.

Dougherty L, Lister S (2011) *The Royal Marsden Hospital Manual of Clinical Nursing Procedures* (8e). Wiley-Blackwell, Oxford.

Downie G, Mackenzie J, Williams A (2000) *Pharmacology and Medicine Management for Nurses* (2e) Churchill Livingstone, London.

Gillon R (1986) *Philosophical Medical Ethics.* John Wiley, Chichester.

Griffith R, Griffiths H, Jordan S (2003) Administration of medicines part 1: the law and nursing. *Nursing Standard* **18**(2): 47–54, 56.

Hyde L (2008) Legal and professional aspects of IV therapy. In: Dougherty L, Lamb J (eds) *IV therapy in Practice.* Churchill Livingstone, Edinburgh.

Jevon P, Payne E, Higgins D *et al.* (2010) *Medicines Management: a guide for nurses.* Wiley-Blackwell, Oxford.

Jordan S, Griffiths H, Griffith Richard (2003) Administration of medicines part 2: pharmacology. *Nursing Standard* **18**(3): 45–56.

Maguire A, Rugg-Gunn A (1994) Consumption of prescribed and over-the-counter liquid oral medicines in Great Britain and the northern region of England, with special regard to sugar content. *Public Health* **108**(2): 121–-30

Maguire A, Baqir W (2000) Prevalence of long-term use of medicines with prolonged oral clearance in the elderly. *British Dentistry Journal* **189**(5) 267–72.

McKenry L, Salerno E (1998) *Pharmacology in Nursing* (20e). Mosby, St Louis.

Mental Capacity Act (2007) The Stationery Office, London.

Mentes A (2001) pH changes in dental plaque after using sugar-free paediatric medicine. *Journal of Clinical Paediatric Dentistry* **25**(4): 307–12.

National Patient Safety Agency (2007) *Safety in Doses: medication safety incidents in the NHS.* NPSA, London.

National Patient Safety Agency (2009) *Safety in Doses: improving the use of medicines in the NHS.* NPSA, London.

National Patient Safety Agency (2010) *Vaccine Cold Storage.* NPSA, London.

National Patient Safety Agency (2011a) *Diabetes: insulin, use it safely.* A patient information booklet for adults who have diabetes and use insulin. NPSA, London.

National Patient Safety Agency (2011b) *The Adult Patient's Passport to Safer Use of Insulin.* NPSA, London.

NHS Executive (2000) *The Prescription Only Medicines (Human Use).* Amendment (No2) Order 2000 SI No 22899. The Stationery Office, London.

NHS Executive (1988) *Guidelines for the Safe Storage and Handling of Medicines (Duthie report).* NHS Executive, London.

Nursing & Midwifery Council (2005) *Guidelines for Records and Record Keeping.* NMC, London.

Nursing & Midwifery Council (2006) *Standards of Proficiency for Nurse and Midwife Prescribers.* NMC, London.

Nursing & Midwifery Council (2007) *NMC Advice for Delegation to Non-regulated Healthcare Staff.* NMC, London.

Nursing & Midwifery Council (2008) *The Code; Standards of Conduct, Performance and Ethics for Nurses and Midwives.* NMC, London.

Nursing & Midwifery Council (2010) *Standards for Medicines Management.* NMC, London.

Nyholm D (2002) Levodopa pharmacokinetics and motor performance during activities of daily living in patients with Parkinson's disease on individual drug combinations. *Clinical Neuropharmacology* **25**(2): 89–96.

Pratt RJ, Pellowe CM, Wilson JA *et al.* (2007) Epic 2: National evidence based guidelines for preventing healthcare associated infection in NHS hospitals in England. *Journal of Hospital Infection* **65**, Supplement !, 51–64.

Rang HP, Dale MM, Ritter JM, Flower RJ (2007) *Pharmacology* (6e). Churchill Livingstone Edinburgh.

Reid J (2003) Valid consent to surgery. *British Journal of Perioperative Nursing* **13**(7): 288–96.

Resuscitation Council (UK) (2005) *The Emergency Medical Treatment of Anaphylactic Reactions for First Medical Responders and for Community Nurses.* Resuscitation Council, London.

Resuscitation Council (UK) (2008) *Emergency Treatment of Anaphylactic Reactions, Guidelines for Healthcare Providers.* Resuscitation Council, London.

Robinson G (2004) Extended vs. Supplementary Nurse Prescribing. *Prescribing Nurse.* Autumn 2004.

Schmidt L, Dalhoff K (2002) Food-drug interactions. *Drugs* **62**(10): 1481–502

Thomson F (2000) Managing drug therapy in patients receiving enteral and parenteral nutrition. *Hospital Pharmacist* **7**(6) 155–64.

Training, Research & Education for Nurses in Diabetes (Trend, UK) (2010) *Diabetes Care in the UK. The first UK injection technique recommendations.* Trend, London.

Trounce J, Gould D (2000) *Clinical Pharmacology for Nurses (16).* Churchill Livingstone, London.

Watkinson S, Seewoodhary RS (2007) Administering eye medications. *Nursing Standard* **22**(18): 42–8.

Useful web resources

www.dh.gov.uk/en/Healthcare/Medicinespharmacyandindustry/Prescriptions/index.htm
www.mhra.gov.uk
www.nurseprescriber.co.uk
www.prodigy.nhs.uk

Moving and handling

Introduction

Manual handling is defined in the Manual Handling Operations Regulations 1992 (as amended 2002) as:

> Any transporting or supporting of a load (including the lifting, putting down, pushing, pulling, carrying or moving thereof) by hand or bodily force.

Background evidence

The Health and Safety Executive says that moving and handling injuries account for 40% of work-related sickness absence and that around 5000 moving and handling injuries are reported in healthcare each year (HSE 2011).

Anecdotal evidence suggests that an everyday part of the community nurse's role is the manual handling of patients. For example:

- performing, hoisting and assisting patients in activities of daily living
- adjusting the patient's position
- the moving and repositioning of a patient to prevent the need for prolonged periods of bending or stooping when carrying out clinical procedures, e.g. venepuncture, dressing changes, administration of medicines and urethral or suprapubic catheterisation.

Where community nurse involvement in manual handling procedures is unavoidable, the primary objectives should be to reduce the risk of injury or harm and the promotion of both patient and practitioner comfort and safety at all times (Dougherty & Lister 2011).

This chapter can only give an overview of the complex practice of manual handling in the community nursing setting; full guidance on the handling of people can be found in *The Guide to the Handling of People* (Smith 2011).

The legal aspects of manual handling

The law relating to the moving and handling of patients is based on the Health and Safety at Work Act 1974 (HSWA; UK Government 1974).

The HSWA places a duty on the employer to provide a safe working environment for both employees and others. It is an 'enabling' Act, allowing for other regulations on specific health and safety topics to be made under that Act.

The following regulations are relevant to manual handling tasks for community nurses.

- The Management of Health and Safety at Work Regulations 1999.
- Manual Handling Operations Regulations 1992 (as amended 2002).
- Provision and Use of Work Equipment Regulations 1998.
- Lifting Operations and Lifting Equipment Regulations 1998.

Full details of all these regulations and their guidance can be found on the HSE website (www.hse.gov.uk/healthservices/moving-handling.htm).

Consent

There is both a legal and a professional requirement for all nurses to obtain a patient's consent before carrying out any treatment, procedure or care (DH 2007; NMC 2008a). Consent, on behalf of an adult patient

District Nursing Manual of Clinical Procedures, First Edition. Edited by Liz O'Brien.
© 2012 Blackwell Publishing Ltd. Published 2012 by Blackwell Publishing Ltd.

who has capacity, can only be given by another person in emergency situations (DH 2005, 2007; NMC 2008a, 2008b).

Where possible, written consent should be obtained for manual handling procedures that are complex or require the use of equipment; however, where this is not possible other forms of consent are acceptable and valid (NMC 2008b; Dimond 2011) (*see* Assessment and communication).

If, following a full explanation of the planned manual handling intervention, including any necessary equipment to be used, the patient declines to give consent, e.g. for the use of a hoist, the community nurse should not comply with the patient's wishes if by doing so it will place the patient, colleagues and/or others at risk of harm or injury (NMC 2010). In these circumstances the community nurse should:

- offer the patient further information and advice
- discuss the potential outcome of the decision with the patient
- inform the patient of any restrictions placed on the planned intervention as a result of their decision
- discuss and negotiate specific aspects of the planned intervention that can be safely provided by community nursing staff
- advise the patient that they are able to change their decision at any time
- clearly document all discussions and subsequent decisions and actions in the appropriate patient records (NMC 2009).

Risk assessment

Health and safety legislation requires that risk assessments are carried out, and this is especially so with regard to manual handling. The HSE (2011) says that moving and handling risk assessments help identify where injuries could occur and what to do to prevent them. It also says that to undertake effective risk assessment within a patient's home the community nurse must have received formal training and possess a level of knowledge, skills and awareness necessary for such complex handling activities. A patient's home may present clinical and environmental risks and hazards outside that of other healthcare work places.

Wherever there is a need to undertake manual handling of any description a risk assessment must be carried out (RCN 2003; HSE 2011; Smith 2011).

A comprehensive risk assessment should identify all actual and potential risks and hazards to the patient, nursing staff and other members of the multidisciplinary team. To reduce risk and determine the extent of

concern about a particular problem the community nurse should consider the following factors.

- Does the problem place any staff at risk?
- Is the problem met frequently or rarely?
- Is the problem likely to cause a major injury?

(Tracy & Tarling 1998)

A comprehensive assessment can be achieved using a generic manual handling tool or framework using the mnemonic LITE that incorporates the following factors.

1 The **L**oad: what is it that has to be handled? Is it the patient or equipment? Is it light or heavy? Is it an awkward shape, etc.? If the load is a patient, are there any factors that should be considered, e.g. ataxia, dementia, amputation, learning disability, claustrophobia, pain?
2 The **I**ndividual's capability: has the person doing the manual handling received appropriate manual handling training? Are they fit and well and competent to undertake the task?
3 The **T**ask: where has the item or patient to be moved to? What is the distance and what is in the way?
4 The **E**nvironment: what environment is this task to be done in – is there furniture in the way? Is it hot or cold? Are there any hazards such as slippery floors, height restrictions, frayed or long pile carpets, pets or small children that may get in the way?

(HSC 1998)

Assessment of a manual handling procedure
Assessment of a manual handling procedure in the home may identify the need to implement control measures, e.g. the removal of items of furniture from the area or the introduction of manual handling equipment. In this instance all recommendations should be clearly explained and discussed with the patient and their family in order to obtain consent prior to implementing any changes (NMC 2008b; Smith 2011). The assessment should not only identify the risks and hazards that are present, but also potential control measures to reduce these to the lowest possible level (RCN 2003; HSE 2011; Smith 2011). The assessment should not focus solely on the procedure but should also contain assessment of the knowledge, skills and capabilities of those who will be carrying out the procedure/manoeuvre.

In situations where the patient, or their family, is reluctant to accept recommendations, or where risks to both patient and nursing staff remain high, nurse managers or a manual handling advisor should be informed and should assist in negotiations (NMC

202

2008a, 2010). Where agreement cannot be reached withdrawal of the district nursing service may need to be considered.

The outcome of the assessment should be recorded in the relevant documentation and contain, for example:

- a description of the task
- the identified risks (**LITE**)
- the risk score/level
- the measures in place to control the risk/s
- any further measures required
- the patient's mobility status, including specific elements of the manoeuvre they are able to do independently or assist with
- a description of the manual handling equipment and techniques to be used
- where slings are to be used the number/position of loops to use should be stated, and if possible these should be marked
- the number of staff needed to carry out the manoeuvre and any special instructions or requirements
- the date of assessment
- the review date
- signature of assessor

(RCN 2003; HSE 2011; Smith 2011)

For examples of areas that should be considered in a generic risk assessment see Smith (2011) or RCN (2003), which is available at www.rcn.org.uk/data/assetts/pdffile/0008/78488/000605.pdf

Control measures
The level of risk depends on the patient's ability to assist in the moving and handling procedure and the environment. For medium to high risks, all or some of the following control measures should be discussed with the patient, and significant other, and where appropriate implemented.

- Carers or nursing staff to place knee(s) on bed or floor to reduce stooping when attending to a patient.
- Provide low stool/seat for carers and nursing staff.
- Provide appropriate mobility aids, e.g. wheeled Zimmer frame, wheeled trolley, walking stick(s), wheelchair.
- If the height of the patient's own bed cannot be adjusted with, for example, bed raisers, an adjustable height single hospital bed should be provided.
- Provide a hoist or sliding board for transfer to/from bed.
- Provide a fabric sliding aid or a hoist for moves up/down bed.
- Provide a fabric sliding aid for turning in bed.

- Provide a one-way sliding aid to stop the patient's bottom from sliding forward while seated in a chair or sliding down when in bed.
- Patient should temporarily remain in bed until equipment is available.
- Where possible provide extra staff.

(RCN 2003; Smith 2011)

Training

All employers have a duty to provide training that includes practical supervision to assess competency, and regular updates for those staff involved in the manual handling of patients (UK Government 1974; HSE 1992). It is important to remember that all bank and agency staff should also receive training in organisational policies and procedures during their induction (DH 2006). Areas that should be covered in moving and handling training include:

- risk factors and assessing risk
- manual handling regulations
- up-to-date local policies
- control measures to reduce risk
- how to carry out a risk assessment and complete documentation
- the need to involve local staff
- advice on where to go for further help and advice
- a demonstration of handling aids.

(RCN 2003)

Training should be carried out in a dedicated area that is equipped with a range of equipment and aids reflecting those available to staff in the community. In addition to formal structured training, staff should receive continued supervision, training and support in the workplace, and this should be carried out by competent practitioners (BackCare 1999).

It is essential that all training records are accurately maintained. These can be used by employers to demonstrate fulfilment of their legal requirement to provide adequate training, also for healthcare standard assessments. They can also be used by nursing staff as evidence of reaching specific core dimensions of their knowledge and skills framework (KSF), for example health, safety and security, and quality, during yearly performance reviews. Training records should include:

- name of staff attendee
- name of instructor
- date
- location
- duration

203

- course contents
- equipment and techniques practised
- copies of printed information given out
- notes of warnings given, e.g. banned lifts.

(Tracy & Tarling 1998)

Evidence suggests that even with correct instruction in lifting techniques, repeated manual handling can result in cumulative strain (RCN 2003; Work & Health Research Centre 2007). Therefore it is important to ensure that the development and implementation of safer working practices and policies is a priority, and training should be viewed as a way to limit and prevent unsafe practice. For up-to-date and in-depth details on essential training topics see Smith (2011).

Manual handling equipment

When considering the use of manual handling equipment it is essential that the community nurse takes the following into account.

- The needs and abilities of the patient.
- The needs and abilities of the nursing team, carers and all family members that may be involved in its use.
- The need to promote health and safety.
- The need to remove/reduce risks, including those within the home environment.

There are a number of other factors that may also need to be taken into consideration.

- There are several different types of hoists – full, standing, mobile, ceiling.
- Tissue viability/pressure relief – if a patient has a dynamic air mattress because of a high Waterlow score, manual handling can become more difficult as the patient often finds it more difficult to assist with manual handling when lying on an air mattress.
- Each piece of equipment should be checked for wear and tear/breakages/faults before using, especially slings.
- The type of full hoist sling currently being used should be reviewed regularly to ensure it is still the most appropriate one for the patient. Patients may be provided with more than one type of sling for different tasks.
- Use of mobile hoist considerations: type of flooring, ceiling height, ceiling light fittings, space to use the hoist (alongside other equipment, e.g. whatever the person is being hoisted on to and off), space to store

the hoist when not in use, plug availability, if the hoist is not being used with a hospital bed, is there enough room to get the legs of the hoist under the bed? Can the hoist get close enough to the piece of furniture the patient is being hoisted into/out of (i.e. a sofa may not be able to be used).

- As the equipment provider/prescriber, that professional has a duty of care to ensure that risk assessments, servicing, etc., are addressed.
- Address any complex manual handling issues to your expert in the field in your trust.

Where a patient is being discharged home, e.g. from a secondary care setting, assessment of their manual handling needs and discussion with family ward staff and relevant members of the multidisciplinary team should take place prior to discharge. This is essential to selecting the most appropriate equipment (*see* Chapter 4). For patients with complex needs it may also be necessary for the hospital occupational therapist or physiotherapist and community staff to undertake a joint home-based assessment (*see* Chapter 4).

If the patient is to continue receiving a rehabilitation programme when at home it is important that they become familiar with the equipment, gain confidence with its use and that relatives, where appropriate, also become familiar with its use prior to discharge. Where relatives are using equipment provided by community services unsupervised by nursing staff, or assisting with moving and handling procedures, training must be provided and documented. Documentation should also include discussion about the unsupervised use of any equipment being at the patient and their family's own risk.

Loan equipment

The loans service accessed by community nurses should supply a comprehensive range of manual handling equipment. However, as each organisation is individually responsible for procurement or the management of a service level agreement with equipment loan suppliers, the types and availability of equipment may differ. See Table 9.1 for examples of equipment; this should be used in conjunction with manufacturer's instructions, local policies and guidelines, and where relevant with advice from a moving and handling advisor and/or occupational therapist. If appropriate equipment is not available to meet the needs of a patient a clinical incident form should be completed and the manager informed.

All equipment should be supplied with the appropriate instructions for use; these should be interpreted by

Table 9.1 Examples of equipment

Patient need	Choice of equipment	Description of equipment
For patients who have difficulty moving or turning in bed	Variable posture bed. Electrically powered and controlled, for example Profile bed	These can be used with or without a pressure relief mattress, to reposition the patient without them having to be manually turned. The height can be altered to prevent the clinician/user stooping or bending
	Low friction rollers. Manually operated	These are made of a length of material, which has either been stitched to form a continuous roller or is folded in a similar way so that the inside surfaces of the roller easily slide against each other
For patients who have difficulty getting their legs into bed	Powered leg lifters	These are powered devices that attach to the bed frame and require the patient to sit on the edge of the bed with their feet on the floor in front of the device. The platform rises through an arc of 90°, lifting the legs of the user to a position just beyond the horizontal, level with the mattress
	Rope leg lifters	These are lengths of rope with a loop at one end. The patient places their foot into the loop and this enables the patient to move the leg in an upwards position
	Inflatable air sac	These air sacs gently inflate to raise legs
For patients who need help to sit up	Monkey pole	The majority have a floor-standing cantilever gate attached. A handle hangs from the given height to enable the patient to pull themself up
	Rope ladders	These either fit to the floorboard, the bed frame or both. The patient pulls on the ladder to help themself into a sitting position
	Pull straps	Similar function to rope ladder
	Grab handles	These grab rails are firmly fixed in place to allow the patient to obtain a firm grip. The patient uses the grab rail to pull on to help them sit up or turn over in bed
	Mattress inclinators/variators. Electrically powered. Used with standard divan bed	Powered devices. Raised they can form a backrest. The use of this item will reduce the need for the carer to manually assist the person to sit forward. There are two types: 1 Placed under the mattress at the bed head. Work best with foam-filled mattresses 2 Placed on top of the mattress with a foam pad on top
	Pillow lifters	These rest on top of the mattress and raise the patient in bed to the sitting position
	Variable posture bed	These beds are made up of sections. Each section can move independently
For patients who have difficulty getting out of bed	Variable posture bed. Electrically powered and controlled, for example the Profile bed	The patient or nurse/carer pushes the button to adjust the tilt of the bed, mattress and pillows The Profile bed can help or aid the patient into a sitting position. By pulling on a strategically positioned grab rail or lifting pole the patient may be able to manoeuvre their bottom to the edge of the bed. Once in position the patient, if able to weight bear, can be eased into the standing position
	Hand blocks	If hand blocks are placed on either side of the patient they can, by pushing down on the blocks, raise themself several centimetres from the bed. This enables the patient to change their position

(Continued)

205

Table 9.1 (*Continued*)

Patient need	Choice of equipment	Description of equipment
Standing up from a sitting position	Variable height bed	Raising the height to enable patient to sit on edge of bed with feet touching the floor
	Bed leg raisers	These can be placed under the legs of the bed to raise the height. They are not suitable for divan beds because of their lack of stability
	Adjustable height bed	To adjust height these beds can be controlled manually or electrically, up or down, to make standing easier
	Appropriate chair: height and width	The height of a chair seat can determine how easy it is to stand and sit. The internal dimensions of the chair should be tailored to the size of the user to ensure adequate support and comfort. A seat too low will be more difficult to get out of and will direct pressure towards the pelvis rather than distributing it evenly along the thighs. In some areas you may have to involve an occupational therapist
For patients who have difficulty rising to a standing position but have enough upper body strength to pull themself up, are able to weight bear, not confused and can follow instructions	Standing hoist. It is recommended that two people should carry out this procedure when using this equipment	The patient holds on to the hoist arms while placing their feet on the foot plate with knees resting against the knee plate. The sling is positioned well down the patient's back. The patient is pulled into the standing position, as the hoist rises
For patients unable to independently move	Electrically powered hoist. It is recommended that two people should carry out this procedure when using this equipment	A tracking system is attached to the ceiling or upper walls, or is mounted on high pillars. The patient can be moved from a position directly under the track. Correct use of sling is important to achieve optimum function, independence, comfort and dignity for patient. The sling is placed on patient and then attached to the hoist by loops
		Lifting is achieved by pressing on the remote control to move the patient upwards, sideways or downwards
	Manual hoist. It is recommended that two people should carry out this procedure when using this equipment	This allows transfer of the patient from one point to another from any position. Correct use of sling is important to achieve optimum function, independence, comfort and dignity for patient
		The sling is placed on the patient, and then attached to the hoist by loops. Lifting is achieved by winding a handle, hydraulic pump or by battery power

NB Manufacturers' instructions and recommendations should be followed at all times.

the community nurse and incorporated into the manual handling assessment and individualised patient care plan. To ensure user competency, where necessary the community nurse should provide training in the correct use of the relevant equipment and information and advice to staff and carers. This should be recorded in the relevant nursing documentation (NMC 2008a; Smith 2011).

Specialist equipment

Where specialist equipment is required an occupational therapist (OT) must carry out an assessment. This may be undertaken as a joint home assessment with the community nurse at any stage during an episode of care. See Chapter 4 for further information regarding OT involvement and home adaptations.

Examples of specialist equipment that may only be supplied on the assessment and instruction of an occupational therapist include:

- bath seat/bath lift/shower board
- perching stool
- toilet raiser/free-standing toilet frame/grab rails
- grab/hand rails/stair rails
- trolley/Buckingham caddy
- wheeled walking frame/outdoor walkers/sticks
- wheelchair/glideabout commode
- Roho cushion.

Cleaning of equipment

The appropriate decontamination of equipment is an essential element in infection control procedures (MHRA DB 2006) (*see also* Chapter 6). Therefore it is essential that all equipment provided for use in the home is supplied with up-to-date maintenance records and cleaning instructions.

In general, if hoists and handling aids are kept clean and dry, bacteria will be unable to multiply (Wilson 2006). However, if it does become soiled most equipment can be cleaned with soap and water or detergent (BackCare 1999). Manufacturers' instructions for cleaning equipment are usually provided and these should be incorporated into local guidelines. Where fabric hoist slings are being used, a minimum of two should be provided as this enables the slings to be rotated for washing and being kept 'socially' clean. Patients living in residential care homes should each have their own slings. The slings should be clearly labelled with the patient's name, and to prevent cross-infection should not be used with other patients (Smith 2011).

Table 9.1 gives some examples of other considerations regarding the use of equipment, while Smith (2011) gives in-depth details on all aspects of manual handling equipment.

Conclusion

The management of manual handling procedures in the home environment can be complex and diverse; therefore the sensitive use of communication skills is essential for negotiation and securing patient cooperation and consent.

To maintain competency, and enable full implementation of the ergonomic and biomechanical principles for safe manual handling, it is essential that community nurses receive continuous, up-to-date training, education and supervision in:

- manual handling techniques/assessment
- risk management
- the range of equipment available and its appropriate use
- local and statutory policy, guidelines and requirements.

A team approach should be used to develop a shared, individualised, care plan that incorporates and respects the wishes and abilities of the patient. The care plan should clearly identify all necessary manoeuvres and instructions, and also reflect the findings of the manual handling and risk assessment, e.g. any control measures that must be implemented prior to or during the procedure to reduce/remove actual and potential risks or hazards.

The community nursing team should review and, where necessary, modify all manual handling procedures at each visit and document this in the patient care plan and nursing documentation.

Procedure guideline 9.1 **Guideline for manual handling of patients in the community: general principles**

Equipment

Patient nursing documentation, including manual handling/risk assessment
Appropriate manual handling equipment
Single-use apron
Single-use gloves (where appropriate)

Nursing action	Rationale
1 Where appropriate facilities are available wash and dry hands. Alternatively cleanse hands with anti-bactericidal alcohol-based hand rub	To prevent the risk of cross-infection/contamination
2 If the patient is known to the service review nursing documentation and current care plan	To update knowledge of patient and maintain patient safety
3 Carry out/review the manual handling and patient's nursing needs assessment, explaining and discussing each aspect with the patient	To ensure that nursing care can be carried out safely or, where relevant, to update prior knowledge of the patient and planned care
	To enable the patient to ask questions
	To alleviate any fears or concerns the patient may have
	To ensure that the patient understands the planned care and individual roles within the manual handling procedure
	To obtain informed consent (DH 2007)
4 If the patient is unknown to the service a full comprehensive assessment must be carried out prior to undertaking the procedure	To identify potential contraindications and or cautions to carrying out the procedure
	To determine if a second nurse is required to assist with the procedure
	To maintain patient safety
5 Where appropriate, clearly record all necessary information in the relevant documentation, e.g. the patient's ability to help with the procedure, which loops should be used on hoist sling	To ensure all staff undertaking the procedure understand the plan of action and coordinate their actions correctly
	To ensure patient and staff safety
6 Prepare the area by moving away any unwanted obstacles, e.g. chairs or coffee table	To provide a safe work space
	To enable ease of movement
If two handlers are carrying out the procedure/ manoeuvre, where necessary the bed should be moved away from the wall or any obstruction	To ensure handler and patient safety, e.g. during rolling/ turning manoeuvres
7 Explain the procedure/manoeuvre to the patient, detailing each step and the equipment to be used	To ensure that the patient understands the plan of care and individual roles within the manual handling manoeuvre
	To offer the patient reassurance and alleviate any fears and concerns
	To gain patient cooperation

Procedure guideline 9.1 **Guideline for manual handling of patients in the community: general principles** *(cont'd)*

Nursing action	Rationale
8 Select appropriate equipment as detailed in the patient care plan	To ensure that the patient is moved with the least amount of effort
	To maintain the safety of both the patient and handlers
	To ensure maximum comfort for the patient
9 Cleanse hands with anti-bactericidal alcohol-based hand rub and apply single-use apron and gloves	To prevent the risk of cross-infection
NB Non-sterile gloves may be used for relevant elements of the procedure/manoeuvre	
10 Assist the patient into the desired position	To enable care to be carried out.
If two handlers are involved one should coordinate the procedure	To promote patient comfort
	To ensure that the handlers' effort is exerted at the same time to prevent unequal strain
	To maintain patient and handler safety
11 Following the manual handling manoeuvre check that the patient is comfortable	To evaluate the effectiveness of the methods and equipment used
12 Remove, clean and store all equipment used in accordance with manufacturer instructions and or local policy/guidelines	To reduce the risk of contamination
	To maintain a safe environment for the patient, nursing staff and others
13 Return any moved items of furniture to their original position	To maintain a safe environment for the patient by restoring any furniture moved to its usual place
14 Remove and dispose of used apron and gloves in accordance with infection control procedures and local policy/guidelines (see Chapter 6)	To prevent the risk of crossinfection
	To promote the safety of others
15 Where appropriate facilities are available wash and dry hands. Alternatively cleanse hands with anti-bactericidal alcohol-based hand rub	To prevent the risk of cross-infection
16 Record the procedure undertaken in the patient records detailing any problems/difficulties that may have arisen	To maintain patient safety (NMC 2009)
	To aid continuity of care
	To maintain the safety of community nursing staff and others that may be involved in the future manual handling of the patient

209

References and further reading

BackCare (1999) *Safer Handling of People in the Community*. Back-Care, Middlesex.

Department of Health (2006) *Health and Safety Management*. Department of Health, London, www.dhsspsni.gov.uk/health_safty_06.doc (last accessed 07 October 2011).

Department of Health (2007) *The Mental Capacity Act, 2005, Code of Practice*. The Stationery Office, London.

Dimond B (2011) *Legal Aspects of Nursing* (6e). Pearson Education, Essex.

Dougherty L, Lister S (eds) (2011) *The Royal Marsden Manual of Clinical Nursing Procedures*. Wiley-Blackwell, Oxford.

Fletcher B (2003) *Evidence-based Patient Handling: tasks, equipment and interventions*. Routledge, London.

Health and Safety Commission (1998) *Manual Handling in the Health Service* (2e). HSE, Books, Sudbury.

Health and Safety Executive (1992) *Manual Handling Operations Regulations as Amended 2002 Guidance on Regulations*. HMSO, London.

Health and Safety Executive (1999) *Management of Health and Safety at Work Regulations*. HMSO, London.

Health and Safety Executive (2001) *Handling Home Care, HSG 225*. HSE, London. www.hse.gov.uk/healthservices/moving-handling.htm (last accessed 7 October 2011).

Health and Safety Executive (2011) *Moving and Handling in Health and Social Care*. HSE, London, www.hse.gov.uk/healthservices/moving-handling.htm (last accessed 10 October 2011).

Medicines and Healthcare products Regulatory Agency (2006) *Managing Medical Devices*. MHRA, London, www.mhra.gov.uk/Publications/Safetyguidance/DevicesBulletins/CON2025142

National Institute for Occupational Safety and Health (1991) *A Work Practice Guide for Manual Lifting*. Publication no. 81-122. DHHS (NIOSH), Cincinnati.

Nursing & Midwifery Council (2007) Mental capacity act advice sheet. NMC, London.

Nursing & Midwifery Council (2008a) *The Code: standards of conduct, performance and ethics for nurses and midwives*. NMC, London.

Nursing & Midwifery Council (2008b) Consent advice sheet. NMC, London.

Nursing & Midwifery Council (2009) *Record Keeping*. NMC, London.

Nursing & Midwifery Council (2010) Environment of care advice sheet. NMC, London.

Pheasant S, Stubbs D (1991) *Lifting and Handling – An Ergonomic Approach*. The National Back Pain Association Thorn – EMIUK Rental, London.

Royal College of Nursing (2003) *Manual Handling Assessment in Hospital and Community*. RCN, London.

Ruszala S (2010) *Moving and Handling People: an illustrated guide*. Clinical Skills, London.

Sander R (2002) Handling and moving: helping people with vascular dementia. *Nursing Older People* **14**(1): 20–6.

Smith J (ed.) (2011) *The Guide to the Handling of People* (6e). BackCare, Middlesex, www.backcare.org.uk (last accessed 7 October 2011).

Tracy M, Tarling C (1998) The management responsibility. In: *The Guide to the Handling of Patients* (4e), pp. 63–72. National Back Pain Association and Royal College Nursing, Middlesex.

United Kingdom Government (1974) *Health and Safety at Work etc. Act*. HMSO, London.

United Kingdom Government (2005) *Mental Capacity Act*. HMSO, London.

Wilkinson R (2000) *The Human Rights Act and Practical Guide for Nurses*. Whurr Publishers, London.

Wilson J (2006) *Infection Control in Clinical Practice*. Ballière Tindall, London.

Work and Health Research Centre (2007) *Manual Handling Investigation of Current Practices and Development of Guidelines*. Research Report 583. HSE, London.

10

Nutritional support

Introduction

A diet that is balanced in nutrients is recognised as essential for maintaining health. During periods of ill health requirements may change, but the need for nutrients does not. However, in healthcare this is an area that is often neglected in daily practice (McWhirter & Pennington 1994; RCP 2002; BAPEN 2006).

Background evidence

Understanding what constitutes a balanced diet in health and illness is essential in planning nutritional support. Dietary reference values (DRV) for food, energy and nutrients for the UK (COMA 1991) provide guidance on the estimated average requirements (EAR) and reference nutrient intake (RNI) for a population, but are of little use in providing practical advice for practitioners. The Balance of Good Health (FSA 2001) provides a pictorial representation of a balanced diet with references to different food groups (Figure 10.1). It can be applied to different cultures by substituting different foods in the identified proportions.

It is assumed that provided an individual consumes a range of foods from each of the groups identified, in the appropriate quantities, the amount of macro- and micronutrients consumed will be sufficient to meet the needs of that individual (Tables 10.1 and 10.2). In addition to the dietary intake, at least 2 litres of fluid needs to be consumed each day. This can be either in the form of liquids (teas, juice or water) or as a component of the food eaten (all foods except those that are dried contain water in varying amounts). In encouraging the consumption of a balanced diet the Food Standards Agency (FSA 2001) recommend a daily reduction in total food intake and an increase in the consumption of:

- bread
- pasta
- rice
- potatoes
- fruit and vegetables (a minimum five portions).

A portion of fruit or vegetables is approximately the amount that can be held in one hand. Alternatively the amounts listed in Table 10.3 can be used.

In our daily lives we have a constant need for energy for cellular function and body activity. Energy is measured in kilojoules (Box 10.1). The amount of energy required will reflect body size, age and activity levels. During periods of growth, as in childhood, energy expenditure is high relative to body size. In periods of ill health, energy demand can change; the extent of this change will vary according to the severity of the illness (Webb 2002). Energy requirement is measured using Megajoules (MJ) and this can be calculated by multiplying the basal metabolic rate (BMR) by the estimated physical activity level. A physical activity level of 1.49 for women and 1.78 for men is considered to reflect the lifestyle of most adults in the UK (SACN 2009). This factor is suitable for people who do little physical activity at work or in their leisure time (Table 10.4). If energy intake matches energy expenditure, then body weight, in adulthood, will remain stable. In healthcare, repeated measurement and recording of body weight over time is a good indicator of whether the energy requirement has been met (Webb 2002).

Foods contain varying amounts of energy dependent on their composition. For example, foods containing a large proportion of fat are more energy dense than those containing carbohydrates. Carbohydrates predominantly provide a source of glucose, which is then available as an energy substrate for immediate use. The

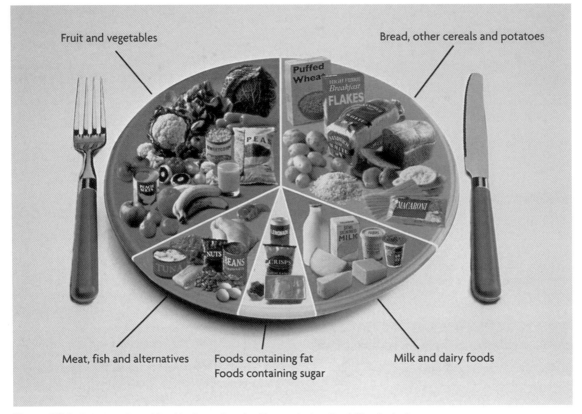

Fruit and vegetables

Bread, other cereals and potatoes

Meat, fish and alternatives   Foods containing fat   Milk and dairy foods
Foods containing sugar

Figure 10.1 Balance of good health. Reproduced with permission Food Standards Agency.

212

more refined (processed) the carbohydrate the more readily available the glucose is.

The consumption of complex carbohydrates as found in fruits, vegetables and cereals, and a reduction in refined carbohydrates containing large proportions of simple sugars, such as confectionary, is recommended (DH 2009).

Fats are more energy dense than carbohydrates and provide a source of energy for immediate use as well as essential fatty acids for cell function, and the fat-soluble vitamins A, D, E and K.

Dietary energy intake in excess of that required by the body is stored as triacylglycerols in adipocytes (Mann & Truswell 2002).

Nutritional status and health

Changes in nutritional status can impact on health. In the developed world, dietary adequacy, the provision of adequate amounts of energy and nutrients, is taken for granted and nutrient deficiencies are only associated with specific groups, for example:

- individuals with chronic health problems
- people with alcohol and drug addiction
- individuals at the extremes of social and economic disadvantage
- older adults.

(Guigoz *et al.* 2002)

There are also an increasing number of health issues that are shown to be influenced by diet:

- hypertension
- type 2 and type 1 diabetes
- heart disease
- cancer.

(NHS Cancer Plan 2000; DH 2000, 2001a, 2001b, 2005)

Table 10.1 Macronutrients in the diet

Macronutrient	Type	Dietary source	Use	Notes
Carbohydrates	Monosaccharides – glucose, fructose	Found in refined food products and fruits	Source of energy for the body – supplies glucose	Can increase blood glucose quickly
	Disaccharides – sucrose, lactose, maltose	Found in milk	Readily converted to glucose to provide energy	Some people are deficient in lactase and cannot digest lactose. Undigested lactase leads to abdominal pain and cramps
	Polysaccharides starch – amylopectin, amylose, modified food starches	Important in diet, include root vegetables, cereals and legumes	Complex carbohydrates that can help to keep blood glucose levels stable as glucose is only released slowly into the bloodstream	Arrangement of amylose and amylopectin in starch granules makes them difficult to digest. This structure is changed when heated in water – gelatinisation making them easy to digest. Rate of digestion depends on extent of cooking (size of particles), ratio of amylose to amylopectin and amount of cellulose (fibre)
	Non-starch polysaccharides, resistant starch and oligosaccharides	Found in cabbage, swede, lentils, onions	Resistant to digestion and pass into the colon where they are fermented by commensal bacteria	Leads to production of short chain fatty acids, which help to maintain health of colonocytes and as an energy substrate
Fats – 95% dietary fat, triglyceride	Saturated fatty acids	Found in animal fats	Contributes to energy supply	Excess stored as triglyceride in adipose tissue. Diets high in saturated fatty acids increase the risk of obesity and heart disease
	Monounsaturated fatty acids	Found in olive oil, rape seed oil	Important component of healthy diet	
	Polyunsaturated fatty acids	Two types – omega 3 and omega 6. Omega 3 found in oily fish, omega 6 found in plant oils	Also known as essential fatty acids and are important in health as they are linked to many cellular functions	Known to influence inflammatory processes

(Continued)

213

Table 10.1 (Continued)

Macronutrient	Type	Dietary source	Use	Notes
Proteins RNI 0.75 g/kg body weight. This requirement can also be expressed as % of total energy – 7–8% of total energy intake. Western diets normally contain 15% of total energy	Proteins contain differing amounts of amino acids. Amino acids are important for meeting cells' needs. They are divided into two groups – the non-essential (dispensable) and essential (indispensable. Non-essential amino acids: alanine, arginine, asparagines, aspartate, glutamate, glycine, glutamate, proline, serine. Essential amino acids: histidine, isoleucine, leucine, lysine, methionine, phenylalanine, threonine, tryptophan, valine. If one of these is lacking then it will be impossible to maintain nitrogen balance	Meat, fish and dairy products are important sources of dietary protein. However, cereal products count for a significant proportion in the Western diet. Meat and meat products 36%; cereal products 23%; fish 6%; milk and dairy 17%. Proteins can be classed by their biological value – the proportion of the protein retained (used) by the body. Proteins that are completely usable include eggs and human milk. Biological value (BV) of 0.9. Mixing proteins increases the BV of a food. Rice pudding, bread and cheese	Proteins are essential for cell growth, replication and cellular activity. The amount of protein required will reflect age and health. In ill health protein requirements can increase, e.g. patients with increased amounts of exudates and infection	Proteins in the body are continually being broken down and replaced This continued breakdown (catabolism) of proteins creates the requirement for dietary protein, as proteins are lost through body secretions or are utilised as body fuels. Using of proteins for 'fuel' indicates that dietary intake of 'energy' is inadequate
Vitamins – organic compounds. Small amounts required for normal metabolic function	Vitamin A – fat-soluble, beta-carotene, retinol	Found only in animal sources and a variety of carotenes (yellow/red/green vegetables). Carotenes metabolised in GI tract to produce retinol	Vision and cell differentiation	Deficiency of vitamin A is major cause of vision defects in developing world
	Vitamin D – fat-soluble. Is really a hormone	Synthesised in the skin by the action of ultraviolet light	Acts as a steroid hormone. Increases transport of calcium across mucosal membrane	Older people who are housebound or who do not go outside very much are at increased risk of deficiency and developing osteomalacia
	Vitamin E – fat-soluble. Two compounds: tocopherol, tocotrienols	Widespread in diets that contain fats/oils	Limits oxidative damage of polyunsaturated fatty acids (PUFA)	No deficiency states known except in cases such as cystic fibrosis
	Vitamin K – fat-soluble	Phylloquinone – found in green leafy vegetables Menaquinones –synthesised by intestinal bacteria	Required for clotting cascade	Action blocked by warfarin
	Vitamin B_1 thiamine – water-soluble	Cereal products	Needed for metabolism and conduction of nerve impulses	Beri-beri – long-term deficiency seen in developing countries leading to muscle weakness and atrophy due to damage in peripheral nervous system

Vitamin	Source	Function	Deficiency/notes
Vitamin B_2 riboflavin – water-soluble	Milk and milk products	Metabolism of metabolic fuels	Deficiency widespread across the world. Signs include cracking at corners of the mouth and lips
Niacin – water-soluble. Nicotinic acid. Nicotinamide	Cereals. Synthesised from tryptophan	DNA repair mechanisms, controlling intracellular calcium	Deficiency leads to pellegra, characterised by a rash when skin is exposed to sunlight and depressive psychosis
Vitamin B_6 – water-soluble	Meat, whole grain cereals	Co-enzyme in metabolism, amino acids, glycogen phosphorylase in muscle, regulation of steroid hormones	Deficiency rare, but toxicity can damage nerves. Anecdotal use in PMS
Vitamin B_{12} – water soluble	Only found in animal sources, can be produced by bacterial fermentation. Active form not produced by yeast	Metabolic reactions, function linked to that of folic acid	Deficiency leads to pernicious anaemia. In elderly atrophic gastritis reduces absorption of vitamin B_{12} in 10–30% of older people
Folic acid – water-soluble	Green leafy vegetables, liver	Wide range of metabolic reactions. Closure of neural tube	Linked to role of vitamin B_{12}. Deficiency leads to alterations in cells of bone marrow, red blood cells, neural tube defects. Folic acid supplementation will mask haematological signs of vitamin B_{12} deficiency and may exacerbate irreversible neurological damage
Vitamin C, ascorbic acid – water-soluble. Difficult to establish adequacy. Reference intakes range from 30 to 80mg/day. At intakes above about 100mg the body's capacity to metabolise vitamin C is saturated	Found in fruit and fruit juices. Must be consumed as part of the diet	Metabolic reactions of proline and lysine in the synthesis of collagen	Deficiency leads to scurvy. This has been seen in elderly patients in the UK

216

Table 10.2 A selection of micronutrients in the diet

Micronutrient	Name	Source	Action	Notes
Minerals Inorganic elements of diet Deficiencies more likely to occur in a large population consuming food from one region where the soil may be deficient in a mineral Many minerals can be toxic if consumed in excess	Calcium	Main sources are milk and cheese Absorbed in the presence of vitamin D	Important for bone /teeth health Important in cell function, e.g. muscle contraction	Deficiency of vitamin D leads to rickets Plasma calcium levels are regulated
	Iron	Found in red meat (haem iron) and green leafy vegetables (non-haem iron) Only about 10% of consumed iron is absorbed. It is more easily absorbed from an animal source	Important function in haemoglobin as allows transportation of oxygen	Can only be absorbed in a reduced form Fe^{2+}; vitamin C reduces iron and increases rate of absorption Stored in cells bound to ferritin, leaves cells bound to transferrin Phytate (in plants), tannic acid (in tea) and calcium reduce iron absorption Supplementation may not benefit those with high iron stores
	Zinc	Found in a wide range of foods	Zinc is widely used in more than 100 different enzyme pathways Involved in the receptor proteins of steroid hormones, thyroid hormones, calcitrol and vitamin A Acts on an integral part of proteins that initiate gene transcription within DNA	Deficiency states rare, but absorption is inhibited by phytate. Excess consumption of water can 'wash out' zinc and reduce levels. Zinc supplement may reduce copper status, impair immune responses and decrease plasma high-density lipoproteins (HDL)
	Selenium	Found in many foods, such as brazil nuts	Functions in many different enzyme pathways, including those involved with thyroid hormones, insulin, antioxidant	Need only 75 µg/day, excessive intakes are toxic and the WHO recommends that an intake of no more than 200 µg be taken

Table 10.3 Rough guide to portion sizes. Adapted from the Food Standards Agency (2011)

Vegetables – raw, cooked, canned, bottled or frozen	2–3 tablespoonfuls
Salad leaves	1 dessert bowl
Grapefruit/avocado pear	½ fruit
Apples, bananas, oranges and similar fruit	1 fruit
Plums and similar size fruits	2 fruits
Grapes, cherries and berries	1 cupful/handful
Fresh fruit salad, stewed canned fruit	2–3 tablespoonfuls
Dried fruit	½–1 tablespoonful
Fruit juice	1 glass – 150 ml

Table 10.4 Estimated energy requirements. Adapted from COMA (1991)

Estimated average requirements (EAR), MJ/day (Kcal/day)

Age	Males		Females	
19–50 years	10.60	(2220)	7.72	(1845)
51–59 years	10.60	(25550)	8.10	(1900)
60–64 years	9.93	(2380)	7.99	(1900)
65–74 years	9.71	((2330)	7.96	(1900)
74+ years	8.77	(2100)	7.61	(1810)

Box 10.1 Measurement of energy

Joules are the SI unit for energy. 1 J is a very small amount of energy. In nutrition the kilojoule (kJ) or megajoule is used (MJ). In many texts the kilocalorie is still used.

1 kcal = 4.184 kJ

- morbidity (Arnaud-Battandier *et al.* 2004; Oliver 2005)
- infection (Wild *et al.* 2010)
- delayed recovery following hip-fractures (Bruce *et al.* 2003; Eneroth *et al.* 2005)
- delayed healing of pressure sores (Stratton 2003).

The impact of malnutrition in the community is an increasing pressure on the use of healthcare resources, therefore it is important to identify people who would benefit from active nutritional care (Edington *et al.* 2004). Furthermore by providing nutritional care in the community it is suggested that admission rates may be reduced and patient well being improved (Guest *et al.* 2011).

Malnutrition

Evidence of malnutrition has been shown in the National Diet and Health Surveys of both the young and the old (National Diet and Health Survey for England 2011). The BAPEN nutritional screening survey (2010) identified that on admission to hospital and care homes, one in three people were malnourished and that malnutrition originated within the community. Researchers found that one in six older adults in institutions were underweight (BMI < 20), and although in the community this ratio was reduced, a number of older adults were also malnourished. It was also noted that older adults living in institutions were more likely to be deficient in vitamin C, thiamine, folate, vitamin B_{12} and vitamin D (National Diet and Health Survey for England 2011).

It is suggested that a weight loss of >10% increases the risk of malnutrition (Stratton *et al.* 2003). This amount of weight loss may also be linked to prognostic indicators in end of life care and increase the risk of, for example:

Identifying patients at risk of malnutrition (initial nursing assessment)

Assessing nutritional status or the risk of malnutrition relies on a range of different approaches with no single method considered to be a 'gold standard'.

Successful nutritional assessment depends on the systematic use of basic nursing skills. For example:

- observation
- questioning the patient accurately about dietary habits
- measuring and recording the patient's statistics accurately
- interpreting laboratory data
- using a valid and reliable nutritional assessment/ screening tool
- taking appropriate actions, e.g. referral to the community dietician and/or speech and language

therapist (CSALT), liaison with the patient's GP regarding supplements and diagnostic tests.

(Peddler 1998)

Community nurses are involved in the assessment of their patients in order to identify need and plan appropriate care. As part of the initial patient assessment the British Association of Parenteral and Enteral Nutrition recommends that four key questions should always be asked

- Have you unintentionally lost weight in the past 3 months?
- Have you been eating less than usual?
- What is your usual weight?
- How tall are you?

(Lennard-Jones 1995)

This initial nursing assessment may also identify other factors that can contribute to changes in nutritional status (Table 10.5).

Physical assessment and observation of clinical signs can also identify a range of specific nutrient deficiencies or indicate underlying conditions that may contribute to a change in the patient's nutritional status (Table 10.6). The National Institute for Health and Clinical Excellence (NICE) recommend that assessment and nutritional screening should take place on initial registration at a general practice and when there is clinical concern (NICE 2006).

Assessment of dietary intake

Nursing assessment frameworks often include a component that considers dietary intake. Asking individuals or their carers what is normally eaten and in what quantities can indicate the adequacy of the diet, but this relies on the respondent having a good memory. A more formal approach is to consider recording dietary intakes over a specific period of time, such as the previous 24 hours, or keeping a food diary (Mann & Truswell 2002).

In completing a written record of the patient's dietary intake the community nurse must consider the following areas.

- Asking the patient to identify their normal eating patterns indicating when and where they eat.
- Encouraging the patient to talk about all the food and drink they are consuming by asking them to

Table 10.5 Factors that contribute to a change in nutritional status

Influencing factor	Rationale
Social situation	
Living alone	These factors can make shopping, storing and cooking of food more difficult with an over-reliance on cheaper and processed foods. As a consequence the range of nutrients within the diet can be reduced and the diet less well balanced
Social isolation	
Low socioeconomic group	
Poor education	
Poverty	
Psychological	
Bereavement	Eating is a social activity and we generally eat as part of a group. Sudden changes, such as losing a spouse, can lead to changes in dietary intake. Depression and anxiety can influence food choices as individuals can eat excessively or reduce intake completely. Loss of memory and confusional states will also reduce food intake, as cues for eating are lost. Not recognising signs of hunger and losing awareness of food or how to use eating utensils can lead to inappropriate consumption of non food items or altered eating behaviour
Depression	
Anxiety	
Mental impairment	
Physiological	
Changes in eating/dietary intake	Many illnesses influence the ability to eat, swallow, digest and utilise nutrients. Alterations to taste, poor dental/oral hygiene will reduce appetite. Reduction in mobility/dexterity can influence ability to shop and prepare food. Drug–nutrient interactions can also alter nutrient and/or drug bioavailability (see Table 10.19)
Diagnosis	
Polypharmacy	
Physical impairment	
Ageing process	
Multiple pathology	
Cancer	
Dry oral mucosa	
Poor-fitting dentures	
Tooth decay	

Source: Pirlich et al. 2005.

describe what they have eaten at the previous mealtime. For example, 'What did you eat and drink when you woke up this morning?' 'What did you eat for your breakfast?' 'Did you have anything to eat and drink after breakfast but before your lunch?'

Table 10.6 Examples of clinical signs/symptoms that may indicate nutritional deficiency. Adapted from Webb G (2002)

Sign/Symptom	Deficiency
Loose-hanging clothes, wasted appearance, loose-fitting rings and watches	Energy/protein deficiency
Loss of hair pigment. Hair falls out easily	Protein/energy deficiency in children
White 'foamy' spots on the cornea	Vitamin A
Dry and infected cornea	
Oedema	Protein
Dermatitis	Niacin
Loss of peripheral sensations	Thiamin (vitamin B_1)
Spongy, bleeding gums	Vitamin C
Bowed legs	Vitamin D
Confusion	Water, niacin
Easy bruising	Vitamin C, K
Pale conjunctiva	Iron
Atrophic tongue	Iron, vitamin B_{12}, folic acid, riboflavin
Angular stomatitis	Iron, riboflavin

- Where possible, suggesting that the patient or their carer measure food portions using standard household measures such as spoonfuls and cups.
- Asking the patient to include any supplements that they might be taking, including vitamins and minerals.

Assessment of swallowing

Following an initial assessment a more detailed assessment of swallowing may be required. In many care settings nurses are being trained using an identified screening tool to complete an initial swallowing (dysphagia) screen prior to referral to the CSALTs (Figure 10.2) (Perry 2001; Dangerfield & Sullivan 2002; SIGN 2004). In completing the tool it is important that local protocol gives guidance about when to refer to the CSALT team. Training in the use of a screening tool and regular clinical updates is essential to maintain competency and update knowledge.

Following a referral to the CSALT, where relevant the patient will be given a list of foods that should be avoided and advice about modifications to food consistency. Changing the consistency of food can be achieved by mashing, liquidising or, if using fluids, adding a maize starch substance such as 'Thick and Easy', which is added in measured amounts to liquids (food and drinks) to achieve the required thickness. The community nurse may play an essential role in supporting patients and/or carers in the use of thickening agents and adherence to the advice given. 'Thick and Easy' is available on FP10 (GP10 in Scotland).

Screening for swallowing difficulties
Early identification of swallowing difficulties is essential to ensure the appropriate nutritional support is given. Patients at risk of suffering from dysphagia include those with:

- cerebral vascular accidents (CVA)
- motor neurone disease
- multiple sclerosis
- dementia
- Parkinson's disease
- tracheostomy
- laryngectomy
- head/neck surgery (or those receiving radiotherapy to these areas)
- head/neck tumours.

Some of the signs and symptoms that may indicate a patient is having problems with swallowing include:

- drooling and loss of lip seal
- impaired chewing, poor control of food in the mouth
- pocketing of food between the mouth and gums, mouth odour
- difficulty in initiation of swallowing; delayed or slow swallowing
- coughing, choking, nasal regurgitation
- wet-sounding voice, repeated throat clearing
- food sticking in the throat, regurgitation, heartburn, chest pain
- chronic chest infection
- weight loss.

(Wieseke *et al.* 2008; Nazarko 2010)

Nutritional risk screening tools

Nutritional risk screening tools have been developed to assist the assessment process by providing a quick

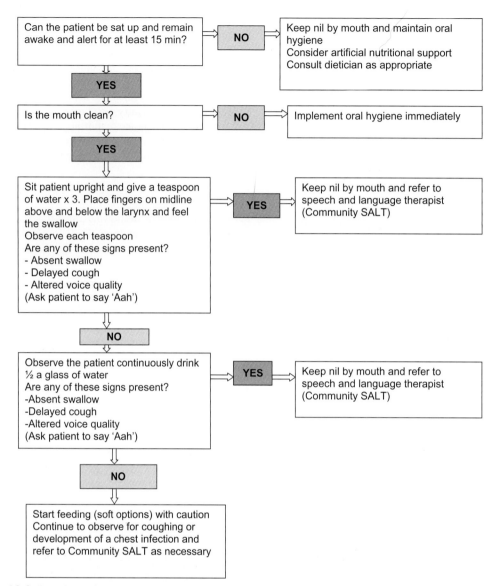

Figure 10.2 Example of a swallowing screen. Adapted from SIGN 78 2004.

method of identifying nutritional risk. There are a number of tools available, many of which contain elements derived from anthropometry (Webb 2002). However, few have been validated and their reliability can be questioned (Mackintosh & Hankey 2001).

In completing a nutritional screening tool it is important that each component is completed, a score identified and the appropriate action taken. Most tools now include a list of actions to be taken with given scores;

these range from monitoring and encouraging dietary intake to use of supplements and referral to the community dietetics department.

MUST screening tool

In 2003, the European Society for Parenteral and Enteral Nutrition (ESPEN) produced guidelines for nutritional screening in community, hospital and elderly care settings. It is suggested that the MUST system has a high degree of reliability and validity when screening patients for under nutrition (ESPEN 2003; Stratton *et al.* 2004). Furthermore its use in the UK within the community setting is now recommended (BAPEN 2003a).

Malnutrition screening tool (MST)

The malnutrition screening tool (MST) was developed for use in the community setting (Ward *et al.* 1998). During its development, validity and reliability in identifying those patients at risk of malnutrition was demonstrated. The questions used within this tool have been adopted by many Trusts in the production of their tools.

Mini nutritional assessment tool (MNA)

This tool has been designed for the specific assessment of older adults (Vellas *et al.* 1999). In its development it was validated by three consecutive studies, which demonstrated its reliability in 93% of cases.

Anthropometric assessment

Weight

Weight gain or loss (except when dieting) is not generally rapid; therefore in health, an individual's weight tends to remain stable for long periods of time. Routine weighing of a patient is of use in the community to identify times when weight loss or gain is excessive. Total body weight loss of more than 5% in 3 weeks or 10% in 3 months is considered excessive.

In older adults, excessive weight loss correlates with an increase in morbidity and mortality (Omran & Morley 2000a).

In the community, weighing patients can be difficult, but whenever possible a weight should be obtained. In weighing patients it is recommended that:

- the same scales are used each time
- patients are weighed wearing similar layers of clothing and that this is documented.

Waist circumference

If it is not possible for the community nurse to obtain a patient's weight, measuring waist circumference is an acceptable alternative and can be a useful aid to assessment.

- A waist circumference greater than 94 cm in men and 80 cm in women indicates that no further weight should be gained.
- A waist circumference greater than 102 cm in men and 88 cm in women is indicative of obesity and weight loss is required.

(Kushner & Blatner 2005)

Central adiposity (fat deposition around the waist) is linked to:

- heart disease
- hypertension
- type 2 diabetes.

(NHS Cancer Plan 2000; DH 2000, 2001a)

Body mass index (BMI) – Quetelet's index

The BMI is the most widely used method of predicting body mass (fat and lean mass) in adults. However, it is suggested that this should be used with caution when assessing older, frail patients as the index/tool was derived from studies using younger, well individuals (Elia & Lunn 1997).

Using this method the BMI is calculated by dividing the patient's weight, in kilograms, by their height in metres squared, and the result is then compared with standard figures (Box 10.2).

$$BMI = \frac{weight\ (kg)}{height\ (m^2)}$$

Height should be recorded in the standing position by using a standometre or portable anthropometre. Where patients have severe curvature of the spine or are unable to stand the height can be estimated from calculating the knee height, ulna length or demi-span.

Box 10.2 BMI and its relationship to weight

BMI	
BMI < 19	Underweight
BMI 20–25	Normal range
BMI 26–30	Overweight
BMI 31 and over	Obese

A patient would be considered malnourished if they had any of the following:

- BMI less than 18.5kg/m^2
- BMI less than 20kg/m^2 and unintentional weight loss greater than 5% within the past 3–6 months
- Unintentional weight loss greater than 10% within the past 3–6 months.

(NICE 2006)

If neither height nor weight can be obtained then BMI can be estimated by measuring the mid upper arm circumference (MUAC).

- If MUAC is <23.5 cm, BMI is likely to be <20kg/m^2
- If MUAC is >32.0 cm, BMI is likely to be > 30kg/m^2 (BAPEN 2003b).

Estimation of height using knee height
Knee height is recorded while the patient is sitting, using a tape measure from the knee to the floor. The estimated height is then calculated by the following equations:

$$(2.03 \times \text{knee height [cm]}) - (0.04 \times \text{age [yr]} + 64.19)$$
$$= \text{height of a man}$$

$$(1.83 \times \text{knee height [cm]}) - (0.24 \times \text{age [yr]} + 84.88)$$
$$= \text{height of a women}$$

Estimation of height using demi-span
The estimation of height using the demi-span is considered acceptable in the assessment of body mass index and is considered a practical approach for estimating height in the community (Hirani & Mindell 2008). The demi-span is the distance from the web of the fingers (between middle and ring finger) and the sternal notch, measured using a non-stretch measuring tape, when the subject's arm is held horizontally.

Further information on how to estimate height using alternative measures is available online from BAPEN (www.bapen.org.uk/must_nutrition_screening.html).

Diagnostic tests

There are many biochemical tests that can be undertaken including the following.

- Testing of the blood/urine for ketones and glucose may be useful. Ketones alone, without an increase in glucose, can indicate periods of time with inadequate food intake. Changes in blood glucose can indicate how well diabetes is controlled or the impact of an acute illness.
- Serum albumin. This is a measure of long-standing protein energy malnutrition (PEM). Hypoalbuminaemia can be predictive of anergy (inadequate energy intake), sepsis and malnutrition (Goodinson 1987). However, serum albumin is not a good indicator of nutritional status in physically frail elderly (Kuzuya *et al.* 2007).
- Serum iron tests measure whether iron levels are too low. A low level may be indicative of iron deficiency anaemia or an iron storage disorder, and it can also be predictive of low iron intake.

It is essential to remember that biochemical tests alone are not recommended for assessment of a patient's nutritional status. Any test/s undertaken must be used in conjunction with a full nursing assessment and nutritional screen (Omran & Morley 2000b).

Referral to the community dietetic department

Community nurse caseloads contain a number of patients living with long-term diseases/conditions. Therefore it is essential that community nurses have the knowledge and competence necessary to be able to offer patients and/or carers ongoing nutritional advice and support. Indicators for when to make a timely and appropriate referral to the community dietician/local dietetic department for assessment/reassessment should also be an integral component of case management and care planning. This is particularly important when a patient is being discharged from an acute setting with enteral feeding, as it may take up to 7 days to organise the delivery of equipment and feed (NCCAC 2006). Prompt referral will also ensure that the overall strategy for nutritional support is focused on:

- meeting the individual needs of the patient
- preventing unnecessary admissions to hospital due to exacerbation of long-term conditions/diseases
- improving outcomes for the patient
- improving a patient's ability to function
- improving a patient's quality of life.

(NHS Cancer Plan 2000; DH 2000, 2001a, 2001b, 2005; Chatterjee 2005)

To aid the accurate assessment of a patient referred to the dietician and prevent repetition of diagnostic tests, the community nurse should, with the patient's consent, provide the following information:

- name, age and diagnosis
- previous medical history
- medications (prescribed and over the counter)
- name of GP and contact details
- weight history, current weight and height
- results from nutritional screening tool
- results from swallowing screening tool
- results from any biochemical tests taken
- outcomes of any strategies already tried, e.g. advice and encouragement regarding food choices, fortification of food and supplementation of the diet
- details of referral to any other members of the multiprofessional team, including speech and language therapy or occupational therapy.

Wound healing

Wound healing is closely associated with nutritional status, yet there is limited evidence to support active nutritional support in reducing complications or improving wound healing (Wild *et al.* 2010).

Some micronutrients have been associated with wound healing (Table 10.7) and patients with leg ulcers may benefit from active nutritional support. In general the community nurse should advise patients to eat a healthy, balanced diet.

Coronary heart disease

Obesity and hypertension are associated with the development of coronary heart disease (CHD) and dietary

Table 10.7 Micronutrients and their role in wound healing (Biesalski 2010)

Nutrient	Action	Rationale	Advice
Vitamin C	A water-soluble antioxidant that is essential in the hydroxylation of proline and lysine in the synthesis of collagen	Vitamin C use increases with acute illness, stress and injury Smokers generally have a requirement that is twice that of non-smokers	Encourage an increase in fruit and vegetable intake within the diet Suggest drinking fruit juice as this can help fluid intake as well as vitamin C intake. Avoid grapefruit juice if the patient is also taken cardiac drugs
Vitamin A	Important for cellular differentiation and proliferation. Enhances the inflammatory response Increases the release of growth factors, which are important in wound healing	Patients with a severely reduced appetite may have an inadequate intake	Suggest an increase in the consumption of dairy products, eggs and liver (if appropriate)
Zinc	An essential component of a number of enzyme pathways including those in the formation of collagen	Zinc deficiency can occur as a result of diarrhoea, diuretic use, laxatives, enteral and parenteral nutrition Iron tablets can compete with zinc in the diet for absorption and contribute to deficiency states	Dietary sources include red meat products and unrefined cereals. Generally added to breakfast cereals
Iron	It is important in the transportation of oxygen by haemoglobin and as a factor in collagen hydroxylation	Elderly patients are more at risk of iron deficiency due to reduced dietary intake and changes in the GI tract	Iron is widely found in both animal and green vegetable products, but its availability is limited. Iron supplementation may be appropriate if the appetite is poor. Patients on iron tablets should be encouraged to take these with orange juice to increase absorption and to avoid taking them with food or tea, which reduces absorption

223

Table 10.8 Dietary advice in the management of coronary heart disease

Dietary advice	Rationale
Encourage a healthy balanced diet	Eating a healthy balanced diet should enable a reduction in the consumption of fats and refined carbohydrates
If BMI 25 or more advise patient to lose weight giving the following advice:	Obesity increases the level of circulating triglyceride, increasing the level of low-density lipoproteins, which contribute to an increased risk of CHD
Reduce total fat intake by removing all visible fat from meat products	Obesity also increases peripheral resistance increasing the risk of hypertension
Remove skin from chicken	
Measure oils and fats when cooking	
Use low-fat spreads	Low-fat food products can help patients to lose weight as part of a diet but patients need to remember that they still contain fat and should not eat them to excess
Use skimmed milk and low-fat dairy products	
Reduce intake of refined carbohydrates such as cakes, biscuits and sweets	Excess energy consumed in the form of carbohydrates is stored as triglycerides in the body, increasing the risk of obesity
Reduce intake of processed foods such as meat pies, sausages and pizzas	Processed foods can contain 'hidden' amounts of fats
Increase exercise/activity	Increasing exercise increases energy expenditure (see Table 10.4) and can help patients to lose weight
Reduce salt intake:	Patients with hypertension can benefit from restricting their salt intake. A reduced level of salt (sodium) reduces fluid retention and as a consequence may reduce blood volume and blood pressure
Replace salt in cooking with pepper and herbs	
Do not add additional salt at the table	
Avoid processed foods that contain salt such as ham, bacon, preserved foods, pizzas, canned vegetables, pickles, canned and packet soup, meat and yeast extracts, stock cubes, biscuits and foods containing monosodium glutamate.	
Avoid salt substitutes	Salt substitutes should be avoided as they can increase consumption of other electrolytes such as potassium. Patients may consume more than recommended to achieve a 'salt' taste
Eat monounsaturated and polyunsaturated fats as part of a balanced diet by:	Most patients with CHD need to reduce their total fat intake, but fats contain essential fatty acids (EFA) and are beneficial in the diet and can help in the management of CHD. By consuming oily fish and rapeseed oil and olive oil consumption of EFA can be maintained even though total fat intake is reduced.
including oily fish such as mackerel, herring and salmon in the diet	
using rape seed/olive oil instead of butter/lard in cooking	
Read food labels	By reading food labels people can become more aware of the food they are consuming and what ingredients are contained within them. Many processed foods contain hidden amounts of salt, fat and sugar

224

advice is an important component in the care management of the patient (Table 10.8).

Disorders of the gastrointestinal tract (GI tract)

Patients with disorders of the GI tract may require support from the community nurse to follow dietary advice or regimens prescribed. In other situations patients may report symptoms that can be managed by the community nurse (Table 10.9).

Diabetes mellitus

Diabetes mellitus is classified into two broad groups type 1 and type 2. Diet is an important component in the management of both type 1 and type 2 diabetes, and dietary advice is essential to reduce the risk of

Table 10.9 GI tract disorders, common symptoms and dietary advice

Disease/ condition	Symptom/s	Advice/action	Rationale
Dyspepsia (indigestion)	Nausea, heartburn, discomfort, epigastric pain	Avoid foods such as onions, cucumbers, peppers, raw vegetables and coffee	These foods have been associated with adverse reactions leading to discomfort
		Eat small frequent meals, taking a snack at bedtime.	Food in the stomach stimulates the production of bicarbonate rich pancreatic secretions, which neutralises acid in the duodenum
		Avoid nicotine, aspirin and highly spiced food.	These substances are known to cause gastric irritation
Early Dumping syndrome (30 min after consumption of food)	Faintness, sweating, epigastric discomfort and giddiness after consumption of food	Eat small regular, dry meals	Rapid gastric emptying is triggered by distension of the stomach
		Take drinks between meals and not with meals	Fluids empty more quickly than solids
		Avoid foods that worsen symptoms	Individuals may find that certain types of food precipitate the symptoms these should then be avoided. Care must be taken that the diet remains balanced without any major food groups removed
Late Dumping syndrome (1–1½h after consumption of food)	Faintness, sweating, confusion – similar to that of hypoglycaemia	Avoid sugar and sugar-containing foods. Eat carbohydrates in the form of starch-containing foods such as bread or pasta	Sugar and sugar-containing foods increase blood glucose levels quickly. Eating starch-containing foods slows down the rate at which blood glucose increases
Irritable bowel syndrome (IBS)	Abdominal pain, diarrhoea, constipation, passing mucus, flatulence, nausea and vomiting, and bloating	Try to eat a diet that is as varied as is possible	Excluding too many food groups will lead to an imbalanced diet and may lead to nutrient deficiencies
		Avoid certain foods that are known to aggravate symptoms	Certain foods such as green peppers are thought to trigger abnormal colonic responses, which lead to symptoms
		Increase intake of non-starch polysaccharides by increasing fruit, vegetable and pulse consumption	Non-starch polysaccharides are important in maintaining the 'health' of the colon by providing substrates for bacterial fermentation. Abnormal fermentation has been linked to IBS (Bosaeus 2004; Bennett & Talley 2002
Constipation	Altered pattern of defecation, hard pellet-like stools, abdominal pain, confusion, excess straining	Suggest drinking a glass of water with each meal as well as regular drinks throughout the day. Eat more tinned, frozen or fresh fruit. Choose whole grain or cereal enriched breakfast cereals such as Weetabix, Puffed Wheat, Shredded Wheat and All Bran	Patients who are dehydrated can become constipated as more fluids are absorbed from the colon
			Increasing the consumption of foods containing non-starch polysaccharides and cellulose increases faecal mass. This in turn increases peristalsis. Adding bran to the diet can be unpalatable and not all patients will be able to maintain a high bran diet
		If constipation is secondary to the use of opiates, in the management of chronic pain, consider the use of an appropriate aperients as well as including, where appropriate, the advice listed above	Opiates reduce peristalsis and can lead to constipation. Encouraging an increase in fluids, fruit and vegetables may not be possible due to the underlying illness and inability to eat

225

Table 10.10 Dietary advice for patients with type 1 and type 2 diabetes

Dietary advice	Rationale
Increase consumption of fruit and vegetables that contain complex carbohydrates, reduce intake of refined carbohydrates found in highly processed foods such as biscuits and confectionary	50–55% of the energy intake should be in the form of polysaccharides and non-starch polysaccharides (NSP) that are found in fruit and vegetables. Polysaccharides and NSP contain viscous fibres that slow down glucose absorption leading to a gradual rise in blood glucose levels
If overweight, encourage the patient to lose weight by reducing energy intake and increasing activity levels	Increasing consumption of fruit and vegetables as part of a balanced diet can also reduce energy intake (Barker 2002)
	80% of patients who are diagnosed as having type 2 diabetes are overweight or obese at diagnosis. Losing weight and maintaining a steady weight, whether they require insulin, oral hypoglycaemic or no treatment is essential for optimum diabetic control (Lamont *et al.* 2005)
Encourage the patient to be aware of the impact different carbohydrate food sources have on blood sugar levels	Carbohydrate foods do not all have the same effect on blood glucose levels. The glycaemic effect is determined by many factors, including the presence of fats and proteins and whether the food is processed. Foods that have a lesser effect on blood glucose (low glycaemic index) include pulses, pasta, raw fruit and milk. Foods that have a greater effect on blood glucose (high glycaemic index) include white bread, fruit juices, biscuits and sweet fruits such as strawberries
Reduce total fat consumption and encourage the patient to be more aware of the types of fat consumed	A diet that is high in fat is more likely to lead to obesity. The type of fat consumed can also impact on the effectiveness of insulin and contribute to the overall diabetic management. The percentage of fat in the diet should not exceed 30–35% of the energy requirements, and of that fat consumed, 20–25% should be derived from monounsaturated and polyunsaturated fatty acids. These are found in olive oil, rapeseed oil and fish oils (NHS 2011)
	Patients with diabetes mellitus (type 1) have a greater risk for CHD; reducing fat intake may reduce subsequent arterial disease

complications associated with uncontrolled blood sugar, for example:

- retinopathy
- peripheral neuropathy
- glaucoma
- atherosclerosis.

Type 1 diabetes can occur at any age but is more common in the young. In all cases the condition is treated by the administration of insulin and by diet.

Type 2 diabetes generally occurs in later life, but an increasing number of young adults are presenting with the condition. Patients may be treated by diet, diet and oral medication, or diet and insulin therapy. Obesity, in all ages, increases the risk of type 2 diabetes.

All patients diagnosed with diabetes mellitus will need to be monitored and reviewed by a dietician. The community nurse will also play a leading role in informing and empowering the patient regarding diet and individual needs in line with the diabetes quality standards (NICE 2011).

The principles of dietary advice are based on encouraging healthy eating with an awareness of how foods impact on blood glucose levels. Patients should be advised to avoid buying special 'diabetic' products (Table 10.10).

Cancer

Many patients living with cancer would benefit from nutritional support (van Bokhorst de van der Schueren 2005; Bozzetti 2011). For those being cared for or supported at home by community nurses, it is important that, where relevant, the community dietician is included as part of the multidisciplinary team (MDT).

Malnutrition in patients with cancer can occur due to a range of factors. These include the following.

- The position of the tumour, as this may interfere with the patient's ability to eat and swallow (head/neck) or digest and absorb nutrients (upper GI tract and accessory organs).
- The effects of chemotherapy, which can lead to changes in taste, anorexia, nausea, vomiting,

Table 10.11 Dietary advice for patients with cancer

Advice	Rationale
Administer anti-emetics, analgesia and aperients as appropriate	Nausea and sickness, pain and constipation can all reduce the appetite and decrease food intake
Encourage small meals, prior to treatments, avoiding foods for which there is a taste aversion	Many patients will expect to feel nauseous following chemotherapy and radiotherapy; eating a small meal in advance can ensure dietary intake is maintained. Some patients will feel better if they eat following their treatment, even if they initially feel nauseous
Avoid foods that have bitter and acid tastes such as those found in some fruits and meats	Acidic fruits and meat proteins are most susceptible to taste alteration, with patients describing them as metallic
Avoid foods that are too hot or cold	Extremes of temperature can alter the taste and the enjoyment of food
Avoid foods that have a strong odour	Overpowering odours of some foods may cause nausea
Avoid spicy foods	Spicy foods can exacerbate oral discomfort and may cause nausea
Eat small meals at frequent intervals, offer foods that are enjoyed rather than stick to a rigid diet	Eating small meals more frequently can increase dietary intake over a day and reduce feelings of nausea and bloating. A healthy balanced diet is often less important in the care given to patients with cancer, the emphasis being to encourage eating and enjoyment of food
Use subcutaneous fluids where fluid intake is limited	When a patient is unable to take oral fluids in sufficient quantity subcutaneous fluids can be administered

anaemia, ulcers in the mouth (including oral thrush and stomatitis), constipation and fatigue.
- The effects of radiotherapy, depending on the site can lead to sore mouth and dry throat, changes to taste, fatigue, anorexia, nausea and vomiting, intestinal obstruction and colitis.
- Tumour-induced cachexia due to the presence of circulating cytokines (Argilés et al. 2005).

Planned nutritional support for patients with cancer can improve tolerance to treatment and increase resistance to infection. However, intensive support, via enteral or parenteral routes is not always appropriate and should be discussed with the patient, their family and the MDT before being commenced.

Cachexia

This is a complex condition, characterised by extreme weight loss and wasting, caused by the presence of cytokines in the circulation. Although commonly associated with cancer, in particular prostate and some lung cancers, this condition can also occur in chronic inflammatory disorders such as chronic lung disease, chronic heart disease and auto immune deficiency syndrome (AIDS).

Cancer cachexia is associated with:

- an increase risk of complications
- loss of skeletal muscle and visceral proteins

- lipolysis
- nausea
- anorexia
- fatigue
- weight loss.

(Stephens and Fearon 2008)

In this situation specific dietary advice is difficult to give, therefore the community nurse will need to adopt a sensitive, sympathetic approach and plan care that recognises the needs of both the patient and, where relevant, carer. For example:

- distress caused by an inability to eat
- potential feelings of nausea
- loss of enjoyment from eating.

The community nurse can also play an active role in providing nutritional support by giving practical advice (Table 10.11).

Patients with weight loss/ loss of appetite

Weight loss or loss of appetite can occur for a range of reasons:

- illness/disease for example coronary heart disease (CHD), chronic lung disease and diabetes

227

Table 10.12 A nourishing diet – dietary advice for patients with weight loss or reduced appetite

Dietary advice	Rationale
Eat little and often, have three meals daily as well as 2–3 snacks between meals. Snacks can include sandwiches spread with butter, mayonnaise or both and containing cold meat, fish, cheese, boiled egg or peanut butter. Toast with butter and tinned fish, beans, eggs, tinned pasta and/or cheese. Bread and butter with fish fingers, kippers or smoked haddock	The aim of the dietary advice is to increase the energy (calorie) intake. If a patient has a small appetite each mouthful of food needs to contain more energy (calories). Consuming a diet that is very high in fruit and vegetables, while containing vitamins, minerals and complex carbohydrates will also make somebody feel full, and energy intake may remain low
Encourage the use of milk and milky drinks including hot chocolate, Horlicks, Build-up and Complan	Milky drinks are more economical than commercial supplements and are often better tolerated by patients. Encouraging drinks also increases the fluid intake
Suggest adding 2–4 tablespoons of milk powder (e.g. Marvel) to a pint of full cream milk and use this in place of ordinary milk in drinks, cereals, soups, sauces and puddings	Adding milk powder to milk increases the energy (calorie) content without changing the taste
Add grated cheese to savoury foods	Increasing the energy intake (kilojoules/kilocalories) will help to increase or to maintain weight
Add double cream, custard, evaporated milk, thick and creamy yoghurt, sugar, honey or fruit to puddings and cereals	
Fry vegetables in oil, butter or ghee	
Have extra puddings during the day	
Encourage the patient to have at least one hot meal per day	Elderly frail patients who do not have at least three hot meals each week are more likely to suffer from malnutrition

- cancer
- depression
- reduced mobility/dexterity, which makes shopping or cooking difficult
- constipation
- bereavement
- low income.

(DiMaria & Amelia 2005)

Following a holistic assessment and identification of the probable cause (*see* Chapter 1) the community nurse should plan a programme of nursing interventions in partnership with the patient, and if appropriate carer, that focuses on, for example:

- minimising or treating the identified cause, e.g. referral to the GP for diagnostic testing.
- the prescribing of appropriate medication/s
- advising on the appropriate and correct self-administration of medication
- referral to the community dietician, physiotherapist/ occupational therapist
- improving the patient's food and fluid intake
- encouraging a diet high in calories (energy) and protein
- patient/carer education.

A nourishing diet (Table 10.12) should contain plenty of kilojoules/calories (energy) and protein, and may contain proportionally less fruit and vegetables. In very frail patients with a small appetite it is better to encourage adequate energy intake, as micronutrients can be supplemented through multi-vitamin tablets. As weight is gained appetite increases; at this stage increasing the consumption of fruit and vegetables will restore the balance of the diet. The community nurse should regularly monitor and record the weight of patients with weight loss or reduced appetite and liaise with the GP as appropriate.

If patients are finding it difficult, but are able to cook for themselves, they should be encouraged to continue to prepare their own meals with the use of appropriate aids supplied by the occupational therapist, e.g. perching stool or adapted equipment. Alternatively most supermarkets now offer a wide range of frozen, chilled or packet ready meals, there are also council-run meals-on-wheels services available and some private companies offer home delivery of ready-prepared frozen meals.

If the cause of the patient's weight loss/loss of appetite is due to depression or social isolation, where appropriate, it may be beneficial to the patient to be offered information and contact details for:

- local voluntary organisations
- local luncheon/social clubs
- local religious/cultural groups.

Where under nutrition is associated with low income or restricted mobility, the community nurse should obtain consent from the patient to make a referral to the local social services department for assessment.

Patients who are overweight

If a patient has a sudden onset of weight gain it is essential that they seek advice from their GP as investigations may be necessary to rule out any underlying cause, e.g. an underactive thyroid gland or malignancy.

Overweight people are often very aware of their weight, and many of them will have tried diets before with little or no success. However, achieving even a modest weight loss, of approximately 10% of total body weight at a rate of 1–2 kg per week, can have a positive impact on health. This may also be more achievable than aiming for a goal weight that is desirable for an individual's height.

When supporting patients with a weight-loss programme, the community nurse should discuss strategies sensitively (Table 10.13) and, where appropriate, refer to the community dietician when there are complex needs and/or specific advice and support is necessary. They should also offer health education and advice on increasing physical activity; this may include referral to the community physiotherapist for assessment and advice and suggesting the following activities to the patient:

- standing and walking a few steps around a room
- stting in a chair and lifting the legs alternatively off the floor, 10 times
- stretching arms above the head and then bringing them down, 10 times
- where possible, going outside and walking briskly for 5 min.

Obesity

In recent years the proportion of the population in England that is obese or overweight has been rising. The NHS Information Centre (2011) suggest that 23.1% of men and 24.8% of women are obese. In 2004, the highest prevalence of obesity was noted in ethnic minority groups, with 25% of Black Caribbean men and Irish men and 38% of Black African women categorised as obese.

Health concerns associated with obesity include:

Table 10.13 Dietary advice for patients attempting to lose weight

Dietary advice	Rationale
Suggest patients use smaller plates to serve food	Reducing the size of the plates can reduce the volume of food consumed by reducing portion sizes
Identify normal eating pattern and behaviours	To establish what types of food and the pattern of eating will enable the community nurse to identify ways of reducing food intake that does not involve radical changes in lifestyle
Discourage snacking between meals; if snacking is habitual, suggest fresh fruit and vegetables (celery, carrot, apples) as an alternative to biscuits and cakes	By reducing the amount of snacks between a meal, energy (kilojoules/kilocalories) intake should decrease. Excessive consumption of some fruits and vegetables such as bananas, grapes and avocado that are relatively high in energy (kilojoules/kilocalories) can lead to weight gain.
Increase the proportion of fruit and vegetables eaten with each meal whilst reducing the proportion of fatty or processed foods	By consuming more fruits and vegetables, total energy intake can be reduced.
Remove all visible fats from meat products, use low-fat products where possible, grill food instead of frying, measure oil when cooking	Fat is energy dense (high in kilojoules/kilocalories) and by reducing total fat intake total energy) kilojoule/kilocalorie intake will reduce

- increased risk of developing type 2 diabetes
- high blood pressure
- heart disease
- cancer
- reduced mobility
- poor healing of leg ulcers
- social isolation.

Nutritional support in the home

During the past 30 years, providing nutritional support to people in their own home has expanded rapidly. Elia *et al.* (2001) estimate that in the year 2000 nearly 20 000

229

people in the UK had home enteral tube feeding (HETF). Since then the British Artificial Nutrition Survey (BANS) has reported a reduction in new registrants during the period 2008–9. Of those receiving HETF, 1 in 6 were suffering from some form of malignancy. A similar fall was noted in the number of new patients receiving home parenteral nutrition (HPN) with a total of 148 new registrants being recorded in 2009. This reduction is thought to reflect the need to gain consent for registration and may not reflect the true numbers receiving HETF or HPN (BANS 2010).

In 2001, it was noted that of those receiving home nutritional support:

- 60% were over 60 years of age
- 51% were housebound
- 59% required total help with home enteral feeding.

(Elia *et al.* 2001)

The most common form of artificial nutritional support in the community is the provision of manufactured supplement or sip feeds. It has been calculated that for every one person receiving enteral tube feeding, 12 people are in receipt of a supplement or sip feed (Stratton & Elia 2007).

Oral nutritional supplements and sip feeds

In recent years expenditure on oral nutritional supplements (ONS; manufactured products consumed in addition to dietary intake) has increased. Within the community setting it is suggested that the prescribing of oral supplements is often without appropriate assessment or review (Stratton & Elia 2007). An audit undertaken by one PCT looking at the prescribing of supplement and sip feeds found that following consultation with a dietician:

- 34% of prescriptions were stopped
- 28% of supplements were changed to a lower dose
- 91% of patients required at least one review by a dietician.

(Panico 2002)

The use of oral supplements and sip feeds is of value for patients at high risk of malnutrition and who are not eating well, for example those living with chronic obstructive pulmonary disease (COPD), cancer, cystic fibrosis, Crohn's disease and also older or frail patients. However, it appears that there is no clear evidence of their benefit, which suggests the need for further research in this area within the community setting (Stratton & Elia 2007). Oral nutritional supplements are consumed in addition to a patient's normal dietary

Table 10.14 Dietary advice to patients receiving nutritional supplements (Panico 2002)

Dietary advice	Rationale
Supplements should be taken in addition to, not instead of meals	The prescribed supplements have been prescribed to increase energy and nutrient intake by supplementing but not replacing meals
Advise the patient to take them between meals or after a meal	If they are taken just before a meal they will make the patient feel full, reducing their total food intake
If patients find them difficult to drink from the carton, suggest they empty them into a cup	Older patients may find using a straw more difficult than drinking out of a cup
Advise the patient that they must consume the correct number of supplements each day	By consuming the prescribed amount they will meet their nutritional goal of increasing nutrient intake
If the patient does not like the taste, try serving them at a different temperature, e.g. keep some in the fridge or heat them up	Changing the temperature can improve and change the flavour. The dietician will be able to give you more advice on this. Many manufacturers provide recipes for the use of supplements. If a patient is having supplements for a long period of time (more than about 4 weeks) they may suffer from taste fatigue and require alternative flavours to be prescribed

intake. Sip feeds refer to 'complete' meal replacements, where patients are not consuming food, but rely on manufactured feeds. To ensure that individual patient needs are met it is recommended that both ONS and sip feeds are prescribed and monitored by a community dietician (Table 10.14).

When providing nursing care and/or support to patients in their home receiving nutritional support it is important that the process is managed and co-ordinated by the community nurse.

The role of the community nurse is to:

- provide support and education for the patient and their carer
- advise about storage and usage of the supplement or feed

Table 10.15 Nutritional supplements (on prescription) per 200 ml carton unless otherwise stated. Adapted from the NPF Nurse Prescribing Formulary (http://bnf.org/bnf/bnf/current/search.htm?q=nutritional%20supplements)

	Kcals	Protein (g)	Manufacturer
High energy			
Calshake (90 g sachet plus 240 ml full cream milk)	598	12.00	Fresenius Kabi
Clinutren 1.5	300	11.2	Nestle
Ensure Plus (220 ml)	330	13.75	Abbott Nutrition
Fresubin Energy	300	11.2	Fresenius Kabi
Fortifresh (yoghurt drink)	300	12.00	Nutricia
Fortisip	300	12.00	Nutricia
Resource Shake (175 ml)	300	8.9	Novartis
Scandishake (85 g sachet plus 240 ml full cream milk)	598	12.00	SHS International
Savoury (need to be heated)			
Ensure (250 ml)	250	10.00	Abbott Nutrition
Fresubin Energy	300	11.2	Fresenius Kabi
Fortisip	300	12.00	Nutricia
Puddings			
Clinutren Dessert (125 g)	160	12.00	Nestle
Formance (113 g)	170	4.0	Abbott Nutrition
Forticreme (125 g)	201	12.5	Nutricia
Resource Dessert (125 g)	200	6.00	Novartis
Standard			
Clinutren ISO	200	7.6	Nestle
Ensure (250 ml)	250	10.00	Abbott Nutrition
Fresubin	200	7.6	Fresenius Kabi
With fibre			
Enrich (250 ml)	256	9.4	Abbott Nutrition
Enrich Plus	305	12.5	Abbott Nutrition
Fresubin Energy Fibre	300	11.3	Fresenius Kabi
Fortisip Multifibre	300	12.00	Nutricia
Resource Fibre	300	8.9	Novartis
Fruit juice			
Clinutren Fruit	250	11.2	Nestle
Enlive (240 ml)	300	9.6	Abbott Nutrition
Fortijuice	300	8.0	Nutricia
Provide Xtra	250	7.5	Fresenius Kabi

- monitor the effectiveness of the supplement or feed
- liaise with the GP and community dietician.

There are many different supplements and sip feeds available on prescription FP10 (GP10 in Scotland) and they can be found in Appendix 7 of the Community Practitioners Formulary (CPF). Some Trusts may also have a recommended list of nutritional supplements and sip feeds supplied by local dietetic departments (Table 10.15 Table 10.16).

Home enteral tube feeding

Home enteral tube feeding (HETF) can be used effectively as a sole source of nutrients or as a supplement to food intake within the community. The decision to

Table 10.16 Prescribing supplement and sip feeds (Elia & Stratton 2001)

Principle	Rationale
Complete nursing assessment and nutritional screening tool	Nutritional supplements should only be prescribed following assessment and treatment of the underlying cause of malnutrition and when dietary interventions alone have been unsuccessful
Identify a nutritional plan of care that identifies supplements prescribed. Supplements should be prescribed in the numbers needed, for a set period of time with an outcome identified	Resources spent on nutritional supplements have increased in recent years with little evidence of their effectiveness
All patients prescribed nutritional supplements should be referred to a state registered dietician (SRD)	The SRD can advise on further dietary manipulation and nutritional supplements most appropriate to the individual
The brand of supplement and named flavours should be included on the prescription	Each different flavour is charged as a separate item, if 'various flavours' are requested then an item will be charged for each flavour available
If after dietary advice and use of supplements/sip feeds there is no improvement in condition seek further advice from the SRD	The SRD will be able to offer further dietary advice and suggest appropriate changes to the prescribed supplements

start HETF should only be made following consultation and discussion with the patient (if possible), the family and the healthcare team. As a medical treatment, consent is required from competent patients, prior to the commencement of tube feeding (BAPEN 2005).

Its use may enable patients to gain weight and improve their quality of life. In all cases where the patient will be receiving a complete feed via a feeding tube, referral to the community dietetic department is essential to ensure the appropriate feed is prescribed and that nutritional status is monitored.

The most common routes used for enteral tube feeding in the community include:

- nasogastric (NG)
- percutaneous endoscopically placed gastrostomy (PEG)
- radiologically inserted gastrostomy (RIG)
- jejunostomy.

(Table 10.17)

Types of feeding tube
The type of tube available will depend on the manufacturer the local Trust has contracted with. The giving sets (plastics) are not available on prescription and will be funded by either the commissioning group, dietetic department, community nursing budget or directly by the local health authority. Feeding tubes come in a range of styles depending on the manufacturer and can be made from silicone, polyvinyl chloride (PVC) or polyurethane.

It is important that the feeding tube is compatible with the giving sets (plastics) and pumps, usually supplied by the feed manufacturer. When a patient is transferred from one locality to another, it is important that the type of feeding tube is documented and compatible giving sets and pumps provided.

Nasogastric (NG)
In general, NG tube feeding is recommended for short-term feeding 2–4 weeks (NCCAC 2006). A fine-bore feeding tube should be used because it is less likely to cause complications such as:

- gastritis
- oesophageal irritation
- rhinitis.

NG feeding via fine-bore feeding tubes has been the most common method of providing complete nutritional support (Table 10.18). However, recent concern about the dangers of misplaced tubes has led to guidance being issued by the National Patient Safety Agency (Dougherty & Lister 2011; NPSA 2011). If there are locally agreed guidelines, policy and procedures in place, community nurses can insert fine-bore feeding

Table 10.17 Good practice in providing home enteral tube feeding (HETF) (NICE 2003)

Principle	Rationale
Ensure referral has been made to community dietetic team (see local protocol)	The community dietetic team will ensure that the correct feed is prescribed and delivered to the patient. In HETF the giving sets (plastics) and pumps will be provided by a specific manufacturer and delivered to a patient's own home
Discuss with the patient and/or carer (if appropriate) their involvement in HETF. Ensure that the patient and their carers have relevant contact telephone numbers, are familiar with the equipment, and are happy with the arrangements for feeding and the provision of equipment	It is important that the patient and their carers (if applicable) are happy with the provision of HETF. Patients and their carers need to have relevant contact numbers in case of problems that can occur at any time of the day or night
Prior to discharge from hospital the patient and/or carer, if appropriate, should have been taught how to care for the tube and administer feeds	Many patients/carers will be actively involved in ensuring feeds are administered. If this is not appropriate the community nursing team will be actively involved in the provision of HETF
Unopened feed and equipment should be stored in a cool, dry place. If stored outside in garden sheds or garages during the winter, make sure it does not freeze. Avoid stacking against radiators. Rotate stock to ensure it doesn't go out of date	The feed and equipment will be delivered and require storage. Referral to the manufacturer's instructions will ensure that the feed remains safe. Feed will have limited shelf life and it is important that it is used before it goes out of date
Opened packages of feed can be stored in a fridge for 24 hours	Once opened, feed should be used within 24 hours to minimise bacterial contamination. It can be stored in a household fridge, but care needs to be taken that other food products do not contaminate it

tubes following appropriate training and assessment of competency.

Risk management of a NG tube being used to provide nutritional support in the community is extremely important to maintain both patient and practitioner safety. This is of particular importance in relation to tube position (NPSA 2011). It is recommended that a multidisciplinary risk assessment is completed and documented before discharge from an acute hospital into the community (NPSA 2011). All incidences of misplacement where feeding into the lung has occurred is classed as a 'never event' in England and must be reported both locally and nationally (NPSA 2011).

Gastrostomy
A gastrostomy is recommended where it is anticipated that feeding will be medium to long term in duration, and where sufficient nutrients can be absorbed from the gastrointestinal tract. Placement of the tube will be either:

- percutaneous endoscopically (PEG) or
- radiologically inserted (RIG).

The tube is held in position by one of the following:

- flange
- flexible dome
- inflated balloon
- pigtail.

A gastrostomy tube may be replaced with a silicone button that is flush with the patient's skin (Table 10.19); the site will require cleaning and the button must be turned at least weekly (Thomas & Bishop 2007). This is increasingly becoming the most common route for enteral feeding for a period greater than 6 weeks, as the problems associated with misplacement of a NG tube can be avoided.

Jejunostomy
A jejunostomy tube is placed into a loop of the jejunum and may be the first choice of intervention for example where the patient has:

- delayed gastric emptying
- undergone upper gastrointestinal surgery.

(Table 10.19)

Table 10.18 Nasogastric (NG) feeding tubes

Type of tube	Insertion/position of tube	Use	Length of time in situ	Advantages	Disadvantages
Fine-bore feeding tube 6–9 Fg PVC	Nasogastric (NG)	To supplement oral intake or to provide route for a complete feeding regimen	<6 weeks	More comfortable than a wide-bore tube	If used for too long they tend to harden as the plasticisers (which give tube flexibility) leach out in the acid environment of the stomach
Fine-bore feeding tube 6–9 Fg polyurethane	Nasogastric (NG)	To supplement oral intake or to provide route for a complete feeding regimen	<6 weeks	More comfortable than a wide-bore tube. Remains flexible for longer	More expensive
Rigid wide-bore 10–18 Fg PVC	Nasogastric (NG)	To provide nutritional support for patients at risk of pulmonary aspiration	<6 weeks	Minimises the risk of pulmonary aspiration	Patients should be converted to a fine-bore feeding tube as soon as gastric emptying is established
Fine-bore feeding tube 6–9 Fg 100–120 cm long	Nasoduodenal (ND) Nasojejunal (NJ)	For feeding below the pyloric sphincter	<6 weeks	Can be used for patients with reduced gastric volume or gastric stasis	Tubes are placed either radiologically or endoscopically

The community nurse's role in the provision of HETF

The active and planned involvement of an appropriately trained community nurse can help to improve the patient experience of HETF and help lessen its impact on everyday life (Howard *et al.* 2006).

Community nurses play an important role in ensuring that HETF is successfully and safely achieved by:

- providing patient and carer education regarding the feed, its storage and administration
- acting as a point of contact and support for the patient and their carers
- monitoring the patient's health status and nursing needs, e.g. weight, skin integrity
- where necessary setting up feeds for administration, disconnecting plastics, monitoring the position of the feeding tube and flushing; alternatively supporting the patient and or carer to do this safely
- liaising with the community dietician and patient's GP
- initiating prescriptions.

Important areas for the community nurse to consider in their management of HETF include:

- monitoring the patient's nutritional status prior to and during the period of HETF as this will provide baseline information to assess the outcome of the nutritional support interventions
- considering the psychosocial needs of the patient; this is central to the provision of HETF as HETF can impact on the quality of life
- identifying those patients who are at risk of infection and initiating and monitoring control measures to minimise risks
- ensuring that the patient's oral health is maintained; good oral hygiene at the commencement and throughout HETF can prevent problems occurring later.

Education and training

All qualified community nursing staff who support patients/carers with enteral feeding or undertake the procedure on behalf of the patient should have undergone formal training and assessment of competency that reflects current NPSA recommendations (NPSA 2011).

This is of particular importance in relation to NG tube position, therefore it is essential that all

Table 10.19 Gastrostomy/Jejunostomy feeding tubes

Type of tube	Insertion/position of tube	Use	Length of time in situ	Advantages	Disadvantages
Percutaneous endoscopic gastrostomy (PEG)	Stoma formed and trans-abdominal feeding tube positioned using endoscopy, held in place with a flange of flexible dome	Long-term supplement or complete feeding of patients	Can be left in situ for up to 2 years	Better tolerated by patient for long-term feeding	If PEG is displaced needs admission to endoscopy unit for replacement
Balloon gastrostomy tubes	Initial formation of stoma through endoscopy	Permanent complete feeding of a patient	Can be left in situ for up to 2 years	Following initial placement tube can be replaced by an appropriately trained, competent community nurse or carer (see local protocol). Commonly low-profile button feeding tubes are used	Where an appropriately trained person is unable to replace the tube then admission to hospital will be required for tube replacement
Radiological inserted gastrostomy tube (RIG)	Position under radiological guidance and local anaesthetic	Long-term supplement or complete feeding of patients	Can be left in situ for up to 2 years		Needs admission to radiological unit for replacement
Jejunostomy endoscopic gastrostomy feeding tube (JEG)	Inserted in hospital using a jejunostomy kit, which positions a polyurethane catheter into a loop of the jejunum	Used in patients following gastric surgery or in a situation where there is delayed gastric emptying	Depending on the condition of the patient	Allows the continued feeding of a patient without the need of using parenteral feeding	Needs admission to hospital for placement

235

community nursing staff involved in the patient's package of care have the appropriate level of knowledge skills and understanding (NPSA, 2011). Training should include:

- use of equipment
- testing the level of acidity and use of pH indicator strips
- correct pH levels, i.e. 1–5.5
- the effects of medication on pH level
- tube measurement and markings
- problem solving, what action to take if, for example, aspirate is not obtained
- when it is not safe to commence the feed
- when it is necessary to check or recheck tube position, i.e. following an episode of retching, coughing or vomiting, as the tube may have become displaced
- when to seek medical advice

- when to transfer the patient to the A&E department.

(NPSA 2011)

The NPSA 2011 state that the whoosh test, acid/alkaline tests using litmus paper or interpretation of the appearance of aspirate should never be used to confirm nasogastric feeding tube position as these tests are unreliable.

Enteral feeds

The manufacturer of the feed plays an important role in HETF by for example:

- ensuring prompt and reliable delivery of feeds
- providing appropriate plastics
- providing and maintaining the pumps

- providing ongoing support to both the patient and the community nurse, including contact numbers and home visits
- providing a comprehensive home care service
- providing training for the community nurses in the use of pumps and principles of HETF.

(Howard 2011)

A small number of HETF patients might be in receipt of a specific feed that is individually formulated from a local hospital pharmacy; in those instances the supply of the feed will depend on local protocol, although the giving sets and pumps will still be provided by a manufacturer.

Types of feed
The type of feed that a patient is prescribed by the community dietician will reflect the individual patient's identified need and the function of the gastrointestinal tract. Feeds are most commonly made from:

- proteins
- carbohydrates
- fats
- vitamins, minerals and trace elements.

These are polymeric feeds and are balanced to meet individual needs. They are normally suitable for vegetarians and vegans. If a patient has a specific dietary restriction due to religious/cultural beliefs advice can be obtained from the manufacturer of the feed.

Some patients will not tolerate nutrient feeds that contain whole proteins. In such cases they will be prescribed elemental or peptide feeds (digested proteins). These feeds provide protein in the form of amino acids and peptides, which are of use when digestion and absorption are impaired (Barker 2002).

Administration of feeds
Enteral feeds can be administered as:

- a bolus
- intermittently via gravity or a pump
- continuously via a pump
- dripped by gravity or pump mechanism.

In the community setting the most common method used is intermittently via a pump.

Table 10.20 Good practice for setting up a feed for administration via a feeding tube. Adapted from NICE 2003

Action	Rationale
Effective hand decontamination using soap and water or alcohol handrub, should be carried out before starting feed preparation	Reduces bacterial load on the skin and reduces risk of feed contamination. Enteral feeds provide a perfect medium for bacterial growth. Although normal food and diets are not sterile, limiting bacterial contamination is important
Use pre-packaged, ready-to-use feeds in preference to feeds requiring decanting, reconstitution or dilution	Using ready to use feeds is easier within the community setting
If decanting, reconstituting or diluting feeds a clean working area should be prepared and equipment dedicated for enteral feed use used	
If reconstituting a feed, refer to manufacturer's instructions. Feeds are normally reconstituted using cooled boiled water or freshly opened sterile water using a non-touch technique	
Minimal handling and no-touch technique should be used to connect the administration tubes (plastics) to the enteral feeding tube	Bacterial contamination can occur if the feed is left open for an extended period of time
Plastics and feed containers are for single use and must be discarded after each feeding session	
Ready-to-use feeds may be given for a whole session, up to a maximum of 24h	Reconstituted feeds are of greater risk of contamination as they are opened prior to administration
Reconstituted feeds should be administered over a maximum of 4h	Feeds are prescribed by the volume administered over a set period of time, which ensures nutrient requirement is met
Start feed (after checking position of feeding tube) to ensure correct volume of feed is administered over the specified period of time	

236

The potential advantages of HETF for a dependent patient and the community nurse include the following.

■ It enables measured amounts of feed to be delivered within a specified time for example a 12/24-hour period.
■ It enables the establishment of a feeding pattern that reflects the patient's needs, e.g. overnight in order for the patient to participate in other activities and lead a more normal life during rest periods when the feed is not administered (Barker 2002).
■ It enables the community nurse to plan daily activities around a specific planned visit time for an individual patient.

Disadvantages include the following.

■ Potential risk of gastrointestinal disturbances.
■ Overnight feeding may not be possible where a 24-hour community nursing service is not provided. If problems arise during the night the patient may need to attend the local A&E department.
■ Potential risk of aspiration if the patient lies down (Scolapio 2007).

Nutrient/drug interactions and home enteral tube feeding

There are currently no medications licensed for administration via enteral feeding tubes, however it is recognised that in certain circumstances there are no alternative options available for some patients. Interactions between nutrients and drugs can cause serious adverse reactions, toxicities, nutritional deficiencies or occlusion of the feeding tube. Older adults and those undergoing long-term drug therapies are at particular risk. Also taking over-the-counter medications (OTC) along with prescription drugs increases the potential risk of problems occurring. The community nurse can play an important role in minimising the risk of drug related complications through:

■ patient/carer education about when and how to take medications
■ advising patient/carers to consult the pharmacist before purchasing OTC medications.

It is recommended that wherever possible medications should not be administered via a feeding tube (BAPEN 2004). Issues to be considered prior to a decision being reached regarding administration via this route include the following.

■ Is the medication slow release or enteric-coated?
■ Is there an alternative formulation of the medication available?
■ Is there an alternative route for administration of the medication?
■ Can the medication be crushed/opened?

Where there is a change in the patient's medication/s or large volumes to be administered, the community nurse should seek advice from the community pharmacist (see local protocol) prior to administration via an enteral feeding tube. For a list of some common drugs and their reactions with enteral feeds see Tables 10.21 and 10.22. There are some medicines that should never be crushed or opened these include:

237

Table 10.21 Drug–nutrient interactions

Drug classification	Generic name (Trade name)	Nutrients that may be affected	Patient teaching points
Antibiotics	Tetracycline	Riboflavin (B_2), vitamin C	Take on an empty stomach 1 hour before or 2–3 hours after meals
			Don't take milk or other dairy products and supplements within 1 hour before or within 2 hours after drug dose
			Avoid iron products and zinc
			Eat citrus fruits, baked potatoes, broccoli and whole-grain enriched breads and cereals
Anticoagulant	Warfarin	Need consistent vitamin K intake	Eat a consistent amount of foods containing vitamin K, e.g. spinach, liver and cabbage
Anti-hypertensive drug	Hydralizine	Vitamin B_6	Avoid natural liquorice and monosodium glutamate (MSG)
			Take the oral form with meals to increase absorption
			Eat whole-grain enriched breads and cereals, leafy vegetables

(Continued)

Table 10.21 *(Continued)*

Drug classification	Generic name (Trade name)	Nutrients that may be affected	Patient teaching points
Anti-inflammatory analgesic	Aspirin	Vitamins B$_{12}$ and C, folic acid, iron	Take with food or a large glass of water or milk Eat whole-grain enriched and cereals, citrus fruits, baked potatoes, broccoli, organ meats (e.g. heart, liver). Drink fruit juice
Anti-lipaemic drug	Cholestyramine (Questran) Colestipol (Colestid)	Folic acid, vitamins A, D, K	Take with food or milk. Eat a high-fibre diet Eat green leafy and deep yellow vegetables, citrus fruits and broccoli Drink low-fat milk
Anti-psychotic drug	Thioridazine (Mellaril) and other phenothiazines	Vitamin K	Take on an empty stomach 1 hour before or 2–3 hours after meals Eat green leafy vegetables
	Chlorpromazine (Thorazine),	Folic acid, vitamin D	Take with food or milk Eat citrus fruits and broccoli Drink extra milk
Anti-seizure drug	Phenytoin (Dilantin)	Vitamins B$_6$, D, niacin	Take with food if gastrointestinal irritation occurs Avoid fish, cheese, alcohol and chocolate Eat whole grain enriched breads and cereals, organ meats, leafy vegetables and citrus fruits Drink milk
	Primidone (Mysoline)	Vitamins B$_6$, D, niacin	Take with food if gastrointestinal irritation occurs Avoid alcohol Eat whole-grain enriched breads and cereals, organ meats, leafy vegetables and citrus fruits Drink milk
Diuretics	Furosemide (Lasix), hydrochlorothiazide	Folic acid, potassium, zinc, magnesium	Take with food or milk Eat bananas, nuts, baked potatoes Drink orange juice and milk
Gastrointestinal drug	Antacids	Folic acid, thiamine, calcium, phosphate	Eat whole-grain enriched breads and cereals, leafy vegetables, citrus fruits and dairy products Drink milk
Non-steroidal anti-inflammatory drugs	Indomethacin	Iron, vitamin B$_{12}$	Take with food or milk Eat deep yellow vegetables and organ meats
Steroid	Prednisone	Folic acid, thiamine, vitamin D, calcium	Take with food or milk Eat low-sodium diet Eat whole-grain enriched breads and cereals, leafy vegetables, citrus fruits and dairy products Drink milk Check potassium levels

Table 10.22 Examples of drug interactions with enteral feeds. Adapted from Thomson *et al.* 2000

Medication	Type of interaction	Community nurse action
Ciprofloxacin	Absorption decreased by a possible 25% due to interaction with feeds. Chelation with ions in tap water	Stop enteral feed for 1 hour before and 2 hours after administration of medication
		Liquids should not be diluted further
		Use sterile water if dissolving tablets
		Discuss need for alternative medication
Hydralazine	Decreased absorption and concentration	Monitor changes in blood pressure
Penicillin V	Unpredictable absorption	Stop enteral feed for 1 hour before and 2 hours after after administration of medication
		Consider alternative, e.g. amoxycillin
Sucralfate	Binds to protein in the feed	Use alternatives because enteral feed would need to be stopped for 12 hours each day
Theophylline	Absorption decreased by up to 70%; metabolism increased	Stop enteral feed for 1 hour before and 2 hours after after administration of medication
Phenytoin	Binds to feeding tube (or to proteins and electrolytes in feeds)	Consider parenteral therapy
	Inadequate dissolution due to viscosity of liquid and the acid nature of enteral formulae	Give phenytoin as a single dose during a break in the feeding regimen
		Stop enteral feed for 2 hours before and 2 hours after after administration of medication
	Decreased transit time	
Warfarin	May interact with vitamin K content of feed	Monitor international normalised ratios (INR) closely or use parenteral heparin

- modified release such as verapamil, propranolol, nifedipine and tramadol
- enteric coated such as diclofenic, aspirin, naproxen and sulphasalazine
- hormonal, cytotoxic, steroidal such as tamoxifen, methotrexate and dexamethasone
- nitrate such as Glycerol trinitrate, Isorbide mononitrite and Isorbide dinitrite.

(BNF 2011)

If medications are to be administered via a feeding tube, the tube must be flushed prior to and after administration of the medication with at least 30 ml of drinking or cooled boiled water. If more than one medication is to be given, each should be given separately and the tube flushed with 5–10 ml of water between each drug (Wright 2002). Guidance on how to prepare medications for administration via an enteral feeding tube is given in Table 10.23.

Liquid medicines are not always the best way to give drugs via feeding tubes because:

- some syrups, e.g. ranitidine syrup, contain large amounts of sorbitol. A dose of sorbitol between 7.5 g and 30 g can cause abdominal cramps and diarrhoea
- many liquid preparations are designed for use in children so are of low strength and large volumes may be required, e.g. paracetamol suspension
- the liquid may be thick and viscous and not flow easily through a fine-bore feeding tube, e.g. paracetamol suspension
- not all suspensions can be diluted to reduce their viscosity, e.g. lansoprazole sachets.

Problems associated with HETF

Problems associated with HETF can lead to disruption of the feeding regimen and further compromise the nutritional status of the patient. Common problems include nausea, diarrhoea and tube blockage. Prompt action by the community nurse can reduce their impact and ensures that HETF continues (Table 10.24).

Table 10.23 How to administer medicines via a feeding tube

Action	Liquid medication	Dispersible tablet	Tablet or capsule
Step 1	Shake the mixture or suspension to evenly disperse the drug	Mix with 10–15 ml of freshly boiled and cooled water	If there is no alternative crush tablet or open capsule and mix with 10–15 ml of freshly boiled and cooled water
Step 2	Draw up into 50 ml oral syringe		
Step 3	Flush feeding tube with 30 ml of drinking water or freshly boiled and cooled water		
Step 4	Administer each drug separately, flushing the tube with 5–10 ml of water between each medication Flush syringe with water between each administration of a drug		
Step 5	Flush the feeding tube with 30 ml of drinking water or freshly boiled and cooled water after administration is complete		
Step 6	Record the administration of each medication and the amount of fluid administered		

Table 10.24 Problem solving – complications associated with HETF

Complication	Cause	Action	Rationale
Feeding tube blocked	Failure to flush tube appropriately	Flush tube with water at regular intervals	Removes traces of feed/medication from the wall of the tube
	Administration of medications that are incompatible with the feed/or crushed tablets which block tube	Use pancreatic enzymes by adding contents of Pancrex V capsule dissolved in 1–2 ml water and flush through the tube	Use drugs in appropriate form for administration via a feeding tube. Pancrex V is normally prescribed as a supplement for patients with cystic fibrosis as it aids the digestion of fats, proteins and carbohydrates. As an enzyme it can help to unblock a tube that has been inadequately flushed (check local protocol)
NG tube feeding tube displaced	Irritation, coughing, confusion, vomiting and nausea, retching	Give appropriate medication to alleviate coughing/nausea and vomiting If irritation – reassess and consider alternative route; seek advice from the community dietician	If a feeding tube is displaced there is often a delay in recommencing the feed. Nutritional requirements may not be met as a consequence. Some patients cannot tolerate the tube in their throat. If the tube is removed then reconsider the appropriateness of the route
Gastrostomy tube displaced (balloon retained)	Balloon not inflated to correct size	Check inflation of balloon. If tube falls out insert clean, sterile tube into stoma (spare gastrostomy tube), and contact local hospital (check local protocol) If appropriately trained, replace balloon retained feeding tube.	The stoma can begin to close within about 2 hours, inserting a tube into the stoma will prevent closure and make repositioning of feeding tube easier Balloon retained gastrostomy feeding tubes can be replaced by an appropriately trained community nurse. If not trained contact local hospital (see local protocol)
Gastrostomy tube displaced (flange retained)	Confusion	If tube falls out insert clean, sterile tube into stoma (spare gastrostomy tube), and contact local hospital (check local protocol) Contact local hospital for reinsertion of feeding tube (see local protocol)	The stoma can begin to close within about 2 hours. Inserting a tube into the stoma will prevent closure and make repositioning of feeding tube easier

Table 10.24 (Continued)

Complication	Cause	Action	Rationale
Tube leakage	The tube or Y-adapter at the end of the PEG may be cracked	Replace the Y-adapter or fit another one beyond the crack in the tube The adapter should be carefully fitted, as a good seal is essential to maintain the inflation of the internal retention bumper (check manufacturers guidelines	A leaking tube is distressing to the patient and their carers (where applicable). It can cause the skin to become sore and reduces the amount of feed administered
Infection or exudates around the stoma site	Fixation device is too loose and feed/gastric juices are leaking	Observe site daily for pain, erythema, pus or skin breakdown Check that fixation device is fitted correctly At first signs of infection send a swab to bacteriology for culture and sensitivity Administer appropriate systemic antibiotics if required. Avoid use of topical antibiotics	If the stoma site becomes infected the continuation of HETF may be compromised and the patient's nutritional needs will not be met
	Reduced standards of hygiene in the home	Commence cleaning the site at least twice daily with soap and water or saline. Apply povidone iodine to the site. This can be used for up to 7 days	Cleansing the site can reduce the bacterial load. Povidine iodine creams and ointments should not be used as they can loosen the fixator device
		Avoid dressings if at all possible, but if leakage is excessive, a small dry dressing can be applied and changed at least twice daily	A moist environment will encourage bacterial growth
	The tube may have started to disintegrate	Check the integrity of the tube and contact the endoscopy department (see local protocol) for replacement of tube	Over time the tubes disintegrate, although tubes can be left in situ for up to 2 years, some tubes may need to be replaced sooner
Overgrowth of granulation tissue	Fixation device may be too tight	Check the position of the fixation device and that it can move in and out about ¼ inch (check with manufacturer's guidelines) Ensure tube rotation as per manufacturers guidelines Persistent over granulation may require treatment under the supervision of the tissue viability nurse, nutrition nurse or other appropriately trained person (see local protocol)	If the fixation device is too tight this can cause excessive inflammation which can lead to over-granulation of the stoma site
Diarrhoea	Intolerance to the feed	Slow down feeding regimen and refer to community dietician	The concentration of the feed, can lead to increased peristalsis and diarrhoea
	Prolonged use of antibiotics	Use pre/probiotics, prophylactic administration of *Saccharomyces boulardii* capsules	Antibiotics can cause gastric upsets due to changes in the commensal bacteria in the colon. Pre/probiotics have been shown to reduce incidence of diarrhoea.
	Contamination of feed Enteral administration of magnesium/electrolytes	Check method for setting up and administrating feed	Poor handwashing technique, failure to use clean procedure can contaminate the feed
Constipation	Inadequate fibre in the diet	Refer to GP, contact community dietician Contact community dietician	Many feeds come with added fibre, which can alleviate constipation
	Inadequate fluids in the diet	Increase clear fluid or water administered via enteral feeding tube	Feeds are concentrated within a volume of liquid. Additional fluid may be required to ensure fluid balance is maintained

241

Home parenteral nutrition (HPN)

Home parenteral nutrition is considered a specialised service as defined by the specialist services national definitions. All patients receiving HPN will have their care initiated and managed by secondary care. In recent years the age group receiving HPN has risen, with 14.1% of new registrations being between the ages of 71 and 90, and 5.8% of new registrations residing in nursing homes (Elia *et al.* 2001). BAPEN (2003) estimate that 500 HPN patients are being treated at home at any one time, but due to under-reporting this figure may be as high as 600. Evidence suggests that the use of HPN in the community has increased (BAPEN 2003) and that most patients are able to manage their feeding and care; however, between 1996 and 2001 it is estimated that those requiring help has increased from 8.9% to over 21.7% (BAPEN 2003).

A minority of patients will be unable to manage independently and their care will be provided by a carer, family member, local community nurses or specialist nurses employed by a home care company. Community nurses who become involved in supporting patients with HPN must ensure that they:

- have appropriate training about HPN, management of the intravenous access and the provisions of feeds
- work closely with the community dietician and specialist unit that is supporting the patient and also, where applicable, the carer to ensure that support and advice is continuous and ongoing.

Conclusion

The majority of patients on a district nursing caseload will be able to maintain their nutritional status through oral intake. However, for some, additional or artificial support via other routes may be necessary to optimise body function and composition and prevent, for example, delay in recovery from illness or wound healing.

As with all aspects of nursing practice the basis for ensuring that an individual's nutritional needs are met is dependent on comprehensive patient assessment, subsequent reassessments and effective multidisciplinary care planning.

Procedure guideline 10.1 **Guideline for checking position of NG feeding tube (daily, prior to the administration of a feed or medications following** **episodes of retching, vomiting or coughing)**

Equipment

Alcohol handwash/gel
Disposable non-sterile gloves
Disposable apron
Sterile 50 ml oral syringe
pH indicator strips pH range 0–6 or 1–11 in graduations of 0.5
50 ml fresh drinking water (if patient is immunocompromised cooled freshly boiled water can be used)
Fixing tape

Nursing action	Rationale
1 Where appropriate facilities are available wash your hands or alternatively cleanse with 70% alcohol-based hand rub (in accordance with local policy)	To reduce the risk of cross-infection
2 If the patient is known to the service review nursing documentation and current care plan	To update knowledge of patient and maintain patient safety
3 If the patient is unknown to the service a comprehensive assessment must be carried out prior to undertaking the procedure	To maintain patient safety

Procedure guideline 10.1 **Guideline for checking position of NG feeding tube (daily, prior to the administration of a feed or medications following episodes of retching, vomiting or coughing)** *(cont'd)*

Nursing action	Rationale
4 Explain and discuss the procedure with the patient	To ensure that the patient understands the procedure and gives their valid consent (NMC 2008)
5 Prepare the environment, draw curtains and where necessary obtain patient consent to move furniture	To allow freedom of movement when carrying out the procedure To maintain patient privacy
6 Prepare all necessary equipment	To prevent disruption to the procedure
7 Assist the patient into a comfortable position; this should be sitting as upright as is possible	To ensure patient comfort and facilitate checking position of the feeding tube
8 Where appropriate facilities are available wash your hands or alternatively cleanse with 70% alcohol-based hand rub, (in accordance with local policy	To reduce the risk of cross-infection
9 Apply apron and gloves	To reduce the risk of cross-infection
10 Loosen anchoring tape around nostril/cheek, and check external measurement markings on the NG tube, comparing it with that documented in the care plan	To ascertain that the feeding tube is inserted to the correct point Tubes can be displaced due to peristalsis, regurgitation, vomiting and coughing When a tube is inserted the internal and external amount of feeding tube (total length) must be documented in the patient's care plan (NPSA 2011)
11 Observe the skin around the patient's nostril/cheek	To observe for signs of pressure caused by the tube being anchored in position. Undue pressure caused by the tube may result in pressure sore formation
12 Using fixing tape, anchor NG tube around nostril and on cheek	To secure the tube in place prior to connecting the syringe To reduce the risk of tube movement/displacement
13 Attach the 50 ml oral syringe to the NG tube and gently withdraw gastric contents into the syringe (0.5–1 ml) (Dougherty & Lister 2011) If aspirate not obtained, follow NPSA recommendations (NPSA 2011). If possible reposition the patient on their side, measure the tube and gently inject 10–20 ml of air into the tube and wait for 15–30 min before trying to aspirate (Dougherty & Lister 2011; ECRI 2011)	Using a larger diameter syringe reduces the pressure inside the lumen of the NG tube and reduces the risk of the feeding tube collapsing To enable pH testing to take place To maintain patient safety The insertion of air may clear remaining fluids from the tube Repositioning the patient may alter the position of the tube tip, e.g. away from the stomach wall **NB** To obtain an accurate pH test result a minimum of one hour should have elapsed after the end of feeding or administration of medication, orally or via the NG tube

(Continued)

Procedure guideline 10.1 **Guideline for checking position of NG feeding tube (daily, prior to the administration of a feed or medications following episodes of retching, vomiting or coughing)** *(cont'd)*

Nursing action	Rationale
14 Inject aspirate on to the pH indicator strip	To ascertain the pH of the aspirate and confirm position of the tube
	To maintain patient safety
	If a pH result of less than 5.5 is obtained the NG tube is considered to be appropriately placed and safe to use (NPSA 2011). If the pH result is 6 or above, wait for one hour, aspirate and re-test. If the result remains unchanged or there is any concern regarding a result range of between 5 and 6, the NG tube must not be used because there is a risk that the tube is incorrectly placed (NPSA 2011)
	Locally agreed protocols must be followed as the tube may need to be repositioned, replaced or the position confirmed by X-ray
15 Once the position of the tube has been confirmed as correctly placed, using a clean oral syringe flush the tube with a minimum of 30 ml of cooled boiled water (Dougherty & Lister 2011)	To maintain tube patency
16 Dispose of all used equipment in accordance with locally agreed infection prevention and control policy	To reduce the risk of cross-infection
17 Remove and dispose of apron and gloves in accordance with locally agreed infection prevention and control policy	To reduce the risk of cross-infection
	To prevent contamination
18 Where appropriate facilities are available wash your hands or alternatively cleanse with 70% alcohol-based hand rub (in accordance with local policy	To reduce the risk of cross-infection
19 Assist the patient into a comfortable position	To enhance patient comfort
20 Replace any moved items of furniture to their original position	To maintain a safe environment for the patient by restoring any furniture moved to its usual place
21 Document the outcome in the community nurse record of visits and/or specific charts used. This should include: ■ tube length ■ pH test result ■ skin and nasal condition ■ any further actions taken ■ liaison with other professional	To maintain patient safety
	To ensure continuity of care
	To record findings that may be referred to at subsequent visits
	To ensure accurate and contemporaneous records are kept
	Documentation should provide clear evidence of care planned, decisions made and care delivered (NMC 2008)

Procedure guideline 10.2 **Guideline for gastrostomy tube rotation (flange retained) (daily)**

Equipment

Alcohol handwash/gel
Bowl of warm water
Mild soap
Disposable wash cloths
Towel or disposable wipes for drying
Disposable non-sterile gloves
Disposable apron

Nursing action	Rationale
1 Where appropriate facilities are available wash your hands or alternatively cleanse with 70% alcohol-based hand rub (in accordance with local policy)	To reduce the risk of cross-infection
2 If the patient is known to the service review nursing documentation and current care plan	To update knowledge of patient and maintain patient safety
3 If the patient is unknown to the service a comprehensive assessment must be carried out prior to undertaking the procedure	To maintain patient safety
4 Explain and discuss the procedure with the patient	To ensure that the patient understands the procedure and gives their valid consent (NMC 2008)
5 Prepare the environment, draw curtains and where necessary obtain patient consent to move furniture	To allow freedom of movement when carrying out the procedure To maintain patient privacy
6 Apply apron	To reduce the risk of cross-infection
7 Prepare all necessary equipment	To prevent disruption to the procedure
8 Where indicated offer the patient assistance with removing all necessary articles of clothing	To expose the area of the stoma site
9 Assist the patient into a lying position or as flat as is possible	To ensure that the PEG and stoma site are visible for assessing position and condition
10 Where appropriate facilities are available wash your hands or alternatively cleanse with 70% alcohol-based hand rub (in accordance with local policy)	To reduce the risk of cross-infection
11 Apply gloves	To reduce the risk of cross-infection To prevent cross-contamination
12 Following manufacturer's guidelines, loosen the external fixator device; note the original position of the fixator **If sutures remain in situ to secure the fixator to the patient's abdomen these should not be removed until confirmation is received that they are no longer necessary to maintain the tube position**	Loosening the fixator exposes the stoma for cleaning and assessment

245

(Continued)

Procedure guideline 10.2 **Guideline for gastrostomy tube rotation (flange retained) (daily)** *(cont'd)*

Nursing action	Rationale
13 Clean stoma site with a mild solution of soap and water, rinse and dry thoroughly	To reduce the risk of skin irritation
14 Inspect the skin for signs of redness, swelling, irritation, skin breakdown and leakage	To assess the condition of the skin and stoma site To maintain patient safety
15 Gently push the tube in a little way and rotate 360° then pull back to the original position (check with manufacturer's guidelines)	To prevent tube adhering to the stoma site
16 Retighten the external fixator device so that it lies approximately 2 mm (1/4″) from the skin surface (check with manufacturer's guidelines)	To ensure the feeding tube is positioned securely prior to the commencement of the feed To maintain patient safety
17 Dispose of all used equipment in accordance with locally agreed infection prevention and control policy	To minimise the risk of cross-infection
18 Remove and dispose of gloves in accordance with locally agreed infection prevention and control policy	To minimise the risk of cross-infection To prevent contamination
19 Where appropriate facilities are available wash your hands or alternatively cleanse with 70% alcohol-based hand rub (in accordance with local policy)	To reduce the risk of cross-infection
20 Assist the patient to dress and adjust position	To enable the patient to continue with their normal activities of daily living To maintain patient comfort and dignity
21 Remove and dispose of apron in accordance with locally agreed infection prevention and control policy	To reduce the risk of cross-infection
22 Where appropriate facilities are available wash your hands or alternatively cleanse with 70% alcohol-based hand rub (in accordance with local policy)	To reduce the risk of cross-infection
23 Replace any moved items of furniture to their original position	To maintain a safe environment for the patient by restoring any furniture moved to its usual place
24 Verbally discuss the outcome of the procedure with the patient giving further advice as indicated	To keep the patient informed and reinforce patient knowledge and understanding
25 Document the outcome of the visit in the community nurse record of visits, this should include: the condition of the patients skin, PEG and stoma site	To maintain patient safety To ensure continuity of care To record findings that may be referred to at subsequent visits To ensure accurate and contemporaneous records are kept Documentation should provide clear evidence of care planned, decisions made and care delivered (NMC 2008)

Procedure guideline 10.3 **Guideline for gastrostomy tube rotation (Balloon retained) (weekly)**

Equipment

Alcohol handwash/gel
Bowl of warm water
Mild soap
Disposable wash cloths
Towel or disposable wipes for drying
Non-sterile gloves
Apron
Sterile syringe/s of appropriate volume
Cool boiled water

Nursing action	Rationale
1 Where appropriate facilities are available wash your hands or alternatively cleanse with 70% alcohol-based hand rub (in accordance with local policy)	To reduce the risk of cross-infection
2 If the patient is known to the service review nursing documentation and current care plan	To update knowledge of patient and maintain patient safety
3 If the patient is unknown to the service a comprehensive assessment must be carried out prior to undertaking the procedure	To maintain patient safety
4 Explain and discuss the procedure with the patient	To ensure that the patient understands the procedure and gives their valid consent (NMC 2008)
5 Prepare the environment, draw curtains and where necessary obtain patient consent to move furniture	To allow freedom of movement when carrying out the procedure To maintain patient privacy
6 Apply apron	To reduce the risk of cross-infection
7 Prepare all necessary equipment	To prevent disruption to the procedure
8 Where indicated offer the patient assistance with removing all necessary articles of clothing	To expose the area of the stoma site
9 Assist the patient into a lying position or as flat as is possible	To ensure that the PEG and stoma site are visible for assessing position and condition
10 Where appropriate facilities are available wash your hands or alternatively cleanse with 70% alcohol-based hand rub (in accordance with local policy)	To reduce the risk of cross-infection
11 Apply gloves	To reduce the risk of cross-infection To prevent cross-contamination
12 Following manufacturer's guidelines, attach syringe to the inflation valve of the balloon gastrostomy while holding the feeding tube	Deflating the balloon allows the stoma site to be visualised and the feeding tube to be rotated

247

(Continued)

Procedure guideline 10.3 **Guideline for gastrostomy tube rotation (Balloon retained) (weekly)** *(cont'd)*

Nursing action	Rationale
13 Gently withdraw plunger on the syringe until no more water comes out of the internal balloon	Deflating the balloon allows the stoma site to be visualised and the feeding tube to be rotated
14 Clean site with a mild solution of soap and water, rinse and dry thoroughly	To reduce the risk of skin irritation
15 Inspect the skin for signs of redness, swelling, irritation, skin breakdown and leakage	To assess the condition of the stoma site To maintain patient safety
16 Gently push the tube in a little way and rotate 360° then pull back to the original position (check with manufacturer's guidelines)	To prevent tube adhering to the stoma site
17 Using a clean sterile syringe with cooled boiled water, reinsert the recommended volume of fluid through the inflation valve (check with manufacturer's guidelines)	To reinflate the balloon To ensure the feeding tube is positioned securely prior to the commencement of the feed To maintain patient safety
18 Dispose of all used equipment in accordance with locally agreed infection prevention and control policy	To minimise the risk of cross-infection
19 Remove and dispose of gloves in accordance with locally agreed infection prevention and control policy	To minimise the risk of cross-infection To prevent contamination
20 Where appropriate facilities are available wash your hands or alternatively cleanse with 70% alcohol-based hand rub (in accordance with local policy)	To reduce the risk of cross-infection
21 Assist the patient to dress and adjust position	To enable the patient to continue with their normal activities of daily living To maintain patient comfort and dignity
22 Remove and dispose of apron in accordance with locally agreed infection prevention and control policy	To reduce the risk of cross-infection
23 Where appropriate facilities are available wash your hands or alternatively cleanse with 70% alcohol-based hand rub (in accordance with local policy	To reduce the risk of cross-infection
24 Replace any moved items of furniture to their original position	To maintain a safe environment for the patient by restoring any furniture moved to its usual place
25 Verbally discuss the outcome of the procedure with the patient giving further advice as indicated	To keep the patient informed and reinforce patient knowledge and understanding
26 Document the outcome of the visit in the community nurse record of visits. This should include: the condition of the patients skin, PEG and stoma site	To maintain patient safety To ensure continuity of care To record findings that may be referred to at subsequent visits To ensure accurate and contemporaneous records are kept Documentation should provide clear evidence of care planned, decisions made and care delivered (NMC 2008)

Procedure guideline 10.4 **Guideline for administration of medications via feeding tube**

Avoid the administration of medications via a fine-bore feeding tube as this can lead to an increased risk of tube blockage, drug nutrient interactions and altered drug bioavailability.

Equipment

Alcohol handwash/gel
Sterile 50 ml oral syringe/s
Range of syringe sizes for drug preparation
50 ml fresh drinking water (if patient is immunocompromised cooled freshly boiled water can be used)
Medication in appropriate form
Prescription/administration chart
Tablet crusher (If appropriate)
pH indicator strip (NG tube)

Nursing action	Rationale
1 Where appropriate facilities are available wash your hands or alternatively cleanse with 70% alcohol-based hand rub (in accordance with local policy)	To reduce the risk of cross-infection
2 If the patient is known to the service review nursing documentation and current care plan	To update knowledge of patient and maintain patient safety
3 If the patient is unknown to the service a comprehensive assessment must be carried out prior to undertaking the procedure	To maintain patient safety
4 Explain and discuss the procedure with the patient	To ensure that the patient understands the procedure and gives their valid consent (NMC 2008)
5 Check prescribed drug/s against administration record	To ensure that the correct patient receives: (a) the correct drug (b) the correct dose and strength (c) at the correct time (d) via the correct route
6 Prepare the environment, draw curtains and where necessary obtain patient consent to move furniture	To allow freedom of movement when carrying out the procedure To maintain patient privacy
7 Identify and select all of the medication to be administered and check the expiry date/s	To ensure patient safety and efficacy of treatment
8 Assist patient into a comfortable position sitting as upright as possible	To ensure patient comfort
9 Where appropriate facilities are available wash your hands or alternatively cleanse with 70% alcohol-based hand rub (in accordance with local policy)	To reduce the risk of cross-infection

249

(Continued)

Procedure guideline 10.4 **Guideline for administration of medications via feeding tube** *(cont'd)*

Nursing action	Rationale
10 Prepare all medication to be administered separately. If liquid, then shake the mixture or suspension to evenly disperse the drug, if syrups or thicker liquids mix with an equal amount of water	To ensure patient receives medication on time and in the correct form
If a dispersible tablet, mix with 10–15 ml of freshly boiled cooled water	This method of administration should only be carried out following advice from the community pharmacist regarding appropriateness and bioavailability, as this can be altered
If tablet or capsule then crush tablet or open capsule and mix with 10–15 ml of freshly boiled cooled water	Follow safety instructions if tablet or capsule contains hazardous substances such as cytotoxic drugs
NB Medication should never be added directly to feed	To minimise the risk of interaction (BAPEN 2003)
11 Where appropriate facilities are available wash your hands or alternatively cleanse with 70% alcohol-based hand rub (in accordance with local policy)	To reduce the risk of cross-infection
12 If feed is in progress stop the feed and flush the tube with a minimum of 30 ml of water. If the patient has a jejunostomy tube, sterile water must be used	To clear tube, check patency and minimise the risk of blockage or interactions
	If a jejunostomy is in place sterile water must be used because there is no acidic protection from gastric secretions
NB Feeds may need to be discontinued from between 1–2 hours prior to and following administration	When planning drug administration community pharmacist advice should be sought
13 If administration is via a NG tube tip position must be checked prior to insertion of water and administration of medication (*see* Procedure guideline 10.1)	To confirm tip position
	To maintain patient safety
14 For volumes > than 10 ml administer individual medications via 50 ml syringe	To ensure the patient receives prescribed medication
15 For volumes < 10 ml remove the plunger from a 50 ml syringe and connect the syringe to the feeding tube. Pour the medication to be administered into the barrel of the 50 ml syringe, rinse 10 ml syringe with water and add to the 50 ml syringe barrel	To ensure that the patient receives the prescribed dose of medication (BAPEN 2003)
	To reduce the risk of the tube collapsing
16 If more than one medication is being administered the tube must be flushed with 10 ml of water between each medication (Dougherty & Lister 2011)	To prevent mixing in the tube, drug interactions and the risk of blockage
	To maintain tube patency
17 Flush the tube with at least 30 ml of water on completion of medication administration	To prevent blockage in the tube
18 Dispose of all used equipment in accordance with locally agreed infection prevention and control policy	To minimise the risk of cross-infection
19 Assist the patient to dress and adjust position	To enable the patient to continue with their normal activities of daily living
	To maintain patient comfort and dignity

Procedure guideline 10.4 **Guideline for administration of medications via feeding tube** *(cont'd)*

Nursing action	Rationale
20 Where appropriate facilities are available wash your hands or alternatively cleanse with 70% alcohol-based hand rub (in accordance with local policy	To reduce the risk of cross-infection
21 Replace any moved items of furniture to their original position	To maintain a safe environment for the patient by restoring any furniture moved to its usual place
22 Document the administration of each medication and the volume of fluid administered	To maintain patient safety
	To ensure continuity of care
	To record findings that may be referred to at subsequent visits
	To ensure accurate and contemporaneous records are kept
	Documentation should provide clear evidence of care planned, decisions made and care delivered (NMC 2008)

Procedure guideline 10.5 **Guideline for setting up a feed for administration via an enteral feeding tube**

If feeding via a NG tube the tip position must be checked prior to flushing and commencing the feed (see Procedure guideline 10.1).

Equipment

Alcohol handwash/gel
Sterile plastics (giving set)
Prescribed feed
Feeding regimen
Drip stand
Pump
pH indicator strips (if NG feeding tube refer to guideline)
50 ml oral syringe
50 ml fresh water or cooled freshly boiled water sterile water for immunosuppressed patients and jejunostomy tubes)
Adhesive tape (if NG feeding tube)
Single-use disposable apron

Nursing action	Rationale
1 Where appropriate facilities are available wash your hands or alternatively cleanse with 70% alcohol-based hand rub (in accordance with local policy)	To reduce the risk of cross-infection
2 If the patient is known to the service review nursing documentation and current care plan	To update knowledge of patient and maintain patient safety
3 If the patient is unknown to the service a comprehensive assessment must be carried out prior to undertaking the procedure	To maintain patient safety

(Continued)

Procedure guideline 10.5 **Guideline for setting up a feed for administration via an enteral feeding tube** *(cont'd)*

Nursing action	Rationale
4 Explain and discuss the procedure with the patient	To ensure that the patient understands the procedure and gives their valid consent (NMC 2008)
5 Check prescribed feed against current prescribed regimen and gently shake bag/container	To ensure that the patient receives the correct feed To ensure the feed is evenly mixed and reduce the risk of blockage occurring in the giving set
6 Check expiry date of feed	To ensure that the feed is within date To maintain patient safety
7 Apply apron	To reduce the risk of cross-infection/contamination
8 Assist patient into a comfortable position. Where possible sitting as upright as possible, at an angle of greater than 30°	To ensure patient is comfortable To promote gastric emptying To minimise gastric reflux during the period of the feed
9 Where appropriate facilities are available wash your hands or alternatively cleanse with 70% alcohol-based hand rub, (in accordance with local policy)	To reduce the risk of cross-infection To maintain patient safety
10 Check expiry date and packaging for any damage, and then take the sterile giving set from the package, close the roller clamp	To prevent spillage of feed To maintain patient safety
11 Attach the giving set to the feed	To break the seal on the bag/container
12 Hang the bag/container upside down on the drip stand and open the roller clamp allowing the feed to prime the giving set to the tip	To displace air To prevent air being fed into the patien's stomach Hanging the bag upside down prevents backflow into the feed
13 Following the manufacturer's instructions insert the giving set into the pump	To connect the giving set to the pump in preparation to commence feed
14 Set the pump rate according to the prescribed feeding regimen and manufacturer's instructions	To ensure that the patient receives the feed at the correct rate
15 If feeding via a NG tube use pH indicator strip to check tip position (*see* guidelines on reducing the harm caused by misplaced NG feeding tubes in adults, children and infants; NPSA 2011) see Procedure Guideline 10.1	To maintain patient safety
16 Where appropriate facilities are available wash your hands or alternatively cleanse with 70% alcohol-based hand rub (in accordance with local policy)	To reduce the risk of cross-infection/contamination
17 Attach the 50 ml oral syringe containing 20 ml of water (tap/cooled boiled or sterile) to the feeding tube, inject the water slowly down the tube, remove syringe and discard appropriately	To clear the feeding tube of any debris and ensure the tube is clear
18 Attach the giving set to the feeding tube	To enable the feed to be administered via the correct route

Procedure guideline 10.5 **Guideline for setting up a feed for administration via an enteral feeding tube** *(cont'd)*

Nursing action	Rationale
19 Check the pump rate and start the feed	To ensure that the patient receives the feed at the correct rate over the correct time period
20 Dispose of all used equipment in accordance with locally agreed infection prevention and control policy	To minimise the risk of cross-infection/contamination
21 Remove and dispose of apron in accordance with locally agreed infection prevention and control policy	To reduce the risk of cross-infection
22 Where appropriate facilities are available wash your hands or alternatively cleanse with 70% alcohol-based hand rub (in accordance with local policy)	To reduce the risk of cross-infection
23 If required assist the patient to adjust their position	To maintain patient comfort and dignity
24 Document feed details (start time, rate, amount to be delivered and time feed to be completed)	To ensure that the administration of the feed can be monitored
If via a NG tube external tube length must also be recorded	To maintain patient safety
	To ensure continuity of care
	To ensure accurate and contemporaneous records are kept
	Documentation should provide clear evidence of care planned, decisions made and care delivered (NMC 2008)

References and further reading

Argilés J, Busquets S, López-Soriano FF (2005) The pivotal role of cytokines in muscle wasting during cancer. *International Journal of Biochemistry & Cell Biology*. Available on-line at www science direct.com

Arnaud-Battandier F, Malvy D, Jeondel C *et al.* (2004) Use of oral supplements in malnourished elderly patients living in the community: a politico-economic study. *Clinical Nutrition* 23(5): 1009–15.

BANS (2010) *British Artificial Nutrition Survey*. A report by the British Artificial Nutrition Survey (BANS), a committee of BAPEN (British Association for Parenteral and Enteral Nutrition) Published on www.bapen.org.uk

BAPEN (2003a) *The Malnutrition Universal Screening Tool (MUST)*. BAPEN, Maidenhead.

BAPEN (2003b) *The 'MUST' Explanatory Booklet MAG*. BAPEN, Maidenhead.

BAPEN (2005) *British Association for Parenteral and Enteral Feeding. Ethical and Legal Aspects of Clinical Hydration and Nutritional Support*. BAPEN, Maidenhead.

BAPEN (2011) *Administration of Medications Available*. www.bapen.org.uk/pdfs/d_and_e/de_gp_guide.pdf (last accessed 2011).

Barker H (2002) *Nutrition and Dietetics*. Harcourt, London.

Biesalski H (2010) Micronutrients, wound healing, and prevention of pressure ulcers. *Nutrition* 26(9): 858.

BNF (2011) British National Formulary. Available online at http://bnf.org/bnf/index.htm

van Bokhorst-de van der Schueren MAE (2005) Nutritional support strategies for malnourished patients. *European Journal of Oncology Nursing* 9(Suppl. 2): S74–S83.

Bozzetti F (2011) Nutritional support in oncologic patients: where we are and where we are going. *Clinical Nutrition* (in press).

Bruce D, Laurence I, McGuiness M *et al.* (2003) Nutritional supplements after hip fracture: poor compliance limits effectiveness. *Clinical Nutrition* 22(5): 497–500.

COMA (1991) *Dietary Reference Values for Food, Energy and Nutrients for the United Kingdom* 41. HMSO, London.

Dangerfield L, Sullivan R (2002) Taking the tube. *Nursing Times Supplement* 95(21): 63–6.

Department of Health (2000) *National Service Framework for Coronary Heart Disease*. The Stationery Office, London.

Department of Health (2001a) *National Service Framework for Diabetes*. The Stationery Office, London.

Department of Health (2001b) *National Service Framework for Older People*. The Stationery Office, London.

Department of Health (2005) *National Service Framework for Long Term Conditions*. The Stationery Office, London.

Department of Health (2009) *Complex Carbohydrates*. DH, London.

DiMaria RA, Amelia A (2005) Interventions and assessment can help curb the growing threat of malnutrition. *American Journal of Nursing* **105**(3): 40–50.

Dougherty L, Lister S (2011) *The Royal Marsden Hospital Manual of Clinical Nursing Procedures* (8e). Blackwell Publishing, Oxford.

ECRI (2011) *Understanding Safety, Core Knowledge Diagnostics, Positioning Naso-gastric Feeding Tubes*. ECRI Institute, London.

Eddington J, Kon P, Martyn C (1996) Prevalence of malnutrition in patients in general practice. *Clinical Nutrition* **15**(2): 60–3.

Elia M, Lunn PF (1997) Biological markers of protein energy malnutrition. *Clinical Nutrition* **16**(Suppl. 1): 11–17.

Elia M, Russell CA, Stratton R (2001) *Trends in Artificial Nutrition Support in the UK During 1996–2000*. Committee of the British Artificial Nutrition Survey (BANS), BAPEN, Maidenhead.

ESPEN (2003) ESPEN guidelines for nutritional screening. *Clinical Nutrition* **22**(4): 415–21.

Food Standards Agency (2001) *Balance of Good Health*. DH. London.

Food Standards Agency (2011) www.eatwell.gov.uk/healthydiet/nutritionessentaisl (last accessed July 2011).

Guest F, Panca M, Baeyens JP *et al.* (2011) Health economic impact of managing patients following a community-based diagnosis of malnutrition in the UK. *Clinical Nutrition* **30**(4): 422–9.

Guigoz Y, Vellas B, Garry P (2002) MNA A practical assessment tool for grading the nutritional status of elderly patients. *Facts and Research in Gerentology* **4** (Suppl 2): 15.

Hirani V, Mindell J (2008) A comparison of measured height and demi-span equivalent height in the assessment of body mass index among people aged 65 years and over in England. *Age & Ageing* **37**(3): 311–17.

Howard P, Jonkers-Schuitema C *et al.* (2006) Managing the patient journey through enteral nutritional care. *Clinical Nutrition* **25**(2): 187–95.

Kushner FR, Blatner DJ (2005) Risk assessment of the overweight and obese patient. *Journal of the American Dietetic Association* **105**: S53–S62.

Kuzuya M, Izawa S, Enoki H *et al.* (2007) Is serum albumin a good marker for malnutrition in the physically impaired elderly? *Clinical Nutrition* **26**(1): 84–90.

Lamont E, Muir E, McDonald H, Atkinson J (2005) Taking stock of dietary management. *Diabetes Update* **Spring**: 30–5.

Lennard-Jones JE (1995) *Screening by Nurses and Junior Doctors to Detect Malnutrition When Patients Are First Assessed in Hospital*. BAPEN, London.

Mackintosh M, Hankey CR (2001) Reliability of a nutrition-screening tool for use in elderly day hospitals. *Journal of Human Nutrition & Dietetics* **14**: 129–36.

Mann J, Truswell SA (2002) *Essentials of Human Nutrition* (2e). Oxford University Press, Oxford.

McWhirter J, Pennington C (1994) Incidence and recognition of malnutrition in hospital. *British Medical Journal* **308**(6943): 945–8.

Nazarko L (2010) Rocognising and managing dysphagia. *Nursing and Residential Care* **12**(3): 133–7.

NCCAC (2006) *Nutrition Support in Adults. Oral Nutrition Support, Enteral Tube Feeding and Parenteral Nutrition*. National Collaborating Centre for Acute Care, London. Available from www.rcseng.ac.uk

NMC (2008) The Code. Available online at www.nmc-uk.org/Nurses-and-midwives/The-code/

NDNS (2011) *National Diet and Nutrition Survey. Headline Results from Years 1 and 2 (combined) of the Rolling Programme (2008/09–2009/10)*. NHS, London.

NPSA (2011) *Patient Safety Alert NPSA/2011/PSA022: Reducing the harm caused by misplaced naso-gastric feeding tubes in adults, children and infants*. National Patient Safety Agency, www.nrls.npsa.nhs.uk/alerts

NPSA (2007) *Promoting Safer Measurement and Administration of Liquid Medicines via Oral and Other Enteral Routes*. Available online at www.nrls.npsa.nhs.uk/

NHS Information Centre (2011) Statistics on Obesity, Physical Activity and Diet: England, 2011. NHS IC, London. Available online at www.ic.nhs.uk/statistics-and-data-collections/health-and-lifestyles/obesity

NHS (2011) www.nhs.uk/Livewell/Goodfood/Pages/Fat.aspx

NHS Cancer Plan (2000) *The NHS Cancer Plan*. The Stationary Office, London.

National Institute for Clinical Excellence (2003) *Care During Enteral Feeding. Infection Control – Prevention of Healthcare Associated Infection in Primary and Community Care* (No. 3). Clinical guideline 2. NICE, London.

National Institute for Health and Clinical Excellence (2011) *Quality Standard for Diabetes in Adults*. NICE, London.

Oliver D (2005) Medical input, rehabilitation and discharge planning for patients with hip fractures; Why traditional models are not fit for purpose and how things are changing. *Current Anaesthesia and Critical Care* **16**: 11–22.

Omran ML, Morley JE (2000a) Assessment of protein energy malnutrition in older persons. Part 1 History, examination, body composition and screening tools. *Nutrition* **16**: 50–63.

Omran ML, Morley JE (2000b) Assessment of protein energy malnutrition in older persons. Part II Laboratory evaluation. *Nutrition* **16**: 131–40.

Panico N (2002) *Audit of the prescribing practice for nutritional supplements in primary care. Clinical governance support team*. Eastbourne and County Healthcare [unpublished].

Peddler L (1998) Nursing's nutritional responsibilities. *Nursing Standard* **13**(9): 18–24.

Perry L (2001) Dysphagia: the management and detection of a disabling problem. *British Journal of Nursing* **10**(13): 837–41.

Pirlich M, Schutz T, Kemps M (2005) Social risk factors for hospital malnutrition. *Nutrition* **21**: 295–300.

Scolapio JS (2007) Decreasing aspiration risk with enteral feeding gastrointestinal endoscopy. *Clinics of North America* **17**(4): 711–16.

SIGN 78 (2004) *Management of Patients with Stroke. Identification and Management of Dysphagia*. Scottish Intercollegiate Guidelines Network, NHS Scotland, Edinburgh.

Stephens NA, Fearon KCH (2008) Anorexia, cachexia and nutrition. *Medicine* **36**(2): 78–81.

Stratton RJ, Green LJ, Elia M (2003) *Disease Related Malnutrition: an evidence based approach to treatment.* CABI Publishing, Oxford.

Stratton RJ, Elia M (2007) A review of reviews: a new look at the evidence for oral nutritional supplements in clinical practice. *Clinical Nutrition Supplements* **2**(1): 5–23.

Stratton RJ, Hackston AJ, Price S *et al.* (2004) Malnutrition in hospital outpatients and inpatients: prvalence, concurrent validity and ease of use of the 'Malnutrition Universal Screening Tool' (MUST) for adults. *British Journal of Nutrition* **92**: 799–808.

Thomas W, Rahbarnia A, Kellner M (2010) Basics in nutrition and wound healing. *Nutrition* **26**(9): 862–6.

Van Meyenfeldt M (2005) Cancer associated malnutrition: an introduction. *European Journal of Oncology Nursing* **9**: 535–8.

Vellas B, Guigoz Y, Garry P *et al.* (1999) The mini nutritional assessment (MNA) and its use in grading the nutritional state of elderly patients. *Nutrition* **15**(2): 116–22.

Ward J, Close J, Boaman J (1998) Development of a screening tool for assessing risk of under-nutrition in patients in the community. *Journal of Human Nutrition and Dietetics* **11**: 323–30.

Webb G (2002) *Nutrition: a health promotion approach (2e).* Arnold, London.

Wild T, Rahbarnia A, Keliner M *et al.* (2010) Basics in nutrition and wound healing. *Nutrition* **26**: 862–6.

Wieseke A, Bantz D, Siktberg L, Dilla N (2008) Assessment and early diagnosis of dysphagia. *Geriatric Nursing* **29**(6): 376–83.

Wright D (2002) Swallowing difficulties protocol: medication administration. *Nursing Standard* **17**(14–15): 43–5.

Wright J (2004) Home enteral nutrition. *Journal of Community Nursing* **18**(2). Available online at www.jcn.co.uk/

11

Personal hygiene

Definition

Personal hygiene care is defined as 'the physical act of cleansing the body to ensure the hair, nails, ears, eyes, nose and skin are maintained in an optimum condition. It also includes mouth hygiene, which is the effective removal of plaque and debris to ensure the structures and tissues of the mouth are kept in a healthy condition.' (DH 2010, p.7)

Background evidence

The community nurse needs to use communication and assessment skills to ascertain and respond to the patient's needs and wishes in a respectful and dignified manner. This promotes the individuality of the patient, and involves them in decision making regarding their care.

Carrying out or assisting a patient to meet their personal hygiene needs should not be viewed only as a way of promoting a feeling of comfort and wellbeing, as it also provides the community nurse with an opportunity to assess the patient's actual and potential needs in a number of areas, for example:

■ mobility
■ physical abilities
■ nutritional status
■ skin integrity.

Furthermore, it enables the community nurse to:

■ communicate with the patient
■ listen to any anxieties or concerns the patient may have

■ offer appropriate reassurance, support and guidance
■ reduce the risk of patient social isolation.

Assessment

An holistic assessment enables the community nurse to develop a comprehensive overview of the patient's needs. So it is fundamental that the patient and/or carer is encouraged to provide information on specific needs and requirements, which may dictate care provision and delivery. Although assessment frameworks are useful, it is essential that these are combined with an appreciation of the patient's knowledge and values (Armstrong & Mitchell 2008). The plan of care should be discussed and agreed with the patient, and where necessary, this can be supported by written information (RCN 2004).

As part of the holistic assessment process, the community nurse should also give consideration to the following.

■ The patient's previous experiences and expectations of personal care.
■ The patient's/carer's capability and willingness to be involved in personal care.
■ Consent, confidentiality and autonomy in relation to the professional code of conduct (NMC 2008).
■ Documentation in care records meet professional standards (NMC 2008).
■ Evidence-based policies, procedures and guidance used are up to date.
■ There is co-ordination of service delivery with other health and social care organisations.
■ Diversity and individual needs, inclusive of ethnicity, religion, language, age, gender and sexual orientation (DH 2010, p. 7).

District Nursing Manual of Clinical Procedures, First Edition. Edited by Liz O'Brien.
© 2012 Blackwell Publishing Ltd. Published 2012 by Blackwell Publishing Ltd.

Multicultural needs

Britain is a multicultural society, and the community nurse should be aware that local communities may include individuals and groups of people with differing beliefs, values, perceptions, and religious and spiritual needs. In terms of personal hygiene and cleanliness, it is important that the community nurse recognises and acknowledges that what is acceptable within one culture may not be in another and that preferences may also differ between individuals within a culture.

When planning care, consideration may need to be given to the timing of visits to ensure that the patient's religious customs, prayer and service is not disrupted. The community nursing team may also need to consider who is the most appropriate professional to visit the patient, for example it may not be appropriate for a male nurse to attend female patients and vice versa.

Some examples of specific needs in relation to personal care

Judaism

- Hygiene is central to the way of life, and many religious activities may only be performed in a clean state, handwashing is essential before prayer.
- Once married, orthodox Jewish women cover their hair at all times with a head scarf, and orthodox Jewish men wear a skullcap. The community nurse should not remove these without prior consent.
- The community nurse also needs to be aware that some Jews may not shower on the Sabbath (Saturday) after nightfall (Brooks 2004).

Islam

- Free-flowing running water is essential for washing, therefore the community nurse should consider where possible the use of the shower. The community nurse may improvise using a jug or bowl to simulate running water (Ghazala 2002).
- The community nurse must ensure that patient body exposure is minimal, traditionally Muslim women cover their entire body, concealing their body shape except for the face and hands, and men will cover themselves from the waist to the knee (BBC 2009).
- Significance is placed on the right hand as the 'dominant clean hand' and the left as the 'dirty hand' (Black 2000).

- Some items of jewellery have religious significance, e.g. women may wear bangles and bracelets, which should not be removed without prior consent (Holland & Hogg 2001).

Sikh

- Personal hygiene is extremely important to the Sikh individual. Before food and beverages are taken they may like to brush their teeth and/or wash their hands and face (Gill 2002).
- Significance is placed on the right hand as the 'dominant clean hand' and the left as the 'dirty hand' (Black 2000).
- The community nurse must ensure that patients' body exposure is minimised during the care of personal hygiene as Sikhs value modesty (Singh 2010).
- Sikh men wear a turban and a fresh one is usually tied each day. The community nurse will need to negotiate with the family and/or patient about who will cleanse the hair, scalp and maintain the turban. Women may cover their heads with a scarf known as a duppata (Nesbit 2008). Certain items of jewellery have religious and cultural significance and should not be removed without prior consent (Singh 2010).

Hindu

- Hindus prefer a shower to a bath, and for a Hindu woman their hair is often left uncut (Jootun 2002).
- Significance is placed on the right hand as the 'dominant clean hand' and the left as the 'dirty hand' (Black 2000).
- The community nurse must ensure that patient body exposure is minimal; traditionally Hindu women cover their legs, breasts and upper arms, and men do not expose themselves from the waist to the knee.
- Some jewellery for both men and women have religious significance, they should not be removed without prior consent (Holland & Hogg 2001).
- Married women may have a bindi – this is a spot of vermillion applied to the forehead. This has religious significance and the community nurse should seek guidance from the patient and/or family in regard to re-application of the bindi (Thakrar et al. 2008).

The examples and information above is in no way exhaustive, and the community nurse should seek further advice from specialist sources for any specific

257

care required related to particular faiths, cultures and/or religions.

Manual handling and risk assessment

A risk assessment is a careful examination of what in your work could cause harm to yourself and others (Health and Safety Executive (HSE) (2011).

Prior to carrying out or assisting a patient with personal hygiene a full risk assessment should be carried out and documented in accordance with local policy to ensure that

- Health and safety issues are identified and control measures are put in place.
- The plan of care is realistic and safe for both patient and the community nurse.
- Care provision is managed safely and appropriately.
- The home environment is free from hazards, obstruction and allows ease of movement

(See manual handling chapter).

Conclusion

Community nurses no longer commonly assist patients with bathing or showering unless they have a specific nursing need, for example a dermatological skin condition. Baths can be comforting, relaxing and refreshing (Basavanthappa 2004), but may be difficult to undertake in a patient's own home. Where possible, alternatives should be considered, discussed and negotiated with the patient.

At all times decision making must be guided by the completion of a full risk assessment and local policy (*see* Chapter 9).

To promote patient independence with personal hygiene and enhance patient choice, with the patient's consent, the community nurse should complete a comprehensive assessment to ascertain areas of difficulty (*see* Chapter 1). This will also ensure prompt referral is made to other appropriate community professionals for specialist assessment (e.g. occupational therapist, social services), and thereby enhance the provision of a needs-led care package through the promotion of integrated working partnerships.

Procedure guideline 11.1 **Guideline for bedbathing (general principles)**

This guideline may need to be adapted to reflect Individual patients' personal, religious and cultural beliefs or needs.

Equipment

Clean clothing or nightwear
Clean bed linen as necessary and available
Bowl of hand hot water
Soap and flannels/sponges x 2 – different colours
Towels
Disposable wipes (if appropriate)
Comb
Blanket/large towel to cover patient
Patient's toiletries
Manual handling equipment (where necessary)
Non-sterile single-use gloves x 2 pairs
Disposable single-use apron/s
Protective covering for patient's furniture
Rubbish bag

Nursing action	Rationale
1 Where appropriate facilities are available wash and dry hands. Alternatively cleanse hands with alcohol-based hand rub. Apply disposable apron	To prevent the risk of cross-infection/contamination
2 Read nursing documentation and care plan	To maintain safety by updating practitioner knowledge of the patient

Procedure guideline 11.1 **Guideline for bedbathing (general principles)** *(cont'd)*

Nursing action	Rationale
3 Explain and discuss the procedure with the patient	To enable the patient to express any concerns they may have and gain consent
4 Carry out/review manual handling risk assessment, this should include an environmental assessment	To ensure that health and safety guidelines are adhered to To reduce the risk of injury too patient and nursing team
5 Offer patient the opportunity to use toilet facilities	To ensure patient comfort and prevent disruption to the procedure
6 Collect and prepare all equipment, where necessary protect the patient's furnishings with, e.g. polythene bag, bin liner or tray	To minimise disruption to the procedure and prevent the need to leave the patient unattended To protect patient's furniture
Water for washing should be hand hot	To ensure patient comfort and prevent scalding
7 Draw window curtains and close door	To promote patient privacy and dignity and maintain room temperature
8 Cleanse hands with alcohol-based hand rub and apply apron	To prevent the risk of cross-infection
9 Assist the patient to remove their clothing, if they are unable to do so independently	To ensure patient is kept warm and privacy and dignity is maintained
Cover the patient with large towel/blanket and fold back bedclothes	
10 Ask the patient if they use soap to wash their face. If the patient is able to wash their face with assistance this should be encouraged	To maintain the patient's own routine and promote independence
Place towel across the patient's chest; using a flannel/sponge wash face, ears and neck, rinse well and dry thoroughly	To ensure that the towel is easily accessible Soap can dry the skin and cause irritation
11 Where possible hold the bowl and allow patient to wash and dry their own hands	To promote independence and the feeling of wellbeing
12 Exposing only the area of the body being washed place a towel under the patient's arm that is furthest from you continue to wash, rinse and thoroughly dry the patient's arms and upper body	To maintain patient privacy, dignity and body temperature To keep bed clothes dry To ensure the nearest arm does not become contaminated as the nurse leans over the patient to wash the furthest arm
Where appropriate pay particular attention to skin folds and under breasts	To reduce the risk of infection as skin folds and under breasts if not washed and dried correctly may be prone to an increased risk of fungal infection Washing and drying correctly reduces the risk of skin breakdown
13 Apply toiletries as requested by patient	To reduce body odour, and address patient's individual preferences

(Continued)

Procedure guideline 11.1 **Guideline for bedbathing (general principles)** *(cont'd)*

Nursing action	Rationale
14 Exposing only the area of the body being washed wash the patient's legs following the same process as for arms	To maintain patient privacy, dignity and body temperature To ensure the nearest leg does not become contaminated as the nurse leans over the patient to wash the furthest leg
15 Apply non-sterile gloves	To reduce the risk of cross-infection To reduce the risk of contamination to the practitioner To promote patient comfort
16 Explain to the patient that you are going to wash the genital area offering them the option to do this for themselves. If they are unable to do so expose the genital area and wash using the second flannel/ sponge; disposable wipes may be used where appropriate and available e.g. for menstruating or incontinent patients	To maintain patient dignity and promote independence To reduce risk of cross-infection
For female patients wash from front to back	To reduce the risk of cross-infection
For uncircumcised male patients the foreskin should be retracted during washing and returned to its natural position once the area has been thoroughly dried	To reduce risk of infection and aid patient comfort. If the foreskin is not repositioned the patient is at risk of developing a paraphimosis
Remove and dispose of gloves in accordance with health and safety regulations and local policy	To reduce the risk of cross-infection and contamination of others
17 Ensure that the patient is in a safe position, change the water	To maintain patient safety To reduce the risk of cross-infection To promote patient comfort
18 Keeping the patient covered, gently role them on to their preferred side. Wash, rinse and thoroughly dry shoulders and back with the flannel/sponge previously used to wash the upper part of the body (prepare clean bottom sheet if appropriate)	To maintain patient privacy, dignity and body temperature To maintain patient and practitioner safety
19 Carry out an observational assessment of skin integrity and potential pressure areas	To review and or aid decision making regarding pressure-relieving equipment and the need for protective dressings
20 Apply non-sterile gloves	To reduce the risk of cross-infection To reduce the risk of contamination to the practitioner To promote patient comfort
21 Wash, rinse and thoroughly dry the buttocks and anal area using the second flannel/sponge; disposable wipes may be used where appropriate and available, e.g. for menstruating or incontinent patients	To reduce risk of cross-infection Washing and drying correctly reduces the risk of skin breakdown
Change bottom sheet if required	To promote patient comfort
22 Remove and dispose of gloves in accordance with health and safety regulations and local policy	To reduce the risk of cross-infection and contamination of others

Procedure guideline 11.1 **Guideline for bedbathing (general principles)** *(cont'd)*

Nursing action	Rationale
23 Assist patient with dressing or nightwear	To maintain patient dignity and self-esteem
24 Remake bed	To ensure patient comfort
25 Brush/comb patient's hair if they are unable to do so	To promote patient dignity and self-esteem and promote a positive body image
26 Assist patient into a comfortable position	To enhance patient comfort
27 Dispose of/tidy away all equipment and toiletries, ensure that flannels/sponges are rinsed and the bowl is washed and dried	To reduce risk of cross-infection To ensure the environment is safe and tidy for patient, nurse and carer.
Ask patient/carer where to place towels for drying and where to put used/soiled linen and clothing	To minimise the risk of cross-infection, where necessary store patient toiletries separately
28 Remove and dispose of apron in accordance with health and safety regulations and local policy where appropriate facilities are available wash and dry hands. Alternatively cleanse hands with alcohol-based hand rub	To reduce the risk of cross-infection and contamination of others
29 Complete nursing documentation updating care plan as necessary	To ensure safe continuity of patient care

Procedure guideline 11.2 **Guideline for facial shaving**

Equipment

Bowl of hand-hot water
Flannel
Patient's shaving cream/soap
Disposable razor or electric shaver
After shave/facial moisturiser (where appropriate)
Disposable single-use apron
Towel
Protective covering for patient's furniture

1 Where appropriate facilities are available wash and dry hands. Alternatively cleanse hands with alcohol-based hand rub	To prevent the risk of cross-infection/contamination
2 Read nursing documentation and care plan	To maintain safety by updating practitioner knowledge of the patient
3 Complete/review risk assessment	To ensure health and safety guidelines are adhered to

(Continued)

4 Explain and discuss the procedure with the patient	To ease any anxieties the patient may have and gain patient consent
5 Put on a plastic disposable apron	To reduce the risk of cross-infection
6 Collect and prepare all equipment	To minimise disruption to the procedure and prevent the need to leave the patient unattended
Where necessary protect the patient's furnishings with, e.g. polythene bag, bin liner or tray	To protect patient's furniture
7 Place the patient in a position that allows easy access to their face and avoids the need for the nurse to stoop or bend	To ensure patient is comfortable during the procedure and maintain staff safety
8 Observe patient's face for any spots/moles that need to be avoided	To reduce the risk of nicks or cuts to sensitive areas with the razor that may cause pain/bleeding
9 Place towel around patient's neck	To keep clothing dry
10 **For a wet shave**	To create a lather
Apply shaving cream/soap as per product instruction	
11 Pull the facial skin taut with your non-dominant hand. Begin on one side of the face and work down to the neck area	To ensure the dominant hand holds the razor; non-wrinkled skin is easier to shave and this also minimises the risk of accidental cuts to the skin
	To ensure no area of the face is missed
12 With the razor shave in short strokes following the direction of stubble/hair growth	To prevent discomfort to the patient
13 Clean razor in bowl of water after each stroke	To remove shaved stubble, and prevent the razor from clogging up
14 Once face and neck has been shaved change water and rinse the patient's face using the flannel	To remove excess shaving cream/soap and aid patient comfort
15 Dry face and neck area with towel	To aid patient comfort
16 If appropriate, apply patient's aftershave and/or facial moisturiser	To promote patient wellbeing and self-esteem
17 Assist patient into a comfortable position	To enhance patient comfort
18 Dispose of water, clean and dry bowl	To reduce risk of cross-infection
Put the towel to dry or wash	To ensure the environment is safe and tidy for patient, nurse and carer
Tidy toiletries clean/dispose of razor as appropriate	
19 Remove and dispose of apron. Wash hands and dry well. Alternatively cleanse hands with 70% alcohol-based hand rub	To reduce the risk of cross-infection
20 Complete and where necessary update nursing documentation	To ensure safe continuity of patient care
21 **For shave using an electric razor**	
Follow steps 1–8 above	

22 Pull the facial skin taut with the non-dominant hand. Begin on one side of the face and work down to the neck area	To ensure the dominant hand holds the razor; non-wrinkled skin is easier to shave. To ensure no area of the face is missed
23 With the razor shave in short strokes following the direction of stubble/hair growth	To prevent discomfort to the patient
24 Rinse the patient's face using the flannel and warm water	To freshen face
25 Dry face and neck area with towel	To aid patient comfort
26 If appropriate, apply patient's aftershave and/or facial moisturiser	To promote patient wellbeing and self-esteem
27 Assist patient into a comfortable position	To enhance patient comfort
28 Dispose of water, clean and dry bowl. Put the towel to dry or wash Tidy toiletries clean razor as appropriate	To reduce risk of cross-infection To ensure the environment is safe and tidy for patient, nurse and carer
29 Remove and dispose of apron. Where appropriate facilities are available wash and dry hands alternatively, cleanse hands with alcohol-based hand rub	To reduce the risk of cross infection (*see* Chapter 6)
30 Complete and where necessary update nursing documentation	To ensure safe continuity of patient care

Procedure guideline 11.3 **Guideline for oral care**

Equipment

Clean tray with:
Tumbler of fresh water or mouthwash
Toothbrush or disposable single-use foam sticks
Spittoon/small bowl
Tissues
Toothpaste
Tongue depressor
Torch
Towel
Denture cleanser
Denture pot
Disposable single-use apron
Non-sterile single-use gloves

(Continued)

Procedure guideline 11.3 **Guideline for oral care** *(cont'd)*

Nursing action	Rationale
1 Where appropriate facilities are available wash and dry hands. Alternatively cleanse hands with alcohol-based hand rub	To prevent the risk of cross-infection/contamination
2 Read nursing documentation and care plan	To maintain safety by updating practitioner knowledge of the patient
3 Complete/review risk assessment	To ensure health and safety guidelines are adhered to
4 Explain and discuss the procedure with the patient	To ease any anxieties the patient may have
	To gain patient consent
5 Collect and prepare all equipment	To prevent interruption of the procedure
6 If the patient is able to clean their own teeth/ dentures, ensure they have all the equipment they need	To promote patient independence
7 Cleanse hands with alcohol-based hand rub	To reduce the risk of cross-infection
Put on non-sterile gloves and disposable plastic apron	
8 Assess the patient's mouth (where appropriate remove dentures). You may need to use a torch and/ or tongue depressor	To observe for any ulcers, sores, redness, furred or dry/ cracked tongue. If any of these are noted, it should be documented, and the appropriate action taken
	To aid decision making on whether to use a toothbrush or foam sticks, dependent on the findings of the assessment
	Care should be taken when using a tongue depressor as this may stimulate the gag reflex
	If the mouth is free from sores/ulcers, the patient's toothbrush may be used. If on assessment the patient has, e.g. mouth ulcers or a fungal infection, then the use of foam sticks may be a softer, more appropriate option
9 If using mouthwash solution or tablets, prepare as per manufacturer's instructions	To ensure correct dilution of the product before administering it to the patient
10 Place a towel around the patient's chest and neck area	To keep clothing clean and dry, and to absorb any spittle or secretions from the mouth
11 If the patient is unable to expel spittle and excess secretions into a bowl independently or has dysphasia. The mouth should be cleaned using moistened foam sticks	To aid patient comfort and maintain safety
Use a single rotational short stroke technique	To ensure that debris is removed from the mouth
12 Apply toothpaste to the toothbrush	Toothpaste is a cleansing agent
13 Holding the tooth brush at a 45°angle against the patient's teeth, brush both the inner and outer aspect of the teeth in small single short strokes	To assist in removing plaque from the gums and from between the teeth

Procedure guideline 11.3 Guideline for oral care (cont'd)

Nursing action	Rationale
14 Offer the patient fresh water or mouthwash at regular intervals to rinse mouth	To encourage the removal of residual toothpaste and loosened debris, and to freshen the mouth.
	If toothpaste is used and not rinsed out, it can have a drying effect on the mouth, which may cause a burning sensation
Ensure tissues/towel is near by	To enable excess moisture and secretions to be removed from around the patients mouth
15 Dentures should be removed and cleansed with a toothbrush, cleaning the inner and outer aspect as described in step 13 above. Where necessary cleanse gums with moistened foam sticks or alternatively offer the patient an appropriate mouthwash	To remove debris from dentures and gum areas
	To reduce the risk of oral infection
	To enhance patient comfort
Dentures can be soaked in an appropriate cleansing agent but must be rinsed in fresh water, before giving them back to the patient	Soaking dentures aids the removal of debris and micro-organisms and reduces plaque build up
	Moistened dentures are easier to re-insert into the mouth
	To remove cleansing agent
	To enhance patient comfort
16 Once the teeth or dentures have been cleaned:	To ensure all the equipment is ready for the next time the procedure is carried out.
Clean and dry the equipment used	To prevent the risk of cross-infection
Dispose of used tissues and foamsticks	
Remove towel from the patient, and make sure they are comfortable.	
17 Remove gloves and disposable apron	To prevent the risk of cross-infection
Wash and dry hands thoroughly or alternatively cleanse with alcohol based hand rub	
18 Complete documentation	To ensure safe continuity of patient care

Procedure guideline 11.4 **Guideline for washing a patient's hair in bed**

Equipment

Shampoo/conditioner
Towels – minimum 3
Plastic sheeting or opened bin liner
Washing up bowl or equivalent x 2
Flannel
Jug or large beaker
Hairbrush/comb
Hairdryer
Disposable single-use apron

(Continued)

Procedure guideline 11.4 **Guideline for washing a patient's hair in bed** (cont'd)

Nursing action	Rationale
1 Where appropriate facilities are available wash and dry hands or alternatively cleanse with alcohol-based hand rub	To prevent the risk of cross-infection/contamination
2 Read nursing documentation and care plan	To maintain safety by updating practitioner knowledge of the patient
3 Complete manual handling risk assessment; this should include assessment of the environment	To ensure health and safety guidelines are adhered to
	To ascertain if one or two team members are required to carry out this procedure
	To assess if the patient can be positioned on their back throughout the procedure
	To ensure patient and team member's safety is maintained
4 Explain and discuss the procedure with the patient	To allay any concerns or anxieties the patient may have and to gain patient consent
5 Collect and prepare all necessary equipment	To minimise disruption to the procedure and prevent the need to leave the patient unattended
6 Where necessary adjust bed position and furnishings	To ensure that the area is free of obstruction and allows safe ease of movement
If possible remove headboard; alternatively alter patient's position so that their head is at the foot of bed	To maintain patient and nurse safety
	To promote patient comfort
7 Prepare a bowl of hand-hot water. Place at the side of the patient on the floor. Check that water temperature is suitable for the patient	To maintain patient safety and aid comfort
8 Cleanse hands with alcohol-based hand rub	To reduce the risk of cross-infection
Put on plastic disposable apron	
9 Cover the floor area beneath the patients head with plastic sheeting/towel	To protect floor and furnishings
	To protect the patient's property and to absorb minor splashes of water
Remove the pillow from beneath the patient's head, and place plastic sheeting with towel on top of the mattress under the patients shoulders and head	
Adjust the patient's position, to ensure that their head is just over the edge of the mattress	To enable the nurse to gather all hair for washing
10 Give flannel to patient or second nurse	To enable the patient/nurse to wipe any excess water away, and/or protect eyes from shampoo
11 Place empty bowl, on the floor under the patient's head	To collect water that is poured on to the patient's hair
12 Using a jug or beaker gently pour water over patient's head, continue until hair is wet	Wet hair is needed to lather shampoo
13 When hair is wet massage shampoo gently into hair, as per manufacturer instructions	To cleanse hair and scalp

Procedure guideline 11.4 **Guideline for washing a patient's hair in bed** *(cont'd)*

Nursing action	Rationale
14 Rinse hair with clean water from the bowl, making sure the empty bowl is positioned to collect rinsed water and gently squeeze excess water from hair	Removes shampoo and lather
15 If the patient wishes, apply and rinse conditioner as per manufacturer instructions	Conditioner can act as a detangler
16 Remove wet towel and plastic sheeting from under the patient's shoulders.	To promote patient comfort
17 Place a dry towel around the patient's hair and shoulders and readjust their position	To ensure the patient's safety and comfort To absorb water and protect bedding
18 Remove bowls and dispose of water	To avoid spillage onto patient's flooring
19 Gently towel-dry the patient's hair	To remove excess water
20 Comb/brush patient's hair, if they are unable to do this independently	To remove tangles and style hair to patient's wishes To maintain patient dignity and self-esteem
21 If appropriate, use a hairdryer	To complete hair drying and aid patient comfort
22 Once procedure is complete, assist patient into a comfortable position	To promote patient safety and comfort
Where necessary, replace headboard and readjust position of furniture	To maintain a safe environment for the patient, carer and visitors to the patient's home
23 Put away all used equipment. Hang towels in an appropriate place to dry	To ensure all the equipment is ready for the next time the procedure is carried out
24 Remove and dispose of apron appropriately. Wash hands and dry well or alternatively cleanse with alcohol-based hand rub	To prevent the risk of cross-infection
25 Complete documentation	To ensure safe continuity of patient care

Procedure guideline 11.5 **Guideline for eye care**

If the patient is unable to independently remove and/or insert an artificial eye or contact lenses the community nurse should not attempt to do so unless they are trained and competent in the procedure. For further advice and guidance the community nurse should contact the local or nearest eye hospital or ward.

Equipment

Sterile eye care pack or dressing pack – 1 per eye
Sterile sodium chloride 0.9% for irrigation or sterile water for irrigation
Towel
Non-sterile single-use gloves
Disposable single-use apron

Nursing action	Rationale
1 Where appropriate facilities are available wash and dry hands or alternatively cleanse with alcohol-based hand rub	To prevent the risk of cross-infection/contamination
2 Read nursing documentation and care plan	To maintain safety by updating practitioner knowledge of the patient
3 Explain and discuss the procedure with the patient	To ease any anxieties the patient may have and to gain patient consent
4 Prepare a clean working area/surface	
5 Collect and prepare all equipment, check cleansing fluid to be used is in date and the seal is intact. Discard all damaged or expired equipment	To minimise disruption to the procedure and prevent the need to leave the patient unattended To maintain patient safety
6 Assist patient into a comfortable position with their head slightly tilted back; if necessary provide support with a pillow, place a towel around the patient's neck and shoulders	To allow ease of access to the eye and aid patient comfort To absorb any excess fluid during the procedure
7 Cleanse hands with alcohol based hand rub Apply disposable apron and gloves	To reduce the risk of cross-infection
8 If appropriate, cleanse the uninfected eye first	To reduce the risk of cross-infection
9 The eye should initially be cleansed with moistened gauze with the eyelid closed	To reduce the risk of corneal damage
10 Ask the patient to look upwards, and using a single-stroke method, gently wipe slightly moistened swab across the lower eyelid starting at the inner aspect of the eye	To reduce the risk of cross-infection and aid patient comfort as excess fluid may drip on to patient
Using a new swab each time repeat as necessary for each eye	To prevent the risk of cross-infection and the reintroduction of debris back into the eye

Procedure guideline 11.5 Guideline for eye care (cont'd)

Nursing action	Rationale
11 Ask the patient to look downwards, and using a single-stroke method, gently wipe slightly moistened swab across the upper eyelid starting at the inner aspect of the eye	To reduce the risk of cross-infection and aid patient comfort as excess fluid may drip on to patient
Using a new swab each time repeat as necessary for each eye	To prevent the risk of cross-infection and the reintroduction of debris back into the eye
12 Dispose of swab appropriately after each single use	To reduce the risk of cross-infection
13 Once eyes have been cleansed, dry thoroughly using a dry gauze swab for each eye	To reduce the risk of cross-infection and promote patient comfort
14 Remove towel from patient's shoulders and assist them to readjust their position	To maintain safety and promote patient comfort
15 Remove apron and gloves and dispose of all single-use items in accordance with health and safety regulations and local policy	To prevent the risk of cross-infection/contamination
16 Where appropriate facilities are available wash and dry hands or alternatively cleanse with alcohol-based hand rub	To prevent the risk of cross-infection/contamination
17 Complete documentation and where necessary update documentation	To ensure safe continuity of patient care

NB Where the patient has suffered trauma to the eye or has undergone surgery this procedure should be carried out using an aseptic technique.
For instillation of eye drops, see Procedure guideline 8.5 in Chapter 8.

Procedure guideline 11.6 **Guideline for nail care**

As part of the assessment process the patient's finger nails, toe nails and feet should be visually inspected for signs of, e.g. fungal infections, nail discolouration and cracks or breaks in the skin. The community nurse should not attempt to cut a patient's nails unless they are appropriately trained and competent to do so. For those patients whose nails require cutting or potential specialist treatment, the community nurse should refer to the appropriate professional, e.g. podiatrist or chiropodist, this is particularly relevant for those patients with diabetes. Patients with diabetes should receive education and training regarding the importance of checking their feet and hands on a regular basis and advised regarding the appropriate action to take.

Equipment

Emery board
Nail file
Non-sterile disposable gloves
Plastic single-use apron
Hand bowl
Towel x 1

(Continued)

Procedure guideline 11.6 **Guideline for nail care** *(cont'd)*

Nursing action	Rationale
1 Where appropriate facilities are available wash and dry hands or, alternatively cleanse with alcohol-based hand rub	To prevent the risk of cross-infection/contamination
2 Read nursing documentation and care plan	To maintain safety by updating practitioner knowledge of the patient
3 Complete/review risk assessment	To maintain patient and staff safety
4 Explain and discuss the procedure with the patient	To ease any anxieties the patient may have and to gain patient consent
5 Apply non-sterile gloves and disposable single-use apron	To reduce the risk of cross-infection
6 Assist the patient into a comfortable position; where necessary and possible adjust the bed height or sit facing the patient to carry out the procedure	To allow ease of access to the patient's finger nails and prevent the need for the community nurse to bend or stoop
7 Visually assess fingernails	If nails are too long or have rough edges they may cause skin tears
8 Collect and prepare all equipment	To minimise disruption to the procedure
9 If nails require filing, soak the patient's hands in warm water and dry thoroughly	To soften nails before filing Aids the removal of debris that may be present underneath the finger nails
10 Where necessary file the patient's nails gently with an emery board; where possible remove debris from underneath fingernails using the nail file	To smooth the nail edges and reduce the risk of skin tears
11 If the patient's fingernails require cutting, refer to the appropriate professional	The community nurse should not attempt to cut the nails unless they are appropriately trained To reduce the risk of causing skin nicks and tears that may result in discomfort for the patient or require further treatment
12 Remove and dispose of gloves appropriately	To reduce the risk of cross-contamination
13 Where necessary assist patient into a comfortable position and readjust bed height and any furniture moved	To maintain patient safety To maintain a safe environment for the patient, carer and visitors to the patient's home
14 Remove apron and dispose of single-use items appropriately; put away other equipment used	To reduce the risk of cross-infection
15 Where appropriate facilities are available wash and dry hands or, alternatively cleanse with alcohol-based hand rub	To prevent the risk of cross-infection
16 For toe nails follow steps above adjusting as necessary e.g. soaking feet in warm water	
17 Complete documentation updating as necessary	To ensure safe continuity of patient care

References and further reading

Alibhai-Brown Y (1998) *Caring for Ethnic Minority Elders*. Age Concern England, London.

Armstrong J, Mitchell E (2008) Comprehensive nursing assessment in the care of older people. *Nursing Older People* **20**(1): 36–40.

Basavanthappa B (2004) *Fundamentals of Nursing*. Jaypee Brothers Medical Publishers, New Delhi.

BBC (2009) Hijab [online] www.bbc.co.uk/religion/religions/Islam/beliefs/hijab_1.shtml (last accessed 9 August 2011).

Black P (2000) Practical stoma care. *Nursing Standard* **14**(41): 47–53.

Brooks N (2004) Diversity in medicine. *Clinical Cornerstone* **6**(1): 7–16.

Clay M (2000) Oral Health in Older People. *Nursing Older People* **12**(7): 21–6.

Department of Health (2010) *Essence of Care Benchmarks for Personal Hygiene*. The Stationery Office, Norwich.

Dougherty L, Lister S (eds) (2011) *The Royal Marsden Hospital Manual of Clinical Nursing Procedures*. Wiley-Blackwell, Oxford.

Ghazala S (2002) Nursing with dignity. *Nursing Times* **98**(16): 40–2.

Gill B (2002) Nursing with dignity. *Nursing Times* **98**(14): 39–41.

Gould D (2002) Health related infection and hand hygiene – Part 1. *Nursing Times* **98**(38): 48.

Health and Safety Executive (HSE) (2011) *Five Steps to Risk Assessment*. HSE, London.

Holland K, Hogg C (2001) *Cultural Awareness in Nursing and Health Care*. Arnold, London

Jootun D (2002) Nursing with dignity. *Nursing Times* **98**(15): 38–40.

Kennedy C (2002) The work of the district nurse. *Journal of Advance Nursing* **40**(6): 710–20.

Marsden J, Shaw M (2003) Correct administration of topical eye treatment. *Nursing Standard* **17**(30): 42–4.

Nesbit E (2008) *Sikhism; a very short introduction*. Oxford University Press, Oxford.

Nicoll M, Bavin C, Cronin P, Rawlings-Anderson K (2008) *Essential Nursing Skills*. Mosby, London.

Nursing and Midwifery Council (2008) *The Code: standards of conduct, performance and ethics for nurses and midwives*. NMC, London.

Pearson L, Hutton J (2002) A controlled trial to compare the ability of foam swabs and toothbrushes to remove dental plaque. *Journal of Advanced Nursing* **39**(5): 480–9.

Poxton R (2004) Partnerships made painless: a joined-up guide to working together. *Health and Social Care* **12**(3): 280–2.

Royal College of Nursing (2004) *Patient Information and the Role of the Carer*. RCN, London.

Seinko K (2002) Providing culturally competent health services for ethnic minorities. *Nursing Standard* **16**(48): 38–9.

Singh D (2010) Care of the elderly: a Sikh perspective. *Nursing & Residential Care* **12**(3): 138–9.

Thakrar D, Das R, Sheikh A (eds) (2008) *Caring for Hindu Patients*. Radcliffe, Oxford.

Workman B, Bennett C (2003) *Key Nursing Skills*. Whurr Publishers, London.

Xavier G (2000) The importance of mouthcare in preventing infection *Nursing Standard* **14**(18): 47–51.

12

Syringe driver/pump management and symptom control in palliative care

Definition

Infusion devices administer medication by subcutaneous, intravenous or intrathecal (within the meninges of the spinal cord) routes (Perdue 2004). They are known as ambulatory infusion devices, and are designed to administer a small volume of medication over a set length of time. They include the Graseby syringe drivers and McKinley syringe pump.

Ambulatory pumps fall into two categories.

- **Mechanical devices**, which are usually disposable. They may be gas-powered, driven by an inflatable balloon or spring-loaded (Quinn 2002).
- **Battery-operated pumps**, which use alkaline or rechargeable batteries. They are usually small, can be worn discretely and are often used for ambulant patients. Syringe drivers fall into this category.

Ambulatory infusion devices have been used in the acute sector for pain control and chemotherapy administration, and also in neonatal and coronary care units (Dougherty & Lister 2011). This chapter will focus on the use of infusion devices in palliative and end of life care in the home setting.

Background evidence

In the late 1970s, Dr BM Wright developed a device that would deliver a continuous flow of medication to patients over a 24-hour period. It used a battery-driven syringe to pump medication slowly into the subcutaneous tissue (Mallet & Dougherty 2000).

It quickly became evident that this device would be suitable for use with palliative care patients who were unable to tolerate oral medication, and in the terminal phase of an illness when a patient may become comatose yet still need symptom control. Therefore, although an infusion device may not be suitable for all palliative care patients it should be considered as a means to help deliver symptom control rather than as a last resort method of treatment (Perdue 2004).

Evidence to support this suggests that the administration of single or combination therapies, via syringe drivers, has had a significant impact on increasing patient comfort, for example in the control of symptoms such as:

- pain
- nausea and vomiting
- agitation
- excessive, distressing chest secretions (Mitten 2001).

The NHS Cancer Plan (DH 2000), in conjunction with The Liverpool Care Pathway (LCP) (DH 2008), and Gold Standards Framework (GSF) (Mahmood-Yousuf *et al.* 2008) emphasises the importance of the primary care team in palliative care. Community nurses are part of this team and, as such, will often be the ones to provide the clinical aspects of care to patients and ongoing support to carers and families before and after death. Nationally, access to a specialist palliative care service is available to around 75% of cancer patients,

District Nursing Manual of Clinical Procedures, First Edition. Edited by Liz O'Brien.
© 2012 Blackwell Publishing Ltd. Published 2012 by Blackwell Publishing Ltd.

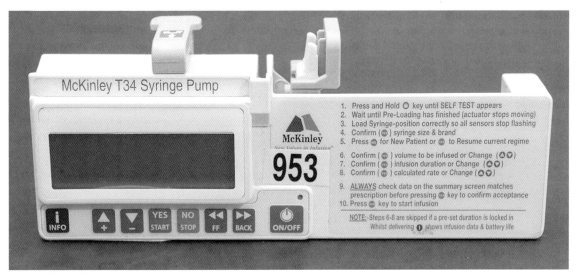

Figure 12.1 McKinley T34 syringe pump (Dougherty and Lister, 2011).

with most patient contact centring on advice and symptom control (St Christopher's Hospice 2001).

The specialist palliative care team may be based in a hospice or hospital and usually consists of a multiprofessional team of doctors, clinical nurse specialists (CNS), chaplain, social workers, welfare officers and others who are trained to address the physical, emotional, psychosocial and spiritual needs of patients and carers (Twycross 1997). They are also a resource to general practitioners (GPs), who remain the primary physician, and community nurses, who remain the primary care providers.

The choice of infusion device will depend on local availability and cost. A number of devices are available, for example the McKinley T34 syringe pump (Figure 12.1) and the Micrel syringe pump (MHRA 2003), the Graseby MS 16A (Figure 12.2) and Graseby MS26 (Figure 12.3) syringe drivers (Trotman & Hami 2003). However, for improved safety reasons many community nursing services and palliative care centres have begun to replace syringe drivers with syringe pumps in response to recommendations made by the National Patient Safety Agency (NPSA) (NPSA 2010).

Education and training

The Nursing and Midwifery Council (NMC) states that nurses must at all times safeguard the interests of

patients by accepting responsibility only for duties for which they are competent and requires them to possess appropriate knowledge, skills and abilities to practise safely without supervision (NMC 2008). Nurses should also be aware that they might not be protected from legal implications if their actions are inappropriate (Medical Devices Agency 2003). There is a high incidence of human error in using infusion pumps (Quinn 2002; MDA 2003), therefore it is essential that specific training in the use of infusion devices, through specialist palliative care units, local educational and development departments, or company representatives is provided. For those who do not use them regularly, updates should be available (MDA 2003).

It is suggested that theoretical knowledge alone is insufficient to use infusion devices safely; rigorous training in theoretical aspects of the device as well as practical application of the theory is essential to prevent adverse incidents (MDA 2003). Ongoing assessment of practitioner competency is also essential to maintain safe practice. This can be achieved through the development of a locally agreed competency framework and/or knowledge skills framework (KSF) that incorporates up-to-date indicators for best practice and clearly sets out the requirements for continuous training and updating. Special considerations need to be taken into account for nurses in the community, for example working in isolation and the difficulty in maintaining competency through clinical practice if infusion devices are used infrequently.

273

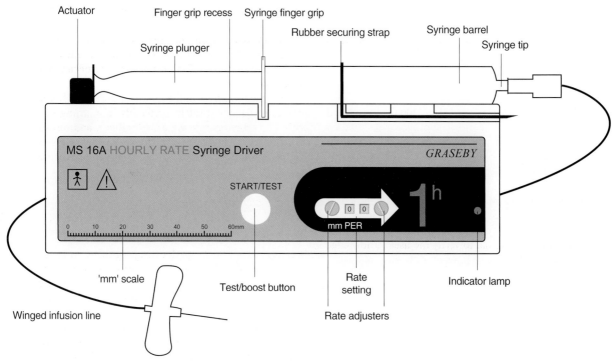

Figure 12.2 Graseby MS 16A hourly rate syringe driver.

274

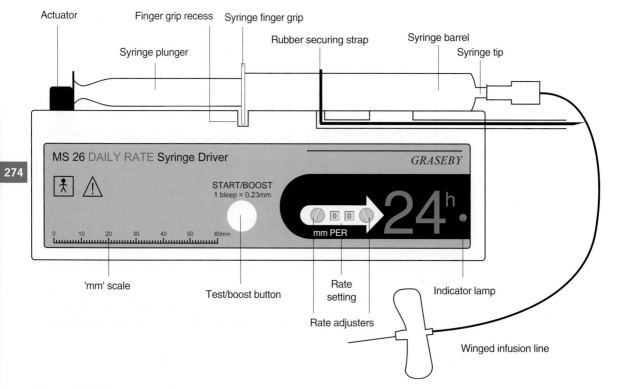

Figure 12.3 Graseby MS 26 daily rate syringe driver.

Each employing community service provider or organisation is obliged by current Health and Safety law to provide training in the correct use of medical devices to ensure safe standards of practice (MDA 2003).

Resources for training

Medical Devices Regulations (MDA 2003) recommend the following.

1 Manufacturers must provide operating and maintenance instructions which should be used when preparing teaching packages for staff.
2 All users should be supplied with a training log to record their continuing professional development.
3 Assessment of competence through local training procedures is essential to verify the user's knowledge and skills in the use of infusion devices.

Prescribing and administering drugs in the community

End of life care requires preparation and forward planning; it is unacceptable for patients to have to wait for a doctor to prescribe or a chemist to dispense medication to relieve distressing symptoms (Sykes & Pace 2003; NMC 2007). The CNS or experienced community nurse can often anticipate patients' needs and organise prescriptions and a record of administration chart before problems arise. Good communication between the community nurses, GP and palliative care team is essential in meeting these needs promptly.

In most cases the local hospice will provide a written prescription and record of administration chart for use with a syringe driver or pump. The record of administration chart should include:

■ the patient's full name and date of birth
■ name and dose of drug administered (and amount wasted if required by local policy)
■ route of administration
■ time of administration, using the 24-hour clock (NMC 2007)
■ condition of infusion site, e.g. no inflammation at canulae site
■ total number of unused ampoules of each controlled drug.

(*See* Chapter 8.)

It can take up to 48 h for a pharmacist to prepare a prescription in the community, therefore it is essential that there is sufficient prescribed medication in the home for several days; this should allow for rescue doses for uncontrolled symptoms. Extra consideration must also be taken to anticipate out of hours, weekends and Bank Holidays, when GP surgeries and pharmacies may be closed.

Once the medicines and equipment are in the home they must be stored safely, preferably in a strong box with a lid (for example a plastic toolbox), and out of sight and reach of small children. A good supply of equipment should always be maintained, and should include:

■ a range of syringes
■ administration sets and canulae
■ sharps box.

Because of the often complex drug regimens and subsequent calculations used for symptom control, it is recommended that a second registrant independently checks the calculation to minimise the risk of errors (NMC 2007). The need for a second registrant in the administration of medicines and controlled drugs in the community should be based on local risk assessment and management strategies (NMC 2007). (*See* Chapter 8.)

The timing of the community nurse visits to renew medication in the syringe is important for avoiding peaks and troughs in symptom control, and it may be necessary to adapt visit times to meet the needs of the patient and their family (NMC 2007).

Using a syringe driver/pump

There are no absolute contraindications to the use of a subcutaneous infusion; however, it is essential to carefully consider the reasons for setting up a syringe driver or pump. In palliative care, it is important that it is not seen as a last resort, but as a way of relieving symptoms (Twycross *et al.* 2002), and the community nurse should explain this to the patient and significant others in order to obtain informed consent (DH 2005) (Table 12.1). This discussion should also include the reasons for use and any potential advantages and disadvantages (Box 12.1).

When parenteral medication is indicated for patients with uncontrolled symptoms it may be given by injection at regular intervals or by syringe driver/pump. These symptoms include:

■ pain
■ nausea and vomiting

275

Table 12.1 Indications for using an infusion device

Problem	Potential cause
Gastrointestinal	
Dysphagia	Oesophageal disease, anxiety Infection, oral thrush
Nausea and vomiting	Chemotherapy, drug-induced, enlarged liver, gastric stasis
Intestinal obstruction	Tumour growth, metastases
Malabsorption	Gluten intolerance, liver disease
Rectal route inappropriate	Local disease, fistula, patient preference
Poor drug absorption (rare)	Defect in small intestine
Physical	
Patient semiconscious or unconscious and unable to swallow	Disease progression
Cachexia, repeated injections cause discomfort	Loss of underlying muscle and fat allodynia
Death rattle in unconscious patient	Build up of chest secretions
Psychological	
Loss of confidence in oral drugs	Inappropriate dosing, poorly controlled symptoms
Erratic drug administration	Non-concordance of patient, difficulty in timing of district nurse visits
Poor symptom control with oral drugs	Anxiety and fear
Terminal restlessness	Pain, agitation, anxiety

Adapted from Trotman & Hami 2003 and Twycross *et al*. 2002.

Box 12.1 Advantages and disadvantages of infusion devices

Advantages

- Avoids the need for 4-hourly injections
- A combination of drugs controls many symptoms
- Avoids peaks and troughs in medication levels; plasma concentrations are stabilised throughout the 24 h (Twycross *et al*. 2002)
- Ensures effective use of resources in terms of community nurse time
- Improved comfort for the patient; subcutaneous access is easy, and the patient does not have to be moved or turned
- Patients can remain ambulant
- Reduces the need for administration of rescue doses once symptoms are controlled.

Disadvantages

- Staff must be trained and regularly updated in their use
- Concerns by patients or carers that it may be a last resort
- Patient dependence on the device
- Inflammation at infusion site
- The warning system will only operate if the pump stops or infusion has finished, it does not warn of cannula displacement or line disconnection (Trotman & Hami 2003)
- Not all drugs can be given subcutaneously
- A daily syringe driver may mean rescue doses of drugs are necessary until symptoms are controlled
- Potential for drug interaction if the prescriber is inexperienced

(Adapted from Twycross *et al*., 2002)

- intestinal obstruction
- excessive secretions in the terminal phase of life.

The syringe driver/pump is especially useful if a variety of drugs are indicated, as most medications can be mixed. This will avoid the need for repeated injections and thus enhance patient comfort.

For a patient who is symptomatic or terminally ill, using a syringe driver/pump means that they can receive a continuous flow of medication over a set period of time, avoiding the peaks and troughs of oral or inject-able medication (Twycross *et al.* 2002).

In the home setting, a careful assessment of the patient's and/or carer's ability to cope with the device must be completed as they will need to share responsi-bility for the care of the syringe driver/pump between

community nurse visits. This will require the commu-nity nurse to provide basic training and education in, for example, the recognition of potential problems and the correct actions to take should they occur.

All relevant contact telephone numbers for the com-munity nurses, including evening and night services, and the local hospice/palliative care team must be left in the patient's home.

Selecting a syringe driver or pump

Graseby MS16A (Figure 12.2)

This device has a blue label and delivers a set number of millimetres (mm) of fluid in one hour. It may be used for a quick infusion over a few minutes (such as dexamethasone in 10 min) or for a slower infusion of up to 24 h (i.e. diamorphine). It is essential to check which type of driver is to be used and document this clearly, as fatal errors have been made where drugs have been over-infused (MDA 2003).

Once the battery is inserted the indicator light flashes every second to confirm the syringe driver is working (Graseby Medical 2002).

Graseby MS26 (Figure 12.3)

This device has a green label and delivers a set number of millimetres of fluid in one day. It may be used to infuse medication over 24 hours or over a period of several days. The indicator light flashes every 25 seconds, which indicates the battery has been inserted and confirms that the syringe driver is working (Graseby Medical 2002).

Parts of the Graseby syringe drivers
Battery, alarm and indicator light

A 9-volt long-life alkaline battery is recommended to power the device. A new battery should last for 50 full syringes; the power is switched off automatically at the end of plunger travel when the syringe is empty. It is essential to have a spare battery available at all times in case of battery failure. If the battery is low, the indicator light (see Figures 12.2 and 12.3) will stop flashing but the battery will continue to power the driver for the duration of the infusion in both types of syringe driver, provided it does not exceed 24 hours (Graseby Medical 2002). Zinc carbon batteries are not recommended as they perform poorly and need to be replaced more often (Graseby Medical 2002). When the battery is inserted the alarm will sound for 15 seconds. Pressing the start/test button on the MS16A and start/boost button on the MS26 stops the alarm, indicating that the syringe driver is ready for use.

The audible alarm will also sound when the syringe is empty or if the infusion set is occluded, the syringe driver stops in both cases. The indicator lamp, which flashes to show that the syringe driver is working, will stop if:

- the battery needs replacing
- the syringe is empty
- the syringe driver has stopped and switched itself off (Graseby Medical 2002).

There is no off switch to stop the syringe driver before the syringe is empty; however, it can be stopped by removing the battery or moving the set rate to 00 (Graseby Medical 2002).

Set rate

The set rate is the rate at which the syringe plunger will be propelled forward by the motor. There is one window for the tens and one for the units. The set rate indicates the distance the plunger will move in **mm per hour for the MS16A** and **mm per 24 hours for the MS26.** Rates from 0 to 99 may be set. A rate adjuster is provided with the syringe driver, but if this is not available, a small screwdriver with a straight blade may be used to move the numbers in the boxes. The numbers should be in the centre of the boxes for accuracy of administration and the set rate should always be checked prior to attaching the syringe driver to the infusion set. Special attention should be paid to the rate setting prior to use when a syringe driver has been returned from servicing, because a number of different rates may have been tested and the driver may have been left at an incorrect rate.

Confusion can arise if rates need to be changed; to minimise the risk of error one type of syringe driver with a fixed rate should be used (Trotman & Hami 2003).

Start/test button MS16A

The syringe driver's safety system must be tested before administering the infusion to the patient. This is done by pressing the start/test button and holding it down, releasing the button starts the syringe driver. If the syringe driver alarm does not sound the system is not safe to use and should be replaced (Graseby Medical 2002).

Start/boost button MS26

The MS26 must be tested just before administration by pressing the start/boost button; releasing the button starts the syringe driver. If the alarm does not sound the system is not safe to use and should be replaced (Graseby Medical 2002). If the start/boost button on the MS26 is held down when the infusion is in progress it activates the boost system. This will administer an extra dose of medication. The quantity of which is determined by the number of beeps (1 beep = 0.23 mm of fluid) (Graseby Medical 2002).

It is not safe practice to use the boost button to administer extra medication as it is difficult to measure the dose given, and it will also increase the dose of any co-therapy in the syringe and could result in overdosage (Twycross et al. 2002).

Using the boost button will also mean that the infusion will finish early and medication will have to be renewed before the next planned community nurse visit time.

Table 12.2 Recognition and causes of syringe pump problems McKinley T34

Alarm type	LCD display	Possible cause	Nursing action
Visual and audible (intermittent beep)	**Syringe displaced**	No syringe loaded in pump/ has been displaced or moved	Check and confirm syringe flanges are in a vertical position and that the syringe is loaded correctly in the pump
			Resume infusion
Visual and audible	**Syringe empty or occlusion**	Infusion line kinked or blocked	Remove occlusion and restart infusion
		Cannula blocked or displaced	Flush or replace cannula as per locally agreed policy
		Maximum actuator travel position reached	Programme end switch off pump
Visual and audible (intermittent beep)	**Pump paused too long**	Keys not pressed for 2 min	Continue with programming pump start infusion or switch pump off
Visual and audible (intermittent beep)	**Near end**	15 min from the end of infusion completion	Prepare new syringe or switch off pump
Visual and audible (intermittent beep)	**End programme**	Infusion completed	Press yes to confirm programme end renew syringe or switch off pump
Visual and audible (intermittent beep)	**Low battery**	30 min of battery remaining	Change battery
Visual and audible	**End battery**	Battery depleted	Change battery

McKinley T34 syringe pump

The McKinley T34 syringe pump (Figure 12.1) is designed to administer medication over a 24-hour period. The pump contains many of the features of a larger syringe pump, but it is small, compact, lightweight and portable, and therefore practical for use in the home care setting. Safety features are an integral part of the pump. For example, by closing the barrel clamp down prior to use and pressing the on/off key to turn the pump on, automatic system checks are performed.

The McKinley T34 has the following key features.

- It is calculated in millilitres per hour as opposed to millimetres per hour.
- When the syringe is loaded the pump detects the size and brand of syringe and this is visible in the display panel.
- The pump will accept 10–50 ml syringes. which can reduce the need for using two devices for larger volumes.
- The pump has three sensors, barrel, collar and plunger.

When labelling the syringe you must ensure that the label is not kinked or bulky under the barrel clamp as this can lead to the incorrect detection of the syringe size.

The alarm will sound for a number of reasons (*see* Table 12.2).

Selection of needle/cannula

Research suggests that the use of a Teflon or Vialon cannula with extension set, as opposed to a needle (butterfly), greatly reduces the need for resiting cannulas and there are fewer incidences of allergic reaction (Dawkins *et al*. 2000; Ross *et al*. 2002). These cannulae are not available on prescription (FP10) but may be purchased through the local community services (depending on purchasing agreements) and are sometimes provided by the hospice involved in the patient's care at home. Although initially more expensive to buy, this type of cannula does have positive benefits for both the patient and community nurse.

Benefits to patients
- Less discomfort through fewer allergic reactions at the cannula site.
- Reduced need for resiting of the device as cannulae last twice as long as metal needles (Ross *et al*. 2002).
- Improved comfort and symptom control, as there is less disruption to the infusion and absorption of medication.

Benefits to the community nurse

- Less time spent on resiting the device, which enables the nurse to focus on being with the patient and their family.
- Less need to re-prioritize daily patient visits for self and other team members to make an unplanned patient visit to resite the more traditional winged infusion set.

Needles should not be used for patients who are allergic to nickel. Reactions to nickel include redness, tenderness and inflammation at the site, which may have the potential to prevent effective absorption of medication. It is important to remember that some types of medication in the syringe driver/pump can also cause similar skin reactions, these include:

- cyclizine
- levomepromazine.

Other less commonly used medications include:

- diclofenac
- methadone
- ketamine.

(Trotman & Hami 2003; Dickman 2010)

Diazepam, prochlorperazine and chlorpromazine may also cause severe reactions, therefore these drugs should never be given subcutaneously (BNF 2011).

Syringe sizes

The choice of syringe used will depend on local availability but it should always be of good quality and the Luer lock type (attached by a twisting action) to avoid disconnection (RCN 2003). It is essential that each new syringe is sterile, the plunger must slide easily in the barrel and the syringe must fit securely into the syringe driver or pump.

The Graseby syringe driver will hold a 5–30 ml syringe (Graseby 2002); as a minimum it is suggested that a 20 ml syringe is used for infusions, as a larger volume of fluid may reduce the risk of adverse site reactions and incompatibility of medication (Dickman 2010). If the volume of fluid exceeds 30 ml best practice suggests that the dose of medication is divided in half and administered over 12 hours. This will mean that evening or night nurses must visit 12 hours later to administer the second half. Where appropriate, an alternative is to ask the prescriber to alter the medication to one with a smaller volume.

Community nurses should be aware that the dimensions of syringes will vary depending on the manufacturer and this is particularly significant when using the

Table 12.3 Suggested syringe sizes and medication volumes for the McKinley T34 syringe pump

Beckton Dickinson luer lock syringe size	Total medication volume drawn up	McKinley T34 pump approximated hourly rate
10 mL	10 mL	0.42 mL/h
20 mL	17 mL	0.71 mL/h
30 mL	22 mL	0.92 mL/h
50 mL	32 mL	1.33 mL/h

Graseby syringe driver. This is because there is variation in the internal diameter of different makes of syringe, for example one make of syringe filled to 48 mm holds 8 ml in volume, while another will hold 9 ml. For this reason the volume of fluid needed must be measured on the syringe driver ruler before drawing up the medication (Figures 12.1 & 12.2).

Unlike the Graseby syringe driver, when the syringe is loaded into the McKinley T34 pump it will automatically detect the size, 10–50 ml, and brand of syringe; this will be visible in the display panel. The pump will also detect the volume of fluid contained in the syringe and calculate the administration rate (Table 12.3).

Priming the extension set

Priming the extension set for both the Graseby syringe driver and McKinley T34 pump is the same. The prepared syringe must be attached to the selected extension set and the set must be primed to the tip of the needle/cannula; this procedure should be done manually and prior to needle/cannula insertion. However, in relation to the Graseby syringe driver there is currently two schools of thought concerning the volume of diluent to be used and the most appropriate method of measurement.

- Prime the set before measuring the volume of fluid in the syringe (Kaye 1994; Graseby 2000). Add extra diluent to compensate; this means that the drug concentration level/s will be less than that prescribed (Mitten 2001).
- Measure the volume prior to priming the set and do not add extra diluent as above. This method ensures that the correct drug concentration levels will be administered, as prescribed, but provision must be made to visit the patient earlier the next day as the infusion will finish early. This method is described in the procedure guideline, but community nurses

should adhere to locally agreed policies concerning this procedure.

As opinion appears to be divided in this matter, it is suggested that a specific policy should be developed for individual areas of practice to provide clarity for community nurses and uniformity of practice within individual community nursing services (Mitten 2001).

Siting the infusion device

The infusion needle/cannula must be inserted into subcutaneous fat to enhance absorption of medication. If the patient is cachectic, the abdomen may be the most suitable site as it generally has the greatest quantity of subcutaneous fat and is central in the body. This will improve absorption if the peripheral circulation is compromised (Mitten 2001) (Figure 12.4).

When siting the infusion device areas to be avoided are:

■ bony prominences
■ joints
■ skin folds
■ lymphoedematous tissue
■ broken skin
■ sites of tumour or infection
■ recently irradiated skin
■ areas of inflammation.

(Mitten 2001; Trotman & Hami 2003)

It is suggested that 1 mg of dexamethasone added to the syringe driver/pump medication may significantly extend the viability of subcutaneous cannulation sites (Reymond *et al.* 2003; Dickman *et al.* 2005).

Protection and positioning of the syringe driver

A clear, strong plastic cover is available to protect both driver and syringe. A cloth holster may be used for ambulant patients so that the syringe driver can be worn comfortably and to prevent it being dropped. Also available are a lock box to prevent tampering and a non-slip base, which may be used to stand the syringe driver on a flat surface for those who are confined to bed.

There is a potential risk of bolus delivery if the device is placed too far above the level of the infusion site and of delivery delay if it is placed too far below (MDA 2003). For example, if the infusion site is the thigh of an ambulant patient, the driver should be positioned around the waist rather than in a shirt pocket.

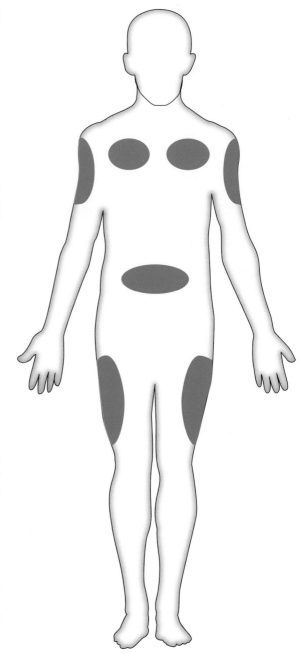

Figure 12.4 Suggested ares for siting an infusion device.

The syringe driver will work effectively at between 10 and 40°C but care should be taken to avoid moving it from a very humid environment to a much cooler one and vice versa (Graseby 2002). The syringe driver is not a sealed unit and condensation may form on the inside, leading to problems with the mechanism. The device should be protected from sunlight by covering it with a cloth cover and prevented from overheating (MDA 2003).

When not in use the syringe driver should be stored in a warm dry place (MDA 2003).

Symptom management

Symptom management is the prime objective of palliative and end of life care but should never be considered in isolation. Disease management, and physical and psychosocial care, of both the patient and family, are equally important as they help to:

- achieve relief from distressing symptoms (Lucas 1998; Watson *et al.* 2009)
- support the patient to adjust and where necessary adapt their lifestyle according to their changing needs
- help the patient's family to adjust.

(Twycross & Wilcock 2001)

Modern medicines can relieve a variety of symptoms; however, it is not always possible to achieve immediate, complete symptom control. To determine, for example, the correct drug/s to be administered and individual doses, it is essential that the community nurse carries out an assessment of the patient and their symptoms every 24 hours. Where indicated, the appropriate syringe driver/pump medication should be increased, for example where rescue (stat) doses of medication have been administered, to aid the control of symptoms (see rescue doses of medication).

Crisis box

If the course of a patient's disease is predictable it is advisable to anticipate the need for injectable medication to enable prompt symptom relief and avoid prolonged discomfort and anxiety for the patient (Sykes & Pace 2003). This can be achieved through the provision of a 'crisis' box, left in the home, which contains:

- a selection of syringe sizes
- cannulae or winged infusion devices and extension sets
- a selection of different needles for drawing up medication and administering rescue (stat) doses
- alcohol swabs for skin cleansing, if recommended by local policies

- semipermeable dressings to secure infusion device once in position
- the appropriate infusion device with a new and a spare battery
- the prescribed medication, including sterile water for injection (or saline if appropriate)
- labels on which to record drugs given, diluent used, time of next syringe change, and set/administration rate (according to local guidelines).

Medication can be prescribed by specialist doctors from the local hospice or by the GP. It may also be prescribed by some specialist nurses who have undergone a non-medical prescribing course giving them prescribing rights within their sphere of competence and in accordance with local policy (*see* Chapter 8).

Pain control

Pain is a very individual experience and is multidimensional in nature, including physical, social, psychological and spiritual elements (Twycross 1997; Lucas 1998; Hanks *et al.* 2009). If the patient is experiencing difficulties in any of these areas they will need to be addressed in order for symptom control to be effective.

Pain thresholds vary considerably from person to person and a patient's perception of pain may be altered by, for example:

- mood
- morale
- the meaning of pain for the patient.

(Twycross & Wilcock 2001)

Many patients with chronic pain or advanced cancer will have been taking an oral opioid, analgesic or anti-inflammatory medication, or a combination of all three. Most drugs used in pain control can be converted into appropriate medication for use in an infusion device (Kaye 1994; Back 2001). However, decision making with regard to the most appropriate medication and dosages is complex, and advice and support should be sought prior to set up (Barclay *et al.* 2002).

Diamorphine

If an opioid is indicated, the morphine derivative diamorphine is the most suitable for use in a syringe driver/pump as it is highly soluble (up to 250 mg dissolves in 1 ml of water) and compatible with many other drugs used in palliative care (Trotman & Hami 2003).

Although it is an effective analgesic, reactions to subcutaneous diamorphine can arise quickly. For example:

281

- where the patient is opioid-naive (not taken opioids before)
- in high doses.
- where the pain may not be opioid responsive
- with rapidly escalating doses.

(Trotman & Hami 2003)

Caution should be also be exercised in diamorphine use with older adults as they may be more prone to toxic reactions, due to less effective clearance by the kidneys. Consequently doses should always be titrated up slowly (Trotman & Hami 2003) (Table 12.4).

The common side effects of diamorphine are, to some degree, predictable (Table 12.4) and in most cases can be minimised by taking preventative measures. For example

- warning patients of potential difficulties while emphasising the benefits of the drug
- encouraging the patient to report new symptoms promptly
- prescribing an anti-emetic to be given via the syringe driver/pump if nausea has been a problem previously
- prescribing a laxative to be given by the most appropriate route, oral or rectal.

In most cases the majority of side effects subside within a week of commencing treatment, but for some patients they may prove more distressing than the original symptoms (Twycross & Wilcock 2001). If the side effects are very distressing for the patient and do not improve quickly, the community nurse should seek advice from the hospice/hospital palliative care team or GP. The effectiveness of pain relief and identified/reported side effects should be reviewed, monitored and documented at each visit; this should also include any actions taken by the community nurse.

NB: It is recommended that opioids other than diamorphine or morphine sulphate should only be used in a syringe driver/pump on the advice of a doctor who is a specialist in palliative care (Dickman *et al.* 2005; Dickman 2010) (Table 12.4).

Converting oral morphine to diamorphine

It is suggested that although most GPs are familiar with the modern management of cancer pain, they appear to be less aware of the drugs used in syringe driver/pumps especially the dose conversion of oral morphine to subcutaneous diamorphine (Barclay *et al.* 2002). There is also anecdotal evidence to suggest that, in general, community nurses are not expected to convert oral medication to subcutaneous without obtaining the appropriate

advice, guidance and support, particularly when setting up an infusion device for the first time.

To convert oral morphine to subcutaneous diamorphine, the total amount of oral analgesic, both opioid and other administered over a 24 hours period, must be taken into consideration. This should include any extra doses of medication used for related breakthrough pain. Care should be taken if additional rescue doses are administered for pain prior to carrying out, for example, bathing or wound management, as it may not be necessary to include these. All drug calculations should be checked prior to conversion, prescribing and administration.

Diamorphine is three times as strong as oral morphine (Back 2001; Twycross 2002) so the total amount of oral morphine should be divided by three to obtain the dose of subcutaneous diamorphine in 24 hours (Watson *et al.* 2011). However, there is considerable variation in the effectiveness of drugs between patients, and with different drugs in the same patient (Gibbs 2000). See Table 12.5 for a guide to commonly used analgesics and their dose equivalents to oral morphine.

NB: Suggested doses are an approximation only.

Morphine sulphate

In recent years there have been some manufacturing problems with diamorphine, and morphine sulphate has become a suitable alternative. An advantage of using morphine sulphate is that it is pre-prepared and this removes the need for reconstitution. However, a disadvantage is that the highest strength available is 30 mg in 1 ml (BNF 2011). This may cause difficulties where the patient is prescribed a high dose of morphine sulphate in combination with other drugs, because this will require a large total fluid volume and consequently a larger syringe, which may impact on device selection.

Morphine sulphate in injection form is twice as strong as oral morphine, therefore to calculate the starting dose in a syringe driver or pump the total oral dose, including any rescue doses, needed in 24 hours should be divided by two (Watson *et al.* 2011) (Table 12.5).

Fentanyl transdermal patches

Transdermal fentanyl causes less constipation, sedation and cognitive impairment than morphine preparations. It is preferred by some patients who dislike oral medication, but may be associated with a higher incidence of nausea and vomiting (Back 2001). Other disadvantages are:

Table 12.4 A guide to medication commonly used in infusion devices in palliative care

Drug and preparation	Type of drug	Usual dose	Indications for use	Potential side effects	Potential adverse reactions	Precautions	Compatible with
Diamorphine 5 mg, 10 mg, 30 mg, 100 mg, 500 mg in powder form, dilute with sterile water for injections	Opioid	5–10 mg/ 24 hours in renal failure; 10 mg/ 24 hours in opioid-naive. No upper limit	Pain, dyspnoea	Nausea, vomiting, anorexia, drowsiness, sedation, constipation, dry mouth. Respiratory depression in large doses	Excess sedation, cognitive dysfunction, confusion, delirium, allodynia, myoclonus	Do not dilute with saline. Increase dose slowly in the elderly. May precipitate with large doses of haloperidol or cyclizine	Haloperidol and cyclizine in usual doses, metoclopramide, midazolam, octreotide, ondansetron, glycopyrronium, levomepromazine
Morphine sulphate 10 mg, 15 mg, 20 mg 30 mg pre-prepared	Opioid	10 mg/ 24 hours in opioid-naive. No upper limit	Pain, dyspnoea	Nausea, vomiting, sedation, anorexia, constipation. Respiratory depression in large doses	Myoclonus	Increase dose slowly in the elderly. May precipitate with large doses of cyclizine	Haloperidol, cyclizine in usual doses, glycopyrronium, levomepromazine
Midazolam (Hypnovel) 10 mg/2 ml	Benzodiazepine	1060 mg/ 24 hours	Muscle stiffness, terminal agitation, intractable hiccups, sedation with amnesia. Drug of choice for convulsions	Sedation. Tolerance, requiring increased dose	Profound sedation		Diamorphine, metoclopramide, levomepromazine, hyoscine butylbromide, dexamethasone, ondansetron
Metoclopramide (Maxolonl) 10 mg/2 ml	Anti-emetic	30–120 mg/ 24 hours	Nausea and vomiting with gastric stasis, partial bowel obstruction	Irritation at injection site	Facial and body spasm	Can crystallise in combination with cyclizine. Discard if it becomes discoloured in the syringe. Do not use in complete bowel obstruction	Diamorphine, levomepromazine, midazolam, dexamethasone, octreotide
Haloperidol (Haldol, Serenace) 5 mg/1 ml	Antipsychotic, anti-emetic	2.5–5 mg/ 24 hours as antiemetic. 10–30 mg for agitation	Nausea and vomiting caused by drugs or hypercalcaemia, intractable hiccups, intestinal obstruction, schizophrenia and other psychoses	Tremor, abnormal face and body movements, restlessness, drowsiness	Hypotension in the elderly		Diamorphine, midazolam, dexamethasone, hyoscine butyl bromide
Cyclizine (Valoid) 50 mg/1 ml	Anti-emetic	100–150 mg/ 24 hours	Nausea and vomiting caused by raised intracranial pressure or bowel obstruction with colic	Irritation at injection site, dry mouth, restlessness, drowsiness	Urinary retention in high doses		Diamorphine, haloperidol, dexamethasone

(Continued)

283

Table 12.4 (Continued)

Drug and preparation	Type of drug	Usual dose	Indications for use	Potential side effects	Potential adverse reactions	Precautions	Compatible with
Ondansetron 4 mg/2 ml, 8 mg/4 ml	Anti-emetic	24–32 mg/ 24 hours	Intractable nausea and vomiting	Constipation, headache, hiccups	Hypersensitivity reactions	Use conventional drugs first, decrease dose in liver disease. Use only when recommended by a palliative care specialist	Diamorphine, metoclopramide, midazolam, glycopyrronium, dexamethasone, octreotide
Levomepromazine (methotrimeprazine Nozinan) 25mg/1ml	Anti-emetic, antipsychotic	6.25–25 mg/ 24 hours as anti-emetic, 25–200 mg/ 24 hours as for agitation	Nausea, vomiting, restlessness confusion, schizophrenia	Drowsiness	Deep sedation in higher doses. In ambulant over-50s, check BP for risk of postural hypotension	Keep drug out of sunlight (may turn purple). Subcutaneous dose is twice as potent as oral dose	Diamorphine, metoclopramide, midazolam
Glycopyrronium (glycopyrrolate Robinul) 200 mcg/1 ml, 600 mcg/3 ml	Antisecretory	600 mcg– 2.4 mg/ 24 hours	Excess secretions in the lungs. Excess secretions in the intestine, associated with bowel colic	Dry mouth, constipation	Urinary retention	Do not combine with dexamethasone	Diamorphine, midazolam, cyclizine, levomepromazine, haloperidol
Hyoscine butylbromide (Buscopan) 20 mg/1 ml	Antispasmodic (relaxes smooth muscle)	60–180 mg/ 24 hours	Bowel obstruction with colic, excess respiratory secretions	Dry mouth, constipation, occasional nausea, vomiting and giddiness. Steatorrhoea	Urinary retention	Do not confuse with hyoscine hydrobromide	Diamorphine, midazolam, metoclopramide, haloperidol, cyclizine, levomepromazine
Octreotide (Sandostatin) 50mcg/1 ml, 100mcg/1 ml, 200 mcg/1 ml	Hormone antagonist	300– 600 mcg/ 24 hours	Large-volume vomiting. Severe diarrhoea to reduce gastro-intestinal secretions	Anorexia, nausea and vomiting, abdominal pain, flatulence, irritation at injection site		Do not combine with cyclizine or dexamethasone	Diamorphine, midazolam, haloperidol, metoclopramide, levomepromazine
Dexamethasone 8 mg/2 ml	Steroid	4–16 mg/ 24 hours	Raised intracranial pressure, nausea, vomiting, dyspnoea (due to tumour-related airways obstruction), pain from nerve compression or hepatomegaly, irritation at injection site	Insomnia, agitation, restlessness, fluid retention, candida. **Prolonged use: facial oedema, mental agitation, diabetes, increased appetite, weight gain, dyspepsia, potential peptic ulceration**	Hypomania, paranoia	Consider using a separate syringe driver/pump as it precipitates with many drugs. Dilute before adding compatible drugs	Diamorphine, metoclopramide, haloperidol, midazolam, octreotide

284

Adapted from Dickman et al. 2005; Twycross et al. 2002; Trotman & Hami 2003; Back 2001; BNF 2009.

Table 12.5 Guide to oral morphine dose equivalents

Drug	Dose	Equivalent 4-hourly oral morphine dose
Codeine	60 mg 4-hourly	7.5 mg
Coproxamol	2 tabs 4-hourly	2.5 mg
Codydramol	2 tabs 4-hourly	2.5 mg
Cocodamol 30/500	2 tabs 4-hourly	7.5–10 mg
Dihydrocodeine	60 mg qds	10 mg
Hydromorphone (palladone)	1.3 mg 4-hourly	10 mg
Hydromorphone (palladone SR)	4 mg bd	10 mg (i.e. 30 mg bd)
Methadone	5 mg (single dose)	7.5 mg
Oxycodone (oxynorm)	5 mg 4- to 6-hourly	10 mg
Oxycodone (oxycontin)	15 mg bd	10 mg (i.e. 30 mg bd)
Tramodol	50 mg qds	10 mg
Fentanyl patch	12 mcg/h	
	25 mcg/h	45–120 mg in 24 hours
	50 mcg/h	120–200 mg in 24 hours
	75 mcg/h	200–300 mg in 24 hours
	100 mcg/h	300–400 mg in 24 hours

NB: After repeated doses of methadone, because of accumulation, doses may appear more potent – seek further information, e.g. from a specialist in palliative care and the Palliative Care Formulary. Adapted from Gibbs 2000.

- its long half-life of 18 hours
- possible increased absorption if the patient is pyrexial or the application site is exposed to external heat (BNF 2011)
- decreased absorption if sweating occurs (Back 2001).

Fentanyl toxicity is subtler than with morphine and may present as:

- vagueness
- drowsiness
- feeling unwell.

(Back 2001)

The patch should be changed every 72 hours (BNF 2011), although 25% of patients have better pain control if they are changed every 48 hours (Back 2001).

If pain control is ineffective the patient may need to be given diamorphine via an infusion device. In this instance it is essential that the specialist palliative care team is contacted for advice about the continued use of the fentanyl patch and to calculate the most appropriate starting dose of diamorphine.

Patients, carers and community nurses should be aware of the risks involved when changing fentanyl patches.

- Discarded patches must always be folded in half to avoid unused medication seeping out.
- They should be disposed of carefully wrapped in the household rubbish or in a sharps box if available.
- Hands should be washed prior to and after application.

Anxiolytics

Patients who are facing death may become anxious and fearful, this may be related to:

- fear of the future
- fear of pain
- anxiety over the separation from loved ones.

As the community nurse usually has more contact with the patient and their family than other health professionals it may be that they are the first person to realise the patient's distress. Symptoms can manifest in a number of ways, for example:

- panic attacks
- poor sleep pattern
- frightening dreams
- worries about being left alone.

If these symptoms are not acknowledged and addressed they can lead to:

- depression
- increased or uncontrolled pain
- the potential for suicide.

(Twycross 1997)

Terminal agitation/acute confusional state

Terminal agitation/acute confusional state is associated with impaired consciousness and myoclonic events

285

(muscle spasms) and is often very distressing for the patient and their family (Dickman *et al.* 2005). If this should occur, the patient will need an urgent reassessment to exclude reversible causes, such as pain, a full bladder or uncomfortable position. If no medical or nursing cause is indicated and the patient's symptoms persist, adding Midazolam to the infusion device medication may reduce these symptoms.

If the patient is delirious haloperidol may need to be considered.

Anti-emetics

The mechanism of nausea and vomiting is complex (Twycross & Wilcock 2001) and it is essential that the community nurse utilises differential diagnosis skills to establish the correct cause.

A full history of the pattern of nausea and vomiting should be taken; this is to establish anticipatory causes and to exclude reversible problems for example:

- constipation
- drug induced
- infection
- dyspepsia
- gastric stasis
- dysuria
- hypercalcaemia (high blood calcium)
- anxiety.

(Twycross & Wilcock 2001)

Prolonged nausea and/or vomiting can be extremely distressing for the patient and will also affect the absorption and efficacy of oral medication being taken. Therefore it may be necessary to add a prescribed anti-emetic to the infusion device medication. For information about individual anti-emetics see Table 12.4.

Drugs used for excess secretions

Respiratory secretions

As the patient's condition deteriorates and periods of consciousness become infrequent, a build-up of fluid may occur in their airway; this is usually due to the patient's inability to cough.

Medication will not dry up secretions already in the lungs (Sykes & Pace 2003), therefore when the noise of excess secretions is heard, the community nurse must act promptly to prevent further secretions entering the lungs and increasing the risk of chest infection.

Glycopyrronium is the suggested drug of choice in the treatment of excessive respiratory secretions because it is three times as potent as hyoscine hydrobromide, which may also cause agitation and a dry mouth (Twycross 1997 cited in Dickman *et al.* 2005; Twycross & Wilcock 2001; BNF 2011)

Intestinal secretions

Octreotide is an anti-secretory drug that reduces production of water and sodium in the intestine and stimulates absorption of water and electrolytes. It is sometimes used in controlling excessive diarrhoea or when large-volume vomiting is a problem (Table 12.4).

Drugs used for intestinal obstruction

A feature of intestinal obstruction is increased gastrointestinal secretions, which can lead to nausea and large-volume vomiting (Dickman *et al.* 2005). Hyoscine butylbromide reduces these secretions and may have an indirect anti-emetic effect (Dickman *et al.* 2005). Hyoscine butylbromide is an effective drug for the relief of colic in intestinal obstruction (partial or complete) and may be most effective when combined with diamorphine, for the continuous element of the pain, and an anti-emetic such as cyclizine (Sykes & Pace 2003) (Table 12.4).

Steroids

Dexamethasone can be an important part of symptom management in patients with raised intracranial pressure caused by brain tumours (Dickman *et al.* 2005). It has a long half-life, so may be given once a day in the morning to prevent insomnia. In its usual dose of 4–16 mg (depending on symptoms) it can be administered via a separate infusion device as it is incompatible with many injectable medications used in palliative care (Dickman *et al.* 2005).

Dexamethasone may also be given as a second line anti-emetic and in large bowel obstruction where there is no contraindication to the use of steroids (Back 2002) (Table 12.4).

Rescue doses of medication

Patients commencing on medication via a syringe driver/pump may not have their symptoms well controlled immediately, therefore it is recommended that rescue medication and its dose, or range of doses, should always be included in the prescription chart.

If the patient is experiencing pain, nausea or agitation, a rescue dose of the relevant prescribed medication may be given at the same time as setting up the infusion device, as it will take some time for the drugs to be absorbed in sufficient quantities to be effective (Trotman & Hami 2003).

Rescue doses may also be given while the infusion device is running if, for example the patient is experiencing:

■ breakthrough pain
■ nausea
■ agitation.

If regular rescue doses are necessary the relevant drug in the infusion can be increased, within the prescribed dose range, at the next syringe change or sooner if symptoms continue to be very poorly controlled.

Rescue doses of diamorphine

A rescue dose of diamorphine is administered once breakthrough pain has started (Davies 2006). The rescue dose of subcutaneous diamorphine is one sixth of the total daily dose, for example, if the 24-hour dose of diamorphine is 60 mg the rescue dose for breakthrough pain would be 10 mg and the effect will last approximately 4 hour (BNF 2011). If this dose of medication is ineffective in relieving pain it may be repeated on the advice of the GP or palliative care team. However, a comprehensive reassessment of the patient's needs should also be carried and consideration given to: (a) increasing the daily subcutaneous dose of diamorphine; (b) commencement of anticipatory non opioid/adjuvant co-therapy (Davies 2006).

There is no maximum dose of diamorphine in palliative care (Trotman & Hami 2003; Dickman *et al.* 2005), but the community nurse must always practise within the limits of the prescribed prescription (NMC 2007) and locally agreed policies, protocols and guidelines.

NB: The boost button on the syringe driver (MS26 only) should not be used at any time to increase medication as it is impossible to calculate with any accuracy the dose given and it will also boost any co-therapy medication in the driver (Trotman & Hami 2003; Dickman *et al.* 2005).

Monitoring

It is not always possible to accurately predict the right dose of drugs needed to control symptoms in patients who are terminally ill, as their medical condition may change quickly, and pain is complex, especially when associated with cancer (Trotman & Hami 2003).

To achieve optimum symptom control the efficacy of the prescribed drug regimen and the patient's condition must be reassessed and documented at each visit to ensure that:

■ symptoms are controlled
■ adverse reactions are identified and promptly treated
■ continuity of care is maintained.

(Mitten 2001)

Discussion with the patient or their relatives is also an essential element of the reassessment as this will:

■ aid the community nurse's decision making about the need for rescue doses of medication
■ inform decision making about the potential need to change the dose or type of drugs in the infusion device.
■ enable the community nurse to update the patient, family or carers and discuss plans for future care and any necessary drug changes.

The following should also be checked/observed and documented.

■ The infusion rate.
■ Measurement of the amount of medication remaining in the syringe (see Graseby syringe driver guideline).
■ Volume remaining (see McKinley T34 syringe pump guideline).
■ Needle/cannula site.
■ Battery level.

Reactions at the infusion site

Many patients experience reactions at the infusion site. These may vary from mild erythema to major inflammation with infection and abscess formation requiring antibiotic therapy or tissue necrosis necessitating the need for specialist practitioner involvement (Trotman & Hami 2003).

Reactions are more likely to occur in patients who:

■ are immunosuppressed
■ have liver or renal failure
■ have severe clotting abnormalities.

(Trotman & Hami 2003)

To minimise the risk of reaction it is recommended that subcutaneous infusion sites are rotated a minimum of every three days, or before if there is pain, erythema or blood at the infusion site (RCN 2003).

If reaction does occur, the community nurse must re-site the infusion and consider the following.

1 Change from a metal needle to a Teflon or Vialon cannula (if appropriate).
2 Dilute the infusion with sterile water for injections using a 20 or 30 ml syringe (Back 2001).
3 Speak to the prescriber to consider changing the medication, especially if those likely to cause reactions are in use. These include less commonly used drugs such as cyclizine, levomepromazine, diclofenac, methadone and ketamine (Trotman & Hami 2003).
4 Seek advice on the use of a low dose corticosteroid such as dexamethasone (Back 2001).
5 Ensure an aseptic technique is used during preparation of medication and connection of the infusion (Trotman & Hami 2003).
6 Ensure the needle or cannula tip is not too shallow (Back 2001).

Ethical issues and consent

The ethics of palliative care are no different from those in all forms of clinical practice, that is:

- to preserve life and relieve suffering
- to respect patient choice (autonomy)
- justice
- non-maleficence
- beneficience.

(Twycross & Wilcock 2001; Beauchamp & Childress 2009)

There is a moral obligation to relieve pain, but also a moral obligation not to cause the patient's death (Randall 2003). When it becomes impossible to preserve life the potential benefits of treatment for the patient balanced against the relief of suffering becomes increasingly important (Twycross 1997; Twycross & Wilcock 2001).

Community nurses are well placed to monitor patients' pain and other symptoms, and the effectiveness of treatment, if an infusion device is in use. Often the community nurse has a unique relationship with the patient and family through their professional caring role at a time when patients are at their most vulnerable and family tensions may become apparent. Continuity of care through the named district nurse and team is invaluable when supporting these patients and their families in the community.

Anecdotal evidence suggests that through this unique professional relationship, the community nurse is often able to affirm to relatives that medication in the infusion device is the equivalent of the drug taken orally, and that the aim of the medication is to control symptoms, and not to lengthen or shorten life.

The aim of palliative care is not to prolong life but to ensure the life that remains is as comfortable and meaningful as possible. Priorities change when the patient is dying, and measures to treat acute problems may contribute to a lingering death and therefore may not be appropriate (Twycross 1997).

If the patient has been assessed as having mental capacity their wishes must be considered of prime importance, so the patient is entitled to give informed consent to treatment or to refuse treatment. Consent must be obtained before treatment or care is given and this includes consent to the use of an infusion device to administer medication (NMC 2008).

It is suggested that two dimensions should be considered when patients are unable to give informed consent or refuse treatment for themselves. These are:

- that relatives know the patient best and are most likely to know their wishes and values
- that healthcare professionals are better placed in knowledge and experience to advise on pain and symptom management (Randall 2003).

However, patients who are confused or have mental health needs can often make rational decisions regarding treatment and may be asked to indicate a preference, having had a simple explanation (Randall 2003) (*see* Chapter 1).

Risk management

The effective use of subcutaneous infusions in any healthcare environment requires the development of policies and procedures that safeguard the patient, practitioner and organisation (Trotman & Hami 2003). The community nurse should consider the manufacturer's instructions for the infusion device they are using, together with local policies and guidelines, to ensure safe practice, prevent errors and encourage practitioners to report incidents without fear of personal reprimand (RCN 2003).

To support this important aspect of risk management community services should have an explicit and clear clinical governance strategy that:

- values practitioner involvement
- clearly identifies lines of accountability and responsibility in reporting procedures
- has transparent investigative procedures for clinical errors and near misses, for example through the use of root cause analysis

288

- closes the loop through the sharing of generalist themes from investigations and provides relevant training and education.

Infusion devices

The use of infusion devices is not without risks to the patient, and nurse errors are common, some of which have resulted in serious harm to patients (MDA 2003).

Between 1990 and 2000, 1495 adverse incidents with all types of infusion pump were reported to the MDA, of these 27% were caused by human error due to:

- inadequate training of relevant staff
- inappropriate local modifications and adjustments to the devices
- poor equipment storage environment
- insufficient servicing and maintenance of equipment (MDA 2003).

In 2003 the MDA also made the following recommendations.

- The introduction of national operational and training standards for users.
- Clearly defined structures for the management of infusion devices (MDA 2003).

The implications of these recommendations for community services suggest that their responsibilities should include:

- the effective use of resources
- establishing transparent lines of responsibility for staff
- the appointment of a medical devices co-ordinator.

It is also strongly recommended that the medical devices co-ordinator should take responsibility for:

- selection and procurement
- development of a unit policy to determine appropriate use, set standards and audit
- risk assessment
- installation and commissioning.
- maintenance
- staff training, assessment and updating
- operational documentation
- development of policies that identify spare infusion devices, control lending out and facilitate recovery of devices both from hospital departments and the community
- ensuring that safety warnings have been acted upon.

(MDA, 2003, p. 10).

In smaller institutions these facilities may not be available on site. In such cases, arrangements should be put in place through a service level agreement (SLA) with a local medical physics department, manufacturer or supplier (MDA 2003).

From January 2005 to June 2010 the NPSA received 175 reports involving ambulatory syringe drivers, eight of which resulted in fatality from over-infusion (NPSA 2010). This has resulted in recommendations regarding the discontinuation of using existing ambulatory syringe drivers that require infusion rates to be set manually beyond December 2011; and the transition to ambulatory devices with additional safety features (NPSA 2010).

Safety checks prior to use

To ensure correct functioning of the infusion device the community nurse must check the following prior to use with each patient.

- All external parts are undamaged.
- There is documentary evidence that cleaning has taken place in accordance with the manufacturer's instructions.
- There is an up-to-date service history for the specific device and that this is in accordance with the manufacturer's instructions and local policy.
- Always ensure that the syringe driver/pump actuator is positioned correctly and is secure (Figure 12.5) (MDA 2003).

Any malfunctioning of the syringe driver should be reported to the manufacturer and MHRA as soon as possible.

Recommendations for the use of syringes in infusion devices

- Always use the type and brand of syringe recommended by the manufacturer and ensure it is sterile prior to use.
- Always check that the plunger is undamaged and runs smoothly prior to drug preparation.
- Never use a defective syringe.
- Remember to prime the set before attaching the infusion to the patient.

Never place tape on the syringe barrel where the securing strap is positioned, as this will obscure the view of the fluid in the syringe. This is important when measuring the amount of fluid left in the syringe to check if the syringe driver is running to time.

When using a syringe driver to prevent free-flow of the infusion the following precautions should also be taken.

289

- Syringe barrel and plunger must be secured correctly.
- Syringe and administration set must be intact and correctly connected.
- The syringe driver must be positioned as closely to the height of the infusion site as possible (MDA 2003).

General suggestions to ensure safe use of syringe drivers
- Check the battery daily when in use by ensuring the light is flashing.
- Avoid the use of mobile phones within 1 metre of the syringe driver to avoid risk of interference.
- Keep the syringe driver dry.
- Do not move a syringe driver from a hot, humid place to a much cooler one or vice versa as performance may be affected.
- Treat with care; wipe with detergent and water at the end of use. Do not immerse in water. Avoid spirits and solvents for cleaning, as the plastic case may become damaged.
- Don't use a syringe driver near strong magnetic fields or it may stop working (see note below).
- Send for annual servicing to a qualified technician (adapted from Graseby 2002).

NB: If the patient is attending the outpatient department, the community nurse should seek advice from the hospital staff regarding the proximity of strong magnetic fields, e.g. MRI scanner, as this may cause malfunction of a syringe driver. If the patient is attending the hospital for an MRI scan, advice should be sought from the palliative care team or GP, as an alternative source of symptom management may be necessary. The community nurse should liaise with the relevant hospital personnel prior to the appointment to ensure they are aware of any actual or potential needs the patient may have. To avoid any complications for the patient and hospital staff, the community nurse patient visit on the day of the hospital appointment should be at a time that will ensure that medication will not need to be renewed during attendance at the appointment.

Reporting adverse incidents

'An adverse incident is any event which gives rise to, or has the potential to produce, unexpected or unwanted side effects involving the safety of patients, users or other persons' (MDA 2003, p. 39).

Adverse incidents may be caused by:

- incorrect prescription
- inadequate instructions for use
- problems with the device itself
- poor servicing and maintenance of the device
- inadequate training
- user errors
- locally initiated adjustments or modifications to the device
- wrong storage environment
- inappropriate management procedures; for example, poor quality syringe selection.

(MDA 2003)

It is the responsibility of the individual community nurse to report adverse incidents to their line manager and medical devices coordinator according to local policies. In accordance with clinical governance guidelines all Trusts should have reporting procedures in place so that significant events can be analysed. Where appropriate, lessons learnt from mistakes and near misses should be implemented through changes in practice, policy or guideline. The Medicines and Healthcare products Regulatory Agency (MHRA) should be informed promptly by telephone, followed up by a written report as soon as possible. Information on serious incidents should be reported as quickly as possible, preferably transmitted via the MHRA's website by email or by fax. For details see useful contacts at the end of the chapter.

When reporting an adverse incident involving an infusion device the community nurse should include the following information.

- The make and model and serial number of the device.
- Brand, size and lot number of the infusion set.
- Brand and size of syringe used.
- The prescribed infusion time and set/infusion rate and the rate it was set at when the incident was discovered/reported.
- The prescribed drugs being used, including dose and expiry date.
- The date and time of the last medication renewal and the amount of fluid left in the syringe when the incident was discovered/reported.
- Other details in connection with the incident, e.g. date, time and names of staff discovering and reporting the incident; the condition and position of the device in relation to the infusion site.
- The consequences of the error for the patient.

■ The immediate nursing action taken by staff discovering the error.

(MDA 2003)

Conclusion

Although the potential difficulties that can arise as a result of using an infusion device may seem daunting to the inexperienced community nurse, with a satisfactory level of training and support, the problems encountered should be minimal. However, keeping up to date and achieving and maintaining competency in the use of the devices may be difficult in the community, as this will depend on the caseload profile and patient needs.

As part of the primary healthcare team, GPs and community nurses are often at the forefront of palliative care. They work in partnership to provide a service that hopes to maintain good symptom control, with input from community nurse specialists, nurse consultants, and hospital and/or hospice palliative care teams. If an infusion device is in use, then daily community nurse visits to change the syringe mean that close links can be forged with both the patient and family.

At this time more than any other, partnership with the patient, family and caregivers is essential to ensure that the patient can live as fully and comfortably as possible. A contented family increases the likelihood of a contented patient (Twycross 1997), and community nurses are well placed to offer appropriate support to the family.

For those patients whose preferred place of death is in their own home, even though symptoms may be severe, the effective use of an infusion device to assist in the control of pain, nausea, vomiting and other potentially distressing symptoms can help them achieve this goal.

Useful contacts

Agenda for change
Website: http://webarchive.nationalarchives.gov.uk/+/
  www.dh.gov.uk/en/Managingyourorganisation/Workforce/
  Paypensionsandbenefits/Agendaforchange/index.htm

Graseby Medical
Colonial Way
Watford
Herts WD24 4LG
Tel: 01923 246434
Fax: 01923 231595
Website: www.graseby.co.uk/index2.php

Medical Devices Agency (MHRA)
151 Buckingham Palace Road
London SW1W 9SZ
Tel: (weekdays 9:00–17:00): 020 3080 6000
Fax: 0203 118 9803
Email: info@mhra.gsi.gov.uk
Website: www.mhra.gov.uk

National Patient Safety Agency (NPSA)
4–8 Maple Street
London W1T 5HT
Tel: 020 927 9500
Fax: 020 7927 9501
Website: www.npsa.nhs.uk

Royal College of Nursing
20 Cavendish Square
London W1G 0RN
Tel: 020 7409 3333
Website: www.rcn.org.uk

Procedure guideline 12.1 **Subcutaneous drug administration via a syringe driver (Graseby MS16A/MS26)**

Identify the make and model of syringe driver you will be using.

For example, the Graseby MS16A is the HOURLY rate model with the rate in mm per hour and has a BLUE label.
The Graseby MS26 is the DAILY rate model with the rate in mm per day and has a GREEN label.

Equipment

Patient prescription, completed and signed by a doctor
Nursing documentation
Drugs and diluent
Luer lock syringe; size to accommodate amount of medication
1 ml syringe if small amount of drug is required (i.e. haloperidol 5 mg/ml if the dose is less than 5 mg)
Needle to draw up drugs
Winged infusion set or Teflon or Vialon cannula and fine bore infusion set
Drug additive label
Syringe driver
9V alkaline battery
Alcohol swab (for skin preparation; RCN 2003)
Transparent film dressing
Sharps bin
A clean surface to work from such as a coffee table, covered for protection.

Nursing action	Rationale
1 Where appropriate facilities are available wash your hands or alternatively cleanse with 70% alcohol based handrub (in accordance with local policy)	To prevent the risk of cross-infection/contamination
2 If the patient is known to the service, review nursing documentation and current care plan	To update the nurses knowledge of the patient To maintain patient safety
3 If the patient is unknown to the service a comprehensive assessment must be carried out prior to undertaking the procedure. This must include the identification of known allergies	To identify potential contraindications and/or cautions To maintain patient safety
4 Explain and discuss the procedure with the patient	To ensure that the patient understands the procedure and gives his/her valid consent

5 Check the following information on the patients prescription:
 	
  a. patient's name
 	
  b. prescription is legible, valid and signed by GP or relevant medical practitioner
 	
  c. drug/s to be administered
 	
  d. drug/s strength and dose to be administered
 	
  e. drug/s have not passed their expiry date
 	
  f. diluent and expiry date
 	
  g. route of administration
 	
  h. date and time of administration
 	
  i. time of last administration
	To ensure that the patient receives the correct prescribed drug/s and dose via the correct route safely
	
	To comply with NMC standards for the administration of medicines

Nursing action	Rationale
6 Check present symptoms and contact hospice staff or GP if necessary	To obtain expert advice in specific situations
7 Prepare the environment	To maintain patient privacy
8 Assemble and prepare all equipment on a clean surface; check that: (a) all relevant seals and packaging are intact and undamaged; (b) all relevant equipment is within the recommended date for use; (c) check that the syringe plunger runs smoothly	To prevent disruption to the procedure To prevent contamination of equipment To maintain patient safety
9 Calculate prescribed drug dose plus diluent	To ensure selection of correct syringe size (which must be 5–30 ml) (Graseby 2002)
10 Where appropriate facilities are available, wash your hands or alternatively cleanse with 70% alcohol based handrub (in accordance with local policy)	To prevent the risk of cross-infection/contamination
11 Draw up medication and enough diluent to ensure the volume is correct, measuring the 'stroke length' in mm on the syringe driver body against the syringe	To ensure correct dilution of drugs and correct volume To maintain patient safety
12 Discard used ampoules/vials and used needles in sharps box	To maintain patient and nurse safety To reduce the risk of needlestick injury
13 Once drawn up make a visual inspection of the fluid in the syringe. Observe for, e.g. cloudiness, particles or any discoloration **NB: If this occurs discard contents and prepare a fresh syringe**	To maintain patient safety To identify potential drug incompatibility
14 Complete and stick the drug additive label to the syringe in accordance with local policy/guidelines. Do not obscure syringe markings	To maintain patient safety To enable other visiting nursing staff to identify: (a) the contents of the syringe; (b) which nurse prepared the drug/s; (c) the time the infusion commenced To enable the amount of fluid remaining in the syringe to be observed at each visit
15 Connect the syringe to the infusion set with a twisting action	To ensure secure connection
16 Gently depress the plunger of the syringe until fluid appears at the tip of the needle/cannula	To prime the infusion set To displace air with fluid To maintain patient safety To ensure that the patient receives the correct drug dose immediately
NB: When the syringe driver is first set up or a new infusion set used, the earlier the infusion will finish. This has implications for the timing of the next community nurse visit to renew medication in the syringe	Delivery time will be reduced as a result of priming the infusion set
17 Set the correct rate setting for the driver as follows	To ensure the infusion is delivered at the correct rate To maintain patient safety

(Continued)

Nursing action	Rationale
18 Setting the correct rate for the Graseby MS16A over 24 hours	
(a) Measure the volume of the fluid to be infused in mm, that is, the stroke length (multiples of 24 are easiest to calculate)	To calculate the set rate
(b) Check the delivery time in hours	To ensure medication is given in the prescribed time
(c) Calculate the rate setting by dividing stroke length in mm by delivery time in hours	To set the correct rate, i.e. 48 mm divided by 24 hours = set rate of 2 mm per hour
(d) Check and if necessary, adjust the set rate on the syringe driver prior to commencing the infusion (see Figure 12.2)	To ensure that the correct dose of drug(s) is infused at the correct rate To ensure patient safety.
19 Setting the correct rate for the Graseby MS26 over 24 hours	
(a) Measure the volume of fluid to be infused in mm, that is, the stroke length	To calculate the set rate
(b) Check delivery time in days	To ensure medication is given in the prescribed time
(c) Calculate the rate setting by dividing the stroke length in mm by the delivery time in days	To ensure accurate administration i.e. 48 mm divided by 1 day = set rate of 48
(d) Check and, if necessary, adjust the set rate on the syringe driver prior to commencing the infusion (see Figure 12.3)	To ensure the correct dose of drug(s) is infused at the correct rate To ensure patient safety
20 Where appropriate facilities are available wash your hands or alternatively cleanse with 70% alcohol based handrub (in accordance with local policy)	To prevent the risk of cross-infection/contamination
21 Apply disposable plastic apron	To prevent the risk of cross-infection/contamination
22 Assist the patient into a comfortable position	To allow easy access to the relevant area To maintain the patient's dignity and comfort
23 Where indicated offer the patient assistance with removing relevant clothing	To expose the appropriate area
24 Remove and dispose of apron in accordance with health and safety regulations and local policy	To prevent the risk of cross-infection
25 Where appropriate facilities are available wash your hands or alternatively cleanse with 70% alcohol based handrub (in accordance with local policy)	To prevent the risk of cross-infection/contamination
26 Select and clean appropriate infusion site with the alcohol saturated swab and allow the area to air dry	To prepare the skin To maximise absorption rate To reduce the risk of infection To prevent stinging on needle/cannula insertion
27 Grasp a fold of skin firmly	To lift subcutaneous tissue
28 Insert the needle at an angle of 45 degrees with the bevel pointing down. When using a cannula remove the stylet place in sharps bin and attach infusion set	To aid absorption of drugs To prevent needlestick injury
29 Loop the infusion line around the site and secure it in place with a clear adhesive dressing	To prevent pulling and displacement of needle/cannula To allow freedom of movement and inspection of the site

Nursing action	Rationale
30 Connect the syringe to the driver by positioning the syringe along the top of the syringe driver, with the finger grips secured in the pump body recess (Figure 12.5)	To place the syringe correctly To secure the syringe and ensure correct functioning
31 Secure the syringe in place with the rubber securing strap (Figures 12.2 & 12.3)	To hold the syringe barrel tightly
32 Gently move the actuator assembly carefully along the lead screw by pressing the white button until it is firmly against the plunger (Figure 12.5) then release the button	To ensure the pump action can start immediately
NB: The plunger must not be pushed forward	**To maintain safety by ensuring that the patient does not receive a bolus dose of medication prior to commencement of the infusion**
33 Insert the battery. The alarm will sound on both models. Press and immediately release the start button (see Figures 12.2 & 12.3)	To test the syringe driver and begin the infusion To start the driver and stop the alarm, both models
Check that the indicator light is flashing both models	To ensure that the syringe driver is functioning correctly
34 Place the syringe driver in the plastic cover and place it at same height as the infusion site	For protection To prevent increased or decreased infusion rate
35 Cleanse hands with bactericidal alcohol hand rub	To reduce the risk of cross-infection
36 Apply disposable plastic apron	To prevent the risk of cross-infection/contamination
37 Assist the patient to dress and help into their chosen position	To maintain patient's dignity and comfort
38 Dispose of all used equipment in accordance with locally agreed infection prevention and control policy	To reduce the risk of cross-infection To maintain the health and safety of self and others
39 Remove and dispose of apron in accordance with health and safety regulations and local policy	To prevent the risk of cross-infection
40 Where appropriate facilities are available wash your hands or alternatively cleanse with 70% alcohol based handrub (in accordance with local policy)	To prevent the risk of cross-infection/contamination
41 Verbally discuss the procedure with the patient and, where relevant, the carer, giving further advice and information as indicated, e.g. explain how to monitor the syringe driver	To support the patient's understanding. To reduce anxiety To increase confidence in managing the syringe driver
42 Give contact telephone numbers for the day, evening and night community nursing service, the hospice and or palliative care team	To maintain patient safety To ensure prompt response to problems or difficulties if they arise To reduce patient/carer concerns
43 Complete all nursing documentation in accordance with locally agreed policy and NMC guidelines. This should include, e.g. drug/s name, batch number, dose, diluents, expiry dates, time infusion commenced, specific patient needs identified	To maintain patient safety To enable continuity of care To maintain practitioner safety Documentation should provide clear evidence of the care or procedure carried out

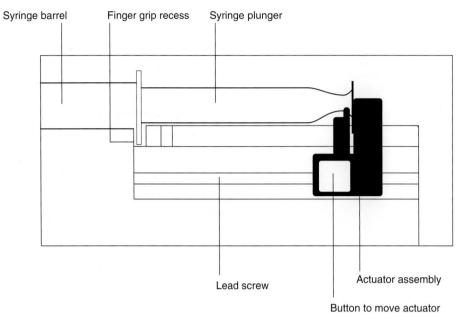

Syringe barrel   Finger grip recess   Syringe plunger

Lead screw

Actuator assembly

Button to move actuator

Figure 12.5 Graseby syringe driver – rear view.

Procedure guideline 12.2 **Subcutaneous drug administration via a McKinley T34 syringe pump**

Equipment

Patient prescription/authorisation chart, completed and signed by a doctor
Nursing documentation
McKinley syringe pump with lockable plastic box
Key for lock box
9V alkaline battery
Drugs and diluent
Luer lock syringe; size to accommodate amount of medication
Needle to draw up drugs
Winged infusion set or Teflon or Vialon cannula and fine bore infusion line
Drug additive label
Alcohol swab (for skin preparation; RCN 2003)
Transparent film dressing
Sharps bin
A clean surface to work from such as a coffee table, covered for protection.

Procedure guideline 12.2 **Subcutaneous drug administration via a McKinley T34 syringe pump** *(cont'd)*

Nursing action	Rationale
1 Where appropriate facilities are available wash your hands or alternatively cleanse with 70% alcohol based handrub (in accordance with local policy)	To prevent the risk of cross-infection/contamination
2 If the patient is known to the service, review nursing documentation and current care plan	To update the nurses knowledge of the patient To maintain patient safety
3 If the patient is unknown to the service a comprehensive assessment must be carried out prior to undertaking the procedure. This must include the identification of known allergies.	To identify potential contraindications and or cautions To maintain patient safety
4 Explain and discuss the procedure with the patient	To ensure that the patient understands the procedure and gives his/her valid consent
5 Check the following information on the patient's prescription: a. Patient's name b. Prescription is legible, valid and signed by GP or relevant medical practitioner c. Drug/s to be administered d. Drug/s strength and dose to be administered e. Drug/s have not passed their expiry date f. Diluent and expiry date g. Route of administration h. Date and time of administration i. Time of last administration	To ensure that the patient receives the correct prescribed drug/s and dose via the correct route safely To comply with NMC standards for the administration of medicines
6 Check present symptoms and contact hospice staff or GP if necessary	To obtain expert advice in specific situations
7 Prepare the environment	To maintain patient privacy
8 Assemble and prepare all equipment on a clean surface; check that: (a) all relevant seals and packaging are intact and undamaged; (b) all relevant equipment is within the recommended date for use; (c) check that the syringe plunger runs smoothly	To prevent disruption to the procedure To prevent contamination of equipment To maintain patient safety
9 Calculate prescribed drug dose plus diluent to total volume (see Table 12.3)	To ensure correct syringe size selection To maintain patient safety
10 Where appropriate facilities are available wash your hands or alternatively cleanse with 70% alcohol based handrub (in accordance with local policy)	To prevent the risk of cross-infection/contamination
11 Draw up drug/s plus diluent to total volume (see Table 12.3)	To prepare drug/s correctly and ensure accuracy To maintain patient safety

(Continued)

*Procedure guideline 12.2 **Subcutaneous drug administration via a McKinley T34 syringe pump** (cont'd)*

Nursing action	Rationale
12 Discard used ampoules/vials and used needles in sharps box	To maintain patient and nurse safety To reduce the risk of needlestick injury
13 Once drawn up make a visual inspection of the fluid in the syringe. Observe for, e.g. cloudiness, particles or any discoloration. **NB: If this occurs discard contents and prepare a fresh syringe.**	To maintain patient safety To identify potential drug incompatibility
14 Complete and stick the drug additive label to the syringe in accordance with local policy/guidelines. Do not obscure syringe markings	To maintain patient safety To enable other visiting nursing staff to identify: (a) the contents of the syringe; (b) which nurse prepared the drug/s; (c) the time the infusion commenced To enable the amount of fluid remaining in the syringe to be observed at each visit
15 Calculate the correct rate setting for the pump	To ensure the infusion is delivered at the correct rate To maintain patient safety
16 Where appropriate facilities are available wash your hands or alternatively cleanse with 70% alcohol based handrub (in accordance with local policy)	To prevent the risk of cross-infection/contamination
17 Connect the syringe to the infusion set with a twisting action	To ensure secure connection
18 Gently depress the plunger of the syringe until fluid appears at the tip of the needle/cannula	To prime the infusion set To displace air with fluid To maintain patient safety To ensure that the patient receives the correct drug dose immediately
NB: When the pump is first set up or a new infusion set used the earlier the infusion will finish. This has implications for the timing of the next community nurse visit to renew medication in the syringe	Delivery time will be reduced as a result of priming the infusion set
19 Apply disposable plastic apron	To prevent the risk of cross-infection/contamination
20 Assist the patient into a comfortable position	To allow easy access to the relevant area To maintain the patient's dignity and comfort
21 Where indicated offer the patient assistance with removing relevant clothing	To expose the appropriate area
22 Remove and dispose of apron in accordance with health and safety regulations and local policy	To prevent the risk of cross-infection
23 Where appropriate facilities are available wash your hands or alternatively cleanse with 70% alcohol based handrub (in accordance with local policy)	To prevent the risk of cross-infection/contamination

Procedure guideline 12.2 **Subcutaneous drug administration via a McKinley T34 syringe pump** *(cont'd)*

Nursing action	Rationale
24 Select and clean appropriate infusion site with the alcohol saturated swab and allow the area to air dry	To prepare the skin
	To maximise absorption rate
	To reduce the risk of infection
	To prevent stinging on needle/cannula insertion
25 Grasp a fold of skin firmly	To lift subcutaneous tissue
26 Insert the needle at an angle of 45 degrees with the bevel pointing down. When using a cannula remove the stylet and attach infusion set	To aid absorption of drugs
27 Loop the infusion line around the site and secure it in place with a clear adhesive dressing	To prevent pulling and displacement of needle/cannula
	To allow freedom of movement and inspection of the site
28 Adjust the pump actuator to the correct syringe length by pressing the **<< FF or >> back button, the barrel clamp arm must be in the down position with no syringe loaded**	To prepare for loading of the syringe
29 Lift the barrel clamp arm of the pump and load the syringe in a position that stops the collar, barrel and plunger sensors flashing	To ensure correct positioning of the syringe
30 When syringe brand and size is correctly confirmed by the pump press the **Yes key** **NB: If the pump detects the incorrect syringe size remove the pump from use and send for servicing** (McKinley)	To ensure correct pump operation
	To maintain patient safety
31 Set a new programme for each medication renewal	To ensure the correct infusion rate is set
	To maintain patient safety by reducing the risk of error
32 Confirm volume and duration on pump display is correct and press yes	To start infusion
33 Press and hold the 'info' key. LED screen displays 'keypad lock' and pump bleeps to confirm the lock is on	To lock the key pad
	To prevent accidental over infusion
	To maintain patient safety
34 Place the pump in the lock box	To maintain patient safety
	To aid protection of the pump
35 Cleanse hands with bactericidal alcohol hand rub	To reduce the risk of cross-infection
36 Assist the patient to dress and help into their chosen position.	To maintain patient's dignity and comfort
37 Dispose of all used equipment in accordance with locally agreed infection prevention and control policy	To reduce the risk of cross-infection
	To maintain the health and safety of self and others

(Continued)

Procedure guideline 12.2 **Subcutaneous drug administration via a McKinley T34 syringe pump** *(cont'd)*

Nursing action	Rationale
38 Where appropriate facilities are available wash your hands or alternatively cleanse with 70% alcohol based handrub (in accordance with local policy)	To prevent the risk of cross-infection/contamination
39 Verbally discuss the procedure with the patient and, where relevant, the carer, giving further advice and information as indicated, e.g. explain how to monitor the syringe pump	To support the patient's understanding To reduce anxiety To increase confidence in managing the syringe pump
40 Give contact telephone numbers for the day, evening and night community nursing service, the hospice and/or palliative care team	To maintain patient safety To ensure prompt response to problems or difficulties if they arise To reduce patient/carer concerns
41 Complete all nursing documentation in accordance with locally agreed policy and NMC guidelines. This should include, e.g. drug/s name, batch number, dose, diluents, expiry dates, time infusion commenced, specific patient needs identified	To maintain patient safety To enable continuity of care To maintain practitioner safety Documentation should provide clear evidence of the care or procedure carried out

Procedure guideline 12.3 **Best practice for observation of the syringe driver during infusion**

Nursing action	Rationale
1 Observe and monitor infusion site for erythema and swelling at each visit	Inflammation slows the absorption rate of medication and can be painful for the patient
2 Check the set rate is correct and corresponds to documentation	To reduce the risk of error and ensure patient safety
3 Use a ruler to measure the amount of medication left in the syringe at each visit and record in the nursing documentation	To maintain patient safety by ensuring the infusion is running to time
4 Check that the syringe is secured in the driver at each visit	To prevent accidental disconnection
5 Monitor symptom control at each visit	To promote patient comfort by assessing the need for rescue doses of medication or an increase in medication in the syringe driver
6 Document findings	To enable comparison of symptoms at the next community nurse visit To maintain patient and staff safety

Problem solving table 12.1 Syringe driver

Problem	Possible cause	Action
Damage to the syringe driver	Through dropping, getting wet or other accidents	Take out of use; must be serviced and checked by a qualified technician
		Ensure relevant documentation is completed
Syringe driver will not start	Battery has run out	Fit new battery
	Start button insufficiently depressed	Press start button again
		Document in patient's nursing records
	Syringe driver faulty	Take out of service, return to manufacturer. Complete relevant documentation
Infusion has finished early	Insufficient fluid in syringe	Prepare a new syringe. Inform patient, GP, hospice and line manager. Complete incident form according to local trust policy and complete patient's nursing documentation
	Wrong alignment of syringe in driver	Ensure finger grip of syringe is in the recess of the syringe driver body and the actuator is firmly against the end of the plunger. Complete all relevant documentation
	Incorrect set rate	Correct error, document in patient records, inform patient and GP. Report to manager and MDA. Complete incident form and reporting procedures according to trust policy
	Priming the line	Plan to visit before 24 hours. A fine bore infusion line 1 m long holds approximately 1 ml of fluid. If the syringe is filled to 8 ml, the infusion will finish approximately 3 h early
Infusion too slow	Incorrect set rate	Rectify error and document in patient records. Inform patient and GP. Report to manager. Complete incident form and reporting procedures according to trust policy
	Inflammation at infusion site.	Remove infusion line and re-site: consider allergy to metal; try Teflon cannula. Consider reaction to drugs. Document in patient's nursing record
	Occlusion in line	Check line for kinks; monitor for signs of crystalisation in line or syringe, report to hospice/ GP and prepare and connect new syringe if indicated. Document problem in the patient's nursing record
Syringe driver has stopped before contents have been discharged	Battery is flat	Fit new battery
	Blocked infusion line	Fit new line. Re-prime the line and ensure visit time is adjusted as the infusion will finish earlier than planned. Document in the patient's nursing record
The syringe driver has stopped, but its light is still flashing	The mechanism for pushing the plunger has worn out. Listen for a faint click when the motor turns a few times (Graseby models)	Stop the infusion and replace the syringe driver. Send faulty syringe driver for servicing. Document in the patient's nursing record
Alarm does not sound when battery inserted	Battery put in the wrong way	Insert the battery the right way round
	Defective syringe driver	Take out of use and send for servicing. Document in the patient's nursing record and in records at the hospice/ community nurse base
Alarm is sounding and does not stop after 15 s		NB: Do not use the syringe driver if the motor does not stop or the alarm does not sound
Cloudy fluid in syringe or presence of crystals in syringe	Incompatible medication, concentration of medication too high	Discard syringe, draw up medication with more diluent and use a larger syringe. If the same occurs, discard syringe and contact the prescriber
		Document in patient records

The Medical Devices Agency (MDA) and the Medicines Control Agency (MCA) merged to form the Medicines and Healthcare products Regulatory Agency (MHRA) in April 2003.
Adapted from Graseby 2002.

References and further reading

Back I (2001) *Palliative Medicine Handbook* (3e). BPM books, Cardiff.

Barclay S, Todd C, Grande G, Lipscombe J (2002) Controlling cancer pain in primary care: the prescribing habits and knowledge base of general practitioners. *Journal of Pain and Symptom Management* 23(5): 383–92.

Beauchamp T, Childress J (2009) *Principles of Biomedical Ethics* (5e). Oxford University Press, New York.

British National Formulary 61 (2011) British Medical Association & Royal Pharmaceutical Society of Great Britain, London.

Dawkins L, Britton D, Johnson I, Higgins B, Dean T (2000) A randomised trial of winged vialon cannulae and metal butterfly needles. *International Journal of Palliative Nursing* 6(3): 110–16.

Davies A (2006) *Cancer Related Breakthrough Pain*. Oxford Pain Management Library (OPML) Oxford University Press, Oxford.

Department of Health (2008) *End of Life Care Strategy: promoting high quality care for all adults at the end of life*. Department of Health, London.

Department of Health (2005) *The Mental Capacity Act: Code of Practice, April (2007)*. The Stationery Office, London.

Dickman A (2010) *Drugs in Palliative Care*. Oxford University Press, Oxford.

Dickman A, Scheider J, Varga J (2005) *The Syringe Driver*. Oxford University Press, Oxford.

Dougherty L, Lister S (eds) (2011) *The Royal Marsden Hospital Manual of Clinical Nursing Procedures* (8e). Wiley-Blackwell, Oxford.

Field D, Clark D, Corner J, Davis C (eds) (2000) *Researching Palliative Care*. Open University Press, Milton Keynes.

Gibbs M (2000) *Guide to Dose Equivalents to Oral Morphine*. St Christopher's Hospice, Sydenham, London.

Graseby Medical Ltd (2002) *MS 16A Syringe Driver, MS 26 Syringe Driver Instruction Manual*. Graseby Medical Ltd, Watford.

Graseby Medical Ltd (1998) *Graseby MS26 & MS16A Syringe Driver Competency Checklist*. Graseby Medical Ltd, Watford.

Hanks G, Christakis NA, Fallon M, Kassa S, Portenoy RK (2009) *Oxford Textbook of Palliative Care Medicine* (4e). Oxford University Press, Oxford.

Kaye P (1994) *A to Z of Hospice and Palliative Medicine*. EPL Publications, Northampton.

Lucas C (1998) *Palliative Care*. Vade Mecum. Princess Alice Hospice, Surrey.

Mahmood-Yousuf K, Munday D, King N, Dale J (2008) Interprofessional relationships and communication in primary palliative care: impact of the Gold Standards Framework. *British Journal of General Practice* 58(549): 256–63.

Mallet J, Dougherty L (2000) *The Royal Marsden Manual of Clinical Nursing Procedures*. Blackwell Science, Oxford.

McCormack P, Cooper R, Sutherland S, Stewart H (2001) The safe use of syringe drivers for palliative care: an action research project. *International Journal of Palliative Nursing* 7(12): 574–80.

McKinley Medical. *McKinley T34 syringe pump: User pocket reference guide*.

Medical Devices Agency (2003) *Device Bulletin. Infusion Systems*. Department of Health, London.

Medicines & Healthcare Products Regulatory Agency (2003) *Evaluation 03117 Micrel Medical Devices*. MHRA, London.

Mitten T (2001) Subcutaneous drug infusions: a review of problems and solutions. *International Journal of Palliative Care Nursing* 7(2): 75–85.

Morgan S, Evans N (2004) A small observational study of the longevity of syringe driver sites in palliative care. *International Journal of Palliative Nursing* 10(8): 405–13.

NHS Cancer Plan (2000) *A Plan for Investment: a Plan for Reform*. Department of Health, London.

National Institute of Clinical Excellence (2003) *Infection Control: prevention for healthcare-associated infection in primary and community care* (Clinical Guidelines 2). NICE, London.

National Midwifery Council (2008) *The Code, Standards of Conduct, Performance and Ethics for Nurses and Midwives*. NMC, London.

National Midwifery Council (2007) *Standards for Medicines Management*. NMC, London.

National Patient Safety Agency (2010) *Rapid Response Report NPSA/2010/RRR019, Gateway ref 14877*. NPSA, London.

Perdue C (2004) The syringe driver – an aid to delivering symptom control. *Nursing Times* 100(13): 32–5.

Quinn C (2002) Infusion devices: risks, functions and management. *Nursing Standard* 14(26): 35–41.

Randall F (2003). In: Sykes N, Fallon M, Patt R (eds) *Clinical Pain Management. Cancer Pain*. Arnold, London.

Randall F, Downie RS (1999) *Palliative Care Ethics* (2e). Oxford University Press, Oxford.

Reymond L, Charles M, Bowman J, Treston P (2003) The effects of dexamethasone on the longevity of syringe driver subcutaneous sites in palliative care patients. *The Medical Journal of Australia* 178: 486–9; www.mja.com.au

Ross J, Saunders Y, Cochrane M, Zepetella G (2002) A prospective, within-patient comparison between metal butterfly needles and Teflon cannulae in subcutaneous infusion of drugs to terminally ill hospice patients. *Palliative Medicine* 16: 13–16.

Royal College of Nursing (2004) *Agenda for Change: Knowledge & Skills Framework*. Nursing Standard Essential Guide 19(12). RCN, London.

Royal College of Nursing (2003) *Standards for Infusion Therapy*. RCN, London.

St Christopher's Hospice (2001) *Minimum Data Sets: National Survey 1999–2000*. St Christopher's Hospice, London.

Sutton and Merton Community Services (2009) *McKinley T34 Syringe Pump Management: guidelines and procedures*. Sutton and Merton Community Services, London.

Sykes N, Pace V (2003) In: Sykes N, Fallon MT, Patt R (eds) *Clinical Pain Management. Cancer Pain*. Arnold, London.

Trotman I, Hami F (2003) In: Breivik H, Campbell W, Eccleston C (eds) *Clinical Pain Management. Practical Applications and Procedures*. Arnold, London.

Twycross, R., (1997) *Introducing Palliative Care*. 4th edition, Radcliffe publishing Ltd, Oxford.

Twycross R, Wilcock A, Charlesworth S, Dickman A (2002) *Palliative Care Formulary*. Radcliffe Medical Press, Oxford.

Twycross R, Wilcock A (2001) *Symptom Management in Advanced Cancer* (3e). Radcliffe Medical Press, Oxford.

Watson M, Lucas C, Hoy A, Black I, Armstrong P (2011) *Palliative Adult Network Guidelines (3e)*. Available on line from www.despatch365.com/palliative

Watson M, Lucas C, Hoy A, Wells J (2009) *The Oxford Textbook of Palliative Care* (2e). Oxford University Press, Oxford.

13

Urinary catheterisation and management

Introduction

Urethral catheters are designed for insertion into the urinary bladder to allow drainage of urine, removal of clots, debris or mucus, or for the instillation of medication (Pomfret 2000a).

Background evidence

The cost of supporting a patient with a long-term urinary catheter in the community for a three-month period is estimated at £2585, a large proportion of this cost arising from the time provided by community nurses (O'Donohue *et al.* 2010).

Urethral and suprapubic urinary catheterisation is commonly performed by community nurses and is carried out for a number of clinical needs, for example:

- to bypass an obstruction, e.g. an enlarged prostate or urethral stricture
- to relieve retention of urine for patients with neurological or spinal injury
- to determine residual urine volumes
- to measure urine output
- acute or chronic urinary retention
- end of life care
- management of urinary incontinence when there is no other option available
- to allow irrigation of the bladder.

(Pomfret 2000a; RCN 2008)

Risk management

All forms of catheter usage present a number of associated risks and it is essential that the community nurse completes a risk assessment prior to undertaking the catheterisation procedure (RCN 2008).

Training and education

Community nurses undertaking all forms of urinary catheterisation must have received formal theoretical training, practice supervision using a model or manikin and a period of mentorship in order to gain knowledge, skill and competency prior to carrying out the procedure with patients (NMC 2008; RCN 2008). A formal update should be accessed by all nursing staff at least every five years (RCN 2008).

Catheter selection

An essential element of successful clinical management of both long- and short-term indwelling catheterisation is the selection of the catheter. Therefore careful assessment and documentation of the patient and their needs and choices should be carried out to establish the most appropriate type of: (a) length; (b) function of the catheter, e.g. intended length of time the catheter is to

District Nursing Manual of Clinical Procedures, First Edition. Edited by Liz O'Brien.
© 2012 Blackwell Publishing Ltd. Published 2012 by Blackwell Publishing Ltd.

remain in situ as this will aid decision making regarding the material; (c) size; (d) balloon capacity; and (e) tip design (Pomfret 2000b). This is to ensure that:

- the catheter selected is appropriate and effective
- complications are minimised
- patient comfort and quality of life are supported.

(Robinson 2001)

Types of catheter

There are two main types of catheter that are generally seen in the community these are:

- Foley with a balloon – these are designed to be retained
- Netalon without a balloon – these are designed for intermittent use.

(Robinson 2009)

Ballooned catheters have two channels running along their length, one to drain urine and the other, which is smaller, to allow water to be instilled to inflate the retention balloon (Table 13.1).

Catheter size

There are a number of complications associated with the use of large-gauge catheters, for example:

- pain, discomfort and bladder irritation (Getliffe 2003b)
- bypassing – the catheter may distend the natural folds of the urethral mucosa so they are unable to close around the catheter and leakage occurs (Rew & Woodward 2001). Bypassing may also occur due to bladder spasm caused by irritation
- pressure ulcers, which may lead to stricture formation and pressure necrosis (Getliffe 2003b; Robinson 2006)
- blockage of paraurethral ducts leading to urethritis, abscess formation (Robinson 2006).

Therefore the most important guiding principle when selecting a catheter is to choose the smallest size necessary to maintain adequate drainage (Getliffe 2003a, 2003b). For example, if clear urine is to be drained, a size 12 Ch should be considered; if debris or clots are present a larger-gauge catheter may be necessary (Pomfret 1996; Robinson 2001). The Charrière (Ch) size denotes the measurement of the outer circumference of the catheter, and this is usually indicated by the colour band found around the inflation valve (Robinson 2006).

Catheter length

Due to the difference in length of the female and male urethra, standard or 'male'-length catheters should only be used for the urethral catheterisation of adult male patients (Figures 13.1 and 13.2). When catheterising adult females, either a standard or female-length may be used, but the shorter length of the female catheter helps to reduce the risk of looping, kinking and pulling (Pomfret 2000a). It may also be more discreet when wearing a skirt or dress. However, it has the potential to cause pressure sores in the groin of wheelchair bound and obese patients, so a standard length catheter may be more appropriate for this type of patient (Pomfret 2000a; Rew & Woodward 2001). Female-length catheters may be considered for supra-pubic use in both male and female patients; however, the standard/male-length should always be used for male catheterisation (Robinson 2008; NPSA 2009a). A female-length catheter is 23–26 cm, and a standard/male-length catheter is 40–44 cm (Dougherty & Lister 2011).

Catheter balloon size and inflation

The size of the balloon refers to the amount of fluid needed to inflate it, for example 10 ml and 30 ml for adult catheters, the 30 ml being designed to aid post-prostatectomy haemostasis by applying pressure on the bladder neck (Pomfret 2000b; Robinson 2001).

Large ballooned catheters can be uncomfortable, for example due to the weight inside the bladder, cause bladder spasm, bypassing of urine and damage to the bladder neck (Pomfret 2000a; Robinson 2001, 2006). The drainage eye of larger balloons also sits higher in the bladder and allows residual urine to collect under the balloon, increasing the risk of infection (Bardsley 2005). Therefore it is recommended that a 10 ml balloon is used for adults to reduce the risk of catheter-related problems (Getliffe 2003b; Robinson 2006).

It is essential that the correct amount of fluid is used to inflate the balloon, as under- or over-inflation can lead to distortion of the balloon and deflection of the catheter tip. Subsequently this may result in irritation of the bladder, causing:

305

- pain
- bladder spasm
- urine bypassing
- mucosal trauma
- catheter expulsion and urethral trauma.

(Robinson 2001)

Over-inflation may also cause the balloon to rupture, leaving fragments in the bladder, which have to be

Table 13.1 Catheter recommended use, material and renewal times

Recommended use	Catheter material	Maximum time in situ
Short term		
These catheters are fairly rigid and have a wide internal diameter which allows for a rapid flow rate. Mainly for intermittent use, although ballooned versions are available. Some PVC catheters without balloons are coated with a hydrophilic coating, which, if immersed in water, lubricates the catheter so no additional lubrication is required. Coated catheters are for single use only; uncoated catheters may be reused by the same patient if correctly cleansed and stored, as these are designed to be washed and reused up to a maximum period of one week (Dougherty & Lister 2008)	Polyvinylcholoride (PVC) or plastic	14 days (Bardsley 2005)
Short term		
This is the softest type of catheter. It is prone to encrustations and is associated with urethral trauma and stricture formation (Pomfret 2000b; Robinson 2001)	Latex	14 days (Bardsley 2005)
It is essential that the community nurse identifies previous or current latex or rubber hypersensitivity during pre-assessment of the patient prior to using this type of catheter (Robinson 2009)		
Short–medium term		
This is a latex catheter that has been bonded with Teflon. The bonding causes the latex to become inert, which subsequently reduces urethral encrustations (Slade & Gillespie 1987) and the absorption of water by the latex core; this minimises the swelling (Ryan-Woolley 1987)	Polytetrarafluroethyylene (PTFE)	14–28 days Robinson 2009
Long term		
This consists of a core latex catheter that has been bonded with silicone to give the catheter very smooth internal and external surfaces. The coating acts in a similar way to a PTFE coating, making the latex inert, and reduces water absorption	Silicone elastomer-coated latex	12 weeks (Bardsley, 2005)
Long term		
The core of this catheter is made of latex bonded with a hydrophilic polymer coating that absorbs a small amount of water. The coating creates a smooth, soft, slippery surface that causes very little urethral irritation and reduces friction on both insertion and withdrawal of the catheter. These catheters are reported as being resistant to bacterial colonisation and encrustations (Nacey & Delahunt 1991; Woollons 1996)	Hydrogel-coated latex	12 weeks (Bardsley 2005)
Long term		
The catheter is latex-free and can be used for patients who have a latex allergy. It is an inert material that is less likely to cause urethral irritation, but due to the crescent-shaped lumen may induce encrustation formation (Pomfret 1996). This type of catheter is more rigid than the latex-cored, consequently some patients may find them uncomfortable (Pomfret 2000a,b). Water in the balloon of all silicon catheters can diffuse; this allows the balloon to deflate and may result in the catheter dislodging or falling out. Checking the balloon infill half-way through the catheter's life span can help to prevent this. (Pomfret 2000a,b)	Hydrogel-coated silicone	12 weeks (Bardsley 2005)

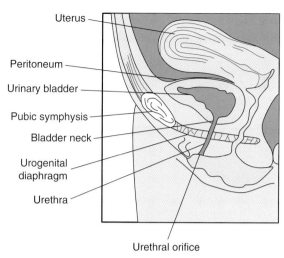

Figure 13.1 The female urethra. (From Bardsley 2005, used with permission)

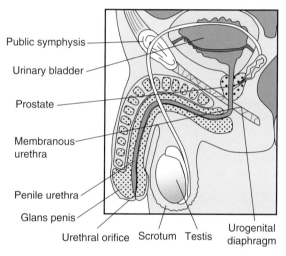

Figure 13.2 The male urethra. (From Bardsley 2005, used with permission)

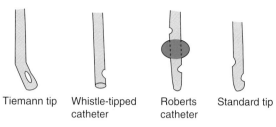

Figure 13.3 Catheter tip design. (Dougherty and Lister 2011)

available that have been designed to overcome specific problems, for example using a tapered-end catheter to negotiate a narrowed urethra (Dougherty & Lister 2011) (Figure 13.3).

Anaesthetic/Lubricating gel

The introduction of a catheter can cause trauma to the urethra and this can increase the risk of infection (Bardsley 2005). To reduce this risk the use of sterile anaesthetic lubricating gel, for example lidocaine hydrochloride, is recommended for both male and female patients both via uretheral and suprapubic routes (MacKenzie & Webb 1995; Tortora & Grabowski 2002; Tanabe *et al.* 2004; Bardsley 2005; Woodward 2005; Pratt *et al.* 2007).

The gel should be instilled into the urethra and left for a minimum of 4 minutes before commencing the catheterisation procedure, in order to anaesthetise and dilate the urethra (NICE 2003). If the procedure is performed too soon after the instillation of the gel, the efficacy of the local anaesthetic will be lost and it will only act as a lubricant (Association for Continence Advice [ACA] 2003).

Caution should be exercised in the use of local anaesthetic gel with, for example, older adults and those patients with cardiac dysrhythmias because under some circumstances systemic absorption may occur (British National Formulary [BNF] 2010).

Suprapubic catheterisation

A suprapubic catheter is inserted through the abdominal wall, above the symphysis pubis, and passed through the detrusor muscle into the bladder (Robinson 2008). The initial procedure is performed under either a general or local unaesthetic and the catheter is secured to the abdomen by either sutures or tape (Robinson 2008). Although there are a number of positive benefits

removed to avoid infection and stone formation (Getliffe 2003b; Robinson 2006).

Sterile water should be used to inflate catheter balloons (Robinson 2006); 0.9% sodium chloride is not recommended because the salt crystals can cause blockages in the inflation channel (Pomfret 2000b; Robinson 2001).

Tip design

The standard catheter tip design is straight, rounded and has two drainage holes. There are several other tips

307

to suprapubic catheterisation, for example there is no risk of urethral associated complications in long-term use, risks associated with the procedure include haemorrhage and intestinal injury (RCN 2008; NPSA 2009b) (Box 13.1). Encrustation of the catheter may cause trauma during removal (Robinson 2008) and altered body image may have a negative psychological impact on the patient, especially if they remain sexually active (Addison & Mould 2000).

For the first 7–10 days following initial suprapubic catheterisation it is essential that a strict aseptic technique is used when cleansing and redressing the cystostomy site (Colpman & Welford 2004).

After this time the site should be healed and the catheter and site can be cleansed during bathing using soap, water and a clean cloth (Colpman & Welford 2004). Once healed, dressings are not essential but may be required by the patient if secretions are present.

Intermittent catheterisation

Intermittent catheterisation involves the periodic introduction of a catheter into the bladder to remove urine; once the bladder is emptied the catheter is removed (see Box 13.2 for advantages and disadvantages).

Long-term use of this procedure is generally associated with patients who are unable to completely empty their bladder, for one of a number of clinical reasons, including the following.

- Neurogenic bladder, which occurs when the neurological control mechanisms of the bladder are damaged, e.g. due to trauma caused by spinal injury or diseases such as multiple sclerosis.
- Hypotonic bladder, this is when the bladder does not contract sufficiently to completely empty.

Box 13.1 Advantages, risks and disadvantages of suprapubic catheterisation

Advantages	Risks and disadvantages
Reduced risk of infection as the bacterial count on abdominal skin is less than around the perineal and perianal areas (Winn 1998; Simpson 2001)	Bowel perforation and haemorrhage at the time of insertion
Urethral integrity is retained, therefore less chance of stricture formation and trauma	Infection, swelling, encrustation and granulation at insertion site
Facilitates a voiding assessment following surgery	Pain, discomfort and or irritation
Allows for the resumption of urethral voiding	
Pain and catheter related discomfort is reduced	Bladder stone formation and possible long-term risk of squamous cell carcinoma
Easier to manage for wheelchair-bound patients	
Increased satisfaction for some patients as independence is increased and sexual intercourse can occur with fewer impediments (Milligan 1999; Colpman & Welford 2004)	Urethral leakage (Addison & Mould 2000)

Box 13.2 Advantages and disadvantages of intermittent catheterisation

Advantages	Disadvantages
Urinary tract complications are minimised (Chai et al. 1995; Bakke et al. 1997)	Increased risk of urethral bleeding and urethritis (Vaidyanathan et al. 1994, 1996)
Bladder function is maintained and continence may be achieved (Bakke & Malt 1993)	Chronic bacteraemia (although not necessarily symptomatic)
Upper urinary tract is protected from reflux	Increase risk of urethral false passage with poor technique (Koleilat et al. 1989)
Reduced risk of urethral trauma, urinary tract infection and encrustation	Unacceptable procedure for some patients, causing psychological distress (Bakke & Malt 1993)
Arguably a reduced need for equipment and appliances compared to stoma care patients	
Improved quality of life (Bakke & Malt 1993). Patients are able to self-care and gain independence	
Increased patient satisfaction (Webb et al. 1990)	
Greater freedom to express sexuality (Getliffe 2003b)	

- Outflow obstruction due to an enlarged prostate or urethral stricture.
- Detrusor dyssynergia when the detrusor muscle contracts but the urethral sphincter does not relax.
- Following surgery for bladder or urethral replacement or reconstruction (e.g. enterocystoplasty or Mitrofanoff formation), and gynaecological surgery (e.g. colposuspension, transvaginal tape TVT).

(Winn 1998; Colpman & Welford 2004; Leaver 2004)

Patients who are suitable for intermittent self-catheterisation (ISC) include those who:

- have capacity to give informed consent to undertake the procedure
- have the ability to understand and learn all aspects of the techniques and procedures involved
- can store urine in their bladder without leakage between catheterisation
- have the dexterity and mobility to position themself and manipulate the catheter
- are motivated and committed to the procedure
- have a competent willing partner or carer who is able to perform the procedure with the patient's consent.

(Colley 1998; Leaver & Pressland 2001; Leaver 2004; NMC 2007; RCN 2008)

It is recommended that a Nelaton catheter is used to carry out intermittent catheterisation. These are available in standard, male and paediatric length and in 6–24 Charrière sizes. They are normally made from PVC, but a non-PVC, chlorine-free catheter and an all-silicone female catheter are also available. It is essential that the manufacturer's instructions and local Trust guidelines and policy are adhered to when using single and reusable catheters for this procedure.

Intermittent catheterisation should be performed as often as necessary to stop the bladder becoming over-distended and to prevent incontinence (Bennett 2002). The frequency of the procedure may vary from weekly, daily or 4–6 hourly, depending on the individual's needs. For patients carrying out ISC at home the procedure may be performed using a clean technique (Wilson 1997; Lapides et al. 2002).

Meatal hygiene

It is suggested that meatal cleansing, when a urinary catheter is in situ, should be carried out as part of the patient's normal personal hygiene routine (Saint & Lipsky 1999; Pratt et al. 2001; Pomfret & Tew 2004;

Wilson 2005). For male patients this involves cleansing the area around the opening of the urethra and under the foreskin, if the patient is not circumcised (Leaver 2007). With female patients this area is located between the labia minoria above the opening to the vagina (Leaver 2007).

Mechanical meatal cleansing should be carried out as part of the patient preparation prior to insertion of a urethral catheter using an aseptic technique and 0.9% normal saline solution (Leaver 2007; Pratt et al. 2007). If the patient is performing ISC, then soap and water is sufficient (Dougherty & Lister 2008).

Drainage systems

Urine drainage bags available on prescription (FP10 in the UK) range from the large 2-litre capacity to 350–750 ml body worn or leg bags. They are available with an integrated tap to enable urine to be drained out of the bag, non-drainable disposable bags and products adapted for wheelchair users. If the patient or carer is able to participate in, e.g. drainage of the bag, it is important that the community nurses accurately assess their manual dexterity in order to select the most appropriate drainage system and tap mechanism.

Leg bags are available in a number of different styles. They vary in shape from oblong to oval, and some have a cloth-like backing for greater comfort. Others are ridged to allow for an even distribution of urine which results in greater conformity of the bag to the leg.

Drainage bag inlet tubes vary in length, with direct fit as well as short, long or adjustable length. The intended position of a leg bag, i.e. to be worn on the patient's thigh, knee or lower leg, and the patient's comfort and preference should dictate which length of tubing is used. Patients may need to trial several different systems before they find the one that suits their needs and lifestyle best and maintains their privacy and dignity.

To increase bag capacity at night a number of leg bags enable a larger 1- to 2-litre bag to be connected via the outlet tap. This also avoids breaking the closed drainage system and reduces the risk of introducing infection (Leaver 2007).

Catheter valves are an alternative to drainage bags. They allow the bladder to fill and empty intermittently, and so mimic normal bladder function (Pomfret 2000b). Catheter valves are suitable for patients who:

- have an adequate bladder capacity
- have the manual dexterity to manipulate the valve
- have good cognitive function.

309

They are inappropriate for patients with uncontrolled detrusor over-activity, ureteric reflux or renal impairment (Fader *et al.* 1997).

To be an effective form of management the selected valve needs to fulfill certain criteria, for example:

- easy to manipulate
- leak-free
- comfortable and inconspicuous.

(Fader *et al.* 1997)

As with all forms of urine drainage systems the manufacturer's recommendations combined with local policy and guidelines must be followed when using a valve.

Infection

The risk of a urinary tract infection increases on average by 5–8% a day during the patient's period of catheterisation, but potential complications such as infection should not be viewed as an acceptable consequence (Crow *et al.* 1988; Mulhall *et al.* 1988; Getliffe 1996; Saint & Lipsky 1999; Tew *et al.* 2005).

There are a number of possible routes through which bacteria can enter the bladder of a catheterised patient:

- intra-luminal, suggested as being caused by contamination of the tap of the drainage bag or catheter disconnection
- periurethral – the migration of bacteria between the walls of the catheter and the urethra
- via the lumen of the catheter
- via the catheter and/or tip during insertion.

(Getliffe 1996; Godfrey & Evans 2000; Madeo & Roodhouse 2009)

Bacteria can colonise the urinary tract without invading the tissues. This is known as bacteriuria and the presence of a urinary catheter provides a good medium for this to occur (Wilson 1997). This is because bacteria adhere to the surface of the catheter, forming a biofilm, and produce polysaccharides that form a thick coating on the surface, called the glycocalyx (Wilson 1997). It is suggested that bacteria in the biofilm are generally less susceptible than their free-living counterparts, making it difficult for antiseptic and antibiotic agents to penetrate (Getliffe 1996; Liedl 2001; Saye 2007). Bacteria in the urine may be successfully killed but may persist in the biofilm and restart the cycle of infection. Consequently, the routine use of bladder irrigation solutions that contain antibiotic or antiseptic components is not advocated (Stickler & Hughes 1999).

There are several points where there is the potential for microorganisms to enter. These include:

- via migration on the inside of the catheter via biofilm
- at the junction between the catheter and drainage tube
- at the outlet of the drainage bag/valve
- at the connection points of the link system
- via the sample port on the drainage bag tubing
- via any puncture of the drainage bag.

(Gould 1994; Wilson & Coates 1996)

To reduce the risk of infection manipulations of the closed system should be kept to a minimum. This includes unnecessary emptying and/or changing of the drainage bag or valve and sample taking (Pomfret 2000a, 2000b). The catheter drainage bag should not be positioned higher than the bladder and it should never be allowed to become over-full as this promotes urine reflux, which is associated with infection (Dougherty & Lister 2008). Before handling catheter drainage systems hands must be decontaminated and a pair of non-sterile gloves should be worn (Pratt *et al.* 2001). An aseptic technique should be used when taking urine samples from the specially designed ports (*see* Chapter 6).

It is suggested that different types of catheter may delay the onset and reduce the risk of infection, for example hydrogel-coated and silver alloy catheters and the Foley pre connected system (Wilson 1997; Saint *et al.* 1998; Neil-Weise *et al.* 2002; Brosnahan *et al.* 2004; Pellowe *et al.* 2004; Godfrey & Fraczyk 2005; Madeo & Roodhouse 2009).

Catheter blockage and encrustations

Catheter blockage is a common problem associated with long-term catheterisation, with approximately half of all catheterised patients at risk (Getliffe 2003a).

Potential causes of catheter blockage include:

- encrustations, which form on the surfaces of the catheter and within its lumen
- detrusor spasm – bladder mucosa closes around the eyes of the catheter because of muscle spasm
- mucosal blockage due to hydrostatical suction resulting from the vacuum effect of urine in the drainage tubing; this sucks the bladder mucosa into the eyes of the catheter
- mucus or debris plugs blocking the lumen of the catheter

- twisted/kinked drainage tubing
- the drainage bag being positioned higher than the level of the bladder
- constipation – stool loaded in the rectum can cause pressure on the catheter lumen and prevent drainage.

(Pomfret 2000b; Simpson 2001; Getliffe 2003a, 2003b; Leaver 2004)

Catheter encrustations consist of mineral salts, magnesium ammonium phosphate (struvite) and calcium phosphate (hydroxyapatite) (Getliffe 2002). The encrusatations build up on the outer surface, balloon and lumen of urinary catheters as a result of urease activity produced by bacteria in the urine (Stickler & Hughes 1999; Liedl 2001). This splits urinary urea into ammonia and carbon dioxide, which increases the alkalinity of urine and subsequently crystals develop and adhere to the catheter (Rew & Woodward 2001).

A number of pre-packaged catheter maintenance solutions are available to dissolve mineral deposits (Table 13.2). However, these should be used with caution because any solution other then saline can cause:

- loss of urethral cells (Getliffe 2003a)
- inflammatory reactions (Getliffe 1996)
- removal of the surface layer of mucosa in the bladder (Getliffe 2002)

Table 13.2 Catheter maintenence solutions

Type of maintenance solution	Active ingredient	Usage
Solution R	6% citric acid	Used to dissolve persistent crystallisation (Getliffe 2002)
Suby G	3.23% citric acid and magnesium oxide	Used to prevent or dissolve crystallisation (Getliffe 2002)
Mandelic acid 1%	Acidic solution pH2	Used to prevent growth of urease-producing bacteria by acidifying the urine (Getliffe 2002)
Chlorhexidine 0.02%	Antiseptic solution	Used to prevent or reduce bacterial growth, in particular *E. coli* (Getliffe 2002)
0.9% sodium chloride	Neutral solution pH7	Used for mechanical flushing to remove tissue debris and small blood clots (Getliffe 2002)

- increased shedding of urethelial cells, although this may also be due to the physical force of the mechanical action of inserting the solution under pressure (Getliffe 2003b).

The purpose of using a maintenance solution is to fill the lumen of the catheter and bathe the tip. To achieve this it is suggested that only 4–5 ml of fluid is necessary (Getliffe 2002). However, such a small amount of fluid would quickly become saturated with minerals. Therefore it is recommended that smaller volumes of solution instilled on a regular basis, for example on alternate days, minimise the potential irritant effects, are effective at reducing encrustations and allow time for repair of the bladder mucosa in between irrigations (Getliffe 2003a, 2003b). An in vitro study by Getliffe *et al.* (2000) found that two sequential wash-outs with 50 ml retained for 15 min were significantly better at removing encrustations than a single 100 ml washout.

Before making the decision to use a catheter maintenance solution the community nurse should undertake an evaluation of the patient, their lifestyle and their current catheter management plan. This should include:

- an assessment of the patient's diet and fluid intake, activity and mobility, standard of hygiene and, where appropriate, the patient or carer's ability to continue to participate in the management plan
- regular testing of urinary pH, e.g. weekly or more frequently if the patient's catheter is prone to block every few days
- catheter history, including length of catheter life before blockage and the identification of any known cause/s of blockage.

(Getliffe 2002)

It is also recommended that between three and five consecutive catheters should be observed to diagnose the cause of any blockage problem (Rew 1999). The tip of the removed catheter should be inspected and the catheter split along its length to observe if encrustations have adhered to its lumen (Rew 1999). Patients can be classed as 'blockers' (regularly developing encrustations that lead to shorter catheter life) or 'non-blockers' (do not routinely block even with prolonged catheter insertion). Therefore it is essential that care for patients is planned on an individual basis in order to establish a catheter history and plan catheter changes in accordance with the patient's needs (Getliffe 2003a, 2003b). For patients in whom there is no clear pattern or identifiable cause of blockage, or for whom catheter changes are traumatic, the use of catheter maintenance solutions may be beneficial in reducing catheter encrustations (Getliffe 1996, 2003b; Rew 2005).

311

Conclusion

While catheterisation is widely recognised as playing an important role in the medical treatment and nursing care of a patient, it is essential to remember that it also present risks to the patient that have the potential to result in serious complications. To minimise these risks community nurses play an essential role in the training, education and monitoring of patients, carers and colleagues.

Procedure guideline 13.1 **Guideline for urethral urinary catheterisation (male)**

Equipment

Sterile catheterisation pack
Single-use sterile gloves
Single-use plastic apron x 2
Single-use waterproof protective pad, e.g. incontinence pad or similar
0.9% sodium chloride solution
Single-use sterile anaesthetic lubricating gel 11 ml syringe
Sterile water
Appropriate urethral catheter (standard length) (Robinson 2006)
Selected drainage system or valve
Catheter bag stand or holder
Sterile 10 ml syringe (depending on balloon size)
Sterile hypodermic needle
Sharps bin
Universal specimen container (where relevant)

Procedure

Nursing action	Rationale
1 Where appropriate facilities are available wash your hands or alternatively cleanse with 70% alcohol-based hand rub (in accordance with local policy)	To prevent the risk of cross-infection/contamination
2 If the patient is known to the service review nursing documentation and current care plan	To update the nurse's knowledge of the patient To maintain patient safety
3 If the patient is unknown to the service a comprehensive assessment must be carried out prior to undertaking the procedure. This must include the assessment of any manual handling techniques required to carry out the procedure, and the identification of any known or potential allergies, e.g. local anaesthetic gel	To identify potential contraindications and or cautions To determine if a second nurse is required to assist with the procedure To maintain patient safety To ensure health and safety regulations are met and maintain practitioner safety
4 Explain and discuss the procedure with the patient	To ensure that the patient understands the procedure and gives their valid consent
5 Prepare the environment, draw curtains and where necessary obtain patient consent to move furniture	To allow freedom of movement when carrying out the procedure To maintain patient privacy

Procedure guideline 13.1 **Guideline for urethral urinary catheterisation (male)** *(cont'd)*

Nursing action	Rationale
6 Assemble all equipment on a clean surface; check that (a) all relevant seals and packaging is in tact and undamaged and (b) all relevant equipment is within the recommended date for use	To prevent disruption to the procedure To prevent contamination of equipment To maintain patient safety
7 Protect the bed with an appropriate disposable waterproof underpad	To protect mattress and bedding from soiling
8 Put on disposable plastic apron	To prevent the risk of cross-infection/contamination
9 Where indicated offer the patient assistance with removing all clothing below the waist	To expose the appropriate area
10 Assist the patient into the supine position with legs extended cover the exposed area of the body with a towel/blanket	To make sure the appropriate area is easily accessible To maintain the patient's dignity and comfort
11 Remove and dispose of apron in accordance with locally agreed infection prevention and control policy	To minimise the risk of cross-infection
12 Where appropriate facilities are available wash your hands or alternatively cleanse with 70% alcohol-based hand rub (in accordance with local policy)	To reduce the risk of cross-infection
13 Put on disposable plastic apron	To reduce the risk of cross-infection
14 Open sterile pack and prepare all equipment on the sterile field. Using an aseptic technique, draw up recommended amount of sterile water, disposing of needle in sharps bin	To maintain patient safety by reducing the risk of introducing micro-organisms into bladder To prevent disruption to the procedure To prevent the risk of needlestick injury to self and others
15 Place catheter into sterile receiver	To prevent disruption to the procedure To maintain patient safety
16 Remove cover that is maintaining patient privacy and place disposable waterproof pad under patient's buttocks and thighs	To ensure patient bedding does not become soiled
17 Cleanse hands with bactericidal alcohol hand rub	Handling outer packs and/or cover may have contaminated hands
18 Put on sterile gloves	To reduce risk of cross-infection
19 Place sterile towels across the patient's thighs and under buttocks	To create a sterile field
20 Inform patient that you are about to start the procedure	To confirm that the patient continues to consent to the procedure being undertaken To promote patient relaxation To gain patient co-operation
21 Wrap a sterile low-linting swab around the penis	To prevent contamination of the nurse's gloves when correctly positioning the penis during the catheterisation procedure

(Continued)

Procedure guideline 13.1 **Guideline for urethral urinary catheterisation (male)** *(cont'd)*

Nursing action	Rationale
22 Using a low-linting swab retract the foreskin, if necessary, and clean the glans penis with 0.9% sodium chloride or sterile water; dry thoroughly	To reduce the risk of introducing micro-organisms into the urinary tract during catheterisation To reduce risk of cross-infection
23 Gently insert the nozzle of the anaesthetic/lubricating gel into the urethra and instil the gel according to manufacturer's instructions to a maximum volume of 10.6 ml. Remove the nozzle and discard the syringe appropriately Apply gentle external massage	Adequate lubrication helps to prevent urethral trauma (Bardsley 2005) Use of an anaesthetic gel helps minimise any discomfort that may be experienced by the patient 10.6 ml is the average volume the male urethra can hold (Bardsley 2005) Anaesthetic lubricating gel is suggested to reduce the risk of catheter insertion-related urinary tract infection (Kambal *et al.* 2004) To disperse gel along the urethra
24 Using the sterile gauze hold the penis behind the glans raising it until it is almost fully extended. Maintain hold until procedure is finished	To prevent glove contamination To prevent the anaesthetic gel from escaping Extension of the penis straightens the urethra and promotes a smoother procedure when inserting the catheter
25 Wait a minimum of 5 mins before starting the insertion procedure (Dougherty & Lister 2011)	To allow the anaesthetic gel to take effect
26 Place the receiver containing the catheter between the patient's legs and ask the patient to relax, e.g. as if he were passing urine or coughing	Straining gently or coughing helps to relax the external sphincter
27 Insert the catheter for 15–25 cm until urine is observed in the receiver	To ensure correct positioning of the catheter; the male urethra is approximately 18 cm long (Bardsley 2005)
28 Resistance may be felt at the external sphincter. A combination of slightly increased traction on the penis and steady gentle pressure on the catheter should be applied. Ask the patient to relax, as in step 25 above	Resistance may be due to external sphincter spasm Straining gently or coughing helps to relax the external sphincter
29 Once the position of the catheter has been confirmed by the presence of urine in the receiver the catheter should be gently advanced to almost bifurcation	Advancing the catheter prior to inflating the balloon ensures it is correctly positioned in the bladder To prevent pain and urethral trauma that may occur if the catheter is positioned in the urethra or bladder neck and the balloon inflated (Getliffe & Dolman 2003; Robinson 2006) To maintain patient safety
30 Attach the syringe containing the correct amount of sterile water and slowly inflate the balloon according to the manufacturer's instructions	To secure the catheter in place
31 If the patient experiences any pain or discomfort during balloon inflation discontinue installation of sterile water immediately. Deflate the balloon and gently advance the catheter a few more centimetres before trying again	To prevent pain and urethral trauma that may occur if the catheter is positioned in the urethra when the balloon is inflated (Getliffe & Dolman 2003) To maintain patient safety

Procedure guideline 13.1 **Guideline for urethral urinary catheterisation (male)** *(cont'd)*

Nursing action	Rationale
32 Once the balloon is fully inflated gently withdraw the catheter until slight resistance is felt	To ensure that the catheter balloon is in the correct position in the bladder
33 Attach the selected drainage system	To facilitate urine collection
Where relevant measure the amount of urine drained and/or collect a urine specimen	To promote patient comfort
	To establish and document an objective baseline record
	To provide the GP with further information, e.g. presence of infection
34 Clean the glans penis with 0.9% sodium chloride and dry thoroughly; where necessary reposition the foreskin	To prevent secondary infections and skin irritation
	To prevent constriction and retraction of the foreskin behind the glans penis, also none as paraphimosis
	To promote patient comfort
	To maintain patient safety
35 Cover exposed area of the patient's body with a blanket/towel	To maintain patient dignity
36 Dispose of all used equipment in accordance with locally agreed infection prevention and control policy	To reduce the risk of cross-infection
	To maintain the health and safety of self and others
37 Remove and dispose of gloves in accordance with locally agreed infection prevention and control policy	To reduce the risk of cross-infection
38 Cleanse hands with bactericidal alcohol hand rub	To reduce the risk of cross-infection
39 Assist the patient to dress and help into their chosen position, e.g. sitting in chair, open curtains	To maintain patient's dignity and comfort
40 Remove and dispose of apron in accordance with locally agreed infection prevention and control policy	To reduce the risk of cross-infection
41 Where appropriate facilities are available wash your hands or alternatively cleanse with 70% alcohol-based hand rub (in accordance with local policy)	To reduce the risk of cross-infection
42 Replace any moved items of furniture to their original position	To maintain a safe environment for the patient by restoring any furniture moved to its usual place
43 Verbally discuss the outcome of the procedure with the patient and where relevant carer, giving further advice as indicated. Where possible this should be supported with written/diagrammatic information	To reinforce verbal information and support patient's understanding
44 The following information should be recorded in the nursing documentation in accordance with local policy and NMC guidelines: (a) date and time of the procedure; (b) rationale for the catheterisation; (c) catheter type; (d) length; (e) size; (f) amount of sterile water instilled to inflate the balloon; (g) selected drainage system; (h) batch number; (i) manufacturer; (j) any difficulties experienced during the procedure; (k) review date; (l) date of next catheter change	To maintain patient safety
	To enable continuity of care
	To maintain practitioner safety
	Documentation should provide clear evidence of the care or procedure carried out

Procedure guideline 13.2 **Guideline for urinary catheterisation (female)**

Equipment

Sterile catheterisation pack
Single-use sterile gloves
Single-use plastic apron
Single-use waterproof protective pad, e.g. incontinence pad or similar
0.9% sodium chloride solution
Single-use sterile anaesthetic lubricating gel
Sterile water
Appropriate urethral catheter standard/female length
Selected drainage system or valve
Catheter bag stand or holder
Sterile syringe (depending on balloon size)
Sterile hypodermic needle
Sharps bin
Universal specimen container (where relevant)

Procedure

Nursing action	Rationale
1 Where appropriate facilities are available wash your hands or alternatively cleanse with 70% alcohol-based hand rub (in accordance with local policy)	To prevent the risk of cross-infection/contamination
2 If the patient is known to the service review nursing documentation and current care plan	To update the nurse's knowledge of the patient To maintain patient safety
3 If the patient is unknown to the service a comprehensive assessment must be carried out prior to undertaking the procedure. This must include the assessment of any manual handling techniques required to carry out the procedure and identification of any known or potential allergies, e.g. local anaesthetic gel	To identify potential contra-indications and or cautions To determine if a second nurse is required to assist with the procedure To ensure health and safety regulations are met and maintain practitioner safety To maintain patient safety
4 Explain and discuss the procedure with the patient	To ensure that the patient understands the procedure and gives their valid consent
5 Prepare the environment, draw curtains and where necessary obtain patient consent to move furniture	To allow freedom of movement when carrying out the procedure To maintain patient privacy
6 Assemble all equipment on a clean surface; check that (a) all relevant seals and packaging is in tact and undamaged, and (b) all relevant equipment is within the recommended date for use	To prevent disruption to the procedure To prevent contamination of equipment To maintain patient safety
7 Protect the bed with an appropriate disposable waterproof underpad	To protect mattress and bedding from soiling
8 Put on disposable plastic apron	To prevent the risk of cross-infection/contamination
9 Where indicated offer the patient assistance with removing all clothing below the waist	To expose the appropriate area

Procedure guideline 13.2 **Guideline for urinary catheterisation (female)** *(cont'd)*

Nursing action	Rationale
10 Assist the patient into the supine position with knees bent, hips flexed and feet resting comfortably apart; cover the exposed area of the body with a towel/blanket	To make sure the appropriate area is easily accessible To maintain the patient's dignity and comfort
11 Remove and dispose of apron in accordance with locally agreed infection prevention and control policy	To minimise the risk of cross-infection
12 Where appropriate facilities are available wash your hands or alternatively cleanse with 70% alcohol-based hand rub (in accordance with local policy)	To reduce the risk of cross-infection
13 Put on disposable plastic apron	To reduce risk of cross-infection from micro-organisms on uniform
14 Open sterile pack and prepare all equipment on the sterile field. Using an aseptic technique, draw up recommended amount of sterile water, disposing of needle in sharps bin	To maintain patient safety by reducing the risk of introducing micro-organisms into bladder To prevent disruption to the procedure To prevent the risk of needlestick injury to self and others
15 Place catheter into sterile receiver	To prevent disruption to the procedure To maintain patient safety
16 Remove cover that is maintaining patient privacy and place disposable waterproof pad under patient's buttocks and thighs	To ensure patient bedding does not become soiled
17 Clean hands with bactericidal alcohol hand rub	Handling outer packs and/or cover may have contaminated hands
18 Put on sterile gloves	To reduce risk of cross-infection
19 Place sterile towels across the patient's thighs and under buttocks	To create a sterile field
20 Inform patient that you are about to start the procedure	To confirm that the patient continues to consent to the procedure being undertaken To promote patient relaxation To gain patient co-operation
21 Separate the labia minora using a low-linting swab. Using a second low-linting swab, the non-dominant hand should maintain labial separation until the whole procedure is complete	To expose the urethral meatus To ensure ease of access to the urethral orifice To reduce the risk of catheter contamination
22 Clean around the urethral orifice with 0.9% sodium chloride using single downward strokes; dry thoroughly	To reduce the risk of introducing micro-organisms into the urinary tract during catheterisation To reduce risk of cross-infection

(Continued)

Procedure guideline 13.2 **Guideline for urinary catheterisation (female)** *(cont'd)*

Nursing action	Rationale
23 Gently insert the nozzle of the anaesthetic lubricating gel into the urethra and instil the gel according to manufacturer's instructions, remove the nozzle and discard the syringe appropriately	Adequate lubrication helps to prevent urethral trauma (Bardsley 2005)
	Use of an anaesthetic gel helps minimise any discomfort that may be experienced by the patient
	Anaesthetic lubricating gel is suggested to reduce the risk of catheter insertion-related urinary tract infection (Kambal et al. 2004)
24 Wait a minimum of 5 mins before starting the insertion procedure (Dougherty & Lister 2011)	To allow the anaesthetic gel to take effect
25 Place the receiver containing the catheter between the patient's legs	To provide a receptacle for urine as it drains
26 Insert the catheter for 5–6 cm in an upwards and backwards direction (Dougherty & Lister 2001)	To correlate to the anatomical structure of the area
If there is any difficulty in visualising the urethral orifice due to vaginal atrophy and retraction of the urethral orifice. With the patient's consent the index finger of the non-dominant hand may be inserted into the vagina and the urethral orifice can be palpated on the anterior wall of the vagina	To position the index finger just behind the urethral orifice. This then acts as a guide so the catheter can be correctly positioned (Jenkins 1998)
27 Advance the catheter 6–8 cm until urine is observed in the receiver	Advancing the catheter prior to inflating the balloon ensures it is correctly positioned in the bladder
	To prevent pain and urethral trauma that may occur if the catheter is positioned in the urethra or bladder neck and the balloon inflated (Getliffe & Dolman 2003; Robinson 2006)
	To maintain patient safety
28 Attach the syringe containing the correct amount of sterile water and slowly inflate the balloon according to the manufacturer's instructions	To secure the catheter in place
29 If the patient experiences any pain or discomfort during balloon inflation discontinue installation of sterile water immediately. Deflate the balloon and gently advance the catheter a few more centimetres before trying again	To prevent pain and urethral trauma that may occur if the catheter is positioned in the urethra or bladder neck when the balloon is inflated (Getliffe & Dolman 2003)
	To maintain patient safety
30 Once the balloon is fully inflated gently withdraw the catheter until slight resistance is felt	To ensure that the catheter balloon is in the correct position in the bladder
31 Attach the selected drainage system	To facilitate urine collection
Where relevant measure the amount of urine drained and/or collect a urine specimen	To promote patient comfort
	To establish and document an objective baseline record
	To provide the GP with further information, e.g. presence of infection

Procedure guideline 13.2 **Guideline for urinary catheterisation (female)** *(cont'd)*

Nursing action	Rationale
32 Clean and thoroughly dry the area with 0.9% sodium chloride	To prevent secondary infections and skin irritation To promote patient comfort To maintain patient safety
33 Cover exposed area of the patient's body with a blanket/towel	To maintain patient dignity
34 Dispose of all used equipment in accordance with locally agreed infection prevention and control policy	To reduce the risk of cross-infection To maintain the health and safety of self and others
35 Remove and dispose of gloves in accordance with locally agreed infection prevention and control policy	To reduce the risk of cross-infection
36 Cleanse hands with bactericidal alcohol hand rub	To reduce the risk of cross-infection
37 Assist the patient to dress and help into their chosen position, e.g. sitting in chair, open curtains	To maintain patient's dignity and comfort
38 Remove and dispose of apron in accordance with locally agreed infection prevention and control policy	To reduce the risk of cross-infection
39 Where appropriate facilities are available wash your hands or alternatively cleanse with 70% alcohol-based hand rub (in accordance with local policy)	To reduce the risk of cross-infection
40 Replace any moved items of furniture to their original position	To maintain a safe environment for the patient by restoring any furniture moved to its usual place
41 Verbally discuss the outcome of the procedure with the patient and where relevant carer, giving further advice as indicated. Where possible this should be supported with written/diagrammatic information	To reinforce verbal information and support patient's understanding
42 The following information should be recorded in the nursing documentation in accordance with local policy and NMC guidelines: (a) date and time of the procedure; (b) rationale for the catheterization; (c) catheter type; (d) length; (e) size; (f) amount of sterile water instilled to inflate the balloon; (g) selected drainage system; (h) batch number; (i) manufacturer; (j) any difficulties experienced during the procedure; (k) review date; (l) date of next catheter change	To maintain patient safety To enable continuity of care To maintain practitioner safety Documentation should provide clear evidence of the care or procedure carried out

Procedure guideline 13.3 **Guideline for changing a suprapubic catheter**

Equipment

Sterile catheterisation pack
Single-use sterile gloves
Non-sterile single-use disposable gloves x 2
Single-use plastic apron
Single-use waterproof protective pad, e.g. incontinence pad or similar
0.9% sodium chloride solution
Single-use sterile anaesthetic lubricating gel
Standard/female length catheter latex or 100% silicone (Robinson 2008)
Sterile water
Selected drainage system or valve
Catheter bag stand or holder
Sterile syringe (depending on balloon size) x 2
Sterile hypodermic needle
Sharps bin

Procedure

Nursing action	Rationale
1 Where appropriate facilities are available wash your hands or alternatively cleanse with 70% alcohol-based hand rub (in accordance with local policy)	To prevent the risk of cross-infection/contamination
2 If the patient is known to the service review nursing documentation and current care plan	To update the nurse's knowledge of the patient To maintain patient safety
3 If the patient is unknown to the service a comprehensive assessment must be carried out prior to undertaking the procedure. This must include the assessment of any manual handling techniques required to carry out the procedure, and identification of any known or potential allergies, e.g. local anaesthetic gel	To identify potential contraindications and or cautions To determine if a second nurse is required to assist with the procedure To maintain patient safety To ensure health and safety regulations are met and maintain practitioner safety
4 Explain and discuss the procedure with the patient	To ensure that the patient understands the procedure and gives their valid consent
5 Prepare the environment, draw curtains and where necessary obtain patient consent to move furniture	To allow freedom of movement when carrying out the procedure To maintain patient privacy
6 Assemble all equipment on a clean surface; check that (a) all relevant seals and packaging is intact and undamaged, and (b) all relevant equipment is within the recommended date for use	To prevent disruption to the procedure To prevent contamination of equipment To maintain patient safety
7 Protect the bed with an appropriate disposable, waterproof underpad	To protect mattress and bedding from soiling
8 Apply disposable plastic apron	To prevent the risk of cross-infection/contamination

Procedure guideline 13.3 *Guideline for changing a suprapubic catheter* (cont'd)

Nursing action	Rationale
9 Where indicated offer the patient assistance with removing all clothing below the waist	To expose the appropriate area
10 Assist the patient into the supine position cover the exposed area of the patient's body with a towel/blanket	To allow easy access to the cystostomy area To maintain the patient's dignity and comfort
11 Apply non-sterile gloves and empty catheter bag; place on the bed next to the patient, or if the patient is using a catheter valve ask them to empty their bladder	To reduce the risk of cross-infection To prepare for procedure To aid patient comfort
12 Remove and dispose of gloves and apron in accordance with locally agreed infection prevention and control policy	To reduce the risk of cross-infection
13 Where appropriate facilities are available wash your hands or alternatively cleanse with 70% alcohol-based hand rub (in accordance with local policy)	To reduce the risk of cross-infection
14 Apply disposable plastic apron	To reduce risk of cross-infection from micro-organisms on uniform
15 Open sterile pack and prepare all equipment on the sterile field. Using an aseptic technique, draw up recommended amount of sterile water disposing of needle in sharps bin	To maintain patient safety by reducing the risk of introducing micro-organisms into bladder. To prevent disruption to the procedure To prevent the risk of needlestick injury to self and others
16 Place catheter into sterile receiver	To prevent disruption to the procedure To maintain patient safety
17 Remove cover that is maintaining patient privacy and place disposable waterproof pad under patient's buttocks and thighs	To ensure patient bedding does not become soiled
18 Clean hands with bactericidal alcohol hand rub	Handling outer packs and/or cover may have contaminated hands
19 Put on non-sterile gloves and where appropriate remove and dispose of dressing on cystostomy site. Observe site for discharge, granulation and inflammation	To reduce risk of cross-infection To detect signs of infection or skin excoriation. If any signs noted, liaise with GP and or specialist nurse
20 Remove and dispose of gloves in accordance with locally agreed infection prevention and control policy	To reduce the risk of cross-infection
21 Where appropriate facilities are available wash your hands or alternatively cleanse with 70% alcohol-based hand rub (in accordance with local policy)	To reduce risk of cross-infection
22 Apply sterile gloves	To reduce risk of cross-infection

321

(*Continued*)

Procedure guideline 13.3 **Guideline for changing a suprapubic catheter** *(cont'd)*

Nursing action	Rationale
23 Inform patient that you are about to start the procedure	To confirm that the patient continues to consent to the procedure being undertaken
	To promote patient relaxation
	To gain patient co-operation
24 Attach a syringe to the inflation valve on the catheter and withdraw the water from the balloon	To deflate the catheter balloon in preparation for removal
	To maintain patient safety
25 Place a finger on the abdomen on each side of the catheter and grip the catheter low at the skin surface (Robinson 2008)	To apply support during removal
	To prepare for catheter removal
26 Apply gentle rotational and steady upward traction on the catheter	To remove the catheter
27 If resistance is felt gently increase force **NB** Resistance may be due to catheter balloon cuff formation (Robinson 2008)	To remove the catheter
28 Observe the catheter for length to ensure it is intact and for the presence of encrustations	To ensure that the catheter is whole and intact
	To plan future catheter care, as encrustations can cause trauma on removal
	To maintain patient safety
29 Dispose of old catheter in accordance with locally agreed infection prevention and control policy	To reduce risk of cross-infection
	To reduce the risk of contaminating sterile working area
	To reduce the risk of environmental contamination
30 Remove and dispose of gloves in accordance with locally agreed infection prevention and control policy	To reduce the risk of cross-infection
31 Where appropriate facilities are available wash your hands or alternatively cleanse with 70% alcohol-based hand rub (in accordance with local policy)	To reduce risk of cross-infection
32 Apply sterile gloves	To reduce risk of cross-infection
33 Cover the areas above and below the cystostomy with sterile towels	To provide a sterile working area
34 Cleanse cystostomy site with 0.9% sodium chloride	To reduce the risk of infection
35 Gently insert the nozzle of the anaesthetic/lubricating gel into the cystostomy and instil the gel according to manufacturer's instructions. Remove the nozzle and discard the syringe appropriately **NB** Extra caution should be taken when using anaesthetic gel because there is a higher risk of systemic absorption via a cystostomy tract (Addison 2000)	Adequate lubrication helps to prevent urethral trauma (Bardsley 2005)
	Use of an anaesthetic gel helps minimise any discomfort that may be experienced by the patient
	Anaesthetic lubricating gel is suggested to reduce the risk of catheter insertion-related urinary tract infection (Kambal *et al*. 2004)

Procedure guideline 13.3 **Guideline for changing a suprapubic catheter** *(cont'd)*

Nursing action	Rationale
36 Wait a minimum of 5 mins before starting the insertion procedure (Dougherty & Lister 2011)	To allow the anaesthetic gel to take effect
37 Introduce the catheter into the cystostomy; a slight resistance may be felt as it passes through the bladder wall	Resistance or pain may indicate that the balloon is in the cystostomy and not the bladder or that the catheter has been pushed into the urethra (Addison 2000)
38 Slowly inflate the balloon, initially with 2.5–3 ml of sterile water, according to the manufacturer's instructions. If resistance to balloon inflation is felt or the patient experiences pain, stop, deflate the balloon, reposition the catheter and re-inflate (Robinson 2008)	To secure the catheter in place To maintain patient safety
39 Gently withdraw the catheter until it is felt against the bladder wall inflate balloon with remaining sterile water (Robinson 2008)	To maintain patient safety
40 Observe for urine drainage into the receiver	To ensure that the catheter is correctly positioned and draining
41 Attach selected drainage system or valve	To facilitate urine collection To promote patient comfort
42 Clean and thoroughly dry the cystostomy area with 0.9% sodium chloride	To prevent secondary infections and skin irritation To promote patient comfort To maintain patient safety
43 Apply dressing to cystostomy area only if a discharge or bleeding is present	To protect the patient's clothing If the cystostomy site is left exposed it aids cleansing as part of normal hygiene routine and the site is easily observed for early detection of any complications
44 Cover exposed area of the patient's body with a blanket/towel	To maintain patient dignity
45 Dispose of all used equipment in accordance with locally agreed infection prevention and control policy	To reduce the risk of cross-infection To maintain the health and safety of self and others
46 Remove and dispose of gloves in accordance with locally agreed infection prevention and control policy	To reduce the risk of cross-infection
47 Cleanse hands with bactericidal alcohol hand rub	To reduce the risk of cross-infection
48 Assist the patient to dress and help into their chosen position, e.g. sitting in chair, open curtains	To maintain patient's dignity and comfort
49 Remove and dispose of apron in accordance with locally agreed infection prevention and control policy	To reduce the risk of cross-infection
50 Where appropriate facilities are available wash your hands or alternatively cleanse with 70% alcohol-based hand rub (in accordance with local policy)	To reduce the risk of cross-infection

(Continued)

*Procedure guideline 13.3 **Guideline for changing a suprapubic catheter** (cont'd)*

Nursing action	Rationale
51 Replace any moved items of furniture to their original position	To maintain a safe environment for the patient by restoring any furniture moved to its usual place
52 Verbally discuss the outcome of the procedure with the patient and where relevant carer, giving further advice as indicated. Where possible this should be supported with written/diagrammatic information	To reinforce verbal information and support patient's understanding
53 The following information should be recorded in the nursing documentation in accordance with local policy and NMC guidelines: (a) date and time of the procedure; (b) rationale for the catheterization; (c) catheter type; (d) length; (e) size; (f) amount of sterile water instilled to inflate the balloon; (g) selected drainage system; (h) batch number; (i) manufacturer; (j) any difficulties experienced during the procedure; (k) review date; (l) date of next catheter change	To maintain patient safety To enable continuity of care To maintain practitioner safety Documentation should provide clear evidence of the care or procedure carried out

Procedure guideline 13.4 **Guideline for collection of a catheter specimen of urine**

Equipment

Sterile single-use gloves
Single-use apron
Swab saturated with isopropyl alcohol 70% x 2
Gate clamp
Sterile syringe and needle
Sharps bin
Universal specimen container (where relevant)
Completed pathology request form (where relevant)

Procedure

Nursing action	Rationale
1 Where appropriate facilities are available wash your hands or alternatively cleanse with 70% alcohol-based hand rub (in accordance with local policy)	To prevent the risk of cross-infection/contamination
2 If the patient is known to the service review nursing documentation and current care plan	To update the nurse's knowledge of the patient To maintain patient safety
3 If the patient is unknown to the service a full assessment should be carried out prior to undertaking the procedure	To maintain patient and practitioner safety

Procedure guideline 13.4 **Guideline for collection of a catheter specimen of urine** *(cont'd)*

Nursing action	Rationale
4 Explain and discuss the procedure with the patient	To ensure that the patient understands the procedure and gives their valid consent
5 Prepare the environment, draw curtains and where necessary obtain patient consent to move furniture	To allow freedom of movement when carrying out the procedure To maintain patient privacy
6 Assemble all equipment on a clean surface; check that (a) all relevant seals and packaging are intact and undamaged, and (b) all relevant equipment is within the recommended date for use	To prevent disruption to the procedure To prevent contamination of equipment To maintain patient safety
7 If no urine is present in the tubing clamp the tubing below the needle sampling port	To obtain an adequate volume of fresh urine for the specimen
8 Cleanse hands with bactericidal alcohol hand rub	To reduce the risk of infection
9 Apply apron and gloves	To reduce the risk of cross-infection/contamination
10 Clean the access port with a swab saturated with 70% isopropyl alcohol and allow to air dry	To reduce risk of cross-infection To prevent contamination of the specimen
11 **Needle sampling port:** insert the needle into the port at an angle of 45° and aspirate the required amount of urine withdraw the needle. Dispose of the needle in sharps bin	To reduce the risk of the needle going straight through the tubing To reduce the risk of a needlestick injury
12 **Needleless sampling port:** insert the syringe firmly into the centre of the needleless port (following the manufacturer's instructions). Aspirate the required amount of urine and disconnect the syringe	To obtain the specimen
13 Place the specimen in a sterile container. Dispose of used syringe in accordance with locally agreed infection prevention and control policy	To prevent contamination of the specimen To ensure safe transportation of the specimen To comply with health and safety regulations
14 Unclamp tubing if necessary	To allow drainage of urine to continue To ensure patient comfort
15 Re-clean the access port with a swab saturated with 70% isopropyl alcohol	To reduce the risk of contamination of the access port To reduce the risk of cross-infection
16 Dispose of all used equipment in accordance with locally agreed infection prevention and control policy	To reduce the risk of cross-infection To maintain the health and safety of self and others
17 Remove and dispose of apron and gloves in accordance with locally agreed infection prevention and control policy	To reduce the risk of cross-infection
18 Where appropriate facilities are available wash your hands or alternatively cleanse with 70% alcohol-based hand rub (in accordance with local policy)	To prevent the risk of cross-infection/contamination

(Continued)

Procedure guideline 13.4 **Guideline for collection of a catheter specimen of urine** *(cont'd)*

Nursing action	Rationale
19 If required assist the patient to adjust their position	To maintain patient's dignity and comfort
20 Label the container clearly with the required patient information and dispatch it with the completed request form to the laboratory (in accordance with local policy/guideline) as soon as possible after sample is taken Complete relevant details on pathology form, e.g. date, time	To ensure that the correct results are received for the correct patient To maintain patient safety To facilitate more accurate results from culture
21 Document the date and time the sample was taken in the patient nursing documentation	To maintain patient safety To enable continuity of care To maintain practitioner safety Documentation should provide clear evidence of the care or procedure carried out

Procedure guideline 13.5 **Guideline for administering a catheter maintenance solution**

Equipment

Sterile dressing pack
Sterile single-use gloves
Non-sterile single-use gloves
Single-use waterproof protective pad, e.g. incontinence pad or similar
Single-use apron
Bactericidal alcohol rub
Absorbent sheet
Prescribed pre-packaged catheter maintenance solution
Administration chart/record
Jug
Lotion thermometer
Sterile drainage bag/catheter valve

Nursing action	Rationale
1 Where appropriate facilities are available wash your hands or alternatively cleanse with 70% alcohol-based hand rub (in accordance with local policy)	To prevent the risk of cross-infection/contamination
2 If the patient is known to the service review nursing documentation and current care plan	To update the nurse's knowledge of the patient To maintain patient safety

Procedure guideline 13.5 **Guideline for administering a catheter maintenance solution** *(cont'd)*

Nursing action	Rationale
3 If the patient is unknown to the service a full assessment should be carried out prior to undertaking the procedure	To maintain patient and practitioner safety
4 Explain and discuss the procedure with the patient	To ensure that the patient understands the procedure and gives their valid consent
5 Prepare the environment, draw curtains and where necessary obtain patient consent to move furniture	To allow freedom of movement when carrying out the procedure To maintain patient privacy
6 Assemble all equipment on a clean surface; check that (a) all relevant seals and packaging are intact and undamaged, and (b) all relevant equipment is within the recommended date for use	To prevent disruption to the procedure To prevent contamination of equipment To maintain patient safety
7 Protect the bed with an appropriate disposable, waterproof underpad	To protect mattress and bedding from soiling
8 Apply disposable plastic apron	To prevent the risk of cross-infection/contamination
9 Where indicated offer the patient assistance with removing all clothing below the waist	To expose the appropriate area
10 Assist the patient into the supine position cover the exposed area of the body with a towel/blanket	To allow easy access to the catheter. To maintain the patient's dignity and comfort
11 Place the maintenance solution container into a jug of warm water and heat to 38°C (use lotion thermometer to confirm water temperature)	To maintain patient comfort To maintain patient safety
12 Cleanse hands with bactericidal alcohol hand rub	To reduce the risk of infection
13 Apply non-sterile gloves and empty catheter bag; place on the bed next to the patient, or if the patient is using a catheter valve ask them to empty their bladder	To reduce the risk of cross-infection To prepare for procedure To aid patient comfort To prepare bladder and catheter for instillation of the catheter maintenance solution
14 Open sterile pack and prepare all equipment on the sterile field, using an aseptic technique	To maintain patient safety by reducing the risk of introducing micro-organisms into bladder. To prevent disruption to the procedure
15 Remove and dispose of gloves in accordance with locally agreed infection prevention and control policy	To reduce the risk of cross-infection
16 Where appropriate facilities are available wash your hands or alternatively cleanse with 70% alcohol-based hand rub (in accordance with local policy)	To reduce the risk of cross-infection/contamination
17 Remove cover that is maintaining patient privacy and place disposable waterproof pad under patient's buttocks and thighs	To ensure patient bedding does not become soiled

327

(Continued)

Procedure guideline 13.5 **Guideline for administering a catheter maintenance solution** *(cont'd)*

Nursing action	Rationale
18 Clean hands with bactericidal alcohol hand rub	Handling outer packs and/or cover may have contaminated hands
19 Apply sterile gloves	To maintain patient safety by reducing the risk of introducing micro-organisms into bladder
	To reduce the risk of cross-infection/contamination
20 Close the clamp on the maintenance solution container tubing, remove security ring on solution container connection port and loosen cover from the connection port	To prepare equipment
	To prevent leakage of solution when connection port is opened
21 Gently squeeze the end of the catheter just above the connection to drainage bag/valve and disconnect. While maintaining pressure on the catheter remove the cover from the connection port on the maintenance solution container and connect it to the catheter; release the pressure on the catheter end	To prevent urine leaking from the catheter
	To prepare for instillation of maintenance solution
22 Open the clamp on the solution container, raise the bag slightly above the level of the bladder and allow the required amount of solution to flow into the bladder. Gentle pressure may be needed initially to start the flow	Rapid instillation of the solution could be uncomfortable for the patient
23 If the solution is to be retained for a period of time, close the clamp on the solution container tubing and place container beside the patient at the level of the bladder	To allow the solution time to act on the bladder/catheter as prescribed
	To reduce the risk of backflow
Re-cover the patient and ensure they are comfortable	To maintain the patient's dignity and comfort
24 When the solution is to be drained, place the container below the level of the bladder open the tubing clamp and allow the solution to drain	To enable gravity to aid drainage
25 When all of the solution has drained out of the bladder close the clamp on the solution tubing, gently squeeze the catheter just above the connection to the solution container. As the solution container is disconnected attach the new drainage bag/catheter valve	To prevent spillage of solution
	To reestablish closed drainage system
	To maintain patient safety
	To maintain patient comfort
26 Cover exposed area of the patient's body with a blanket/towel	To maintain patient dignity
27 Dispose of all used equipment in accordance with locally agreed infection prevention and control policy	To reduce the risk of cross-infection
	To maintain the health and safety of self and others
28 Remove and dispose of gloves in accordance with locally agreed infection prevention and control policy	To reduce the risk of cross-infection
29 Cleanse hands with bactericidal alcohol hand rub	To reduce the risk of infection

Procedure guideline 13.5 **Guideline for administering a catheter maintenance solution** *(cont'd)*

Nursing action	Rationale
30 Where required assist the patient to dress and help into their chosen position, e.g. sitting in chair, open curtains	To maintain patient's dignity and comfort
31 Remove and dispose of apron in accordance with locally agreed infection prevention and control policy	To reduce the risk of cross-infection
32 Where appropriate facilities are available wash your hands or alternatively cleanse with 70% alcohol-based hand rub (in accordance with local policy)	To reduce the risk of cross-infection
33 Replace any moved items of furniture to their original position	To maintain a safe environment for the patient by restoring any furniture moved to its usual place
34 Document the type, batch number and expiry date of catheter maintenance solution administered in the nursing documentation. Also where appropriate record the length of time the maintenance solution was left in situ prior to draining and any complications or problems encountered with the procedure	To maintain patient safety To enable continuity of care To maintain practitioner safety Documentation should provide clear evidence of the care or procedure carried out

Problem solving Table 13.1

Problem	Possible cause	Suggested action
Infection	Poor aseptic technique used during catheterisation Inadequate cleansing or urethral meatus Contamination of catheter tip Breaking closed drainage system Poor techniques used when obtaining urine sample Inappropriate use of bladder maintenance solutions	Obtain a catheter sample of urine Inform GP Review catheter care
No drainage of urine	Incorrect identification of external urethral meatus (female patient)	Check that the catheter has been sited correctly. If the catheter has been inserted in the vagina leave in position to act as a guide, re-identify the urethra and catheterise the patient. Remove the inappropriately placed catheter
	Empty bladder	When changing the catheter, clamp the catheter for 30 mins before the procedure. On insertion of new catheter, urine will drain
	Blocked catheter	Check that tubing is not kinked Check for constipation as pressure on the urethra can block the catheter Check that drainage system is below level of bladder Check tubing not blocked (see below)

(Continued)

Problem solving table 13.1 (cont'd)

Problem	Possible cause	Suggested action
Leakage of urine around catheter (bypassing)	Catheter blocked by encrustations	Use catheter maintenance solutions
		Replace catheter
	Catheter blocked non-encrustations	Raise the level of drainage bag above the level of the bladder to reduce hydrostatic suction and free mucosa from eye of catheter. Flush catheter gently with 20–30 ml 0.9% sodium chloride
	Twisted tubing	Change position
		Unkink tubing
	Bladder spasm due to incorrect size of catheter	Replace with correct size catheter, this would usually be a minimum of 2 ch smaller than the catheter in situ
	Bladder spasm due to large catheter balloon	Replace with catheter with a 10 ml balloon
	Bladder spasm due to hyperirritability	Consider anticholinergic drugs or muscle relaxant
Urethral discomfort	Mechanical distention due to large-gauge catheter	Re-catheterise with smaller gauge catheter
Paraphimosis	Failure to reposition foreskin after catheterisation or catheter toilet	Inform GP
		Always reposition the foreskin
Formation of crusts around urethral meatus	Increased urethral secretions due to irritation of urothelium by the catheter collect at the meatus and form crust	Correct catheter toilet
Unable to deflate balloon	Faulty syringe used to deflate balloon	Replace syringe
	Valve expansion, valve displacement	Use needle and syringe, insert needle in inflation arm just above the valve and aspirate
	Encrustation around balloon will not allow it to deflate	Use catheter maintenance solution to dissolve encrustations
	Inflation channel blocked	Unkink catheter, insert another 2 ml of sterile water to dislodge obstruction **do not** attempt to fill the balloon until it bursts inside the bladder as fragments may be left in the bladder andl may lead to trauma, irritation and infection (Rew & Woodward 2001)

References and further reading

Addison R (2000) Risk assessment in suprapubic catheterisation. *Nursing Standard* 14(36): 1–13.

Addison R, Mould C (2000) Risk assessment in suprapubic catheterization. *Nursing Standard* 14(36): 43–6.

Association for Continence Advice (2003) *Notes on Good Practice*. Association for Continence Advice, London.

Bakke A, Malt UF (1993) Social functioning and general well being in patients treated with clean intermittent catheterization. *Journal of Psychosomatic Research* 37(4): 371–80.

Bakke A, Digranes A, Hoisaeter PA (1997) Physical predictors of infection in patients treated with clean intermittent catheterisations: a prospective 7-year study. *British Journal of Urology* 79(1): 85–90.

Bardsley A (2005) Use of lubricating gels in urinary catheterisation. *Nursing Standard* 20(8): 41–6.

Bennett E (2002) Intermittent self-catheterisation and the female patient. *Nursing Standard* 30(17): 37–42

British National Formulary 60 (2010) BMJ Publishing Group, London.

Brosnahan J, Jull A, Tracey C (2004) Types of urethral catheters for management of short-term voiding problems in hospitalised adults. *Cochrane Database Systematic Review* (1): CD004013.

Chai T, Chung AK, Belville WD, Faerber GJ (1995) Compliance and complications of clean intermittent catheterisation in the spinal cord-injured patient. *Paraplegia* 33(3) 161–3.

Colley W (1998) Catheter care 1. *Nursing Times* 94(23) insert.

Colpman D, Welford K (2004) *Urinary Drainage Systems In Urological Nursing* (3e). Baillière Tindall, London.

Crow R, Mulhall A, Chapman R (1988) Indwelling catheterisation and related nursing practice. *Journal of Advanced Nursing* 13(4): 489–95.

Dougherty L, Lister S (2008) *The Royal Marsden Hospital Manual of Clinical Nursing Procedures* (7e). Wiley-Blackwell, Oxford.

Dougherty L, Lister S (2011) *The Royal Marsden Hospital Manual of Clinical Nursing Procedures, Student Edition* (8e). Wiley-Blackwell, Oxford.

Fader M, Petterson-Brooks R, Dean G (1997) A multicentre comparative evaluation of catheter valves. *British Journal of Nursing* 6(7): 359–67.

Getliffe K (1996) Care of urinary catheters. *Nursing Standard* 11(11): 47–54.

Getliffe K (2002) Managing recurrent urinary catheter encrustation. *British Journal of Community Nursing* 7(11): 574–80.

Getliffe K (2003a) Catheters and catheterizations. In Getliffe K, Dolmen M (eds) *Promoting Continence: a clinical and research resource*. Baillière Tindall, London.

Getliffe K (2003b) Continence care: managing recurrent urinary catheter blockage: problems, promises and practicalities. *Journal of Wound, Ostomy and Continence Nursing* 30(3): 146–51.

Getliffe K, Dolman M (2003) *Promoting Continence: a clinical research resource* (2e). Baillière Tindall, London.

Getliffe K, Hughes FC, Le Claire M (2000) The dissolution of urinary catheter encrustation. *British Journal of Urology* 85(1): 60–4.

Godfrey H, Evans A (2000) Management of long-term catheters: minimising complications. *British Journal of Nursing* 9(2): 74–81.

Godfrey H, Fraczyk L (2005) Preventing and managing catheter-associated urinary tract infections. *British Journal of Community Nursing* 10(5): 205–12.

Gould D (1994) Keeping on tract. *Nursing Times* 90(40): 58–64.

Jenkins SC (1998) Digital guidance of female urethral catheterisation. *British Journal of Urology* 82(4): 589–9.

Kambal C, Chance J, Cope S, Beck J (2004) Catheter associated UTIs in patients after major gynaecological surgery. *Professional Nurse* 19(9): 515–18.

Koleilat N, Sidi AA, Gonzalez R (1989) Urethral false passage as a complication of intermittent catheterization. *Journal of Urology* 142(5): 1216–17.

Lapides J, Diokno AC, Silber SM, Lowe BS (2002) Clean, intermittent self-catheterization in the treatment of urinary tract disease. *Journal of Urology* 167(4): 1584–6.

Leaver RB (2004) Reconstructive surgery for urinary incontinence. In: Fillingham S, Douglas J (eds) *Urological Nursing* (3e). Baillière Tindall, London.

Leaver RB (2007) The evidence for urethral meatal cleansing. *Nursing Standard* 21(41): 39–42.

Leaver R, Pressland D (2001) Intermittent self-catheterisation in urinary tract reconstruction. *British Journal of Community Nursing* 6(5): 253–8.

Liedl B (2001) Catheter-associated urinary tract infections. *Current Opinions in Urology* 11(1): 75–9.

Mackenzie J, Webb C (1995) Gynopia in nursing practice: the case of urethral catheterization. *Journal of Clinical Nursing* 4: 221–6.

Madeo M, Roodhouse AJ (2009) Reducing the risks associated with urinary catheters. *Nursing Standard* 23(29): 47–55.

Milligan F (1999) Male sexuality and urethral catheterisations; a review of the literature. *Nursing Standard* 13(38): 43–7.

Mulhall AB, Chapman RG, Crow RA (1988) Bacteriuria during indwelling urethral catheterization. *Journal of Hospital Infection* 11(3): 253–62.

Nacey JN, Delahunt B (1991) Toxicity study of first and second generation hydrogel-coated latex catheters. *British Journal of Urology* 67: 314–16.

National Institute for Clinical Excellence (2003) *Prevention of Healthcare-associated Infection in Primary and Community Care, Section 3, Urinary Catheterisation*. NICE, London.

National Patient Safety Agency (2009a) *Rapid response report, NPSA/2009/RRR02; Female urinary catheters causing trauma to adult males*. NPSA, London.

National Patient Safety Agency (2009b) *Rapid response report, NPSA/2009/RRR005; Minimising risks of suprapubic catheter insertion (adults only)*. NPSA, London.

Neil-Weise BS, Arend Van der SM, Broek PS (2002) Efficacy of antimicrobial impregnated catheter associated catheters in reducing catheter associated bacteriuria: a prospective, randomised, multicentre clinical trial. *Journal of Hospital Infection* 52(2): 81–7.

Nursing and Midwifery Council (2007) *The Mental Capacity Act, 2005; Code of practice advice sheet*. The Stationery Office, London.

Nursing and Midwifery Council (2008) *The Code: standards for conduct, performance and ethics for nurses and midwives*. NMC, London.

O'Donohue D, Winsor G, Gallagher R *et al.* (2010) Issues for people living with long-term urinary catheters in the community. *British Journal of Community Nursing* **15**(2): 65–70'

Pellowe CM, Pratt RJ, Loveday HP *et al.* (2004) The epic project. Updating the evidence-base for national evidence based guidelines for preventing healthcare-associated infections in NHS hospitals in England: a report with recommendations. *British Journal of Infection Control* **5**(6): 10–16.

Pomfret IJ (1996) Catheters: design, selection and management. *British Journal of Nursing* **5**(4): 245–51.

Pomfret I (2000a) Urinary catheters: selection, management and prevention of infection. *British Journal of Community Nursing* **5**(1): 6–13.

Pomfret I (2000b) Catheter care in the community. *Nursing Standard* **14**(27): 46–52.

Pomfret I, Tew LE (2004) Urinary catheters and associated urinary tract infections. *Journal of Community Nursing* **18**(9): 15–19.

Pratt RJ, Pellowe C, Loveday NP, Robinson N (2001) Guidelines for preventing infections associated with the insertion and maintenance of short-term indwelling urethral catheters in acute care. *Journal of Hospital Infection* **47**(Suppl): S39–S46.

Pratt RJ, Pellowe CM, Wilson JA (2007) Epic 2; national evidence based guidelines for preventing healthcare associated infections in NHS hospitals in England. *Journal of Hospital Infection* **65**(Suppl 1): S1–64.

Rew M (1999) Use of catheter maintenance solutions for long-term catheters. *British Journal of Nursing* **8**(11): 708–15.

Rew M (2005) Caring for catheterised patients. *British Journal of Nursing* **14**(2): 87–92.

Rew M, Woodward S (2001) Troubleshooting common problems associated with long-term catheters. *British Journal of Nursing* **10**(12): 764–74.

Robinson J (2001) Urethral catheter selection. *Nursing Standard* **25**(15): 39–42.

Robinson J (2005) Suprapubic catheterisation: challenges in changing catheters, *British Journal of Community Nursing* **10**(10): 461–4.

Robinson J (2006) Selecting a urinary catheter and drainage system. *British Journal of Nursing* **15**(19): 1045–50.

Robinson J (2008) Insertion, care and management of suprapubic catheters. *Nursing Standard* **23**(8): 49–56.

Robinson J (2009) Urinary catheterisation: assessing the best options. *Nursing Standard* **23**(29): 40–5.

Royal College of Nursing (2008) *Catheter Care, Guidelines for Nurses*. RCN, London.

Ryan-Woolley B (1987) *Urinary catheters, aids for the management of incontinence*. King's Fund Project Paper No 65. King Fund, London.

Saint R, Lipsky BA (1999) Preventing catheter-associated bacteriuria. Should we? Can we? How? *Archives of Internal Medicine* **159**: 800–8.

Saint S, Elimore JG, Sullivan SD *et al.* (1998) The efficacy of silver alloy-coated urinary catheters in preventing urinary tract infection: a meta-analysis. *American Journal of Medicine* **105**(3): 236–41.

Saye DE (2007) Recurring and antimicrobial resistant infections: considering the potential role of biofilms in clinical practice. *Ostomy/Wound Management* **53**(4): 46–52.

Simpson L (2001) Indwelling urethral catheters. *Nursing Standard* **15**(46): 47–54, 56.

Slade N, Gillespie WA (1987) *The Urinary Tract and the Catheter: infection and other problems*. John Wiley, Chichester.

Stickler D, Hughes G (1999) Ability of Proteus mirabilis to swarm over urethral catheters. *European Journal of Clinical Microbiology and Infectious Diseases* **18**(3): 206–8.

Tanabe P, Steinmann R, Anderson J *et al.* (2004) Factors affecting pain scores during female urethral catheterization. *Academic Emergency Medicine* **11**(6): 703–6.

Tew L, Pomfret I, King D (2005) Infection risks associated with urinary catheters. *Nursing Standard* **20**(7): 55–61.

Tortora GA & Grabowski SR (2002) *Principles of Anatomy and Physiology*. John Wiley and Sons, New York.

Vaidyanathan S, Soni BM, Dundas S, Krishnan KR (1994) Urethral cytology in spinal cord injury patients performing intermittent catheterization. *Paraplegia* **32**(7): 493–500.

Vaidyanathan S, Krishnan KR, Soni BM, Fraser MH (1996) Unusual complications of intermittent self-catheterisation in spinal cord injury patients. *Spinal Cord* **34**(12): 745–7.

Webb RJ, Lawson AL, Neal DE (1990) Clean intermittent self-catheterisation in 172 adults. *British Journal of Urology* **65**(1): 20–3.

Wilson J (1997) Control and prevention of infection in catheter care. *Community Nurse* **3**(5): 39–40.

Wilson LA (2005) Urinalysis. *Nursing Standard* **19**(35): 51–4.

Wilson M, Coates D (1996) Infection control and urine drainage bag design. *Professional Nurse* **11**(4): 245–52.

Winn C (1998) Complications with urinary catheters. *Professional Nurse Study Supplement* **13**(5): S7–10.

Woodward S (2005) Use of lubricant in female urethral catheterization. *British Journal of Nursing* **14**(19): 1022–3.

Woollons S (1996) Urinary catheterisation for long-term use. *Professional Nurse* **11**(12): 825–32.

Venepuncture

Introduction

Venepuncture (puncture of a vein) is the act of inserting a needle through the skin into a vein for the purposes of obtaining a specimen of blood or to establish venous access (McCall & Tankersley 2008; Scales 2008).

Indications

Venepuncture can be performed to:

- obtain blood samples for diagnostic purposes
- monitor levels of blood components.

(Dimech *et al.* 2011)

Background evidence

Venepuncture is the most commonly performed invasive procedure and has now become a procedure regularly undertaken by nurses in both hospitals and the community. Hospital nurses became more involved in venepuncture in response to the reduction of junior doctors' hours (Inwood 1996). While this procedure has been performed in the community for a number of years, there has been an increase in the number of community nurses performing venepuncture in response to the General Practitioner General Medical Service's (GP GMS) contracts, commissioning and long-term conditions management. The advantages of providing this service in the community include:

- reducing the need for a patient to visit the hospital or GP
- time efficient
- offering a more holistic approach to care.

The main disadvantage is the lack of immediate access to more experienced colleagues in the event of problems. It must be remembered that venepuncture is a procedure not without complications and should only be undertaken by community nurses who have received both theoretical and practical training (Dimech *et al.* 2011).

Education and training

Any nurse wishing to undertake venepuncture should receive theoretical training in the following aspects of venepuncture:

- anatomy and physiology of the peripheral venous system
- selection of a vein
- selection of equipment
- infection control issues
- health and safety/risk management
- patient's perspective
- use of pharmacological and non-pharmacological methods of reducing anxiety and pain
- how to recognise, minimise and manage complications
- legal and professional/accountability issues.

(Inwood 1996; RCN 2010)

This knowledge can be gained by use of distance learning packs and/or attendance at a study day (Collins *et al.* 2006: Phillips 2011). The practitioner must also undergo a period of supervised practice. This should then be followed by an assessment of:

- practical skills using a competency framework
- knowledge, using a role development workbook, for example, which can facilitate transferability of skills and knowledge (RCN 2010; Phillips 2011).

District Nursing Manual of Clinical Procedures, First Edition. Edited by Liz O'Brien.
© 2012 Blackwell Publishing Ltd. Published 2012 by Blackwell Publishing Ltd.

Anatomy and physiology

The venous system can be divided into deep and superficial veins (Collins 2011). The superficial veins are used for venepuncture because their position enables them to be easily visualised and palpated, therefore making access more likely. The veins usually selected are those of the lower arm and antecubital fossa. Veins of the feet are contraindicated except in children, but may be used by community nurses who are experienced as a last resort for obtaining blood (Weinstein 2007).

There are three layers to the vein:

1 tunica intima
2 tunica media
3 tunica adventitia.

The tunica intima is made up of a single layer of epithelial cells and this layer maintains the blood within the vessel (Hadaway 2010). Any damage done to the intima can result in blood leakage into the tissues. This is more likely to occur when patients are on anticoagulants or are thrombocytopenic (Dimech *et al.* 2011). This is due to the delayed healing of the epithelium making the patient more prone to bruising. It is within this layer that small folds of epithelium are found – these semi-lunar folds are called valves, and by opening and closing momentarily as the blood moves through, help to maintain blood flow back to the heart (Hadaway 2010). Valves can be identified by a small visible bulge within the vessel or can be palpated (Dougherty 2008). They always occur at junctions or at a bifurcation and can affect the venepuncture process by closing when a needle comes into contact with them, thereby preventing blood withdrawal (Hadaway 2010). If the needle goes through a valve the patient will feel pain and this could also result in a through puncture. Therefore valves should be avoided, and if identified, the needle should be inserted just above or a few centimetres below the valve (Dougherty 2008; McCall & Tankersley 2008; Collins 2011; Dimech *et al.* 2011).

The tunica media is the middle layer and is made up of smooth muscle and some elastic fibres (Hadaway 2010). These muscles control constriction and relaxation, and therefore stimuli by trauma or changes in temperature and pressure can lead to venous spasm (Hadaway 2010). It is this layer that is affected if a patient is dehydrated, has low blood pressure or is cold, as it results in collapse of the vein thereby making venepuncture more difficult (Dougherty 2008; McCall & Tankersley 2008; Collins 2001; Dimech *et al.* 2011).

The tunica adventitia is the outer layer and is made up of connective tissue, which surrounds and supports the vessel (Dougherty 2008; McCall & Tankersley 2008; Collins 2001; Dimech *et al.* 2011).

The skin is made up of two layers – the dermis and epidermis. The thickness of the epidermis varies with age and in the older person is very thin and friable; this, combined with the lack of subcutaneous tissue, results in poorly supported vessels (Witt 2011). The dermis is the layer containing the nerves and is sensitive to pressure, temperature and pain (Dimech *et al.* 2011).

The main veins for venepuncture are located in an area of the arm that is anterior to and below the bend of the elbow known as the antecubital fossa (McCall & Tankersley 2008). Within this area are the three median veins. These lie close to the surface making them easy to locate and penetrate with a needle. The first choice for venepuncture is the median cubital vein (*see* Figure 14.1). Ernst (2005) lists four reasons for its suitability for venepuncture:

- *proximity* – closest to the skin and therefore readily accessible
- *immobility* – well supported making venepuncture more successful
- *safety* – puncture poses the least risk to injuring underlying structures
- *comfort* – less discomfort when punctured.

The median cephalic vein (on the radial side crosses in front of the brachial artery) is the second choice, and although harder to palpate, it is fairly well supported by subcutaneous tissue. The third choice is the median basilic vein (ulnar side) (Figure 14.1), which is easy to palpate. However, it is not as well supported by subcutaneous tissue and therefore can roll away from the needle and bruise more easily. Care should be taken as the brachial artery and median nerves lie in close proximity (Ernst 2005; McCall & Tankersley 2008).

Other veins that can be utilised for venepuncture include the following.

- *The metacarpal veins.* They are found on the dorsum of the hand and are formed by the union of the digital veins between the knuckles. They form an arch known as the dorsal venous arch. They are usually easily accessible, but insertion may be painful due to increased nerve endings. Blood flow may also be slower and they are prone to bruising if inadequate pressure is applied on removal of the needle (Hadaway 2010; Dimech *et al.* 2011).
- *The cephalic vein.* This runs along the radial bone (Figure 14.1). It is a large vein and ideal for venepuncture. It is usually visible, straight, can be easily stabilised and has a large lumen. However, the radial artery and nerve lie in close proximity to the vein.

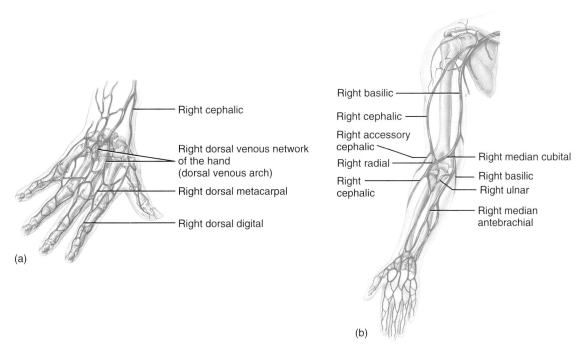

Figure 14.1 (a) Posterior view of superficial veins of the hand. (b) Anterior view of superficial veins. (From Tortora & Derrickson 2009, used with permission)

- *The basilic vein (Figure 14.1).* This runs along the ulnar side of the forearm and has a large lumen. However, it is difficult to position the patient comfortably, awkward to stabilise the vein and often has many valves. It also bruises easily.
- *The digital veins.* These are found along the lateral and distal portions of the fingers. Although they are small they can be used if no other veins are accessible, but they should only be accessed by community nurses experienced in venepuncture.

(Weinstein 2007; Witt 2011)

Selecting a vein

There are two main techniques when selecting a vein:

- inspection
- palpation (Witt 2011).

An inspection is performed on the arms to observe for things such as bruising, phlebitis, multiple punctures, areas of infection, etc. This enables the practitioner to disregard certain areas which are not suitable for venepuncture (Dougherty 2008; Perucca 2010).

Palpation is performed by placing one or two fingers over the vein then pressing lightly, so that on release of the pressure, the elasticity and rebound filling can be assessed. It should be done using the index finger and third forefinger of the non-dominant hand. The thumb should not be used because it has a pulse and is not as sensitive (Dougherty 2008; Perucca 2010; Dimech *et al.* 2011).

Palpation must always be performed before venepuncture in order to ascertain the following:

- the quality and condition of the vein (thrombosed veins may be detected by a lack of resilience and a hard cord-like feeling (Table 14.1)
- depth and direction of the vein
- to identify and avoid valves
- to ascertain if it is an artery (arteries pulsate, veins do not).

(Dougherty 2008; Perucca 2010; Witt 2011)

335

Table 14.1 Characteristics of suitable and unsuitable veins

A suitable vein is one that is	An unsuitable vein is one that is
Bouncy	Hard – this indicates a scarred vein that will not yield blood and may be painful when the needle is inserted
Soft	Thrombosed
Refills after being compressed – indicates that there is good blood flow and the vein is healthy	Thin – makes it difficult to access the vessel and flow may be poor
Visible – especially when a new practitioner is performing procedure as this makes venepuncture easier	Fragile – vein will become easily damaged
Straight	Has undergone multiple punctures – will result in pain for the patient
Has a large lumen	Near any bony prominences, or if infection and/or phlebitis is present – as this could result in pain and further infection
Well supported – the support from the surrounding subcutaneous tissue prevents the vein moving on insertion of the needle	Bruised – will result in pain for patient and may not yield any blood
	Tortuous – harder to access
	Mobile – harder to access and may result in bruising

Improving venous access

There are a number of methods for improving venous access.

Use of a tourniquet

The tourniquet is the key to successful venepuncture (Garza & Becan-McBride 2010) because applying it promotes venous distension. The tourniquet should be placed 3–5 inches above the intended site of venepuncture (Perucca 2010). The distance of the tourniquet from the vein is important, because if it is applied too close, the vein may collapse as blood is withdrawn and if it is too far, it may be ineffective. The tourniquet should be applied and tightened so that the degree of tightness is sufficient to achieve venous filling but not too tight so that it impedes arterial flow (identified by discoloration of the limb and tingling in patient's hand and arm). It can also be applied over a layer of clothing if there is a chance of causing injury or bruising of the skin, e.g. in older people and those on anticoagulants or who have low platelet counts (Dougherty 2008). The patient may also indicate how tight the tourniquet can be pulled. The tourniquet should not remain tightened for longer than 1–2 min, otherwise venous spasm can occur, which makes locating the vein more difficult. It may also result in ecchymosis, and can cause in changes to certain blood levels, such as calcium and potassium, leading to inaccurate blood results (McCall

& Tankersley 2008; Garza & Becan-McBride 2010). There are also certain tests where it is recommended that blood is taken without the use of a tourniquet, e.g. calcitonin (refer to local laboratory guidelines).

Ideally the tourniquet should have a wide elastic strap to prevent pinching of the patient's skin. A variety of tourniquets are available (although a blood pressure cuff may also be used).

- Velcro tourniquets are useful, because they are easy to clean and apply, but they may not fit all arms well enough to achieve good venous filling (Garza & Becan-McBride 2010).
- Quick-release tourniquets allow release of venous pressure and the ability to tighten with one hand. This is helpful as the nurse can release the pressure during the procedure and retighten it without releasing hold of the venepuncture equipment. This may be necessary as prolonged pressure can result in inaccurate blood results. They are usually comfortable and achieve a good fit but have been associated with an increased risk of cross-infection because they are difficult to clean and decontaminate (Golder 2000).

Some tourniquets can be autoclaved or one can be labelled and left with an individual patient, which may be more suitable in the community if a patient requires repeated venepuncture (Lavery & Ingram 2005; Garza & Becan-McBride 2010). There is now a move to use single-use disposable tourniquets due to the risk of cross-contamination, although this does have cost implications (Franklin *et al.* 2007; Garza & Becan-McBride 2010; RCN 2010).

Gravity

The act of lowering the limb below the level of the heart increases the blood supply and can help to aid venous filling (Weinstein 2007).

Opening and closing the fist

Asking the patient to open and close their fist a few times also aids venous filling. However, patients should not be encouraged to vigorously pump as it causes haemoconcentration leading to erroneous test results (McCall & Tankersley 2008).

Gentle tapping or stroking

This can aid venous filling, but 'slapping' or vigorous tapping can result in venous spasm, discomfort for the patient and, in some cases, bruising of the vessel before venepuncture has even been performed (Springhouse 2002).

Heat

This is an effective method for improving venous access. The patient can place their arm into a bowl or sink of warm water for approximately 5 min following assessment of veins and prior to performing the procedure. To prevent scalding, the temperature of the water must be checked with the patient before the arm is submerged (Lenhardt *et al.* 2002: Dougherty 2008; Dimech *et al.* 2011; Witt 2011).

GTN patch/gel (glycerol trinitrate)

A number of studies have shown the benefit of using GTN to aid venous filling. GTN can be applied as a patch or gel to increase vasodilatation, which results in improved accessibility of a vein. However, this must be prescribed by the patient's GP prior to use and needs to be applied for 10–15 min prior to venepuncture. Patients may suffer from side effects, although these are usually only headaches, which resolve on removal of the GTN patch/gel (Hecker *et al.* 1983; Michael & Andrew 1996; BNF 2011).

Issues that influence venous access

There are a number of considerations that can influence the success of the procedure. Assessment and knowledge of the patient will help the community nurse in ascertaining these and aid in decision making about vein selection.

Age of the patient

The young and older people have similar veins, in that they are often small and thin. In the case of older people, they also have more friable skin with little subcutaneous support that makes the veins more mobile and also more likely to bruise. Older people may also have a more sluggish venous circulation that can result in a slow venous return and distension, making blood sampling difficult (Witt 2011).

Nutritional status

Patients who are malnourished often have very obvious veins, but again there is little subcutaneous tissue and therefore little support. The veins may also be friable. Patients who are obese may have healthy veins, but they are often deep and difficult to palpate, and in this group of patients the most accessible veins are those found in the antecubital fossa or the metacarpal veins (Dimech *et al.* 2011).

Medical history

Reduced venous access will occur in those who have had:

- an amputation
- lymphoedema
- a cerebrovascular accident (CVA) as the affected limb will have reduced muscle tone and venous circulation and so the non-affected limb should be used
- a mastectomy (the arm on the side of the unaffected breast should be used)
- some surgical procedures or the presence of a haemodialysis shunt.

(Lavery & Ingram 2005; Dougherty 2008; Witt 2011)

Prescribed medication

Patients who are on anticoagulants or long-term steroids will have more fragile veins, be more prone to bruising and require longer application of pressure following removal of the needle to ensure that bleeding has stopped (Dougherty 2008).

Physical condition of the patient

Patients who are dehydrated, in shock or hypothermic will all have poor peripheral venous circulation making the process of finding a vein more difficult. This can lead to a sluggish blood flow, resulting in inadequate blood samples (Dimech *et al.* 2011).

Skill of the practitioner

It has been well documented that the skill of the practitioner can have an impact on the whole procedure and that skilled practitioners have been found to cause less pain and anxiety in patients (Ernst 2005; Dougherty 2008; Dimech *et al.* 2011). There may be no problems with a patient's veins, but if the practitioner does not appear to be confident and competent the patient may become anxious and this is turn will result in reduced venous circulation and accessible veins (Dougherty 1994).

Selection of equipment

Blood collection systems

There are a number of different devices available for obtaining blood samples (Table 14.2). Nevertheless, the selection of the needle and system must be based on the needs of the patient, number of samples required, the size and location of the vein, and the experience of the practitioner (Dougherty 2008; Dimech *et al.* 2011). All blood collection needles come in a range of gauge sizes and lengths, and are sterile, disposable and designed for single use only (Garza & Becan-McBride 2010). The commonest system used in most hospitals and community settings is the vacuum blood collection system. This system consists of a plastic holder that contains or is attached to a sterile disposable double-ended needle. One needle is inserted into the patient and the other is covered in a rubber sheath and sits within the plastic holder. Once the needle is in the vein, the rubber topped lid of the blood sample bottle is pushed on to the needle within the holder and the rubber sheath covering the shaft of the needle is forced back, allowing blood to flow into the blood sample bottle (Dojcinovska 2011). Whichever system is used, the community nurse must be confident and competent in its use (NMC 2008b; Hyde 2011).

Unless it contains a safety activation needle, the needle and syringe is no longer a recommended method of obtaining blood samples due to its high risk of blood contamination and needlestick injury (Garza & Becan-McBride 2010). Therefore nurses who are not familiar with other systems should gain further training before using them (Dojcinovska 2011). This will enable them to always use the safest methods for venepuncture. They should also make a case for the provision of safety systems to further reduce the risk of needlestick injury (NHS Employers 2007; EU Directive 2010; RCN 2010).

Blood bottles

Blood bottles are available in different sizes, require different volumes and can be purchased in glass or unbreakable plastic (Garza & Becan-McBride 2010). Colour-coding of the bottle tops indicates the presence and type of additives. All bottles have expiry dates and it is important that these are checked, because if they have expired this can affect either the vacuum or the results of the tests (McCall & Tankersley 2008). The type of bottle used for certain tests may differ depending on the needs of the laboratory; an example guide can be found in Table 14.3, but this may vary between laboratories. It is important to fill bottles to the allotted line, because bottles that are over- or under-filled can result in inaccurate results, e.g. clotting screen (McCall & Tankersley 2008). Once the sample has been obtained the bottles should be inverted five or six times to mix the blood with the additive. It is important not to shake the bottle vigorously because this will result in damage of cells and inaccurate results. The order in which the blood sample bottles are used may vary between manufacturers, and it is recommended that the manufacturer's instructions are followed (Dojcinovska 2011). This is in order to reduce the risk of contamination of the specimen by additives from other bottles, which may interfere with analysis (*see* Table 14.3; Becton Dickinson 2003).

Specimen handling and transportation

From the moment the blood enters the sample bottle, its cellular and chemical components are subject to the effects of time, temperature and light (Ernst 2005). Therefore procedures to protect samples from deterioration during transportation and storage of samples must be maintained, especially if testing is delayed (Ernst 2005; Jansen *et al.* 1997). The Health and Safety Executive (2003) recommend that blood samples should be placed in a rigid container that is washable (or autoclavable), leakproof and labelled with a biohazard label. This container should be stored in the boot of a car during transportation and not exposed to extremes of temperature. Samples must be delivered to laboratories promptly to prevent sample deterioration and subsequent inaccurate results. Time frames for samples, from sampling to analysis, depend on the type of sample and the general requirements of the local laboratory. Some samples can be stored in a refrigerator designated for clinical use (in a clinic or health centre) to extend stability times, e.g. full blood count (Ernst 2005). However, coagulation studies and biochemistry samples must be analysed within 4 h (Ernst 2005).

Table 14.2 Types, advantages and disadvantages of venepuncture equipment

Device	Gauge sizes	Advantages	Disadvantages
Needle and syringe	25g–19g	This is a readily available and cheap method of venepuncture. Most nurses know how to assemble the equipment together and use it	This is the most hazardous method of venepuncture as it increases the risk of needlestick injury, and where a vacuumed bottle is used it is not good practice to remove the top from the bottle and decant blood in from a syringe as it may result contamination by blood splash or spill, and once in the laboratory the top could dislodge from the bottle during analysis. The correct size syringe needs to be selected according to the volume of blood required, making it cumbersome if 50–60 ml syringes have to be used. Difficulty in manipulating the syringe can result in trauma to the patient's vein and cause discomfort
Vacuum blood collection system	23, 22 and 21g A standard 21g needle should be used to obtain the sample as it is quick and fewer cells are damaged. However, a 22g needle may be used if the vein is small or fragile	This is a closed system of blood sampling so there is very little risk of blood spillage and less risk of needlestick injury as blood is vacuumed directly into sample bottles (removing the need to decant blood) and exact volumes are obtained. It is readily available in most health centres in the community and is relatively cheap Safety needles are now also available	The practitioner will not know if they have been successful in entering the vein until the first bottle is applied to the system The vacuum system may be less easy to manipulate if the needle is not in the vein The suction can cause collapse of smaller veins It is important to remove the last bottle from the holder prior to removing the needle or it can result in a backflow of blood from the needle. This in turn can lead to the contamination of the practitioner When the nurse first starts practising venepuncture, it may be difficult to change the bottles without moving the needle within the patient's vein (causing trauma and possible bruising)
Winged infusion devices ('butterflies') This system comprises a steel needle, a pair of flexible wings and plastic tubing. The wings enable the device to be grasped during insertion	25, 23, 21, 19g A standard 21g needle should be used to obtain sample as it is quick and fewer cells are damaged. However, a 23g needle can be used if the vein is small or fragile. A 25g needle is too small to use for blood sampling as it damages the cells	These are easy to use and there is immediate verification of a successful venepuncture. They are also easier to hold and manipulate. As the bottles are changed further from the patient there is no trauma to the vessel. They are useful for large volumes of blood or in small, fragile or awkward veins. They are also available with a safety shield	They are more expensive and not always readily available except for certain groups of patients

(Dougherty 2008; McCall & Tankersley 2008; Dimech *et al.* 2011)

339

Table 14.3 Example of blood sample bottle, their order and their uses

Order of bottles	Colour of bottle top	Volume	Test
1	Blood culture bottles	5–10 ml	Infections
2	Red	6 ml	Serum samples, e.g. thyroid function tests, B_{12}
3	Pink	6 ml	Cross-match
4	Blue	2.7–4.5 ml	INR clotting screen
5	Green or gold	6 ml	Biochemistry (urea and electrolytes, liver function tests)
6	Purple	3 ml	Full blood count
7	Black	1 ml	ESR
8	Grey	3 ml	Glucose

(Becton Dickinson 2003)

Safety of staff

It is recommended that well-fitting, clean, non-sterile gloves are worn during the venepuncture process (RCN 2010). The wearing of gloves will not prevent needlestick injury; however, they will protect the practitioner from blood contamination by splashing or spillage (NHS Employers 2007; RCN 2010). Gloves will also reduce the amount of contamination in the event of a needlestick injury, as it has been found that blood is wiped off a needle as it passes through a glove (Mitchell-Higgs 2002; Hart 2011).

Wherever possible community nurses should use safety venepuncture needles and sampling systems. These devices have been designed to reduce the risk of needlestick injury. Some require the safety system to be activated by the nurse, while others are self-activated on removal of the needle (RCN 2010).

All sharps should be disposed of immediately into a designated sharps container. The community nurse should take one into the patient's house if the patient does not have a sharps container. If it is to remain in the house then the sharps box should be kept above floor level and out of reach of children or pets, with the lid closed but not permanently sealed (Stevenson 1997). Once filled to the recommended level, they should be labelled with the date and point of origin, e.g. clinic or primary care trust reference code (Stevenson

1997) and disposed of appropriately. All contaminated equipment and waste should be placed into a yellow clinical waste bag and disposed of according to local policy.

In the event of a blood spillage, this should be dealt with according to local policy with an approved disinfectant (Hart 2011). A number of commercial kits are available for use in health centres and clinics (Stevenson 1997). In the home, a dilute solution of domestic bleach or hot soapy water can be used with the patient's permission (Stevenson 1997) (*see* Chapter 6 for further details).

Infection control issues

To prevent and/or reduce the risk of infection, hands should be washed prior to commencing the venepuncture process, and if this is not possible an alcohol-based hand gel should be used as an alternative (*see* Chapter 6).

The literature concerning skin cleansing prior to venepuncture is controversial. For example, Lieffers and Mokkink (2002) suggests that the person must be socially clean and if not then the area should be washed with soap and water. However, others state that the area should be cleaned with a 70% alcohol solution that is applied for a minimum of 30 seconds and allowed to air dry (Dimech *et al.* 2011; Hart 2011). This latter method of skin cleansing may be more applicable now with the increase in antimicrobial resistant strains of micro-organisms such as methicillin-resistant *Staphlococcal aureus* (MRSA). While certain groups of patients may be more vulnerable and require more intensive skin cleansing, for example patients with cancer, older people and people who are immunocompromised, if there is no clear guidance regarding who falls into these categories it is better to clean the skin with an alcohol-soaked swab (Fraise & Bradley 2009). When taking blood cultures, the DH (2010) guidance is to use chlorhexidine 2% on the skin and to clean the top of the blood culture bottles.

Patients' perspective of venepuncture

There are few people who are truly needlephobic, but it is still an anxiety-provoking procedure (Dougherty 1994). There are many aspects that can influence the patient experience of venepuncture and these should be taken into consideration in order to minimise patient anxiety and increase the incidence of a successful venepuncture for example (Dougherty 2011).

Age and gender

A study carried out by Coates *et al.* (1983) showed that women under the age of 40 undergoing chemotherapy were more anxious about having a needle inserted, and tended to feel faint more often than men. Furthermore the literature suggests that younger people will have fears or anxieties when undergoing procedures involving a needle (Agras *et al.* 1969). Anecdotally, it also appears that young men are more at risk of vasovagal reactions during venepuncture.

Previous experiences

It is suggested that a person's previous experiences affects how they may react towards that procedure thereafter (Ost 1991). Many phobias result from previous bad experiences, therefore it is important to take the time to ascertain if patients have been subjected to previous difficult venepunctures and what the problems were. Then the community nurse can work in partnership with the patient to try to resolve some of the fears and anxieties and where necessary, seek advice from an appropriate professional, e.g. GP.

Result of the blood test

For some patients it is not the act of inserting a needle into their vein but the potential results of the blood test that evoke anxiety. This is because the test may identify a disease or confirm that their condition is deteriorating (Dougherty 2011).

Information and consent

Some patients may have little or no idea of what venepuncture actually involves, therefore it is important to ensure they receive a full explanation about the procedure, potential complications (such as bruising) and if necessary are shown the equipment. This will enable them to give full and informed consent (Dougherty 2008). This is usually obtained as verbal consent, although specialist blood tests, e.g. genetic or HIV testing, may require written consent (Lavery & Smith 2008; Scales 2008).

Reducing pain during venepuncture

There are a number of methods for reducing pain. These include injectable or topical local anaesthetics, as well as use of relaxation techniques, distraction and anxiolytics (Moureau & Zonderman 2000). The use of local anaesthetics has been advocated to reduce pain and anxiety (Dougherty 2008; Moureau & Zonderman 2000) and these can be applied as a cream/gel or given as an intradermal injection. These must be prescribed by the GP or hospital doctor prior to use and the community nurse must be competent to administer the anaesthetic (NMC 2008a).

The most commonly used local anaesthetic creams are EMLA (eutectic mixture of local anaesthetics – lidocaine and prilocaine) and Ametop (topical amethocaine). These are applied to the skin 30–60 min prior to venepuncture and covered with an occlusive dressing. EMLA can cause vasoconstriction, making venepuncture more difficult. Ametop has been shown to be more effective than EMLA because it causes significantly less vasoconstriction (Browne *et al.* 1999). However, application can result in an erythematous rash if left in situ longer than the recommended time (BNF 2011).

Intradermal lidocaine 1% can be slowly injected around the vein. However, it should be used with caution due to its potential for a local skin reaction, tissue damage and inadvertent injection of drug into the vascular system. It can obliterate the vein (Perucca 2010; INS 2011) and is therefore not recommended for routine use (Perucca 2010).

This drug needs to be prescribed and the community nurse must be competent regarding its administration and able to deal with any complications and monitor the patient following the procedure, especially if the patient lives alone.

Legal and professional issues

The Nursing & Midwifery Council Code (NMC 2008b) states that nurses should ensure that they maintain knowledge and skills when taking on an expansion to their role. Nurses undertaking venepuncture in the community setting should be supported by their managers and provided with the correct training and updates on new equipment and techniques (Hyde 2011).

There should be policies and procedures in place to guide the community nurses practice. First, criteria should be set for the number of attempts at venepuncture that a nurse may make before passing on to a more experienced colleague. Second, parameters concerning the minimum number of venepunctures the community nurse should perform within a set period of time in order to maintain their skills should be defined within local policies based on best practice. The nurse is professionally accountable for maintaining their skill and knowledge (Lavery & Smith 2008; Hyde 2011). This is now even more relevant as there is an increase in the number of nurses involved in litigation cases related to venepuncture injuries (Dougherty 2003; McConnell & MacKay 1996).

Problem solving

Missed vein

This often occurs when a practitioner first practises venepuncture. It usually results from inserting the needle to the side of the patient's vein.

Prevention
- Careful selection of vein.
- Good anchoring during insertion.

Action
- Explain to the patient what has occurred during the procedure.
- Carefully withdraw the needle a few millimetres and realign the needle into the vein, but check with the patient for any discomfort. If it begins to hurt or any bruising is noticed, then remove the needle immediately and select an alternative vein (Dougherty 2008; Morris 2011).

Blood stops flowing

This can be caused by the following.

- A through puncture – the needle entered the vein, blood flowed, then the needle was advanced too far and punctured the posterior wall of the vein.
- A valve – the needle is up against a valve and stops the flow of blood.
- A faulty bottle – there is no vacuum in the bottle.
- Venous spasm – the vein has gone into spasm due to mechanical irritation caused by the needle or length of time the tourniquet has been applied.
- Vein has collapsed – due to the vacuum in the bottle, especially if in a small thin vein.

Prevention
- Check for location of valves prior to insertion of needle and avoid where possible.
- Ensure that blood bottles are in date.
- Do not leave tourniquet on too long.
- Insert the needle at the correct angle and do not over advance.
- Where possible try to avoid thin small veins.

Action
- Explain to the patient what has occurred during the procedure.
- Through puncture – release the tourniquet and remove the needle.
- Valve – withdraw the needle slightly to move it away from valve.
- Change bottles in case there is a fault with the vacuum.
- Venous spasm – release the tourniquet, wait for a few minutes and then reapply tourniquet and wait for venous filling.
- Gently stroke the vein above venepuncture site (Dougherty 2008; Morris 2011) .

Hitting an artery

This can be identified by the emergence of bright red, sometimes pulsating blood. The patient will usually complain of a sharp pain.

Prevention
- Always palpate the vessel first; arteries tend to be placed more deeply than veins and pulsate, but it could be an aberrant artery. This is an artery that is located superficially in an unusual location (Weinstein 2007).
- The community nurse should have knowledge of where arteries are likely to be located.
- Do not insert the needle at too sharp an angle.

Action
- Release tourniquet and remove the needle immediately.
- Apply pressure to the site with a gauze swab for at least 5 mins.
- Ensure bleeding has stopped before applying dressing.
- Do not reuse the arm for venepuncture for at least 24 hours.
- Explain to the patient what has occurred during the procedure.
- Instruct the patient to inform the nurse if bruising occurs or there is pain and/or numbness in the arm/hands.
- Inform the GP.
- Complete a critical incident form and fully document the incident and action taken in the patient's records.
- Follow-up visits to check the patient and venepuncture site should be considered based on individual patient's needs (Dougherty 2008; Morris 2011).

Touching a nerve

Nerve pain is characterised by a sharp shooting pain, the location is dependent on which nerve has been touched, but the patient often complains of pain shooting into first finger and thumb, and along the length of the arm.

Prevention

- The community nurse should have knowledge of where nerves are located.
- Not inserting the needle too deeply, at too sharp an angle or 'probing' around if unable to locate the vein.
- Avoid the wrist and lower cephalic veins where possible (Roth 2004).

Action

- Release tourniquet and remove the needle immediately.
- Explain to the patient what has happened.
- Instruct patient to inform the nurse if the pain and/or numbness in the arm/hands continues to get worse or does not resolve within 24–48 hours.
- Inform the GP.
- Complete a critical incident form and fully document the incident and action taken in the patients records.
- Follow-up visits to check the patient and venepuncture site should be considered based on individual patient's needs (Dougherty 2008; Morris 2011).

Haematoma

This is characterised by bleeding into the tissues resulting in a hard swelling.

Prevention

- Choosing the most appropriate vein and the smallest device necessary.
- The community nurse should apply adequate pressure (Godwin *et al.* 1992) and the patient should be advised not to bend the arm following removal of the needle (Dyson & Bogod 1987).
- Removing the tourniquet immediately in the event of a through puncture.
- Knowledge of which patients are at a greater risk of bruising.

Action

- Release tourniquet and remove needle if bruising occurs during the venepuncture.
- Apply pressure to the site for as long as necessary to stop bleeding, i.e. anything from 1 min or longer.
- Elevate the affected limb.
- Apply ice to the site if available.

- Explain to the patient what has occurred during the procedure.
- Suggest where possible the patient obtains hirudoid cream or arnica to help reduce bruising. These can both be purchased from the chemists.
- Instruct patient to inform the nurse if the bruising gets worse or if they develop any numbness in the arm/hands.
- Inform the GP.
- Complete a critical incident form and fully document the incident and action taken in the patients records.
- Follow-up visits to check the patient and venepuncture site should be considered based on individual patient's needs (Dougherty 2008; Morris 2011).

Vasovagal reaction

This is characterised by initial sweating and pallor, and results in loss of consciousness.

Prevention

- Knowledge of patient history, e.g. if felt faint or fainted in the past during venepuncture.
- If there is a known risk of fainting, if possible lay patient down while carrying out venepuncture.
- If there is a known risk of a vasovagal reaction ask a colleague to visit with you.

Action

- Attempt to lay patient down or put their head between their knees.
- Check pulse and blood pressure.
- Reassure patient.
- Inform the GP.
- Complete a critical incident form and fully document the incident and action taken in the patient's records.
- Follow-up visits to check the patient and venepuncture site should be considered based on individual patient's needs (Dougherty 2008; Morris 2011).

Conclusion

The procedure of venepuncture may appear to be an easy one and certainly if taught correctly it can be quickly mastered. However, it is not without its hazards both for the patient and the practitioner. Therefore it is vital that community nurses maintain their competency through regular updating of their knowledge and constant practice of their skills. In this way they can provide their patient with a high standard of care and at the same time practise safely to prevent any harm to the patient, themselves and their colleagues.

Procedure guideline 14.1 **Guideline for venepuncture**

Equipment:

Tourniquet
Needle
Plastic shell
Appropriate vacuumed specimen bottles
Cleaning solution/impregnated swabs
Low-linting gauze swabs
Sterile adhesive plaster or appropriate dressing
Completed specimen requisition forms
Non-sterile gloves
Alcohol-based hand gel (as necessary)

Procedure

Nursing action	Rationale
1 Where appropriate facilities are available wash and dry your hands thoroughly or alternatively cleanse with 70% alcohol-based hand rub (in accordance with local policy)	To reduce the risk of cross-infection
2 If the patient is known to the service review nursing documentation and current care plan	To update knowledge of patient and maintain patient safety
3 If the patient is unknown to the service a full comprehensive assessment must be carried out prior to undertaking the procedure	To identify potential contraindications and/or cautions To determine if a second nurse is required to assist with the procedure To maintain patient safety
4 Verbally and where possible visually explain and discuss the procedure with the patient. Written consent should be obtained from the patient and documented prior to carrying out the procedure	To ensure the patient understands the procedure, assessing their capacity in making a decision to consent (Mental Capacity Act 2005) To ensure that the patient can make an informed choice (NMC 2008) to give valid written consent To aid the identification of potential contraindications and/or cautions To maintain patient safety Patient information reduces anxiety To gain co-operation and consent
5 Wash hands or cleanse with an alcohol-based hand rub	To minimise the risk of infection
6 Assemble all required equipment on a clean tray, table or surface	To ensure time is not wasted and to prevent necessity of returning to the surgery or clinic to collect any missing items
7 Ask patient if they have any preferences regarding site, etc.	To involve patient and give them a feeling of control; this may in turn reduce anxiety
8 Place the patient's arm in a comfortable position, well supported on the arm of a chair or on a pillow or a cushion	To ensure patient comfort and to facilitate venous access

Procedure guideline 14.1 **Guideline for venepuncture** *(cont'd)*

Nursing action	Rationale
9 Ensure that the community nurse is in a comfortable position	To prevent trauma to the community nurse's back
10 Apply the tourniquet and inspect the arm for areas of infection, bruising or oedema	To encourage venous filling and to observe for any areas that should be avoided
11 If veins are not easily found, then use other methods such as gravity, heat, etc.	To encourage venous filling
12 Palpate the veins and select the most appropriate vein for the venepuncture	To select the most appropriate vein and to identify any valves, arterial pulse, and to ascertain the condition and direction of the vein
13 Release the tourniquet	To prevent patient discomfort, venous spasm and inaccurate blood results
14 Select and assemble the correct needle gauge size and the type of equipment most suitable for obtaining the sample from the patient, e.g. a winged infusion device in a small vein	To ensure success and to reduce risk of vein trauma
15 Wash hands or cleanse with an alcohol-based hand rub	To minimise the risk of infection
16 Apply gloves	To prevent possible contamination of the community nurse
17 Reapply the tourniquet	To encourage venous filling
18 Clean the skin using 70% alcohol swab for 30 seconds and allow the skin to dry	To minimise the risk of infection, to ensure disinfection has occurred and to prevent pain on insertion of the needle
19 Do not repalpate the skin over the selected vein once it has been cleaned	To maintain asepsis and minimise the risk of infection
20 Remove needle guard from needle only when ready to use and inspect needle for any barbs	To maintain sterility and to prevent any trauma to patient
21 Anchor vein using the thumb of the non-dominant hand by pulling the skin taut	To maintain stability of the vein and to prevent trauma to the patient
22 Check the needle is bevel side up	To prevent trauma to the vein and pain to the patient
23 Holding the shell in the dominant hand, insert the needle smoothly at an angle between 10 and 40°	To reduce pain, which occurs if the community nurse is hesitant in inserting the needle; angle is decided by depth of vein – too shallow and the needle will not enter the vein, too deep and the needle will go through the vein
24 Gently release anchoring and apply the first bottle	To obtain the required blood sample
25 Once the bottle is full, gently remove the bottle and apply additional bottles if required	To prevent trauma of needle moving when removing and applying bottles
26 Gently invert bottles with additives 5–6 times	To ensure the additives are mixed with the blood
27 Once all samples have been taken, release the tourniquet	To allow venous emptying

345

(Continued)

Procedure guideline 14.1 **Guideline for venepuncture** *(cont'd)*

Nursing action	Rationale
28 Gently remove the needle and then apply the swab with pressure to the venepuncture site	To prevent trauma to the patient and vein; if pressure is applied during needle removal it can causes dragging along the intima of the vein resulting in pain
29 Do not resheath the needle but dispose of it immediately into the sharps container	To reduce risk of needlestick injury
30 Maintain pressure on the venepuncture site until bleeding has ceased, usually about a minute, but this may be longer if the patient is prone to bleeding	To ensure that haemostasis has occurred and bruising has been avoided
31 Remove gloves and dispose appropriately	To follow correct guidance for disposal of waste
32 Apply a plaster or appropriate dressing to venepuncture site	To cover puncture site and prevent leakage and contamination of the site
33 Dispose of clinical waste appropriately	To ensure safe disposal and prevent reuse of equipment
34 Wash hands or cleanse with an alcohol-based hand rub	To minimise the risk of infection
35 Label bottles with patient details and transport to locally agreed collection point, e.g. GP surgery, clinic or health centre	To ensure the specimens from the right patient are delivered to the laboratory
36 Document the outcome of the procedure on the community nurse record of visits	To maintain patient safety To ensure continuity of care. To ensure accurate and contemporaneous records are kept Documentation should provide clear evidence of care planned, decisions made and care delivered (NMC 2009)

(Dougherty 2008; Nicol *et al.* 2008; de Verteuil 2011; Dimech *et al.* 2011).

References and further reading

Agras S, Sylvester D, Olivean D (1969) The epidemiology of common fears and phobias. *Comprehensive Psychiatry* **10**(2): 151–7.

Becton Dickinson (2003) *Performing Venepuncture, Guidance.* Becton Dickinson, Oxford.

British National Formulary (2011) British Medical Association and Royal Pharmaceutical Society of GB, London.

Brown J, Larson M (1999) Pain during insertion of peripheral intravenous catheters with or without intradermal lidocaine. *Clinical Nurse Specialist* **13**: 283–5.

Browne J, Awad I, Plant R *et al.* (1999) Topical ametocaine (Ametop) is superior to EMLA for intravenous cannulation. *Canadian Journal of Anesthesia* **46**: 1014–18.

Carlson K, Perdue MB, Hankins J (2010) *Infection Control in Infusion Therapy in Clinical Practice* (2e). WB Saunders, Pennsylvania, pp. 126–40.

Coates A, Abraham S, Kaye SB *et al.* (1983) On the receiving end: patients' perception of the side effects of cancer chemotherapy. *European Journal of Cancer Clinical Oncology* **19**(2): 203–8.

Collins M *et al.* (2006) A structured learning programme for venepuncture and cannulation. *Nursing Standard* **20**(26): 34–40.

Collins M (2011) Anatomy and physiology. In: Phillips S, Collins M, Dougherty L (eds) *Venepuncture and Cannulation*, pp. 44–67. Blackwell Publishing, Oxford.

De Verteuil A (2011) Procedures in venepuncture and cannulation. In: Phillips S, Collins M, Dougherty L (eds) *Venepuncture and Cannulation*, pp. 131–74. Blackwell Publishing, Oxford.

Department of Health (2010) *Clean Safe Care: taking blood cultures. A summary of best practice.* DH, London.

Dick MJ, Maree SM, Gray J (1992) How to boost the odds of a painless IV start. *American Journal of Nursing* **6**: 49–50.

Dimech A, Witt B, Forsythe C *et al.* (2011) Diagnostic procedures. In: Dougherty L, Lister S (eds) *The Royal Marsden Hospital*

Manual of Clinical Nursing Procedures (8e). Wiley Blackwell, Oxford.

Dojcinovska M (2011) Selection of equipment. In: Phillips S, Collins M, Dougherty L (eds) *Venepuncture and Cannulation*, pp. 68–90. Blackwell Publishing, Oxford.

Dougherty L (2003) The expert witness working within the legal system of the UK. *Journal of Vascular Access Devices* **8**(2): 29–37.

Dougherty L (1994) A study to discover how cancer patients perceive the intravenous cannulation experience. Unpublished MSc thesis, University of Guildford.

Dougherty L (2008) Obtaining peripheral vascular access. In: Dougherty L, Lamb J (eds) *Intravenous Therapy in Nursing Practice* (2e). Blackwell Publishing, Oxford.

Dougherty L (2011) Patients' perspective. In: Phillips S, Collins M, Dougherty L (eds) *Venepuncture and Cannulation*, pp. 281–96. Blackwell Publishing, Oxford.

Dyson A, Bogod D (1987) Minimizing bruising in the antecubital fossa after venepuncture. *British Medical Journal* **294**: 1659.

Ernst DJ (2005) *Phlebotomy for Nurses and Nursing Personnel.* Quality Books, Indiana.

EU Directive (2010) *EU Directive to prevent injuries and infections to healthcare workers from sharp objects such as needle sticks.* www.hse.gov.uk/healthservices/needlesticks/eu-directive.htm accessed (last accessed 28 September 2011).

Fetzer SJ (2002) Reducing venipuncture and intravenous insertion pain with eutectic mxture of local anesthetic: a meta analysis. *Nursing Research* **51**: 119–24.

Fraise AP, Bradley C (2009) *Ayliffe's Control of Healthcare-Associated Infection. A Practical Handbook* (5e). Hodder Arnold, London.

Franklin GE, Bal AM, McKenzie H (2007) Phlebotomy tourniquets and MRSA. *Journal of Hospital Infection* **65**(2): 173–5.

Fry C, Anholt D (2001) Local anaesthetic prior to insertion of a PICC. *Journal of Intravenous Nursing* **24**(6): 404–8.

Garza D, Becan-McBride K (2010) *Phlebotomy Handbook – blood collection essentials.* Prentice Hall, New Jersey.

Godwin PGR, Cuthbert AC, Choyce A (1992) Reducing bruising after venepuncture. *Quality in Health Care* **1**: 245–6.

Golder M (2000) Potential risk of cross infection during peripheral venous access by contamination of tourniquets. *Lancet* **355**: 44.

Hadaway L (2010) Anatomy and physiology related to intravenous therapy. In *Clinical Practice* (2e), pp. 65–97. WB Saunders, Pennsylvania.

Hart S (2011) Infection control and risk management. In: Phillips S, Collins M, Dougherty L (eds) *Venepuncture and Cannulation*, pp. 108–30. Blackwell Publishing, Oxford.

Hecker JF, Lewis GBH, Stanley H (1983) Nitroglycerine ointment as an aid to venepuncture. *Lancet* **1**: 206–4.

Health and Safety Executive (2003) *Guidance on Safe Working and the Prevention of Infection in Clinical Laboratories and Similar.* HSE, Suffolk.

Hyde L (2011) Legal and professional issues. In: Phillips S, Collins M, Dougherty L (eds) *Venepuncture and Cannulation*, pp. 5–15. Blackwell Publishing, Oxford.

Intravenous Nursing Society (2011) *Standards for Infusion Therapy*. INS and BD, USA.

Inwood S (1996) Designing a nurse training programme for venepuncture. *Nursing Standard* **10**(21): 40–2.

Jansen RTP *et al.* (1997) EC4 Essential criteria for quality systems of medical laboratories. *European Journal of Clinical Chemistry and Clinical Biochemistry* **35**(2): 123–32.

Lavery I, Ingram P (2005) Venepuncture: best practice. *Nursing Standard* **19**(49): 55–65.

Lavery I, Smith E (2008) Venepuncture practice and the 2008 Nursing and Midwifery Council Code. *British Journal of Nursing* **17**(13): 824–8.

Lenhardt R, Seybold T, Kimberger O *et al.* (2002) Active hand warming eases peripheral intravenous catheter insertion. *British Medical Journal* **325**: 409–12.

Lieffers MA, Mokkink HG (2002) Disinfection of the skin prior to injections does not influence the incidence of infections: a literature study. *Nederlands Tijdschrift voor Geneeskunde* **146**(16): 765–7.

McCall RE, Tankersley CM (2008) *Phlebotomy Essentials* (3e). Lippincott Williams & Wilkins, Philadelphia.

McConnell AA, Mackay GM (1996) Venepuncture: the medicolegal hazards. *Postgraduate Medical Journal* **72**: 23–4.

Medical Devices Agency (2000) *Single Use Medical Devices: implications and consequences of reuse.* DB 2000 (04), London.

Mental Capacity Act (2005) www.legislation.gov.uk/ukpga/2005/9/contents (last accessed 28 September 2011).

Michael A, Andrew M (1996) The application of EMLA and glycerol trinitrate ointment prior to venepuncture. *Anaesthesia and Intensive Care* **24**: 360–4.

Mitchell-Higgs N (2002) *Personal protective equipment – improving compliance.* All points conference. Safer Needles Network, London.

Morris W (2011) Complications in venepuncture and cannulation. In: Phillips S, Collins M, Dougherty L (eds) *Venepuncture and Cannulation*, pp. 155–222. Blackwell Publishing, Oxford.

Moureau N, Zonderman A (2000) Does it always have to hurt? *Journal of Intravenous Nursing* **23**(4): 213–19.

NHS Employers (2007) Needlestick injury. In: *The Healthy Workplaces Handbook*, pp. 1–24. NHS Employers, London.

Nicol M, Bavin C, Bedford-Turner S, Cronin P (2008) Intravenous therapy – venepuncture. In: *Essential Nursing Skills* (3e). Mosby, London.

Nursing & Midwifery Council (2008a) *Standards for Medicines Management.* NMC London

Nursing & Midwifery Council (2008b) *The Code. Standards of conduct, performance and ethics for nurses and midwives.* NMC, London.

Nursing & Midwifery Council (2009) *Record Keeping: guidance for nurses and midwives.* NMC, London.

Ost LG (1991) Acquisition of blood and injection phobia and anxiety response patterns in clinical patients. *Behavioural Research and Therapy* **101**(11): 68–74.

Perucca R (2010) Obtaining vascular access. In: *Clinical Practice* (2e), pp. 338–97. WB Saunders, Pennsylvania.

Phillips S (2011) The learning experience. In: Phillips S, Collins M, Dougherty L (eds) *Venepuncture and Cannulation*, pp. 16–43. Blackwell Publishing, Oxford.

Quick Reference Guide 5 (1999) *Venepuncture* **13**: 36.

347

Roth D (2004) Risks of vascular access/infusion therapy malpractice litigation: factual data. *Journal of Vascular Access* **9**(4): 230–2.

Royal College of Nursing (2010) *Standards for Infusion Therapy*. RCN, London.

Scales K (2008) A practical guide to venepuncture and blood sampling. *Nursing Standard* **22**(29): 29–36.

Springhouse Corporation (2002) *Intravenous Therapy Made Incredibly Easy*. Springhouse Lippincott Williams & Wilkins Philadelphia, Chapters 2 and 3.

Stevenson B (1997) Venepuncture. *Community Nurse* **October**: 21–2.

Tortora GJ, Derrickson B (2009) *Principles of Anatomy and Physiology*, Volume 2 (12e). John Wiley & Sons, New Jersey.

Weinstein S (2007) *Plumers Principles and Practices of Intravenous Therapy* (8e). Lippincott, Philadelphia.

Witt B (2011) Vein selection. In: Phillips S, Collins M, Dougherty L (eds) *Venepuncture and Cannulation*, pp. 91–107. Blackwell Publishing, Oxford.

Wound management

Introduction

A wound is defined as a break in the epidermis or dermis that can be related to trauma or pathological changes within the skin or body (Collins *et al.* 2002). Tissue viability is the ability of tissue to perform its normal function optimally (Collins *et al.* 2002).

The estimated cost to the NHS for the treatment of chronic wounds is said to be between £2.3 billion and £3.1 billion annually, which is approximately 3% of the total NHS healthcare budget (Posnett & Franks 2007). It is suggested that a number of these wounds, for example pressure ulcers, are preventable, and also that with appropriate diagnosis and treatment most wounds can be healed within 24 weeks (Posnett & Franks 2007).

Approximately 50% of community nurses' time is spent on the management of venous leg ulcers (Simon *et al.* 2004).

Background evidence

The role of the nurse in wound management includes the initial and ongoing patient assessment, decision making and treatment planning, and continuous evaluation of selected treatments. To do this, knowledge of the functions and anatomy of the skin and wound physiology is required.

Skin – structure and function

The skin is the largest organ of the body and has a number of functions (Table 15.1). It consists of two main layers, the epidermis and the dermis (Figure 15.1), weighs approximately 3 kg, accounts for 15–20% of a human's total body weight and contains approximately one third of the body's total circulating blood volume

(Herlihy & Maebius 2000). Lying between the epidermis and dermis is a thin layer of protein fibres called the 'basement membrane'. The capillary network that supplies oxygen and nutrients to the overlying epidermal cells lies directly beneath this membrane (Naylor *et al.* 2001).

The thickness of skin varies from 0.05 mm in the tympanic membrane to 6 mm on the soles of the feet (Wysocki 2000). In healthy adults, it is inhospitable to pathogenic organisms, able to withstand a number of mechanical and chemical assaults, and capable of self-regeneration (Parker 2000; Wysocki 2000).

The quality and function of skin is significantly affected by, for example:

- increasing age
- ultraviolet radiation
- alterations to the normal pH (5.5) of skin
- diet
- nutritional status
- medication, e.g. steroids, non-steroidal anti-inflammatory medications (NSAIDs) and antipsychotics (Kudoh 2005).

The effects of ageing on the skin

The ageing process has a detrimental effect on skin and the immunological system and affects the healing process. The resultant effects include the following.

- The sensitivity of the immune system is reduced due to the loss of macrophages and other cells of the immune system; this encourages infection and skin damage.
- Epidermal cells reproduce more slowly and are larger and more irregular in shape. These changes result in thinner, more translucent skin (Herlihy & Maebius 2000).

Table 15.1 Functions of the skin

Protects internal structures	Main protective barrier, preventing damage to internal tissues from physical trauma, ultraviolet (UV) light, temperature changes, toxins and bacteria (Butcher & White 2005)
Regulates fluid and electrolyte retention	Prevents the loss of body fluids and electrolytes necessary to maintain homeostasis (Marieb 2006)
Aids in sensory perception	Contains nerve receptors that are sensitive to pain and pressure that direct the brain to initiate movement by reflex action (Herlihy & Maebius 2000; Wysocki 2000)
Regulates temperature	Aids in the control of body temperature by constricting or dilating the blood vessels within it. The sweat glands produce sweat which stays on the skin allowing the body to cool down (Herlihy & Maebius 2000)
Excretory function	The skin excretes waste products in sweat, which contains water, urea and albumin (Herlihy & Maebius 2000)
Metabolism	When UV light is present, the skin produces vitamin D, which is required for calcium absorption and absorbs medication (Linger 2010)
Communicates through non-verbal cues of facial expression	The skin can convey changes in mood through colour changes such as blushing (Flanagan & Fletcher 2003)

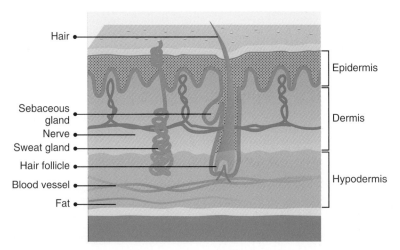

Figure 15.1 Skin structure.

- There is a reduction in sebum secretion and sweating causing dry, coarse, itchy and scaly skin.
- Increase in the incidence of skin problems such as pruritis, dermatitis, squamous cell carcinoma, basal cell carcinoma, blistering diseases, venous leg ulcers and pressure ulcers in older people (Tanj & Phillips 2001).
- Less melanin is produced, which results in paler skin and increased sensitivity to the effects of the sun.
- There is an increased risk of skin cancer and infection (Chandra 1992; Smoker 1999).

- Sensitivity to, for example, pain, heat and pressure is lowered as a consequence of epidermal thinning. This results in a lowered sensory receptor capacity increasing the risk of accidental/unknown injuries and infections (Herlihy & Maebius 2000).
- Sagging and wrinkling appear as skin weakens and the dermis thins by about 20% (Wysocki 1992). Collagen, the foundation for wound healing, is also lost and elasticity decreases, particularly in those areas exposed to the sun.

Table 15.2 Comparison of acute and chronic wounds (Collier 2002). Reproduced by kind permission of James Collier, Registered Nutritionist from www.dietetics.co.uk.

	Acute	**Chronic**
Age of wound	A new or relatively new wound	May develop over time
Healing rate	Heals as anticipated	Healing slow or stopped Fixed in one phase of wound healing
Mode of healing	Typically heals by primary intention	Typically heals by secondary intention
Examples	Surgical and traumatic wounds	Pressure/leg ulcer, diabetic foot ulcer, malignant and dehisced surgical wounds

- The hypodermis becomes thinner making people more prone to pressure damage, bruising and small haemorrhages (Herlihy & Maebius 2000).
- Increased sensitivity to temperature changes due to loss of efficiency of the sweat glands (Herlihy & Maebius 2000). A diminished dermal blood supply may also result in a reduction in the ability to lose heat (Herlihy & Maebius 2000).
- Vascularity decreases in subcutaneous tissue, therefore drugs that are administered subcutaneously are absorbed more slowly.

Physiology of wounds

Wounds are said to be either acute or chronic; acute are those healing as anticipated, and chronic is when they are failing to heal, have become fixed in any one phase of wound healing for a period of 6 weeks. Chronic wounds are associated with complex multiple factors that impede healing (Collier 2002) (Table 15.2). One of the fundamental principles in the effective management of wounds is to identify and, where possible, correct or modify the underlying cause(s) at an early stage.

All wounds may be placed in one of the following categories:

- mechanical – e.g. surgical/traumatic wounds
- chronic – e.g. leg ulcers/pressure ulcers
- burns – chemical or thermal injuries, may be further classified by depth of injury
- malignant – primary lesions such as melanomas.

(Collier 2003)

Wounds may also be classified as partial or full thickness.

A *partial thickness wound* is generally caused through trauma to the dermis; it is shallow in appearance but is often extremely painful for the patient due to exposed nerve endings (Hampton & Collins 2004).

Full thickness wounds include loss of epidermal and dermal layers. In extreme cases this may extend to the subcutaneous layer, muscle layer and bone, for example category 3 and 4 pressure ulcers (Hampton & Collins 2004).

Examples of potential causative factors of acute wounds include:

- skin may be lacerated, torn, burst or crushed (avulsion injury) by external forces
- post surgical
- abscess formation
- extreme heat, e.g. burns or scalds
- cold temperatures, e.g. chilblains
- vascular interruption
- insect bites
- high voltage electricity
- chemical attack.

In all cases of chronic wounds a predisposing factor(s) is responsible for impairing the ability of the body to maintain tissue integrity or heal the wound, for example:

- impaired venous drainage
- impaired arterial blood supply
- co-morbidities
- metabolic abnormalities
- malignant disease
- genetic disorders
- unrelieved mechanical forces.

Wound healing

Wound healing consists of four highly complex, interdependent overlapping phases (Dealey 2005). However, variations in the length of time a wound may take to heal is dependent on a number of influencing factors:

- the cause of the wound
- the degree of tissue damage
- the type of wound healing: primary, secondary, delayed primary or tertiary intention
- correct preparation of the wound bed
- the nutritional status of the patient/malnutrition/obesity (Williams & Leaper 2000)
- the age of the patient
- the patient's health status, e.g. the presence of co-morbidities such as diabetes, vascular/arterial

disease, anaemia or chronic obstructive pulmonary disease
- whether the patient is immunocompromised or suppressed
- malignancy
- infection
- the patient's mobility
- length of hospital stay
- prescribed medication, e.g. steroids, chemotherapy
- the site of the wound
- the efficacy of the blood supply to the wound, e.g. impaired vascularity/ tissue hypoxia
- the general physical and psychological condition of the patient
- the presence of a haematoma
- the presence of slough, infection or a foreign body
- type of primary dressing used and the frequency of dressing changes
- the inappropriate use of cleansing solutions
- the clinical knowledge, experience and expertise of the practitioner
- the ongoing appropriate and effective management of treatment.

(Hampton & Collins 2004; Dealey 2005)

The four main phases of wound healing are:

- the acute inflammatory phase
- the destructive phase
- the proliferative phase
- the maturation phase.

(Hampton & Collins 2004; Dougherty & Lister 2011)

Healing is said to be complete when the skin surface has reformed and the skin has regained most of its tensile strength (Davis *et al.* 1992) (Table 15.3).

Holistic assessment

Prior to treatment planning and wound dressing selection the community nurse must undertake and document a comprehensive holistic patient and wound assessment using an integrated multidisciplinary team approach (*see* Chapter 1). However, ongoing assessment, multiprofessional communication and documentation are essential to the success of treatment plans and care.

Assessment tools

To aid and inform decision making regarding wound management, community nurses must accurately select and use a wide range of evidence-based assessment

tools in conjunction with their clinical knowledge and judgement. For example:

- National Pressure Ulcer Advisory Panel (NPUAP) and European Ulcer Advisory Panel (EPUAP) (Box 15.1)
- classification of diabetic foot ulcers (Wagner 1987) (Table 15.4)
- the Waterlow Risk Assessment Scale (Waterlow 1985) (Figure 15.2)
- nutritional screening, guided by the Malnutrition Universal Screening Tool (MUST) (Exton-Smith 1971; Williams & Leaper 2000; Collier 2008) (*see* Chapter 10).

To optimise wound healing it is essential that patient involvement, education and patient coping strategies are combined with systematic reviews and evaluation of treatment (Price 2005). With the patient's consent the review and evaluation should include the use of photography and the utilisation of a wound assessment tool that incorporates:

- the type and location of the wound
- known allergies, including wound management products and latex
- appearance of the wound bed, e.g. granulating, epithelialisation, slough, necrosis
- wound mapping, e.g. length, width, depth
- level and type of exudate
- odour
- presence and level of bleeding
- wound margins and condition of surrounding skin
- level, type and intensity of pain – this should include at time of dressing change and be carried out using a recognised tool
- review of the use and efficacy of analgesia, including those that may have been bought over the counter (OTC)
- factors that may influence or delay wound healing, e.g. nutritional status, weight, diabetes, COPD, vascular/arterial disease, anaemia, infection
- date and results of relevant diagnostic tests
- details and date of all referrals made to other professionals
- assessment review date
- name/signature and qualification of assessor.

(Naylor *et al.* 2001)

It is not always possible to heal wounds due to the patients underlying aetiology (e.g. in fungating tumours or advanced disease). In this instance palliative care may be the aim, with management of symptoms in a way that is acceptable to the patient.

Table 15.3 Phases of normal wound healing

Phase	Duration	Activity

Inflammatory	0–5 days	■ Injury initiates the essential first step of healing:
		  – Vasoconstriction to reduce blood loss
		  – Release of plasma protein from endothelial cells and platelets for the formation of a platelet plug
		  – Commencement of the clotting process and the formation of a fibrin clot, this also acts as a temporary bacterial barrier and a framework for migrating cells
		  – Vasodilatation to stimulate increased collagen synthesis by fibroblasts and chemotaxis of macrophages
		■ Macrophages initiate angiogenesis and are responsible for:
		  – Attracting fibroblasts into the wound and their multiplication
		  – Stimulating fibroblasts to produce collagen and ground substance
		  – Manufacturing proteins, enzymes and other substances
		  – Breaking down various complex molecules into simple sugars and amino acids to provide local nutrition
		■ Macrophages in conjunction, with monocytes and lymphocytes, orchestrate the activities within the wound and coordinate the processes. In order to achieve this, the wound environment must be warm and moist (Hampton & Collins 2004; Dealey 2005)
		■ Histamine and other mediators for example, growth factor, are released and white blood cells are attracted to the wound via locally dilated blood vessels (Hampton & Collins 2004; Dealey 2005). This causes the signs of inflammation – redness, heat, swelling, pain, loss of function and oedema (Kindlen & Morison 1997)
		■ The overall function of inflammation is to neutralise and destroy any toxic agents at the site of an injury, clear the site of dead and devitalised tissue, to produce growth factors that stimulate the formation of fibroblasts, the synthesis of collagen, the process of angiogenesis and restoration of tissue homeostasis (Kindlen & Morison 1997; Collier 2003)

Destructive phase	1–7 days	■ Active cell population changes to mainly neutrophils and macrophages to:
		  – Clear devitalised tissue
		  – Engulf and digest bacteria
		  – Remove excess fibrin
		  – Produce growth factors
		  – Macrophage stimulation of the production of fibroblasts (Hampton & Collins 2004)
		■ Fibroblasts stimulate cell migration, angiogenesis and are involved in soft tissue growth and regeneration. They are also responsible for most collagen, elastin and fibronectin synthesis and give strength and structure to the repair (Collins *et al*. 2002; Hampton & Collins 2004).
		■ Collagen starts to be laid down and will continue to be modified during the proliferative and maturation stages of healing (Collins *et al*. 2002)

Proliferative phase	3–24 days	■ Fibroblast proliferation ■ Collagen synthesis ■ Angiogenesis ■ Endothelial cell migration ■ Cytokines contribute to the regulation of cellular function and wound repair (Waldrop & Doughty 2000) ■ Myofibroblasts shorten, the wound starts to contract and the edges begin to draw together (Hampton & Collins 2004)
Maturation	14 days onwards (comparability to normal tissue up to one year) (Dealey, 2005)	■ Activity level in this phase is at its highest between 14–21 days (Dealey 2005). ■ There is tissue contraction and re-organisation and synthesis of collagen fibres within the wound, re-epithelialisation occurs ■ Epithelial cells that have remained around the remnants of hair follicles, sebaceous glands, sweat glands and the wound margins divide and migrate over the granulation tissue ■ Myofibroblasts continue to shorten to decrease the size of the wound and bring the edges together (Hampton & Collins 2004) ■ The wound changes colour from red to white as the temporarily increased vascularity of the wound subsides ■ Tensile strength gradually increases as the collagen fibres are reorganised but the resulting scar tissue is never as strong as the original tissue (Kindlen & Morison 1997) **NB** It is estimated that the tensile strength of a wound is only 50% that of normal tissue at three months (Dealey 2005)

Box 15.1 NPUAP-EPUAP Pressure ulcer staging system (2009). Reproduced by kind permission of the European Pressure Ulcer Advisory Panel (EPUAP).

(a) Category/stage I

Intact skin with non-blanchable redness of a localised area usually over a bony prominence. Darkly pigmented skin may not have visible blanching; its colour may differ from the surrounding area.

Further description

The area may be painful, firm, soft, warmer or cooler compared with adjacent tissue. Stage I may be difficult to detect in individuals with dark skin tones. May indicate 'at risk' persons (a heralding sign of risk).

(b) Category/stage II

Partial thickness loss of dermis presented as a shallow open ulcer with a red pink wound bed, without slough. May also present as an intact or open/ruptured serum-filled blister.

Further description

Presents as a shiny or dry shallow ulcer without slough or bruising.* This stage should not be used to describe skin tears, tape burns, perineal dermatitis, maceration or excoriation.

  *Bruising indicates suspected deep tissue injury.

(c) Category/stage III

Full thickness tissue loss. Subcutaneous fat may be visible but bone, tendon or muscle is not exposed. Slough may be present but does not obscure the depth of tissue loss. May include undermining and tunnelling.

Further description

The depth of a Stage III pressure ulcer varies by anatomical location. The bridge of the nose, ear, occiput and malleolus do not have subcutaneous tissue and Stage III ulcers can be shallow. In contrast, areas of significant adiposity can develop extremely deep Stage III pressure ulcers. Bone/tendon is not visible or directly palpable.

(d) Category/stage IV

Full thickness tissue loss with exposed bone, tendon or muscle. Slough or eschar may be present on some parts of the wound bed. Often include undermining and tunnelling.

Further description

The depth of a Stage IV pressure ulcer varies by anatomical location. The bridge of the nose, ear, occiput and malleolus do not have subcutaneous tissue and these ulcers can be shallow. Stage IV ulcers can extend into muscle and/or supporting structures (e.g. fascia, tendon or joint capsule) making osteomyelitis possible. Exposed bone/tendon is visible or directly palpable.

The information below may be useful to community nursing staff however, these categories are only used in the United states of America.

(e) Suspected deep tissue Injury

Purple or maroon localised area of discoloured intact skin or blood-filled blister due to damage of underlying soft tissue from pressure and/or shear. The area may be preceded by tissue found to be painful, firm, mushy, boggy, warmer or cooler as compared to adjacent tissue.

Further description

Deep tissue injury may be difficult to detect in individuals with dark skin tones. Evolution may include a thin blister over a dark wound bed. The wound may further evolve and become covered by thin eschar. Evolution may be rapid, exposing additional layers of tissue even with optimal treatment.

(f) Unstageable

Full thickness tissue loss in which the base of the ulcer is covered by slough (yellow, tan, grey, green or brown) and/or eschar (tan, brown or black) in the wound bed.

Further description

Until enough slough and/or eschar is removed to expose the base of the wound, the true depth, and therefore stage, cannot be determined. Stable (dry, adherent, intact without erythema or fluctuance) eschar on the heel serves as 'the body's natural (biological) cover' and should not be removed.

Table 15.4 Classification of diabetic foot ulcers (Wagner 1987). Reprinted with kind permission of Slack Incorporated.

Grade 0: No ulcer in a high-risk foot

Grade 1: Superficial ulcer involving the full skin thickness but not underlying tissues

Grade 2: Deep ulcer, penetrating down to ligaments and muscle, but no bone involvement or abscess formation

Grade 3: Deep ulcer with cellulitis or abscess formation, often with osteomyelitis

Grade 4: Localised gangrene

Grade 5: Extensive gangrene involving the whole foot

WATERLOW PRESSURE ULCER PREVENTION/TREATMENT POLICY
RING SCORES IN TABLE, ADD TOTAL. MORE THAN 1 SCORE/CATEGORY CAN BE USED

BUILD/WEIGHT FOR HEIGHT	◆	SKIN TYPE VISUAL RISK AREAS	◆	SEX AGE	◆	MALNUTRITION SCREENING TOOL (MST) (Nutrition Vol. 15, No.6 1999 - Australia)		
AVERAGE BMI (20–24.9)	0	HEALTHY	0	MALE	1	A HAS PATIENT LOST WEIGHT RECENTLY	B WEIGHT LOSS SCORE	

ABOVE AVERAGE BMI (25–29.9)	1	TISSUE PAPER DRY OEDEMATOUS CLAMMY, PYREXIA DISCOLOURED	1 1 1 1	FEMALE 14–49 50–64 65–74	2 1 2 3	YES - GO TO B
						NO - GO TO C
						UNSURE - GO TO C
						       AND
						      SCORE 2
							0.5 – 5kg –1
							5 – 10kg –2
							10 – 15kg –3
							> 15kg –4
							UNSURE –2	

OBESE BMI > 30	2	GRADE 1	2	75–80	4	C – PATIENT EATING POORLY/LACK OF APPETITE		
BELOW AVERAGE BMI > 20 BMI = WT(kg)/ HT (m)^2	3	BROKEN/SPOTS GRADE 2–4	3	81+	5	NO – SCORE 0	YES – SCORE 1	
CONTINENCE	◆	MOBILITY	◆	SPECIAL RISKS				
COMPLETE/ CATHETERISED	0	FULLY RESTLESS/FIDGETY	0 1	TISSUE MALNUTRITION		◆	NEUROLOGICAL DEFICIT	◆
URINE INCONT.	1	APATHETIC	2	TERMINAL CACHEXIA	8		DIABETES, MS, CVA	4–6
FAECAL INCONT.	2	RESTRICTED	3	MULTIPLE ORGAN FAILURE	8		MOTOR SENSORY	4–6
URINARY + FAECAL INCONTINENCE	3	BEDBOUND e.g. TRACTION CHAIRBOUND e.g. WHEELCHAIR	4 5	SINGLE ORGAN FAILURE (RESP, RENAL, CARDIAC)	5		PARAPLEGIA (MAX OF 6)	4–6
				PERIPHERAL VASCULAR DISEASE	5		MAJOR SURGERY OR TRAUMA	
SCORE				ANAEMIA (Hb < 8)	2		ORTHPAEDIC/SPINAL	5
10+ AT RISK				SMOKING	1		ON TABLE > 2 HR$^+$	5
15+ HIGH RISK							ON TABLE > 6 HR$^+$	5
20+ VERY HIGH RISK				MEDICATION				
				CYTOTOXICS, STEROIDS, ANTI-INFLAMMATORY MAX OF 4				

Figure 15.2 The Waterlow risk assessment score (1985). Printed with the permission of Mrs Judy Waterlow MBE SRN RCNT www.judy-waterlow.co.uk.

Pain

Effective pain management is a fundamental part of wound healing and it is essential that the community nurse recognises that pain can negatively impact on a patient's quality of life, for example the patient may experience:

- social isolation
- restricted mobility
- stress
- anxiety
- insomnia
- depression.

Pain assessment should include the following.

- The actual pain felt by the patient, including at the time of dressing change.
- The patient's perception of pain.
- The physical, psychological and emotional effects that the patient's experience is having on their normal daily activities and the process of wound healing.

(Nemeth *et al.* 2003; Dealey 2005; Price 2005) (Figure 15.3)

It is suggested that the effective management of pain during wound dressing-related procedures is possible through a combination of:

- accurate assessment
- suitable dressing choices
- individualised analgesic regimens
- skilled wound management.

(European Wound Management Association [EWMA] 2002, 2004)

A number of tools have been developed to support practitioners in the accurate assessment of a patient's pain and its intensity, for example the numerical pain scale (Figure 15.4) and the pain faces scale (Figure 15.5).

Nutritional needs

Nutrition plays an essential role in both the prevention and management of wounds and pressure ulcers.

PAIN DIMENSIONS

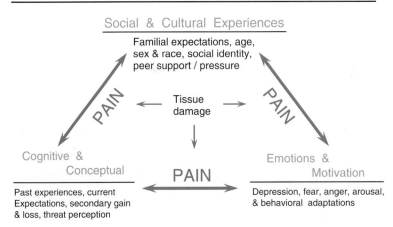

Figure 15.3 Pain dimensions (www.scinfo.org/PAINN2002/sld042.htm). © The Sickle Cell Information Center/J Eckman.

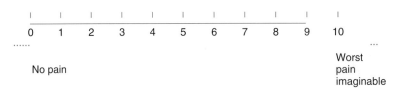

Figure 15.4 Numerical pain scale indicated for use with adults and children over 9 years (McCaffery & Beebe 1999). Reproduced by permission of Elsevier (Mosby).

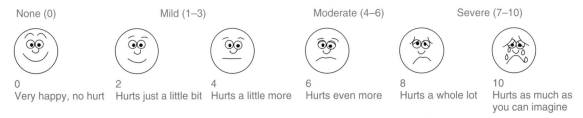

Figure 15.5 Pain faces scale (Wong *et al*. 2001). Reproduced by kind permission of Elsevier (Mosby).

Malnutrition and certain nutritional deficiencies compromise the wound-healing process and increase the risk of pressure ulcer development (Lewis 1997) (Table 15.5).

A thorough assessment using the MUST nutritional assessment tool is important for all patients with wounds, particularly older adults (Thomas & Bishop 2007) (*see* nutritional support Chapter 10).

The European Pressure Ulcer Advisory Panel (EPUAP 2003) suggests that an individual may require a minimum of:

- 30–35 kcals per kg body weight per day
- 1–1.5 g protein per kg body weight per day
- 1 ml fluid per kcal per day.

For further advice *see* Chapter 10.

Other nutritional considerations include the following.

- *Overweight and high-fat diet*: have been linked with the development of venous and arterial ulcers (TVS 2004). Obesity can also cause an individual to

Table 15.5 Wound healing, tissue viability and pressure sores (Thomas, 2007)

Nutrient	Function	Effects of deficiency
Protein	Required for synthesis of new tissue	Slow wound healing exacerbating loss of protein via exudate from wound site
		Tissue of poor tensile strength
		Oedema
Fat and carbohydrate	Required to prevent dietary or tissue protein being Loss of fat stores providing padding between bone carbohydrate used as an energy source	Loss of fat stores providing padding between bone and skin
	Fatty acids have a key role in cell membrane synthesis	Impaired immunocompetence
Vitamin A	Improves cell mediated immunity	Increase in wound infections
	Antioxidant (β-carotene) effect	
	Fibroplasia and epithelialisation	Decreased epithelialisation rate
	Improves collagen synthesis/cross-linkage	Decreased collagen synthesis/cross linking
Vitamin B complex	Coenzymes for energy metabolism	Impaired immunity
	Cofactor for collagen deposition/cross-linkage	
	White blood cell/antibody formation	
Vitamin C	Protection of metalloenzymes from oxidation	Decreased neutrophil/monocyte chemotaxis
	Neutrophil superoxide production	
	Proline and lysine hydroxylation	Impaired local bactericidal activity
	Collagen synthesis	
	Collagen cross-linkage	Wound dehiscence
	Angiogenesis	Increased capillary fragility
Vitamin E	Quenches free radical production	Excessive amounts may also be detrimental to wound healing, increasing fibrosis and risk of haemorrhage
	Prevents oxidation of membrane PUFAs	
Vitamin K	Coagulation	Coagulopathies
		Increased haemorrhage risk
		Increased haematoma formation
Iron	Prevents anaemia	Tissue ischaemia
	Optimises tissue perfusion	Impaired collagen cross-linking
	Promotes collagen synthesis	Reduced tensile wound strength
Zinc	Cofactor in enzyme systems for: Cell proliferation Membrane stabilisation Protein synthesis Protein, fat and carbohydrate metabolism	Decreased epithelialisation rate Reduced collagen synthesis Impaired wound strength Reduced retinol-binding protein synthesis
Copper	Covalent cross-linkage of collagen fibrils (wound maturation)	(Unlikely)
Manganese	Cofactor in metalloenzymes	(Magnesium can substitute if manganese status poor)
Selenium	Incorporated in glutathione peroxidase enzyme to protect cell from hydrogen peroxide damage	Impaired macrophage function

be more vulnerable to pressure ulcers due to the external pressure exerted on surfaces from excess weight.

- *Underweight*: weight loss and muscle wastage resulting from an inadequate energy intake increase the likelihood of pressure sore development due to a reduction in fat and muscle acting as padding between the bones and skin.
- *Dehydration*: can lead to reduced skin elasticity and increased tissue deformability under pressure or friction (Ryecroft-Malone & McInnes 2001).

Wound management

There are two main theories relating to effective wound management:

- moist wound healing for acute wounds
- wound bed preparation for chronic wounds.

The benefits of moist wound healing include:

- maintenance of moisture balance on the wound surface and prevention of scab formation (this must be managed through correct dressing selection, according to the level of exudate to prevent maceration)
- supports epidermal migration
- encourages the correct adjustment of pH and oxygen levels
- lower incidence of wound-related infection
- reduced level of pain
- reduced risk of injury/disruption to wound through dressing changes
- promotes, where necessary, autolytic debridement.

(Dealey 2005)

Wound bed preparation (WBP) is described as a wound management paradigm based on existing concepts. It is supported by the 'TIME' framework (**t**issue, **i**nfection, **m**oisture and **e**dge), which provides practitioners with evidence based guidance for practice (Collier 2002; Sibbald *et al.* 2003). The aim of WBP is to achieve a stable, healthy, well-vascularised, granulating wound bed using actions appropriate to the management of the chronic wound.

This type of management contains four elements:

- debridement of necrotic tissue, e.g. autolytic or surgical
- effective management of exudate
- correction of bacterial balance
- resolution of damaged epidermal edge.

(Dealey 2005)

Debridement

Debridement describes any method that facilitates the removal of dead tissue, cell debris or foreign bodies from a wound and should only be undertaken by practitioners who have undergone specialist training, e.g. the community tissue viability specialist nurse (NICE 2005).

The purpose of debridement is to:

- determine the extent of the wound and identify any undermining
- remove non-viable tissue
- reduce the bacterial load and minimise risk of local and systemic infection
- allow wound drainage
- reduce odour
- promote healing.

(Edwards 2000)

Types of debridement include the following.

Autolytic

This method of debridement is dependent on the natural processes performed by neutrophils and macrophages and is suggested as being a less invasive approach. The process is enhanced by a moist wound environment which can be accomplished through the use of, e.g. hydrogel, hydrocolloid and semi occlusive dressings (Naylor *et al.* 2001).

Conservative sharp debridement (CSD)

This is the removal of dead tissue, with a scalpel or scissors, above the level of viable tissue (NICE 2005). It provides a fast and effective method of wound debridement; however, nurses should be aware of the other methods of debridement available. The nurse must have the knowledge and ability to select the appropriate method for each wound and apply it correctly. Often a combination of methods will be required to achieve rapid safe debridement. CSD may form part of an ongoing maintenance programme of debridement (Falanga 2004). Debridement is complete when 100% of the wound bed consists of healthy granulation tissue (Vowden & Vowden 1999).

Larval therapy

Lucilia sericata or green bottle larvae are selective, only ingesting necrotic tissue. This method should only be used on softened necrotic/sloughy tissue (Thomas & Jones 1999). The sterile larvae (maggots) are applied to and retained at the wound bed and are used generally in chronic wounds (Hinshaw 2000; NICE 2001). The larvae move over the surface of the wound, secreting a mixture of proteolytic enzymes, which break down necrotic tissue; it is also suggested that these secretions promote wound healing by changing pH levels (Hinshaw 2000). They remove devitalised tissue by this method (the enzymes are neutralised by live tissue) while at the same time ingesting and destroying bacteria.

The larvae produce enzymes that break down necrotic tissue which is described as biosurgical debridement.

Larval therapy is indicated for use on infected and necrotic wounds such as:

- osteomyelitis
- burns
- abscesses
- leg ulcers
- pressure ulcers
- surgical wounds
- diabetic foot ulcers
- malignant fungating wounds.

(Naylor *et al.* 2001; Dougherty & Lister 2011)

It is not advisable to apply larvae to wounds that may connect with vital organs or which contain fistulae (Thomas & Jones 1999).

There are two methods of larvae application.

- BioFOAM dressing. Maggots are sealed within a biofoam dressing, which is a finely woven pouch containing small pieces of foam that aid the growth of the larvae and manage exudate. The dressing can be left in place for up to 5 days (BioMonde 2011a).
- 'Free range' LarvE are applied directly on to the wound and retained within a specialised dressing system. The maggots can be left in place up to 3 days before being removed (BioMonde 2011b).

Topical negative pressure therapy (TNP)

TNP has been found to reduce bacterial colonisation, improve blood flow and promote granulation through the application of negative pressure consistently across the wound bed (Naylor *et al.* 2001). The dressing may be foam or gauze. It is a closed pressure system that is dependent on the maintenance of the vacuum seal to be effective; the pressure can be intermittent or continuous and should be set at a level indicated by the wound type (Dealey 2005; Benbow 2006).

TNP can be used on acute and chronic wounds for example:

- pressure ulcers
- cavity wounds
- diabetic foot ulcers

- venous ulcers
- grafts.

(KCI 2004)

It is contraindicated for use in:

- malignant wounds
- heavily infected wounds
- osteomyelitis (untreated)
- suspected and or unconfirmed fistula
- necrotic tissue (eschar present)
- wounds where there are exposed tendons.

(KCI 2004; Dougherty & Lister 2011)

Caution should also be exercised where the patient is on prescribed anticoagulant therapy and or there is active bleeding of the wound (Benbow 2006).

Wound cleansing

The purpose of wound cleansing is to remove excessive exudate/pus or dead tissue and therefore it should not be considered a routine part of wound management, it should only be undertaken when required, e.g. where excessive exudate is present (Morison 1989). If the wound is clean with little or no exudates, cleansing is contraindicated due to the potential damage caused to granulation and epithelialisation (Morison 1989). Furthermore, if carried out incorrectly, i.e. using cold solutions, or if the dressing procedure becomes protracted, the fall in wound temperature will have a negative effect on cell activity and this will further impact on the wound healing time (Collier 1996b).

In general, sterile 0.9% normal saline warmed to body temperature is suggested as being the safest and most appropriate solution for wound cleansing (Fletcher 1997; Morgan 2000). This should be delivered on to the wound under gentle pressure to produce an irrigation effect, if using Irriclens, the container should be held at least 15 cm from the wound to prevent splash back.

When using non-linting gauze swabs to aid the removal of slough, etc., during the cleansing process, care should be taken not to touch clean, healthy areas of the wound as this may damage regenerating epithelial cells (Rainey 2002).

To reduce the risk of postoperative wound-related infection only sterile normal saline should be used for wound irrigation during the first 48 hours post surgery (NICE 2008). Sterile 0.9% normal saline only should also be used where the patient is, for example, immunosupressed has an acute wound or burn, renal failure or a wound where there is exposed bone, tendon or ligament (NICE 2008).

For chronic wound cleansing, tap water at body temperature is often appropriate (RCN 2006; Dougherty & Lister 2011). A recently updated Cochrane review, from a limited number of research studies that spanned all care settings, found no evidence to suggest that using drinkable, good-quality tap water to cleanse wounds in adult patients increases the risk of infection (Fernandez & Griffiths 2007). However, it is suggested that all actual and potential risk factors along with the severity and extent of the wound are taken into consideration before the decision is made to use a non-sterile cleansing solution.

NB Topical antimicrobials or antiseptics must not be used for wound cleansing (Cooper 2004).

Dressing groups

Anecdotal evidence suggests there is currently an extensive and diverse number of dressing products/treatments available to community nurses on FP10, and that this can sometimes make it difficult to select the correct type. Please see Table 15.6 for the most common wound dressings and treatments used within community nursing. The products listed in the table are grouped under generic names, with some trade names given as examples. This is not an exhaustive table but may be used as a guide to selection.

Examples of potential complications in wound healing

Infection

Infection can be defined as the process by which organisms bind to tissue, multiply and invade tissue, eliciting a marked immune response (Kingsley *et al.* 2004).

The diagnosis of infection is determined by the co-existence of factors within the host:

- the quantity of invading micro-organisms
- the mixture of invading micro-organisms
- the effect of toxins
- the host's immune response.

(Kingsley 2001)

The resulting wound bioburden can range in severity, for example:

- *contamination* – the presence of bacteria without multiplication
- *colonisation* – the presence of bacteria with multiplication but with no host reaction
- *critical colonisation* – described as an imbalance of bacteria in the wound bed that prevents healing and

as with colonisation there is no evidence of a host reaction (Kingsley 2001; Moffatt *et al.* 2007)
- *infection* – the deposition and multiplication of bacteria with a host reaction.

(*see* Figure 15.6) (Ayton 1985)

There is an increased risk of infection if the patient is compromised by:

- age, as the immune system is less efficient
- underlying disease processes, e.g. malignancy and diabetes
- current and previous drug therapy, e.g. steroids or immunosuppressant drugs.

(EWMA 2005)

Although the presence of infection does not necessarily prevent wound healing, it can prolong the process, cause pain and lead to excessive production of scar tissue (Davis *et al.* 1992). It also adversely affects healing in the following ways.

- Infecting organisms compete with the cells in the healing tissue for nutrients and oxygen.
- It discourages fibroblast activity and the production of collagen.
- It promotes the release of lysozymes, which destroy existing collagen.
- It places additional demands on the inflammatory mechanism, which impedes its ability to focus on wound healing.
- It is associated with abscess formation in the wound.

(Davis *et al.* 1992; Dealey 2005)

The common signs and symptoms of infection include:

- pyrexia
- increased or change in the nature of pain
- redness
- heat
- swelling
- large amounts of exudate
- malodour.

However, if a patient has a diabetic foot or ischaemic wound the common signs of infection may be absent as a result of neuropathy and reduced arterial supply (Frykberg 2002). The absence of signs and symptoms may also occur where the patient is taking oral steroids or is immunosuppressed; in both instances delayed wound healing may occur (Dougherty & Lister 2011).

Additional criteria for identifying infection of venous and arterial leg ulcers include:

Table 15.6 Dressings groups

Please refer to manufacturer's recommendations with regard to individual products (Beldon 2006)

Dressings	Description	Advantages	Disadvantages
Activated charcoal dressing	Contain a layer of activated charcoal that traps odour-causing molecules thereby reducing/removing wound odour e.g. Carboflex (ConvaTec)	Easy to apply as either primary or secondary dressing; work immediately to reduce odour	Need to obtain a good seal to prevent leakage of odour; some dressings lose effectiveness when wet
Simple island dressings	Consist of a low-adherent absorbent pad located centrally on an adhesive backing. Simple island dressings are only to be used over wounds closed by primary intention, in other words over a suture line. The dressings have a central pad of cellulose material to absorb any oozing from the suture line during the first 24 hours post-surgery e.g. Primapore (Smith & Nephew), Medipore + Pad (3M), Alldress (Mölnlycke)	Quick and easy to apply; one-piece design negates need for multiple product use; protect the suture line from contamination and absorb exudate/blood	Only suitable for light exudate; some can cause skin damage (excoriation, blistering) if applied incorrectly
Alginates	A textile fibre dressing made from the calcium salt of an alginic acid polymer derived from brown seaweed; contain mannuronic and galuronic acids in varying amounts; available as a sheet, ribbon or packing They form a gel on contact with the wound surface by absorbing exudate and conform to the shape of the cavity e.g. Kaltostat (ConvaTec), Sorbsan Flat (Aspen Medical), Curasorb (Covidien), Algisite (Smith & Nephew).	Provide a moist wound environment; suitable for moderate to heavy exudate; can be used on infected wounds; useful for sinus and fistula drainage; some have haemostatic properties; can be irrigated out of wound with sodium chloride (0.9%). Alginate dressings can be used to lightly fill a cavity but should always be covered by a secondary dressing	Cannot be used on dry wounds or wound with hard necrotic tissue (eschar); sometimes a mild burning or 'drawing' sensation is reported on application; secondary dressing required
Antimicrobials	These topical dressings can be used as primary or secondary dressings and are available as alginates, hydrocolloids, charcoal impregnated and creams	Suitable for chronic wounds with heavy exudate that need protection from bacterial contamination by providing a broad range of antimicrobial activity; can reduce or prevent infection	Cannot be used during radiotherapy, sometimes sensitivity occurs with the use of silver and some skin staining can occur; instructions vary with products and dressings are expensive
Cadexomer bead dressings	Consist of hydophilic beads that contain iodine in powder or paste form, which swell and form a gel on contact with exudate	Useful in the treatment of infected, sloughy and necrotic wounds	Require retaining dressing; may be difficult to apply; caution in using products containing iodine. Should only be used for 3 months at a time. Not suitable for people with thyroid disorders

(Continued)

Table 15.6 (*Continued*)

Dressings	Description	Advantages	Disadvantages
Foams	Produced in a variety of forms, most being constructed of polyurethane foam and may have one or more layers; foam cavity dressings are also available e.g. Allevyn (Smith & Nephew), Mepilex Border (Mölnlycke), Biatain Adhesive (Coloplast), Versiva XC (ConvaTec), Tielle Lite (Systagenix)	Suitable for use with open, exuding wounds; non-adherent and provide a moist, thermally insulated wound environment. They can be used for light, moderate or heavy exuding wounds depending on the product Useful secondary dressings Foam dressings absorb exudate – some lock fluid within the core of the dressing, others transform into a gelling foam. Most foam dressings are available in bordered or non-bordered formats – the latter to be used if the patient has a skin sensitivity to adhesives Foam dressings indicate when they need to be changed through the spreading discolouration that appears on the dressing	May be difficult to use in wounds with deep tracts
Honey	Available as impregnated dressing pads or tubes of liquid honey; most widely used is Manuka honey	Suitable for acute and chronic infected, necrotic or sloughy wounds; provide a moist wound environment; non-adherent; antibacterial; assist with wound debridement; eliminate wound malodour; have an anti-inflammatory effect	Can be messy to use and cause leakage if excess exudate is present; caution in diabetes due to absorption of glucose and fructose
Hydrocolloids	Usually consist of a base material containing gelatin, pectin and carboxymethylcellulose combined with adhesives and polymers; base material may be bonded to either a semi-permeable film or a film plus polyurethane foam; some have an adhesive border Warming the dressing between the hands prior to application aids effective adhesion and makes the dressing more pliable The dressing should exceed the size of the wound by at least 2 cm e.g. Duoderm Signal (ConvaTec), Tegasorb (3M), Nu-Derm (Systagenix)	Suitable for acute and chronic wounds with low to no exudate; provide a moist wound environment; promote wound debridement; provide thermal insulation; waterproof and barrier to micro-organisms; easy to use dressings do not contain moisture, but instead form a 'seal' at the wound surface. This prevents the normal daily evaporation of moisture from the skin	May release degradation products into the wound; strong odour produced as dressing interacts with exudate; some hydrocolloids cannot be used on infected wounds Not recommended for general use on patients with diabetic foot ulcers unless on the recommendation of the diabetic foot clinic or tissue viability department

Hydrogels	Hydrogel dressings contain water but the percentage varies depending on the dressing. However, dressings generally contain between 60 and 70% water, which, with other constituents, is held in a viscous form known as the hydrogel. Alternatively, there are also hydrogel sheet dressings available, which contain less water e.g. intrasite Gel (Smith & Nephew), Nu-Gel (Systagenix), Actiform Cool Hydrogel Sheet (Activa Healthcare)	Hydrogel dressings are applied to wounds containing necrotic or dead tissue. Suitable for light exudate wounds; absorb small amounts of exudate; donate fluid to the dead tissue, softening it and aiding the body's process of autolytic debridement The dressings reduce pain and are cooling with low trauma at dressing changes	Cool the wound surface; use with caution in infected wounds; can cause skin maceration due to leakage if too much gel is applied or the wound has moderate to heavy exudate It is important not to apply excessive amounts of hydrogel as this may cause skin maceration. Any hydrogel dressing should be large enough to cover the wound and at least 3cm of surrounding skin. A hydrogel dressing will require a secondary dressing to hold it close against the wound bed – either a film dressing or a hydrocolloid dressing can be used for this purpose Hydrogel dressings may require changing every 2–3 days and care must be taken not to macerate the surrounding skin with excessive amounts of hydrogel
Hydrofibre	A soft, non-woven dressing composed of 100% hydrocolloid fibres (sodium carboxymethylcellulose); available as sheet or ribbon e.g. Aquacel (ConvaTec)	Suitable for highly exuding wounds. These are white fibrous dressings comprising 100% Hydrofibre (sodium carboxymethylcellulose), which is applied dry. On absorbing exudate it is transformed into a gel-like sheet, maintaining a moist environment, which aids autolytic debridement and promotes angiogenesis. It is used on moderate to heavily exuding wounds and must be changed when fully saturated with exudate	Requires a secondary dressing. Patients may occasionally mention a 'drawing' sensation as the dressing absorbs the exudate. These dressings may occasionally stick to the edges of a wound so it is advisable not to overlap onto the surrounding skin
Vapour permeable films and membranes		Water vapour loss may occur at a slower rate than exudate is generated so that fluid accumulates under the dressing and this can cause tissue maceration. Possibility of adhesive trauma if removed incorrectly; do not contain exudate and can macerate, slip or leak
Skin barrier films/creams	Polyurethane film with a hypoallergenic acrylic adhesive; have a variety of application methods often consisting of a plastic or cardboard carrier e.g. Cavilon No sting barrier film (3M Healthcare), Cavilon Durable barrier cream (3M Healthcare)	Only suitable for shallow superficial wounds; prophylactic use against friction damage; useful as secondary dressing; allow passage of water vapour; allow monitoring of the wound Alcohol-free liquid polymer that forms a protective film on the skin e.g. Mepore Film (Mölnlycke), OpSite (Smith & Nephew), Tegaderm Film (3M)

Sterility	Contamination	Colonisation	Critical colonisation	Infection
Absence of microbes	Presence of microbes but little active growth	Growth and death of microbes kept at safe level by host immune response (healthy balance)	Host defences unable to maintain healthy balance, either too many microbes or too many species in wound base	Host defences overwhelmed, local cellulitis (might lead to bacteraemia, septicaemia and death)
Very brief period following initial surgical incision or thermal trauma	Present soon after initial wounding, progresses quickly to colonisation	Situation normal	Delay in healing	Exacerbation of ulceration
No action:	**Action:**	**Action:**	**Action:**	**Action:**
Situation will not persist in wounds healing by secondary intention	No need to artificially prevent movement to colonisation in wounds healing by secondary intention (possible exception burns of 10 percent plus, patients need admission to specialist centres)	Do not disturb balance (possible exception diabetic foot wounds)	Consider antiseptics to return wound to colonisation, review wound, debride quickly and safely as possible if necrotic tissue/ slough present	Systemic antibiotics +/− antiseptics

Figure 15.6 Methods for dealing with each stage of the infection continuum (Kingsley 2003). Reproduced by kind permission of HMP Communications.

- venous:
  - dull brick red wound bed (indicates β-haemolytic streptococci)
  - blue/green exudate (may indicate *Pseudomonas aeruginosa*)
- arterial:
  - erythema or bluish-purple peri-ulcer of tissues
  - palpable crepitus from gas in soft tissue.

(Cutting *et al.* 2004)

Bacterial sampling
Wound swabs should be taken when you suspect the patient has a clinical infection, and not routinely (Donovan 1998). A clear rationale for swabbing should be identified, and appropriate information completed on the microbiology form, for example:

- patient's name
- date of birth
- GP name and practice bar code number
- swab site
- the name of any antibiotic therapy (current or recent)
- date and time of specimen
- the name of any topical antibacterial preparations currently being used.

Cellulitis
Cellulitis is a bacterial infection that occurs when bacteria invade the soft tissues through small wounds or abrasions on the skin surface or through existing conditions, for example leg ulceration, athlete's foot, insect bites or trauma.

Common sites for cellulitis:

- face
- hands/arms
- lower limbs.

Risk factors include:

- obesity
- trauma to the lower limb
- venous and lymphatic insufficiency
- athlete's foot (tinea pedis)
- diabetes
- peripheral vascular disease.

(Eagle 2007)

Lower leg cellulitis is a commonly seen condition in both primary and secondary care (Eagle 2007), but care should be taken to accurately identify the cause. Prior to commencing treatment it is essential that a differential diagnosis is made to rule out symptoms associated with, for example, venous insufficiency, such as lipodermatosclerosis, deep vein thrombosis, varicose eczema (Moffatt *et al.* 2007), and co-morbidities, for example, acute exacerbation of heart failure.

The clinical symptoms of cellulitis include:

- flu-like symptoms prior to cellulitis developing
- acute pain
- area of hot, tender, erythematous swelling in tissues surrounding an existing wound; this area extends rapidly
- generalised erythematous, tender, swollen limb
- raised white cell count (WCC) and raised C-reactive protein (CRP)
- pyrexia.

NB Although non-specific, nearly all patients have a raised white cell count and elevated ESR or C-reactive protein (CREST 2005).

The first-line treatment of cellulitis should include:

- assessment of the patient's pain
- analgesia
- where possible, elevation of the affected limb
- where the lower leg is affected the patient should be encouraged to do dorsiflexion exercises to improve venous return.

For further information on the management of cellulitis please refer to www.lymphoedema.org/lsn

Types of wound commonly managed by community nurses

Leg ulceration

Leg ulcers are defined as a wound on the lower leg that has failed to heal within the normal healing time of 4–6 weeks (Moffatt *et al.* 2007). Ulceration is a debilitating and painful condition; ulcers may be chronic, recurrent or long term in nature and it has been estimated that the cost to the NHS of treating venous leg ulcers is in the region of £168–198 million per annum (Posnett & Franks 2007). Furthermore it is suggested that with an increasing aging population the prevalence and cost of treatment and management will increase (Douglas, 2001).

There are approximately 40 recognised underlying causes of leg ulceration, the majority of which are said

to be caused by alteration to blood flow or inadequate blood flow (Franks & Moffatt 2007).

Due to co-morbidities, a patient may present with mixed venous/arterial ulcers and therefore have a combination of the signs and symptoms (Sieggreen & Kline 2004; RCN 2006; Franks & Moffatt 2007). As a consequence, errors in the diagnosis of underlying aetiology and the mismanagement of treatment can result in serious complications for the patient (RCN 2006).

Leg ulcers have an impact on social and psychological factors, and the effects on quality of life should not be underestimated (Hopkins 2004). Where possible, the community nurse should take steps to address any concerns or care needs that the patient may have. These may include:

- pain
- impaired mobility
- sleep disturbance
- fear
- anger
- depression
- body image
- embarrassment
- social isolation
- employment.

(Persoon *et al.* 2004; Briggs & Fleming 2007; Souza Nogueira *et al.* 2009)

Patients may also feel self-conscious about wound odour and or how they look, and avoid social situations and communal places (Briggs & Fleming 2007). Clothing or shoes may need to be changed or adapted to cover their legs or fit over bandaging, impacting on body image and self-esteem (Ebbeskog & Ekman 2001). Body image may continue to be problematic for some patients once the ulcer has healed. This is because scarring or skin discolouration on their leg, caused by underlying conditions such as staining or ankle flare, may cause embarrassment (Hawkins & Lindsay 2006). Depression appears to be common among patients with leg ulcers and their perception of their own body image seems to be a major contributory factor (Ebbeskog & Ekman 2001; Hopkins 2004; Persoon *et al.* 2004).

It is also suggested that there is a causal link between clinical depression and delayed healing (Moffatt 2004).

Leg ulcer assessment

Leg ulcer assessment to determine the underlying aetiology is a highly skilled and complex activity and should

365

Table 15.7 Signs, symptoms and characteristics of venous and arterial disease/ulcers (SIGN 1998; RCN 2006)

Signs and symptoms	Arterial disease	Venous disease
Site of ulceration	■ Ulcer formation more common on the foot	■ Ulcer are usually found in the gaiter area
Pain	■ Worse at night when the leg is elevated, and with exercise ■ Rest pain associated with critical ischaemia ■ Intermittent claudication	■ Dull, aching or neuropathic ■ Venous rush pain on rising from bed ■ Relieved by elevation ■ Increases during dressing procedures and on exposure to air
Skin	■ Changes usually found below the ankle of the affected limb/s ■ Cold, white, shiny, hairless and taut ■ Trophic changes to the nails ■ Dependent rubor or 'sunset rubra' (skin of the affected limb changes to a reddish colour on dependence)	■ Changes usually found in the gaiter region of the affected limb/s ■ Ankle flare (dilation of the small vessels) ■ Haemosiderin staining ■ Lipodermatosclerosis (fibrosis) ■ Atrophie blanche (avascular areas of white tissue) ■ Eczema, may be wet, dry, localised or general
Oedema	Often seen when legs are dependent	Worse in the evening reduces with elevation
Toes	Poor capillary refill/cyanosed.	N/A
Veins	N/A	Often distended
Appearance of ulcer	■ Punched-out, deep with extensive tissue loss ■ Typically small in size, distal, with a steep 'rolled edge' ■ Poor perfusion of wound base, pale in colour ■ Often occur over bony prominences ■ Low exudate (level may be higher if infection is present) ■ Bone or tendon may be visible	■ Irregular in shape ■ Shallow, with 'beefy' granulation tissue in the base ■ May be multiple or circumferential ■ High exudate
Pulses	■ Foot pulses absent or difficult to find ■ The ankle/brachial pressure index (ABPI) is less than 0.8 ■ Poor capillary refilling time ■ Patient may complain of intermittent claudication	■ Foot pulses palpable ■ The ABPI is 0.8 or over
Examples of presenting medical/clinical patient history	■ Rheumatoid arthritis ■ Heart disease; stroke; myocardial infarction (MI); transient ischaemic attack (TIA) ■ Peripheral vascular disease ■ Hypertension ■ Cigarette smoking ■ Family history of non-venous ulceration ■ Diabetes ■ Raynaud's syndrome ■ Sickle cell anaemia	■ Varicose veins ■ Proven or suspected deep vein thrombosis (DVT) ■ Surgery or leg fracture/s ■ Family history

only be carried out by a trained, competent practitioner (RCN 2006). The lack of a comprehensive clinical assessment can lead to ineffective and inappropriate treatment, which can cause serious limb damage (RCN 2006). Assessment should include the following.

■ Obtaining the patient's full clinical and lifestyle history, including familial history, mobility status and ankle movement.
■ A full medication history, including prescribed and OTC medication.

- Baseline observations, including weight and urinalysis.
- Consideration of patient risk factors (Table 15.8).
- A physical examination of both lower limbs, irrespective of whether both have ulceration. This should be carried out with the patient in both a lying and standing position.
- Appropriate blood and relevant laboratory tests depending on the patient's clinical history and ulcer presentation.
- Doppler ultrasound (both legs).
- Visual assessment of both the patient and the leg ulcer.
- Clear concise completion of all relevant documentation.

(Elliott *et al.* 1996; Vowden *et al.* 1996; Stevens *et al.* 1997; SIGN 1998; RCN 2006)

The purpose of assessment is to:

- determine the correct aetiology
- establish a differential diagnosis (*see* Tables 15.9 and 15.10)
- aid decision making
- ensure that the appropriate treatment is selected

Table 15.8 Predisposing factors for ulceration (Moffatt *et al.* 2007)

Factor	Effect
Age	Increased risk of arterial disease with increasing age
CVA/TIA	Indicates arterial disease
Hypertension	Indicates arterial disease
MI/Angina/IHD/PVD	Indicates arterial disease
Diabetes	May result in calcification of arteries
Auto-immune disease, e.g. rheumatoid arthritis	Vasculitis and inflammatory ulceration
DVT/phlebitis	Damage to vein valves
Varicose veins (treated or untreated)	Sign of venous hypertension
Orthopaedic or abdominal surgery/Fractured lower limbs/ Trauma to lower limbs	Potential for undiagnosed DVT/ineffective vein valves
Pregnancy	Pelvic congestion causes increased venous pressure in lower limbs
Constipation	Increased pressure on pelvic veins

Table 15.9 Differential diagnosis (Moffatt *et al.* 2007)

	Venous	Arterial	Mixed
Site	Usually gaiter area, near lateral or medial malleolus (but can be anywhere on leg)	Any part of leg, commonly below ankle, toes, heel, foot and lateral aspect of leg. May be multiple small lesions	Could be anywhere on leg/foot depending on the aetiology
Wound bed/edge	Shallow with diffuse edges	Deep with 'cliff edges', 'punched out'	Mix of both
Exudate	Can be highly exuding	Normally very little	Range of exudate level
Oedema	Generalised, worse at end of day	Localised and dependent oedema	Other possible causes of oedema should be investigated and eliminated, e.g. cardiac, renal
Limb	Warm, well-perfused, staining, eczema, ankle flare, atrophe blanche	Usually thinner, colder, pale on elevation, rubor when dependent, shiny, hairless skin	Staining is irreversible so staining can be present with arterial impairment
Varicosities	Often (they may not be always visible)	Unusual	Could be present if the aetiology is mixed arterial and venous disease
Pulses	Present	Reduced/absent	Present or absent
Pain	Usually associated with oedema and infection	Severe intractable pain, usually worse at night/on elevation	Range of pain levels

367

- aid symptom management
- support consistency in approach to treatment.

(Flanagan 2003; RCN 2006; SIGN 2010)

All patients who have a wound on the lower limb for a period of 6 weeks or longer should have a full holistic leg ulcer assessment that includes a doppler ABPI (ankle brachial pressure index (RCN 2006; SIGN 2010).

Vascular assessment
Assessment with Doppler ultrasound is a skilled technique and community nurses should not attempt to undertake this procedure if they have not received training and are not deemed competent (RCN 2006; SIGN 2010). Doppler ultrasound is not a diagnostic indicator – the test should be viewed as a screening tool

Table 15.10 Clinical conditions of leg ulceration (Moffatt *et al.* 2007)

Common clinical conditions	Contributory factors
Venous disease	DVT, family history, primary deep vein reflux, fixed/limited ankle function, obesity
Arterial disease	Atherosclerosis, acute arterial thrombus or embolism, inflammatory vascular disease
Mixed arterial and venous disease	Combination of above
Other clinical conditions	
Trauma	Burns, cuts, pre-tibial lacerations, inappropriate bandaging, IV drug abuse
Haematological	Thalassaemia, polycythaemia, leukaemia, sickle cell anaemia
Metabolic disease	Diabetes mellitus
Neoplastic	Squamous cell carcinoma, basal cell carcinoma, Bowen's disease
Neuropathic	Diabetes mellitus, paralysis, alcoholic neuropathy
Connective tissue diseases	Rheumatoid arthritis, polyarthritis, systemic lupus erythematosus

for arterial disease and an aid to assessment and decision making regarding the most appropriate treatment and management (RCN 2006; SIGN 1998). It must never be used in isolation but as part of a complete assessment that incorporates the patient's clinical history and clinical presentation (RCN 2006; CREST 1998; SIGN 2010). Doppler ultrasound is contraindicated where the patient has or is suspected of having a deep vein thrombosis (Moffatt *et al.* 2007).

The ankle brachial pressure index (ABPI) is a ratio comparing the systolic blood pressure in the upper and lower limbs (Moffatt *et al.* 2007). If arterial function is normal there should be minimal difference, if there is a significant difference this would be indicative of arterial disease (Moffatt *et al.* 2007).

ABPI measurement is an important element in defining a safe level of compression therapy for those patients with venous disease (Vowden & Vowden 2001), therefore it is essential that community nurses perform Doppler ultrasound as an integral part of their assessment.

Calculation of ABPI
The ABPI for each leg is calculated by dividing the highest of the ankle pressures by the higher of the two brachial pressures (Figure 15.7).

Interpretation of ABPI
In the absence of other presenting clinical or medical factors, a patient with 'normal' arterial circulation will have an ankle systolic equal or slightly higher than the brachial systolic, i.e. ABPI of 1.00 or just above (Moffatt *et al.* 2007). Any deficit below 1.00 indicates the degree of arterial insufficiency, i.e. an ABPI of 0.6 means only 60% of the arterial flow is reaching that limb (Stubbing *et al.* 1997). The lower the reading the greater the arterial impairment (Table 15.11). ABPI should be interpreted with caution in patients with diabetes mellitus, as falsely elevated readings can be the result of arterial calcification (Vowden & Vowden 2001; Ruff 2003; Stevens 2004).

Toe brachial pressure index assessment (TBPI)
TBPI assessment is indicated where there is a falsely high ABPI reading as a result of calcification of larger vessels or where pain, the size of the ulceration or gross lower limb oedema makes ABPI measurement impossible (Moffatt *et al.* 2007).

$$\text{Ankle brachial pressure index} = \frac{\text{Highest ankle systolic pressure for each leg}}{\text{Highest brachial systolic pressure}}$$

Figure 15.7 ABPI calculation.

Calculating the TBPI

For this calculation comparison is made between the toe and arm pressures and is calculated in the same way as the ABPI, i.e. TBPI pressure divided by the highest brachial pressure (Moffatt *et al*. 2007).

Interpreting the TBPI

Toe pressures are usually smaller than brachial pressures due to the differences in the size of the arteries assessed and therefore the ratios are also lower. For example:

- TBPI > 0.7 – normal satisfactory peripheral arterial supply (Moffatt *et al*. 2007).
- TBPI < 0.65 – indicative of peripheral arterial insufficiency and the patient should be referred to a vascular surgeon for investigations (Moffatt *et al*. 2007) (see Table 15.12).

As with ABPI assessment, TBPI should be viewed as an aid to assessment and must be interpreted by a trained competent community nurse or tissue viability specialist nurse (TVN) within the context of a full holistic assessment.

Table 15.11 Interpretation of ABPI (Vowden & Vowden 2001; Ruff 2003; Stevens 2004)

ABPI	Level of disease
1.3 or above	May indicate arterial disease or calcification. Seek advice from TVN. A toe Doppler pressure index (TBPI) should be carried out
1.0–1.3	Normal arterial flow. High compression is probably safe in the absence of other contraindications
0.8–1.0	Mild arterial disease but indicates enough blood flow for compression therapy in conjunction with clinical assessment
0.5–0.8	Moderate arterial insufficiency. Seek specialist advice as reduced compression therapy may be safe following specialist guidance **NB** Compression should not be applied
< 0.5	Severe ischaemia – urgent referral to vascular surgeon should be advised. No compression

Management of venous leg ulcers

General skin care surrounding the ulcer is essential to maintain skin integrity (SIGN 2010).

Regular washing of the limb in warm tap water with an emollient, if tolerated, helps to remove excess exudate and reduces the odour from the ulcer (Morison *et al*. 2007). The skin surrounding the ulcer should be coated with a barrier preparation to prevent maceration (SIGN 2010).

It is suggested that varicose eczema affects 37–44% of patients with venous leg ulceration (Dealey 2005). It is typically characterised by a dry, weeping, scaly, erythematous reaction of the skin and the patient may complain of itching or a burning sensation (Dealey 2005). If the patient should develop this it is essential to review all products being used on the patient's legs and the type of gloves used during dressing changes to exclude contact allergies. In cases of severe or acute eczema it is suggested that the first-line treatment should be the correct strength of topical corticosteroids (Cameron 2004) this should be in ointment form as cream contains allergens (Moffatt *et al*. 2007).

Compression therapy

Graduated compression bandaging is used to apply therapeutic graduated compression to the limb, providing the highest pressures (40–50 mmHg) at the ankle in a mobile person (Moffatt *et al*. 2007) reducing gradually to 20–25 mmHg below the knee (Partsch 2003; Moffatt *et al*. 2007). There are several factors that will affect the pressure under the bandage (Figure 15.8).

The aim of compression therapy is to:

- reduce the blood pressure in the superficial venous system
- aid venous return of blood to the heart
- reduce oedema of the limb
- increase the velocity of blood flow within the vessels

Table 15.12 Calculation of TBPI

	Right	**Left**
Brachial	130	138
Toe	104	78
TBPI	0.75	0.56

$$\text{Pressure mmHg} = \frac{\text{Number of layers of bandage} \times \text{tension applied} \times 4620}{\text{Circumference of limb} \times \text{width of bandage}}$$

Figure 15.8 Laplace's law (Moffatt *et al*. 2007).

Table 15.13 Types of graduated compression therapy

Compression therapy system	Bandage components	Pressure achieved
Multi/four-layer (long stretch) **NB** For ankle circumference greater than 25 cm use the K-Three C instead of the K-Plus	K-Soft (ensure correct shaping of leg and protection of vulnerable bony areas; *see* section on distorted limbs) K-Lite (spiral, 50% stretch, 50% overlap) K-Plus (figure of eight application, 50% stretch, 50% overlap) Ko-Flex (spiral application 50% stretch, 50% overlap)	40 mmHg at the ankle
Two-layer compression bandaging kit (K-Two long stretch)	K-Press (spiral application as per manufacturers guidance) K-Tech (spiral application as per manufacturers guidance) Use K-Soft as padding first, if required, for correct shaping of leg and protection of vulnerable bony areas (*see* limb shaping)	40 mmHg at the ankle
Short stretch	Actico (100% stretch, 50% overlap, spiral)	30–40 mmHg at the ankle

- facilitate the action of the calf muscle pump
- improve healing time.

(Moffatt *et al.* 2007)

Graduated multi-component bandaging should be routinely used for the treatment of uncomplicated venous leg ulcers (SIGN, 2010) but must only be applied by a trained, competent practitioner after a full, holistic patient assessment has been carried out (RCN 2006; SIGN 2010).

An appropriate primary dressing should be applied under compression; the first choice being a simple, non-adherent wound contact layer, e.g. NA Ultra (RCN 2006; SIGN 2010). If wounds are large and heavily exuding, a more appropriate dressing will be required to reduce the need for more frequent dressing and bandage changes (*see* Table 15.6).

It is essential to remember that distorted limb shapes, e.g. due to oedema, or inverted champagne bottle-shaped or thin, bony limbs are at high risk of damage from compression bandaging if left unprotected. If the patient has no known allergies, wool padding should be applied to the leg prior to the application of the compression bandage system to achieve a graduated limb shape; making the calf of the leg wider than the ankle (Moffatt *et al.* 2007). Particular attention must be given to vulnerable bony areas that may need extra padding; the ankle circumference must be measured after reshaping of the limb to ensure that the correct bandage system is selected (Moffatt *et al.* 2007) (*see* Table 15.13).

In general an ABPI measurement of < 0.8 is considered an exclusion criteria for the application of compression. However, it is suggested that any clinical decision regarding the application/non-application

Table 15.14 Examples of graduated compression hosiery

Class	British Standard (e.g. Activa)	RAL (German Standard) (e.g. ActiLymph, Mediven)
Liner	10 mmHg	
1	14–17 mmHg	18–22 mmHg
2	18–24 mmHg	23–33 mmHg
3	25–35 mmHg	34–36 mmHg

should not be based solely on the result of this investigation and other clinical factors should also be taken into consideration (Moffatt *et al.* 2007).

Compression hosiery

Hosiery kits have been developed to give a graduated compression that is 35–40 mmHg at the ankle (Moffatt *et al.* 2007) (Table 15.14); where necessary these can be custom made.

Hosiery kits can be used for the following.

- The treatment of venous ulcers where the exudate levels are low and therefore a low-profile dressing can be used.
- Patients with venous disease who are unable to tolerate bandaging or who want to be more self-caring.
- Ongoing management to help prevent recurrence of venous leg ulcers.

(Lindsay 2004)

They should not be used on:

- heavy exudate and large wounds
- large or irregular shape limbs (bandages would be more appropriate)

- patients with small limbs or bony prominences (bandages should be used)
- people with diabetes unless after specialist advice
- patients with arterial disease.

(Lindsay 2004)

Prevention of venous leg ulcer recurrence

In the absence of any significant arterial impairment, lifetime compression therapy (hosiery) is advocated for venous disease (RCN 2006; SIGN 2010).

All patients with a healed venous leg ulcer should have a Doppler ABPI assessment every 6 months to confirm suitability for ongoing compression therapy. This may be extended to 12 months for those patients who, for example, have had a stable ABPI for 2 years (Clinical Knowledge Summaries 2011).

Patients with healed venous ulcers should be fitted with the highest level of compression they can tolerate and safely apply (Moffatt *et al.* 2007).

Management of arterial leg ulcers

The potential for healing arterial ulcers is limited unless the arterial supply to the limb can be improved (Moffatt 2001; Dealey 2005). Consequently the management and treatment should primarily be aimed at restoring and or maintaining blood flow and the avoidance of lower limb amputation.

Palpation of the patient's foot pulses is suggested as being an unreliable indicator of arterial disease (Moffatt & O'Hare 1995). Therefore it is recommended that a Doppler ultrasound should form the basis of arterial assessment to record the patient's ABPI in both legs. If the ABPI is < 0.5, compression therapy *should not* be applied and it is recommended that the patient is referred to a vascular surgeon for further investigations and assessment (RCN 1998; SIGN 1998; Dealey 2005; Vowden & Vowden 1997).

Conservative treatment should include the correct selection of an appropriate dressing, according to the needs of the wound; it may also be appropriate to apply a wool bandage and light retention bandage to help keep the limb warm and encourage perfusion but not to restrict the blood supply to the limb (Stevens 2004; Dealey 2005).

Management of mixed arterial/venous ulcers

As with all leg ulceration, a holistic leg ulcer assessment, correct dressing selection and technique, and skin care is essential. However, for this type of ulcer establishing the most predominant causative factor, i.e. venous or arterial insufficiency, is imperative in determining the most appropriate treatment (Dealey 2005).

In patients with an ABPI measurement of 0.5–0.8, and depending on other presenting clinical signs and symptoms, a reduced level of compression between 15 and 25 mmHg may be appropriate (Marston & Vowden 2003). If there is any element of uncertainty the community nurse should seek advice from the tissue viability specialist nurse and where necessary request a joint visit for patient assessment before applying reduced compression.

It is suggested that a reduced level of compression can be achieved, for example by omitting the third layer of a four-layer bandage system or through the use of various multi-layer bandaging combinations (Dealey 2005; Moffatt *et al.* 2007) (Table 15.15). Concordance with this approach to treatment may be difficult for some patients, particularly if they are experiencing ischaemic pain. Therefore it may be necessary to include night nursing visits to remove the bandages prior to the patient going to bed and early morning visits from the day staff to reapply them. Patient safety is of particular importance when using compression for the treatment of ulcers with mixed aetiology, and careful close monitoring must be strictly adhered to (Dealey 2005).

Where the patient's medical history and clinical signs and symptoms, including an ABPI measurement of < 0.5, indicate that arterial disease is the predominant causative factor, treatment and management should be followed as above.

Table 15.15 Reduced compression (15–25 mmHg) (Dealey 2005; Moffatt *et al.* 2007)

Components	Pressure achieved
K-Soft (ensure correct shaping of leg and protection of vulnerable bony areas)	14–17 mmHg at the ankle
K-Lite (spiral application, 50% stretch, 50% overlap)	
K-Plus (figure of eight application, 50% stretch, 50% overlap)	
K-Soft (ensure correct shaping of leg and protection of vulnerable bony areas.)	18–23 mmHg at the ankle
K-Lite (spiral, 50% stretch, 50% overlap)	
Ko-Flex (spiral, 50% stretch, 50% overlap)	

Diabetic foot ulceration

Foot ulceration in patients with diabetes is most commonly the result of: (a) altered quality of the skin, (b) neuropathic, (c) ischaemic changes or a combination of these factors, i.e. neuroischaemic (Dealey 2005; Moffatt et al. 2007).

Following patient assessment, which should include Semmes-Weinstein monofilament testing (Wiersema-Bryant & Kraemer 2000) (Figure 15.9), it is useful to classify the ulcer for future reference. There are several systems available that classify the ulcer by depth, presence of ischaemia and presence of infection, such as the Wagner Classification of Diabetic Foot Ulcers scale (Wagner 1987) (Table 15.4) and the University of Texas Wound Classification System of Diabetic Foot Ulcers (Lavery et al. 1996).

Wound healing is impeded by diabetes mellitus in many ways that are cumulative in their effects. People living with diabetes:

- have a fivefold increase in the risk of wound infection

- have an impaired inflammatory response resulting in poor quality granulation tissue
- suffer from atherosclerosis and small vessel disease that impairs blood flow and healing
- have reduced pain sensation and proprioception (the perception of impulses from the sensory organs (proprioceptors) that give information about the position and movements of the body (Brown 2001).

(Davis et al. 1992)

Exudate levels in this type of ulcer are minimal, but may increase if an infection is present. However, the signs of infection are often masked due to poor immune function, so careful observation of the affected area and documentation are vital. Documentation must be concise and timely, with photographs and linear measurements, rather than tracings, used to track healing progress as there will usually be little noticeable change in the size of the wound (Dealey 2000). Dressing selection should be those that avoid further skin damage and prevent exudate being left in contact with the skin for any length of time. Infection in the limb of a patient with diabetes must not be ignored and must be referred immediately for medical intervention.

The commonly accepted principles of management and where possible prevention of ulceration includes:

- holistic assessment, including the appropriate use of a 5.07 gauge monofilament (at least yearly) to test for sensory neuropathy
- palpation of foot pulses (a minimum of yearly)
- close monitoring of glycaemic control as hyperglycaemia is associated with infection and poor wound healing (Van den Berghe 2001; Dealey 2005)
- Doppler ultrasound
- the identification of any foot abnormalities and referral to, e.g. a specialist diabetic podiatrist
- prompt treatment of infection
- the assessment of footwear and where necessary referral to an orthotist
- patient education; this should include nutrition, foot hygiene and the need for daily inspection of their skin for broken or cracked areas or redness
- correct toe nail cutting, i.e. straight across
- general skin care and the use of emollients and moisturisers
- monitoring to identify diabetes-associated complications.

(NICE 2004; Dealey 2005; Moffatt et al. 2007)

Relatively minor injuries for those living with diabetes may precipitate ulceration (Watkins 2003), therefore the overarching key to effective management is prevention,

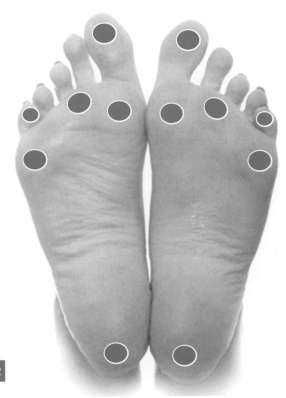

Figure 15.9 Monofilament test areas (McIntosh 2010, © Seattle Group Health Cooperative).

early detection and prompt treatment delivered within a multidisciplinary approach (Edmonds *et al.* 1996).

If the community nurse has any concerns about care and treatment it is recommended that the patient should be referred to a specialist practitioner for further advice, e.g. tissue viability and diabetic specialist nurses.

Pressure ulcers

A pressure ulcer is an area of localised damage to the skin and underlying tissues. They are most commonly found where pressure compresses tissue over a bony or cartilaginous prominence in the body (Collins *et al.* 2002). This can result in tissue necrosis that involves muscle, tendon and bone (RCN 2006). It is suggested that 20% of inpatients, 30% of patients in the community and 20% of people living in nursing and residential homes are affected by pressure ulcers (NPSA 2010).

The NPSA estimates that since 2005, 75 000 safety incidents relating to patients developing pressure ulcers have been received (NPSA 2010); the cost of treating these is said to be in the region of £11 000 to £40 000 per patient, depending on the severity of the ulcer (NPSA 2010). Viewed as a high-risk area, pressure ulcers

have been included in the NPSA National 10 for 2010 programme. The programme aims to reduce the harm caused to patients from pressure ulcers by highlighting prevention, improving reporting and encouraging the sharing of best practice through closer working partnerships (NPSA 2010). This process is further supported by NHS London's serious incident reporting framework for grade 3 and 4 pressure ulcers (NHS London 2011).

The development and treatment of pressure ulcers has considerable implications for both patients and the health service; the most significant being longer hospital stays or community care provision. Consequently, for the patient the effects of this include increased pain and discomfort and a predisposition to systemic illness and, in extreme cases, it may become life threatening (NICE 2001).

There is a large body of evidence regarding, for example, the common sites for pressure ulcer development, those at risk and contributory factors (Table 15.16). However, five key areas have been identified as being most significant:

- immobility
- nutrition

Table 15.16 Examples of common sites and contributory risk factors of pressure ulcer development (Waterlow 1988; Kelly 1994; NICE 2001, 2005; Collins *et al.* 2002; EPUAP 2003; Sciarra 2003)

Common sites	Extrinsic factors	Intrinsic factors	Other risk factors
Sacrum	Pressure or external compression	Extremes of age	Patients that are obese or below average weight
Buttocks		Vascular disease	
Spinal vertebrae	Shear	Reduced mobility or immobility	Incontinent patients (faecal and urinary)
Hips	Friction	Chronic disease	
Heels	Equipment and incorrect moving and handling techniques	Terminal illness	Wheelchair users
Malleoli		Acute illness, e.g. chest infection	Patients that are bed/chair bound
Scapula	Enforced immobility	The co-existence of peripheral neuropathy and microvascular disease increase the risk of damage, e.g. in those with diabetes mellitus	Inability to change position
Top of ears	Sitting for long periods		Older adults
Elbow	Lying in the same position for long periods		Those patients with a poor nutritional/hydration status
		Co-morbidities	Co-morbidity
	Medication, e.g. sedatives, steroids, cytotoxics, anti-inflammatory	Excessive perspiration/skin moisture, e.g. where the patient has a pyrexia	Those with a metabolic disorder
		Wound leakage	Those patients with a malignancy
		Sensory impairment	Immunosuppressed patients
		Level of consciousness	Anaemic patients
		Previous history of pressure damage	The unconscious patient
		Malnutrition	Patients with a spinal injury
		Dehydration	Orthopaedic/medical patients

- perfusion
- age
- skin condition.

(Nixon & McGough 2001)

a) Supine position

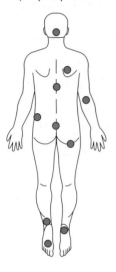

b) Seated position

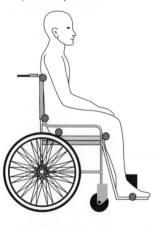

c) Lateral position

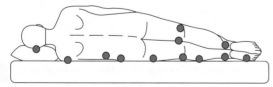

Figure 15.10 Common sites of pressure ulcers (Whiteing 2009). © Royal College of Nursing Publications.

The most common cause of pressure ulcer development is external compression of the soft tissues; this leads to interruption of the circulation to a specific area of the body (Figure 15.10) causing tissue death through ischaemia (Whiteing 2009). The effects of external pressure can be further compounded by, for example, intrinsic factors shear and friction (Sciarra 2003; Dealey 2005; Benbow 2006).

One of the first-line management factors in the prevention of pressure ulcer development is the inspection of each individual patient's skin, focusing on those areas considered to be vulnerable. Risk assessment is also important and should be carried out within 6 hours of contact, regardless of the care setting (NICE 2005). Risk assessment should only be carried out by clinicians who have undergone appropriate training (NICE 2005).

Reassessment of the patient and any relevant equipment being used should form an integral part of community nurses' risk management strategies. This should be carried out using appropriate tools, combined with, for example, photographs and/or calibrated tracings to support clinical judgement and decisions (NICE 2005) (Box 15.1) on initial patient assessment and thereafter a minimum of once weekly or, where indicated, depending on the patient's overall or changing condition (EPUAP 2003; Whiteing 2009). Where there is skin discoloration the blood supply to the affected area should also be assessed using a blanch test (Vanderwee et al. 2007). Other factors that should be taken into consideration with skin discolouration include:

- induration
- warmth
- oedema
- hardness.

(Bethell 2005)

As with all nursing care, contemporaneous, accurate and up-to-date documentation of findings is essential for good communication, evaluation of treatment and management plans (NICE 2005), and continuity of care. The patient's management plan should include the frequency of re-positioning, time spent sitting, the type of mattress/seat cushion used and, when provided, nutritional assessment/supplementation and evaluation of all related interventions (NICE 2005).

Pressure-relieving/reducing equipment
A wide variety of devices are available to help relieve pressure over susceptible areas, e.g. cushions, overlays,

static/dynamic mattresses and replacement beds. The available devices differ in function and complexity and between provider services (NICE 2003). Equipment choice should be based on:

- patient risk assessment
- the severity, cause and location of pressure or ulcer if present
- skin assessment
- the general health of the patient
- the patient's lifestyle and abilities
- critical care needs
- patient acceptability and comfort
- availability of help for re-positioning
- the patient's weight.

It is recommended that all vulnerable patients, including those with a grade 1–2 pressure ulcer, should be nursed at least on a high-specification foam mattress (NICE 2005). Those with a grade 3–4 pressure ulcer should 'have a high-specification foam mattress with an alternating pressure overlay or a sophisticated continuous low-pressure system, for example low air loss, air flotation or viscous fluid mattress' (NICE 2005 p. 3) (Table 15.17). In all cases, the effect on the skin of nursing patients on specialised mattresses should be regularly evaluated. Where indicated, repositioning charts or schedules should be used to guide management and as evidence that care was carried out, and where necessary, specialist advice on equipment, aids and positioning should be sought.

Education and training should be provided regularly to all nursing staff and carers on positioning of the patient, skin cleansing, the use of moisturisers and emollients, and the use of hoists and other patient handling devices to prevent complications caused by shear and friction. It is also essential to be aware of and reiterate that the recommended sitting time for vulnerable patients or those with pressure damage is 2 hours (NICE 2005).

Removal or alleviation of the underlying cause is the foundation of pressure ulcer management and prevention, and this can be achieved by providing the correct support surface, preventing further damage, pain management and optimising the patient's general condition.

International consensus on pressure ulcer prevention and management was reached in 2009 with the subsequent publication of the European Pressure Ulcer Advisory Panel and National Pressure Ulcer Advisory Panel (EPUAP/NPUAP 2009, 2010). Healthcare organisations are currently updating local guidelines to reflect the new guidance.

Skin tears

Skin tears occur mainly from trauma associated with bumping into objects, wheelchair injuries, patient transfers and falls (12.4%) (Payne & Martin 1993). Furthermore, it is suggested that individuals who are dependent on carers for assistance with basic daily activities of living are at high risk of skin tears (Baranoski 2003). The incidence of skin tears increases with age, with a 25% incidence in 60- to 69-year-olds, rising to 45% in people of 85 years and over (Groeneveld *et al.* 2004; Beldon 2006).

In addition to skin changes in older adults, other contributory factors increase an individual's vulnerability to skin tears, for example:

- pre-existing oedema, purpura, or ecchymosis
- the use of corticosteroids for extended periods
- poor nutritional status including dehydration
- dry skin
- poly-pharmacy
- cardiopulmonary disease that results in lower- limb oedema
- acute or long term confusion.

(Payne & Martin 1993)

Skin tears can be classified by the degree of severity and loss of epidermal tissue using the revised Payne-Martin Classification System of Skin Tears (1993) (Table 15.18).

Basic precautions to prevent skin tears include:

- careful positioning and moving techniques to reduce friction and shearing
- education regarding safe patient handling
- padding of bed-rails, wheelchair arms and leg supports
- wearing long sleeves and trousers for protection
- moisturising the skin with creams rather than lotions
- minimising the risk of accidents by, e.g. well-lit environment
- using paper tape or non-adherent dressings; stockinette-type materials to retain dressings rather than tape; foam-stockinette combinations on the arms and legs
- carers and patients must keep their fingernails short
- good nutrition and hydration.

The main aims of treatment for skin tears must be to support healing through providing comfortable, appropriate dressings that optimise the wound environment and do not cause further trauma on removal (Meuleneire 2002).

375

Table 15.17 Examples of pressure relieving equipment

Aid	Indications for use	General comments
Silicone-filled mattress pad/cushion (e.g. Transoft)	Waterlow score of 10 or patients on prolonged bedrest, able to move spontaneously	Relieves pressure by distributing it over a greater area
Roho air-filled mattress/cushions	High- to medium-risk patients, Waterlow 10–15	Interlinked air cells transfer air with movement. Patient can be nursed sitting or recumbent. Non-mechanical. Washable
Alternating pressure beds	High–medium-risk patients, Waterlow 15	Mechanical alteration of pressure. Reduces the frequency of (but not need for) repositioning
Pressure redistributing foam mattress	Moderate risk as above	Two-way multi-stretch foam and flexible covers, less expensive than beds
Dynamic air mattress or low air loss bed	Moderate to high-risk patients, Waterlow 15–20	Equalises pressure and weight and can be programmed to adjust air support to give optimal pressure redistribution
Foam overlay	Foam mattress overlays have been clinically proven to be useful for 'at risk' patients (NHS Centre for Reviews & Dissemination 1995) Useful for Grade 1–2 and up to medium risk dependent on clinical presentation	These overlays should be placed on top of existing mattress. 2–4 inch foam pad of mattress, e.g. Propad with geometrically cut squares. No weight restriction
Fibre-filled static overlay	As for static overlays, these have been shown to be clinically effective for 'at risk' patients Useful for grade 1-2 and up to medium risk dependent on clinical presentation.	These overlays should be placed on top of an existing mattress. Their height is 10 cm and they are constructed of 12 bolsters of siliconised hollow-core polyester fibre covered with a waterproof, vapour-permeable, two-way stretch fabric. Example Spenco. No weight restriction
Foam mattress replacement	Useful for grade 1–3 and up to medium risk dependent on clinical presentation	This mattress is designed to incorporate pressure reduction, comfort, long-lasting durability and support. It is constructed of modular foam that is waterproof, flame retardant and vapour permeable. Example Bodyfoam. No weight restriction
Alternating air-filled overlays (electric alternating mattress)	Patients identified at medium to high risk who can be manually handled or those with pressure ulceration grade 1–4	Air-filled overlays should be placed on top of existing mattress. This product consists of alternating cells, which usually work on a 1 in 2 cycle. The cell size should be greater than 8 cm (3 inch). Patient's weight needs to be keyed into the system. Pump unit should always be visible Weight restriction is up to 22 stone (140 kg) Examples Qualtro, Alpha x cell, Alto (Hillrom)
Bed systems (electrical alternating pressure mattress)	Patients at high risk of developing pressure ulcers and/or patients with existing pressure ulcers grade 2-4. Patients with limited mobility	All systems need an electrical source and will stay inflated if power fails for a limited period of time. The pump can be disconnected for transfer (refer to manufacturer's instructions). The use of plastics, draw sheets, incontinence pads, etc., should be avoided as they render the system less effective. The covering sheet should not be tucked in tightly or be allowed to 'nick up' Nimbus II cells alternate in a 1 in 2, 10-min cycle. Changes in pressure are automatically sensed by system, and air in the cells adjusts to the position/pressure change

Table 15.17 *(Continued)*

Aid	Indications for use	General comments
Low air loss bed	Patients with an existing pressure ulcer grade 2–4. High-risk patients and extremely heavy patients	The system has vapour-closed permeable sacs with their own pressure control panel. The patient's weight can be evenly distributed over the whole surface area. Pressures can be altered for different sections of the patient's body. These systems have temperature control. Patient should be nursed directly on the air sacs
Foam cushions	'At risk' patients	The foam is cut to decrease surface tension and improve pressure relief. Use in both easy chairs and wheelchairs. All cushions should have a washable stretch cover. Example Propad
Roho cushion	Medium to high-risk patients and/or patients with an existing pressure ulcer. Roho cushions are most effective when the patient is sat directly on it	The Roho cushion is a rotation system with air cells interconnected and air-filled bellows incorporated in a foam support. It adapts to the contour of body providing distribution of body weight reducing overall interface pressure. Available in deeper depth for heavier users Must be correctly adjusted for each patient. If the air cells are not correctly inflated this will result in increased pressure No power source is required. Suitable for unusual seating uses. Sheets and covers should be avoided unless provided by the company
Alto seating system	For high-risk patients or those with grade 2–4 pressure ulcers	Operates in conjunction with the Alto mattress replacement system. It adapts to the individual's body contour, ensuring reduced overall interface pressure. The seating system can be disconnected from the air mattress to allow greater patient independence without compromising tissue viability
Repose cushion	Patients assessed as high risk. Appropriate for grade 2 and above, dependent on clinical presentation	The cushion has a combination of two high-technology urethane membranes and provides effective pressure relief due to the multidirectional stretchabilty of the materials. Patient comfort is ensured due to the vapour permeability of the cushion. It is packed in the unique pump, which provides for easy installation to the correct pressure
Flo-tech Solution cushion	Patients assessed at very high risk. Appropriate for grade 3 and above, dependent on clinical presentation	This cushion uses the ultimate combination of a slimmer-shaped foam cushion base and a dual layer of flo-mer polymer sacs. This achieves a superior level of protection for those at very high risk. Can be used in both armchair and wheelchair. Weight restriction 22 stone (140 kg). Example MSS Flo-tech Solution

Table 15.18 Payne-Martin Classification System of Skin Tears (Payne & Martin 1993). Reproduced with permission.

Category I: skin tear can fully approximate wound
A. Linear skin tear – a wound that occurs in a wrinkle or furrow of skin. The epidermis and dermis are pulled apart as if an incision had been made, exposing tissue below
B. Flap-type skin tear – partial thickness wound in which the epidermal flap can be completely approximated or approximated so that no more than 1 mm of dermis is exposed

Category II: skin tear with partial thickness skin loss
A. Scant tissue loss – partial thickness in which 25% or less of the epidermal flap is lost and at least the flap covers 75% or more of the dermis
B. Moderate to large tissue loss – partial thickness wound in which more than 25% of the epidermal flap is lost and more than 25% of the dermis is exposed

Category III: skin tears with complete tissue loss.
A partial thickness wound in which an epidermal flap is present

Procedural guidelines

Community setting

In a patient's home the community nurse does not have access to, e.g. a dressing trolley, and therefore adaptations and creativity are required to ensure that the environment is conducive for the procedure to be carried out. A piece of furniture, e.g. tabletop, coffee table, stool, chair, bed, can be considered as a working field. Where possible the area selected should be cleaned with general household detergent or a damp cloth and be as free from dust as possible. However, in some homes this may not always be possible and consideration should be given to using a plastic sheet, an apron or a procedure sheet under the sterile field as additional protection. The floor should be avoided if possible, and pets should always be removed. In many situations a modified aseptic or 'clean' technique is appropriate (*see* Table 15.19), but it is essential that each individual situation is risk assessed.

Table 15.19 Comparison of aseptic and clean technique

	Aseptic technique	Clean technique
Hand washing	Wash with liquid soap and water and dry thoroughly with paper hand towels	Wash with liquid soap and water and dry thoroughly with paper hand towels
	Where suitable hand washing facilities are not available and hands are visibly clean, alcohol gel can be used	Where suitable hand washing facilities are not available and hands are visibly clean, alcohol gel can be used
Aprons	Disposable plastic. Change between patients and if soiled	Disposable plastic. Change between patients and if soiled
Gloves	Sterile – touching only the inside wrist end. Change if soiled and between removal of soiled dressings and application of new dressings	Non-sterile gloves (latex free). Change if soiled and between removal of soiled dressings and application of new dressings
Dressing field	Sterile dressing pack to lay out dressings. Place sterile sheet under limb/wound area to prevent transfer of bacteria	Clean sheet, sheet from sterile gloves or paper towel to lay out dressings. Clean towel or disposable sheet/apron under patient's limb/wound area
Wound cleansing	Sterile normal saline. Pat dry with sterile gauze/sterile paper towel	Wash the lower legs in a clean bucket lined with a plastic bin liner (the bucket should be cleaned with general purpose detergent and dried thoroughly after use)
		Tap water may be used to irrigate wounds
		Pat surrounding area dry with clean gauze / paper towel
		Patients may wish to shower instead
Dressings	If gauze/dressing pad is required as secondary dressing it must be sterile	Sterile/non sterile gauze or dressing pad can be used as secondary dressing
Instruments, e.g. scissors and forceps	These must be sterile single-use only	
Tapes and probes	Sterile probes and measures from sterile dressing pack to be used only	Sterile probes to measure depth of wound
		Disposable tape measures to be used when measuring leg circumference

Clean technique

The aim of using a clean technique is to reduce the potential introduction of viable micro-organisms to a susceptible site and to prevent the transfer of organisms to other sites, service users or staff. A risk assessment should be completed to ensure that this technique is appropriate for the procedure. A clean technique differs from an aseptic technique, as the use of sterile equipment and the environment are not as crucial as would be required for asepsis. The non-touch technique is incorporated as part of a clean procedure, i.e. the ends of sterile connections should not be touched with other items that could contaminate a susceptible site.

It is acceptable to use non-sterile gloves and tap water (suitable for drinking) for irrigation of chronic wounds, e.g. leg ulcers, traumatic wounds (RCN 2006; Fernandez & Griffiths 2007; Dougherty & Lister 2011).

Procedure guideline 15.1 **Guideline for aseptic technique wound dressing**

Equipment

Sterile dressing pack
Single-use sterile gloves
Single-use non-sterile gloves
Single-use plastic apron x2
0.9% sodium chloride solution
Receptacle containing water at body temperature
Primary and where appropriate secondary dressing
Appropriate tape (to secure dressing in place)
Other equipment, e.g. sterile scissors/probe, bandage (when indicated)

Nursing action	Rationale
1 Where appropriate facilities are available wash and thoroughly dry your hands or alternatively cleanse with 70% alcohol-based hand rub (in accordance with local policy)	To prevent the risk of cross-infection/contamination
2 If the patient is known to the service review nursing documentation and current care plan	To update the nurse's knowledge of the patient To maintain patient safety
3 If the patient is unknown to the service a comprehensive assessment must be carried out prior to undertaking the procedure. This must include the assessment of (a) manual handling techniques required to safely carry out the procedure and (b) known or potential allergies	To identify potential contraindications and or cautions To determine if a second nurse is required to assist with the procedure To maintain patient safety To ensure health and safety regulations are met and maintain practitioner safety
4 Explain and discuss the procedure with the patient	To ensure that the patient understands the procedure and gives their valid consent
5 If the wound is painful or the patient experiences pain at dressing changes, analgesia may be required. The timing of administration should be arranged with the patient prior to the visit if possible	To prevent pain during dressing renewal To ensure patient comfort To reduce the risk of patient distress and anxiety

379

(Continued)

Procedure guideline 15.1 **Guideline for aseptic technique wound dressing** *(cont'd)*

Nursing action	Rationale
6 Prepare the environment, draw curtains and where necessary obtain patient consent to move furniture	To allow freedom of movement when carrying out the procedure To maintain patient privacy
7 Assemble all equipment on a clean surface; check that (a) all relevant seals and packaging are intact and undamaged, and (b) all relevant equipment is within the recommended date for use	To prevent disruption to the procedure To ensure equipment has not been damaged or contaminated To maintain patient safety
8 Put on disposable plastic apron	To prevent the risk of cross-infection/contamination
9 Where indicated offer the patient assistance with removing any necessary items of clothing	To expose the appropriate area
10 Assist the patient into a comfortable position covering any unnecessary exposed areas of the patient's body with a towel/blanket	To make sure the appropriate area is easily accessible To maintain the patient's dignity and comfort
11 If indicated apply non-sterile gloves, e.g. where outer/secondary dressing is soiled	To prevent the risk of cross-infection To maintain nurse safety
12 Where necessary remove outer/ secondary dressing and loosen tape/edges of primary dressing	To facilitate access to the wound site To prevent trauma to the wound bed during removal
13 Remove and dispose of apron (and gloves) in accordance with locally agreed infection prevention and control policy	To minimise the risk of cross-infection
14 Where appropriate facilities are available wash and thoroughly dry your hands or alternatively cleanse with 70% alcohol-based hand rub (in accordance with local policy)	To reduce the risk of cross-infection
15 Put on disposable plastic apron	To reduce the risk of cross-infection
16 Open sterile pack and prepare all equipment on the sterile field, using an aseptic technique	To maintain patient safety To prevent disruption to the procedure To reduce the length of time the wound is exposed during dressing renewal
17 Cleanse hands with bactericidal alcohol hand rub	Handling outer packs may have contaminated hands
18 Insert a hand into the sterile plastic bag supplied in the dressing pack and gently remove the primary wound dressing, inverting the bag on removal	To reduce the risk of cross-infection To maintain the safety of self and others
19 Position the bag as close as possible to the dressing area	To ensure the safe disposal of all clinical waste
20 Place the container of sodium chloride solution in the receptacle containing water at body temperature	To prevent a fall in wound temperature, as this will have a negative effect on cell activity and will further impact on the wound healing time (Collier 1996b)

Procedure guideline 15.1 **Guideline for aseptic technique wound dressing** *(cont'd)*

Nursing action	Rationale
21 Carry out a visual assessment of the wound using the principles of the 'TIME' framework (*see* p. 358)	To evaluate the efficacy of current wound management
	To aid decision making regarding changes to treatment plan
	To enable the accurate documentation of the stage of wound healing
	To enable the early identification of infection and or associated problems, e.g. maceration
22 Cleanse hands with bactericidal alcohol hand rub	To reduce the risk of cross-infection
	To reduce the risk of wound infection
23 Apply sterile gloves	To reduce the risk of wound infection
	To maintain the safety of both nurse and patient
24 If indicated, gently irrigate the wound with the warmed 0.9% sodium chloride solution (Morgan 2000)	Wound cleansing should only be carried out if there is excessive exudates, pus or dead tissue present
	Gentle irrigation should be used to reduce the risk of trauma or damage to granulating cells
	NB If the wound is clean with little or no exudates, cleansing is contraindicated due to the potential damage caused to granulation and epithelialisation (Morison 1989)
25 If necessary, sterile non-linting gauze swabs may be used to gently aid the removal of slough, etc., during the cleansing process	To remove excessive exudate, pus or dead tissue
	NB When using non-linting gauze swabs care should be taken not to touch clean, healthy areas of the wound as this may damage regenerating epithelial cells (Rainey 2002)
26 Apply an appropriate primary wound dressing (*see* Table 15.6 for examples) and secure in place	To produce an environment that is appropriate and conducive to the stage of wound healing
	To promote wound healing
27 Apply secondary dressing as indicated, e.g. where there is excessive exudate/leakage	To maintain patient dignity and comfort
	To prevent soiling of, e.g. patient clothing, bedding
28 Remove and dispose of gloves in accordance with locally agreed infection prevention and control policy	To reduce the risk of cross-infection
29 Secure all dressing in place with an appropriate system, e.g. tape, bandage	To prevent dressing from slipping
	To maintain wound coverage
	To prevent trauma to the wound
	To maintain patient safety and comfort
30 Cleanse hands with bactericidal alcohol hand rub	To reduce the risk of cross-infection
31 Assist the patient to dress and help them into their chosen position	To maintain patient's dignity and comfort

(Continued)

*Procedure guideline 15.1 **Guideline for aseptic technique wound dressing** (cont'd)*

Nursing action	Rationale
32 Remove and dispose of apron and all single use equipment in accordance with locally agreed infection prevention and control policy	To reduce the risk of cross-infection To maintain the health and safety of self and others
33 Where appropriate facilities are available wash your hands or alternatively cleanse with 70% alcohol-based hand rub (in accordance with local policy)	To reduce the risk of cross-infection
34 Replace any moved items of furniture to their original position, open curtains	To maintain a safe environment for the patient by restoring any furniture moved to its usual place To restore the patient's environment
35 Verbally discuss the outcome of the procedure with the patient and where relevant carer, giving further advice as indicated	To support the patient's understanding To reduce any potential patient concerns/anxieties
36 Complete all relevant documentation, e.g. progress notes, wound chart (see Holistic assessment for further guidance)	To maintain patient safety To enable continuity of care To maintain practitioner safety Documentation should provide clear evidence of the care or procedure carried out
37 Liaise with GP as indicated	To update on patient progress To maintain continuity of care and treatment

Procedure guideline 15.2 **Guideline for renewing a negative pressure wound therapy dressing (VAC system) (aseptic technique)**

Equipment

Sterile dressing pack
Single-use sterile gloves
Single-use non-sterile gloves
Sterile single-use forceps
Sterile single-use scissors
Single-use plastic apron
0.9% sodium chloride solution
Receptacle containing water at body temperature
Clamp
Negative pressure wound therapy pump unit
Negative pressure canister and tubing
Negative pressure dressing pack
Appropriate non adherent wound contact layer
Skin barrier product, e.g. Cavilon

Procedure guideline 15.2 **Guideline for renewing a negative pressure wound therapy dressing (VAC system) (aseptic technique)** *(cont'd)*

Nursing action	Rationale
1 Where appropriate facilities are available wash and thoroughly dry your hands or alternatively cleanse with 70% alcohol-based hand rub (in accordance with local policy)	To reduce the risk of cross infection
2 If the patient is known to the service review nursing documentation and current care plan	To update the nurse's knowledge of the patient To maintain patient safety
3 If the patient is unknown to the service a comprehensive assessment must be carried out prior to undertaking the procedure. This must include the assessment of (a) manual handling techniques required to safely carry out the procedure and (b) known or potential allergies	To identify potential contraindications and or cautions To determine if a second nurse is required to assist with the procedure To maintain patient safety To ensure health and safety regulations are met and maintain practitioner safety
4 Explain and discuss the procedure with the patient, giving clear explanations	To ensure that the patient understands the procedure and gives their valid consent To reduce any concerns or anxieties the patient may have
5 If the wound is painful or the patient experiences pain at dressing changes, analgesia may be required. The timing of administration should be arranged with the patient prior to the visit if possible	To prevent pain during dressing renewal To ensure patient comfort To reduce the risk of patient distress and anxiety
6 Prepare the environment, draw curtains and where necessary obtain patient consent to move furniture	To allow freedom of movement when carrying out the procedure To maintain patient privacy
7 Put on disposable plastic apron	To reduce the risk of cross-infection
8 Where indicated offer the patient assistance with removal of clothing and assist the patient into a comfortable position covering any unnecessary exposed areas of the patient's body with a towel/ blanket	To make sure the appropriate area is easily accessible To maintain the patient's dignity and comfort
9 Assemble all equipment on a clean surface; check that (a) all relevant seals and packaging are intact and undamaged, and (b) all relevant equipment is within the recommended date for use	To prevent disruption to the procedure To ensure equipment has not been damaged or contaminated To maintain patient safety
10 Where appropriate facilities are available wash and thoroughly dry your hands or alternatively cleanse with 70% alcohol-based hand rub (in accordance with local policy)	To reduce the risk of cross-infection
11 Open sterile pack and prepare all equipment on the sterile field, using an aseptic technique	To maintain patient safety To prevent disruption to the procedure To reduce the length of time the wound is exposed during dressing renewal

383

(Continued)

Procedure guideline 15.2 **Guideline for renewing a negative pressure wound therapy dressing (VAC system)** *(aseptic technique) (cont'd)*

Nursing action	Rationale
12 Cleanse hands with bactericidal alcohol hand rub	Handling outer packs may have contaminated hands
13 Apply non-sterile gloves	To reduce the risk of cross-infection
14 Where necessary clamp the tubing and disconnect it from the canister tubing. Any fluid remaining in the canister tubing should be allowed to drain into the canister	To prevent spillage of body fluid
15 Switch off pump, clamp canister tubing	To prevent spillage of body fluid
16 Dispose of canister in accordance with locally agreed infection prevention and control policy	To reduce the risk of cross-infection To maintain the safety of self and others
17 Remove the occlusive film as directed by the manufacturer's instructions	To prevent damage to the skin
18 Gently remove the foam dressing from the wound	To reduce the risk of trauma or damage to granulating cells To reduce the risk of patient pain
19 Remove and dispose of gloves	To reduce the risk of cross-infection To prevent contamination
20 Place the container of sodium chloride solution in the receptacle containing water at body temperature	To prevent a fall in wound temperature as this will have a negative effect on cell activity and will further impact on the wound healing time (Collier 1996b)
21 Carry out a visual assessment of the wound using the principles of the 'TIME' framework (*see* Wound management, p. 358)	To evaluate the efficacy of current wound management To aid decision making regarding changes to treatment plan To enable the accurate documentation of the stage of wound healing To enable the early identification of infection and or associated problems, e.g. maceration
22 Cleanse hands with bactericidal alcohol hand rub	To reduce the risk of cross-infection
23 Apply sterile gloves	To reduce the risk of wound infection To maintain the safety of both nurse and patient
24 If indicated gently irrigate the wound with the warmed 0.9% sodium chloride solution (Morgan 2000)	Wound cleansing should only be carried out if there is excessive exudate, pus or dead tissue present Gentle irrigation should be used to reduce the risk of trauma or damage to granulating cells **NB** If the wound is clean with little or no exudates, cleansing is contraindicated due to the potential damage caused to granulation and epithelialisation (Morison 1989)
25 If necessary, sterile non-linting gauze swabs may be used to gently aid the removal of slough, etc., during the cleansing process	To remove excessive exudate, pus or dead tissue (Dealey 2005) **NB** When using non-linting gauze swabs care should be taken not to touch clean healthy areas of the wound as this may damage regenerating epithelial cells (Rainey 2002)

Procedure guideline 15.2 **Guideline for renewing a negative pressure wound therapy dressing (VAC system)** *(aseptic technique) (cont'd)*

Nursing action	Rationale
26 Remove and dispose of gloves, cleanse hands with bactericidal alcohol hand rub	To reduce the risk of cross-infection
27 Apply sterile gloves	To reduce the risk of wound infection
28 Using the sterile scissors cut the wound therapy foam to the exact size and shape of the wound and place into the cavity	To guarantee optimal negative pressure therapy (Beldon 2006)
29 Where the wound bed is fragile, bleeding or granulating and there is reduced exudates, a non-adherent wound contact layer should be placed under the foam (see manufacturer's recommendations)	To prevent trauma to the wound bed when removing the negative pressure foam To reduce pain/discomfort
30 If the skin surrounding the wound is macerated, a non-alcohol-based barrier product, e.g. Cavilon, should be applied and left to air dry prior to occlusive film application	To reduce the risk of further trauma and skin breakdown To reduce patient discomfort To ensure adhesion of film
31 Using the sterile scissors cut the occlusive film to size ensuring there is a minimum border from the foam edges of 3–5 cm, apply film over the foam **NB** Care should be taken not to compress the foam into the wound	To achieve a complete seal To guarantee optimal negative pressure therapy (Beldon 2006) To prevent wound bed damage
32 Using the sterile scissors carefully cut a hole in the film approximately 2 cm in diameter, leaving the foam intact. The position of the hole should be where the tubing, once attached, will not cause external pressure to any area of the patient's body	To enable the tubing to be attached To enable a complete seal to be achieved To prevent pressure injury to the patient To promote patient comfort
33 Attach the TRAC pad to the film ensuring that the hole in the film is at the centre of the elbow joint	To achieve the correct seal
34 Click the canister into place in the pump	To correctly position the canister
35 Attach the dressing and canister tubing together Open clamps	To ensure correct pump operation To prevent pump alarm function
36 Remove and dispose of gloves, cleanse hands with bactericidal alcohol hand rub	To reduce the risk of cross-infection
37 Press the pump 'power' button, instructions will be displayed on screen. The level and type of pressure therapy must be set in accordance with the instructions from the prescribing clinician	To ensure that the pressure is set at a level indicated by the wound type (Dealey 2005; Benbow 2006)
38 Press 'Therapy on/off' button	To start the pump
39 Dispose of all single-use equipment in accordance with locally agreed infection prevention and control policy	To reduce the risk of cross-infection To maintain the health and safety of self and others

385

(Continued)

Procedure guideline 15.2 **Guideline for renewing a negative pressure wound therapy dressing (VAC system)** *(aseptic technique) (cont'd)*

Nursing action	Rationale
40 Cleanse hands with bactericidal alcohol hand rub	To reduce the risk of cross-infection
41 Assist the patient to dress and help them into their chosen position	To maintain patient's dignity and comfort
42 Remove and dispose of apron and all single-use equipment in accordance with locally agreed infection prevention and control policy	To reduce the risk of cross-infection
43 Where appropriate facilities are available wash your hands or alternatively cleanse with 70% alcohol-based hand rub (in accordance with local policy)	To reduce the risk of cross-infection
44 Replace any moved items of furniture to their original position, open curtains	To maintain a safe environment for the patient by restoring any furniture moved to its usual place
	To restore the patient's environment
45 Verbally discuss the outcome of the procedure with the patient and where relevant carer, giving further advice as indicated	To support the patient's understanding
	To reduce any potential patient concerns/anxieties
46 Complete all relevant documentation e.g. progress notes, wound chart (*see* Holistic assessment for further guidance)	To maintain patient safety
	To enable continuity of care
	To maintain practitioner safety
	Documentation should provide clear evidence of the care or procedure carried out
47 Liaise with GP as indicated	To update on patient progress
	To maintain continuity of care and treatment

Procedure guideline 15.3 **Guideline for removal of staples (aseptic technique)**

Equipment

Sterile dressing pack
Single-use sterile gloves
Single-use plastic apron x 2
0.9% sodium chloride solution
Appropriate primary and secondary dressing, where indicated
Appropriate tape (to secure dressing in place if required)
Sterile singlesuse staple remover
Sterile adhesive skin tapes

Nursing action	Rationale
1 Where appropriate facilities are available wash and thoroughly dry your hands or alternatively cleanse with 70% alcohol-based hand rub (in accordance with local policy)	To prevent the risk of cross-infection/contamination
2 If the patient is known to the service review nursing documentation and current care plan	To update the nurse's knowledge of the patient To maintain patient safety
3 If the patient is unknown to the service a comprehensive assessment must be carried out prior to undertaking the procedure. This must include the assessment of (a) manual handling techniques required to safely carry out the procedure and (b) known or potential allergies	To identify potential contraindications and or cautions To determine if a second nurse is required to assist with the procedure To maintain patient safety To ensure health and safety regulations are met and maintain practitioner safety
4 Explain and discuss the procedure with the patient	To ensure that the patient understands the procedure and gives their valid consent
5 Prepare the environment, draw curtains and where necessary obtain patient consent to move furniture	To allow freedom of movement when carrying out the procedure To maintain patient privacy
6 Assemble all equipment on a clean surface; check that (a) all relevant seals and packaging are intact and undamaged, and (b) all relevant equipment is within the recommended date for use	To prevent disruption to the procedure To ensure equipment has not been damaged or contaminated To maintain patient safety
7 Put on single-use plastic apron	To prevent the risk of cross-infection/contamination
8 Where indicated offer the patient assistance with removing any necessary items of clothing	To expose the appropriate area
9 Assist the patient into a comfortable position covering any unnecessary exposed areas of the patient's body with a towel/blanket	To make sure the appropriate area is easily accessible To maintain the patient's dignity and comfort
10 If indicated, apply non-sterile gloves, e.g. where outer/secondary dressing is soiled	To prevent the risk of cross-infection To maintain nurse safety
11 Where necessary remove outer/secondary dressing and loosen tape/edges of primary dressing	To facilitate access to the wound site

387

(Continued)

Procedure guideline 15.3 **Guideline for removal of staples (aseptic technique)** *(cont'd)*

Nursing action	Rationale
12 Remove and dispose of apron (and gloves) in accordance with locally agreed infection prevention and control policy	To minimise the risk of cross-infection
13 Where appropriate facilities are available wash and thoroughly dry your hands or alternatively cleanse with 70% alcohol-based hand rub (in accordance with local policy)	To reduce the risk of cross-infection
14 Put on disposable plastic apron	To reduce the risk of cross-infection
15 Open sterile pack and prepare all equipment on the sterile field, using an aseptic technique	To maintain patient safety To prevent disruption to the procedure To reduce the length of time the wound is exposed during dressing renewal
16 Cleanse hands with bactericidal alcohol hand rub	Handling outer packs and or cover may have contaminated hands
17 Insert a hand into the sterile plastic bag supplied in the dressing pack and gently remove the primary wound dressing, inverting the bag on removal	To reduce the risk of cross-infection To maintain the safety of self and others
18 Position the bag as close as possible to the dressing area	To ensure the safe disposal of all clinical waste
19 Carry out a visual assessment of the wound	To identify potential complications, e.g. infection, areas of gaping To aid decision making regarding the procedure To maintain patient safety
20 Cleanse hands with bactericidal alcohol hand rub	To reduce the risk of cross-infection To reduce the risk of wound infection
21 Apply sterile gloves	To reduce the risk of wound infection To maintain the safety of both nurse and patient
22 If indicated, gently irrigate the wound with the warmed 0.9% sodium chloride solution (Morgan 2000)	Wound cleansing should only be carried out if there is excessive exudates, pus or dead tissue present
23 If necessary, sterile non-linting gauze swabs may be used to gently aid the removal of, e.g. encrustations and to dry the surrounding skin	To enhance the removal of staples To reduce the risk of infection To aid patient comfort To maintain patient safety
24 With the staple remover in the dominant hand, gently insert the lower piece (V-shaped) under the centre of the staple at an angle of 90° and gently squeeze the handles together	To fully open the staple The 90° angle of the staple remover will ensure ease of removal To reduce the risk of patient pain/discomfort

Procedure guideline 15.3 **Guideline for removal of staples (aseptic technique)** *(cont'd)*

Nursing action	Rationale
25 If there is any gaping of the suture line post staple removal, sterile adhesive skin tapes should be applied in accordance with the manufacturer's instructions An appropriate primary dressing should be applied (*see* Table 15.6 for examples) **NB** Wound monitoring will need to continue until healing has taken place	To provide additional support to the suture line and promote healing To reduce the risk of infection To maintain patient comfort To maintain patient safety
26 Dispose of all single-use equipment in accordance with locally agreed infection prevention and control policy	To reduce the risk of cross-infection To maintain the health and safety of self and others
27 Remove and dispose of gloves in accordance with locally agreed infection prevention and control policy	To reduce the risk of cross-infection
28 Where appropriate secure dressing in place with tape or bandage	To prevent dressing from slipping To maintain wound coverage To prevent trauma to the wound To maintain patient safety and comfort
29 Cleanse hands with bactericidal alcohol hand rub	To reduce the risk of cross-infection
30 Assist the patient to dress and help them into their chosen position	To maintain patient's dignity and comfort
31 Remove and dispose of apron and all single-use equipment in accordance with locally agreed infection prevention and control policy	To reduce the risk of cross-infection
32 Where appropriate facilities are available wash your hands or alternatively cleanse with 70% alcohol-based hand rub (in accordance with local policy)	To reduce the risk of cross-infection
33 Replace any moved items of furniture to their original position, open curtains	To maintain a safe environment for the patient by restoring any furniture moved to its usual place To restore the patient's environment
34 Verbally discuss the outcome of the procedure with the patient and where relevant carer, giving further advice as indicated	To support the patient's understanding To reduce any potential patient concerns/anxieties
35 Complete all relevant documentation, e.g. progress notes, wound chart (*see* Holistic assessment for further guidance)	To maintain patient safety To enable continuity of care To maintain practitioner safety Documentation should provide clear evidence of the care or procedure carried out
36 Liaise with GP as indicated	To update on patient progress To maintain continuity of care and treatment

Procedure guideline 15.4 **Guideline for removal of sutures (aseptic technique)**

Equipment

Sterile dressing pack
Single-use sterile gloves
Sterile single-use forceps
Single-use plastic apron x 2
Sharps bin
0.9% sodium chloride solution
Appropriate primary and secondary dressing, where indicated
Appropriate tape (to secure dressing in place if required)
Sterile single-use suture removal pack or stitch cutter
Sterile adhesive skin tapes

Nursing action	Rationale
1 Where appropriate facilities are available wash and thoroughly dry your hands or alternatively cleanse with 70% alcohol-based hand rub (in accordance with local policy)	To prevent the risk of cross-infection/contamination
2 If the patient is known to the service review nursing documentation and current care plan	To update the nurse's knowledge of the patient To maintain patient safety
3 If the patient is unknown to the service a comprehensive assessment must be carried out prior to undertaking the procedure. This must include the assessment of (a) manual handling techniques required to safely carry out the procedure and (b) known or potential allergies	To identify potential contraindications and or cautions To determine if a second nurse is required to assist with the procedure To maintain patient safety. To ensure health and safety regulations are met and maintain practitioner safety
4 Explain and discuss the procedure with the patient	To ensure that the patient understands the procedure and gives their valid consent
5 Prepare the environment, draw curtains and where necessary obtain patient consent to move furniture	To allow freedom of movement when carrying out the procedure To maintain patient privacy
6 Assemble all equipment on a clean surface; check that (a) all relevant seals and packaging are intact and undamaged, and (b) all relevant equipment is within the recommended date for use	To prevent disruption to the procedure To ensure equipment has not been damaged or contaminated To maintain patient safety
7 Put on disposable plastic apron	To prevent the risk of cross-infection/contamination
8 Where indicated offer the patient assistance with removing any necessary items of clothing	To expose the appropriate area
9 Assist the patient into a comfortable position covering any unnecessary exposed areas of the patient's body with a towel/blanket	To make sure the appropriate area is easily accessible To maintain the patient's dignity and comfort

Procedure guideline 15.4 **Guideline for removal of sutures (aseptic technique)** *(cont'd)*

Nursing action	Rationale
10 If indicated, apply non-sterile gloves, e.g. where outer/secondary dressing is soiled	To prevent the risk of cross-infection To maintain nurse safety
11 Where necessary remove outer/secondary dressing and loosen tape/edges of primary dressing	To facilitate access to the wound site
12 Remove and dispose of apron (and gloves) in accordance with locally agreed infection prevention and control policy	To minimise the risk of cross-infection
13 Where appropriate facilities are available wash and thoroughly dry your hands or alternatively cleanse with 70% alcohol-based hand rub (in accordance with local policy)	To reduce the risk of cross-infection
14 Put on disposable plastic apron	To reduce the risk of cross-infection
15 Open sterile pack and prepare all equipment on the sterile field, using an aseptic technique	To maintain patient safety To prevent disruption to the procedure To reduce the length of time the wound is exposed during dressing renewal
16 Cleanse hands with bactericidal alcohol hand rub	Handling outer packs and or cover may have contaminated hands
17 Insert a hand into the sterile plastic bag supplied in the dressing pack and gently remove the primary wound dressing, inverting the bag on removal	To reduce the risk of cross-infection To maintain the safety of self and others
18 Position the bag as close as possible to the dressing area	To ensure the safe disposal of all clinical waste
19 Carry out a visual assessment of the wound	To identify potential complications, e.g. infection, areas of gaping To aid decision making regarding the procedure To maintain patient safety
20 Cleanse hands with bactericidal alcohol hand rub	To reduce the risk of cross-infection
21 Apply sterile gloves	To reduce the risk of wound infection To maintain the safety of both nurse and patient
22 If indicated, gently irrigate the wound with the warmed 0.9% sodium chloride solution (Morgan 2000)	Wound cleansing should only be carried out if there is excessive exudates, pus or dead tissue present
23 If necessary, sterile non-linting gauze swabs may be used to gently aid the removal of, e.g. encrustations, and to dry the surrounding skin	To enhance the removal of staples To reduce the risk of infection To aid patient comfort To maintain patient safety

(Continued)

Procedure guideline 15.4 **Guideline for removal of sutures (aseptic technique)** *(cont'd)*

Nursing action	Rationale
24 Using the sterile forceps lift the loose end of the suture material closest to the knot, pull gently upwards away from the skin	To prepare the suture for removal
25 While maintaining slight tension on the suture, insert the stitch cutter under one end, as close to the skin as is safely possible, and cut through	To enable the correct positioning of the stitch cutter To enable the suture to be safely removed To prevent the risk of procedure-related infection
26 Remove the suture by applying slight counter skin pressure using, e.g. the flat side of the stitch cutter Gently pull the suture towards the cut side	To minimise patient pain and or discomfort To prevent the external suture material from being pulled through the wound To prevent the risk of infection
27 If wound healing appears inconsistent, remove alternate sutures and liaise with the patient's GP	To maintain patient safety
28 If there is any gaping of the suture line post suture removal, sterile adhesive skin tapes should be applied in accordance with the manufacturer's instructions An appropriate primary dressing should be applied (*see* Table 15.6 for examples) **NB** Wound monitoring will need to continue until healing has taken place	To provide additional support to the suture line and promote healing To reduce the risk of infection To maintain patient comfort To maintain patient safety
29 Place stitch cutter into sharps bin and dispose of all used equipment in accordance with locally agreed infection prevention and control policy	To reduce the risk of cross-infection To maintain the health and safety of self and others
30 Remove and dispose of gloves in accordance with locally agreed infection prevention and control policy	To prevent the risk of cross-infection
31 Where appropriate, secure dressing in place	To prevent dressing from slipping To maintain wound coverage To prevent trauma to the wound To maintain patient safety and comfort
32 Cleanse hands with bactericidal alcohol hand rub	To reduce the risk of cross-infection
33 Assist the patient to dress and help them into their chosen position	To maintain patient's dignity and comfort
34 Remove and dispose of apron and all single-use equipment in accordance with locally agreed infection prevention and control policy	To reduce the risk of cross-infection
35 Where appropriate facilities are available wash your hands or alternatively cleanse with 70% alcohol-based hand rub (in accordance with local policy)	To reduce the risk of cross-infection

Procedure guideline 15.4 Guideline for removal of sutures (aseptic technique) (cont'd)

Nursing action	Rationale
36 Replace any moved items of furniture to their original position, open curtains	To maintain a safe environment for the patient by restoring any furniture moved to its usual place
	To restore the patient's environment
37 Verbally discuss the outcome of the procedure with the patient and where relevant carer, giving further advice as indicated	To support the patient's understanding
	To reduce any potential patient concerns/anxieties
38 Complete all relevant documentation, e.g. progress notes, wound chart (*see* Holistic assessment for further guidance)	To maintain patient safety
	To enable continuity of care
	To maintain practitioner safety
	Documentation should provide clear evidence of the care or procedure carried out
39 Liaise with GP as indicated	To update on patient progress
	To maintain continuity of care and treatment

Procedure guideline 15.5 **Guideline for performing a Doppler ultrasound assessment**

Equipment

Doppler ultrasound with an 8 MHz probe (Beldon 2010)
Sphygmomanometer
Blood pressure cuff/s suitable for the size of the patient's ankles and arms
Cling film
Ultrasound gel
Single-use plastic apron
Clinical waste bag
Single-use non-sterile gloves
Equipment for the decontamination/cleansing of reusable medical devices (as per locally agreed infection prevention and control policy/guidelines)
Other equipment necessary to carry out post-procedural wound dressing

NB Prior to carrying out the procedure a risk assessment should be completed. If there are any concerns, e.g. the presence of thrombosis, the Doppler must not be performed advice should be sought and appropriate investigations completed.

Nursing action	Rationale
1 Where appropriate facilities are available wash and thoroughly dry your hands or alternatively cleanse with 70% alcohol-based hand rub (in accordance with local policy)	To prevent the risk of cross-infection/contamination
2 If the patient is known to the service review nursing documentation and current care plan	To update the nurse's knowledge of the patient
	To maintain patient safety

(Continued)

Procedure guideline 15.5 **Guideline for performing a Doppler ultrasound assessment** *(cont'd)*

Nursing action	Rationale
3 If the patient is unknown to the service a comprehensive assessment must be carried out prior to undertaking the procedure. This must include the assessment of (a) manual handling techniques required to safely carry out the procedure and (b) Known or potential allergies	To identify potential contra-indications and or cautions To determine if a second nurse is required to assist with the procedure To maintain patient safety To ensure health and safety regulations are met and maintain practitioner safety
4 Explain and discuss the procedure with the patient giving clear explanations of what they may experience during the assessment	To ensure that the patient understands the procedure and gives their valid consent To reduce any concerns or anxieties the patient may have
5 Prepare the environment, draw curtains and where necessary obtain patient consent to move furniture	To allow freedom of movement when carrying out the procedure To maintain patient privacy
6 Put on disposable plastic apron	To prevent the risk of cross-infection/contamination
7 Prepare the patient Pre-procedural analgesia may be required Where indicated offer the patient assistance with removing necessary items of clothing Assist the patient into a supine position, head supported by one pillow, cover any unnecessary exposed areas of the patient's body with a towel/ blanket. If the patient is unable to lie in this position they should lie as flat as is comfortably possible with legs elevated **NB** The patient should remain in this position for approximately 10–20 min prior to the procedure	To minimise pain/discomfort during the procedure To expose the appropriate areas and allow ease of access during the procedure To minimise gravitational influences (Beldon 2010) To maintain patient comfort and dignity
8 Assemble all equipment on a clean surface	To prevent disruption to the procedure
9 Cleanse hands with bactericidal alcohol hand rub	To reduce the risk of cross-infection
10 Select the correct size blood pressure cuff and apply to the arm in the normal manner	An incorrect cuff size may produce an inaccurate result, e.g. if the artery cannot be compressed
11 Locate the brachial artery using the fingers; once located apply a pea-sized amount of ultrasound gel to the area	To prepare the area for probe use as this will produce a more accurate result than a stethoscope Ultrasound gel is an effective conductor of sound An excessive amount of gel may make it difficult to maintain probe position
12 Switch on the Doppler	To enable the assessment to begin
13 Hold the Doppler probe at an angle of 45–70° and gently move it over the area (Beldon 2010). If no pulse is heard adjust the angle of the probe	To obtain the clearest sound
14 While holding the probe in the correct position inflate the blood pressure cuff until the sound of the pulse disappears. Slowly deflate the cuff until the pulse can be heard again, document the result	To obtain the systolic pressure

Procedure guideline 15.5 **Guideline for performing a Doppler ultrasound assessment** *(cont'd)*

Nursing action	Rationale
15 Repeat steps 10–14 above on the patient's second arm	To obtain the systolic pressure
	The higher of the two brachial readings should be used in the calculation of the ABPI
16 Locate two of the four pedal pulses using the fingers; once located apply a pea-sized amount of ultrasound gel to the area.	To identify the correct areas for probe placement
	To prepare the area for probe use as this will produce a more accurate
Dorsalis pedis	Ultrasound gel is an effective conductor of sound
Peroneal	An excessive amount of gel may make it difficult to maintain probe position
Posterior tibial	
Anterior tibial	
(Beldon 2010)	
17 Apply the correct size blood pressure cuff to the patient's non-ulcerated leg, just above the malleoli	An incorrect cuff size may produce an inaccurate result, e.g. if the artery cannot be compressed
	Placing the cuff just above the malleoli produces a more accurate signal (Vowden & Vowden 2001)
18 Hold the Doppler probe at an angle of 45–70° and gently move it over the area (Beldon 2010). If no pulse is heard adjust the angle of the probe	To obtain the clearest sound
19 While holding the probe in the correct position inflate the blood pressure cuff until the sound of the pulse disappears. Slowly deflate the cuff until the pulse can be heard again, document the result. Repeat procedure for second identified pulse	To establish Doppler result
	The higher of the two readings should be used for the ABPI calculation
20 Cleanse hands with bactericidal alcohol hand rub	To reduce the risk of cross-infection
21 Place a protective cover under the patient's leg, apply gloves and remove the patient's wound dressing	To prevent soiling of the patient's bed/furniture
	To enable the Doppler assessment to be carried out
22 Cleanse the area and surrounding skin as necessary and apply a covering of cling film over the ulcer	To remove excessive exudate/pus
	To promote patient dignity and comfort.
	To prevent contamination of blood pressure cuff and reusable equipment
23 Dispose of all soiled equipment in clinical waste bag and remove gloves	To prevent cross-infection
	To protect the health and safety of self and others
24 Cleanse hands with bactericidal alcohol hand rub	To reduce the risk of cross-infection
25 Repeat steps 16–19 above	To establish Doppler result in the patient's second limb
	The higher of the two readings should be used for the ABPI calculation
26 Remove blood pressure cuff from the patient's limb and assist them into their chosen position	To enhance patient comfort

395

(Continued)

Procedure guideline 15.5 **Guideline for performing a Doppler ultrasound assessment** *(cont'd)*

Nursing action	Rationale
27 Where appropriate facilities are available wash and thoroughly dry your hands or alternatively cleanse with 70% alcohol-based hand rub (in accordance with local policy)	To prevent the risk of cross-infection/contamination
28 Prepare all necessary equipment, apply gloves and carry out wound dressing	To produce an environment that is appropriate and conducive to the stage of wound healing To promote wound healing
29 Dispose of all single-use equipment in accordance with locally agreed infection prevention and management policy	To reduce the risk of cross-infection To maintain the health and safety of self and others
30 Remove and dispose of gloves in accordance with locally agreed infection prevention and control policy	To prevent cross-infection To protect the health and safety of self and others
31 Assist the patient to dress and help them into their chosen position	To maintain patient's dignity and comfort
32 Apply gloves and decontaminate all reusable equipment in accordance with local policy/guidelines	To prevent cross-infection To protect the health and safety of self and others
33 Remove and dispose of gloves, apron and all single-use equipment in accordance with locally agreed infection prevention and control policy	To reduce the risk of cross-infection
34 Where appropriate facilities are available wash your hands or alternatively cleanse with 70% alcohol-based hand rub (in accordance with local policy)	To reduce the risk of cross-infection
35 Replace any moved items of furniture to their original position, open curtains	To maintain a safe environment for the patient by restoring any furniture moved to its usual place To restore the patient's environment
36 Verbally discuss the outcome of the procedure with the patient and where relevant carer, giving further advice as indicated	To support the patient's understanding To reduce any potential patient concerns/anxieties
37 Calculate the ABPI (*see* Figure 15.7)	To aid decision making about treatment plan, e.g. the use of compression bandaging or hosiery, liaison with the patient's GP to discuss results and referral to vascular consultant, where indicated
38 Complete all relevant documentation, e.g. ulcer assessment form, progress notes, wound chart (see relevant sections for further guidance)	To maintain patient safety To enable continuity of care To maintain practitioner safety Documentation should provide clear evidence of the care or procedure carried out

References and further reading

Ayton M (1985) Wounds that won't heal. *Nursing Times* **81**: 16–19.

Baker SR, Stacey MC, Sing G et al. (1992) Aetiology of chronic leg ulcers. *European Journal of Vascular Surgery* **6**: 245–51.

Baranoski S (2001) Skin tears: staying on guard against the enemy of frail skin. *Nursing Management* **32**: 25–32.

Baranoski S (2003) How to prevent and manage skin tears. *Advances in Skin and Wound Care* **16**: 268–70.

Barnett A (1992) Prevention and treatment of diabetic foot ulcers in diabetic patients in a multidisciplinary setting. *Foot and Ankle International* **16**(7): 388–94.

Beldon P (2006) Topical negative pressure dressings and vacuum assisted closure. *Wound Essentials* **1**: 110–14.

Beldon P (2010) Performing a Doppler assessment: the procedure, technical guide. *Wound Essentials* **5**: 87–90.

Benbow M (2000) Mixing and matching dressing products. *Nursing Standard* **14**(49): 56–62.

Benbow M (2006) An update on VAC therapy. *Journal of Community Nursing* **20**(4): 28–32.

Bergstrom N, Braden BJ, Laguzza A, Holman V (1987) The Braden scale for predicting pressure sore risk. *Nursing Research* **36**: 205–10.

Bethell E (2005) Wound care for patients with darkly pigmented skin. *Nursing Standard* **20**(4): 41–9.

BioMonde Ltd (2011a) BioFoam. www.biomonde.com/product/productBiofoam (last accessed 25 August 2011).

BioMonde Ltd (2011b) Frequently asked questions. www.biomonde.com/product/productFAQ (last accessed 25 August 2011).

Bliss M (1990) Editorial – Preventing pressure sores. *Lancet* **335**: 1311–12.

Boulton AJM (1994) Diabetic medicine. *Diabetic Medicine* **11**(1): 5.

Boulton AJM (1996) The pathogenesis of diabetic foot problems: an overview. *Diabetic Medicine* **13**: S12–S17.

Bridel-Nixon J (1997) Other chronic wounds. In: Morison M, Moffatt C, Bridel-Nixon J, Bale S (eds) *Nursing Management of Chronic Wounds*, pp. 221–4. Mosby, London.

Briggs M, Fleming K (2007) Living with leg ulceration: a synthesis of qualitative research. *Journal of Advanced Nursing* **59**(4): 319–28.

British Association for Parenteral and Enteral Nutrition (2006) *Malnutrition Universal Screening Tool*. www.bapen.org.uk/pdfs/must/must_full.pdf (last accessed 7 February 2008).

British Heart Foundation (1999) *Peripheral Arterial Disease. Patient information book*. British Heart Foundation, London.

Brown JAC (ed.) (2001) *Pears Pocket Medical Encyclopaedia*. Little, Brown & Company, London.

Butcher M, White R (2005) The structure and functions of the skin. In: White R (ed.) *Skin Care in Wound Management: assessment, prevention and treatment*, pp. 1–16. Wounds UK, Aberdeen.

Cameron J (1995) The importance of contact dermatitis in the management of leg ulcers. *Journal of Tissue Viability* **5**(2): 52–5.

Cameron J (2004) What I tell my patients about eczema and venous leg ulcers, *British Journal of Dermatology Nursing* **8**(2): 12–13.

Clark M, Defloor T, Bours G (2004) A pilot study of the prevalence of pressure ulcers in European hospitals. In: Clark M (ed.) *Recent Advances in Tissue Viability*. Quay Books, Salisbury.

Clinical Knowledge Summaries (2011) Leg ulcer – venous – management. www.cks.nhs.uk/leg_ulcer_venous/management/quick_answers/scenario_healed_venous_leg_ulcer#311993006 (last accessed 25 August 2011).

Clinical Resource Efficiency Support Team (1998) *Guidelines for the Assessment and Management of Leg Ulceration*. CREST, Belfast.

Clinical Resource Efficiency Support Team (2005) *Guidelines on the Management of Cellulitis in Adults*. www.gain-ni.org/Library/Guidelines/cellulitis-guide.pdf (last accessed 20 October 2011).

Collier M (1996a) Leg ulceration: overview of causes and treatment. *Nursing Standard* **10**(31): 49–51.

Collier M (1996b) The principles of optimal wound management. *Nursing Standard* **10**(43): 47–52.

Collier M (2002) Wound bed preparation. *Nursing Times* **98**(2) NT Plus-Wound Care (supplement)

Collier M (2003) Understanding wound inflammation. *Nursing Times* **99**(25): 63–4.

Collier J (2008) Nutrition and wound healing. *Dietetics*. www.dietetics.co.uk/article-nutrition-wound-healing.asp (last accessed 12 February 2008).

Collins F, Hampton R, White R (2002) *The A-Z Dictionary of Wound Care*. Mark Allen Publishing, Wiltshire.

Cooper R (2004) A review of the evidence for the use of topical antimicrobial agents in wound care. World Wide Wounds. www.worldwidewounds.com/2004/february/Cooper/Topical-Antimicrobial-Agents.html (last accessed 25 August 2011).

Cutting KF, White RJ, Mahoney P, Harding KG (2005) Clinical identification of wound infection: a Delphi approach. In: *EWMA Position Document: Identifying criteria for wound infection*. Medical Education Partnerships, London.

Dale JJ, Callam MJ, Ruckley CV et al. (1983) Chronic ulcers of the leg: a study of prevalence in a Scottish community. *Health Bulletin* (Edinburgh) **41**: 310–14.

David JA, Chapman RG, Chapman RG, Lockett B (1983) *An Investigation of the Current Methods used in Nursing for the Care of Patients with Established Pressure Sores*. Nursing Practice Research Unit, Middlesex.

Davis M, Dunkley P, Harden RM et al. (1992) *The Wound Programme*. Centre for Medical Education, Dundee.

Dealey C (2000) *The Care of Wounds*. Blackwell Publishing, Oxford.

Dealey C (2005) *The Care of Wounds: a guide for nurses* (3e). Blackwell Publishing, Oxford.

Diabetes Care and Research In Europe (1989) The St. Vincent Declaration. *1st Meeting of St Vincent Declaration Diabetes Action Programme*. St Vincent, Italy, 10–12 October.

Dickerson J (1995) The problem of hospital-induced malnutrition. *Nursing Times* **92**(4): 44–5.

Doherty DC, Morgan PA, Moffatt CJ (2006) Role of hosiery in lower limb lymphoedema. Lymphoedema Framework. *Template for Practice: compression hosiery in lymphoedema*. Medical Education Partnerships, London. www.lymphnetz.de/assets/

397

files/pdf%20englisch/compression-hosiery-in-lymphoedema.
pdf (last accessed 25 August 2011).

Donovan S (1998) Wound infection and wound swabbing. *Professional Nurse* **13**(11): 757–9.

Dormandy JA, Ray S (1996) The natural history of peripheral artery disease. In: Tooke JE, Lowe GDO (eds) *Textbook of Vascular Medicine*, pp. 162–75. Arnold, London.

Dougherty L, Lister S (2011) *The Royal Marsden Hospital Manual of Clinical Nursing Procedures* (8e). Wiley-Blackwell, Oxford.

Eagle M (2007) Understanding cellulitis of the lower limb. *Wound Essentials* **2**: 34–44.

Ebbeskog B, Ekman S-L (2001) Elderly peoples' experiences. The meaning of living with venous leg ulcer. *EWMA Journal* **1**(1): 21–3.

Eckman JR (2010) Sickle pain is a pain: management of crisis in the 21st century. Powerpoint presentation. Sickle Cell Information Centre, http://scinfo.org/health-care-providers/

Edmonds ME, Boulton A, Buckenham T *et al.* (1996) Report of the Diabetic Foot and Amputation Group. *Diabetic Medicine* **13**(9 Suppl 4): S27–S429

Elliott E, Russell B, Jaffrey G (1996) Setting a standard for leg ulcer assessment. *Journal of Wound Care* **5**(4): 173–5.

Enoch S, Harding K (2003) Wound bed preparation: the science behind the removal of barriers to healing. *Wounds* **15**(7): 213–29.

European Pressure Ulcer Advisory Panel (1998) *Pressure Ulcer Treatment Guidelines*. www.epuap.org/gltreatment.html (last accessed 12 February 2008).

European Pressure Ulcer Advisory Panel (2003) *Pressure Ulcer Prevention Guidelines*. www.epuap.org.uk

European Pressure Ulcer Advisory Panel and National Pressure Ulcer Advisory Panel (2009, 2010) *Prevention and Treatment of Pressure Ulcers: quick reference guide*. National Pressure Ulcer Advisory Panel, Washington, DC.

European Wound Management Association (2002) *Pain at Wound Dressing Changes*. Medical Education Partnerships, London.

European Wound Management Association (2004) *Minimising Pain at Wound Dressing-related Procedures. A consensus document*. Medical Education Partnerships, London.

European Wound Management Association (EWMA) (2005) Position Document: *Identifying Criteria for Wound Infection*. Medical Education Partnerships, London.

Exton-Smith AN (1971) Nutrition of the elderly. *British Journal of Hospital Medicine* **5**: 639–45.

Faber WR, Michels PPJ, Maats B (1993) The neuropathic foot. In: Westerhot BE (ed.) *Leg Ulcers: diagnosis and treatment*. Elsevier, Amsterdam.

Falanga V (2000) Classifications for wound bed preparation and stimulation of chronic wounds. *Wound Repair and Regeneration* **8**: 347–52.

Falanga V (2002) Wound bed preparation and the role of enzymes: a case for multiple actions of therapeutic agents. *Wounds* **14**(2): 47–57.

Falanga V (2004) The chronic wound: impaired healing and solutions in the context of wound bed preparation. *Blood Cells Molecules and Dieases* **32**(1): 88–94.

Fernandez R, Griffiths R (2002) Water for wound cleansing. *Cochrane Database of Systematic Reviews 2002*, Issue 4. Art. No.: CD003861. DOI: 10.1002/14651858.CD003861.pub2

Field FK, Kerstein MD (1994) Overview of wound healing in a moist environment. *American Journal of Surgery* **167**(1A): S2–S6.

Finegold S (1982) Pathogenic anaerobes. *Archives of Internal Medicine* **142**: 1988–92.

Flanagan M (2003) Improving accuracy of wound measurement in clinical practice. *Ostomy/Wound Management* **49**(10): 28–40.

Flanagan M, Fletcher J (2003) Tissue viability: managing chronic wounds. In: Booker C, Nicol M (eds) *Nursing Adults: the practice of caring*. Mosby, St Louis.

Fletcher J (1997) Wound cleansing. *Professional Nurse* **12**(11): 793–6.

Foster A (1999) Diabetic ulceration. In: Miller M, Glover D (eds) *Wound Management. Theory and Practice*, pp. 72–83. NT Books, London.

Fowkes FGR (1992) Smoking, lipids glucose intolerance and blood pressure as risk factors for peripheral atherosclerosis compared with ischaemic heart disease in the Edinburgh Artery Study. *American Journal of Epidemiology* **135**: 331–40.

Fowkes FG, Housely E, Cawood EH *et al.* (1991) Edinburgh Artery Study: prevalence of asymptomatic and symptomatic peripheral artery disease in the general population. *International Journal of Epidemiology* **20**: 384–92.

Franks P, Moffatt C (2007) Leg ulcers. In: *Skin Breakdown. The Silent Epidemic*, pp. 28–32. Smith & Nephew Foundation, Hull.

Frykberg RG (2002) Diabetic foot ulcers: pathogenesis and management. *American Family Physician* **66**(9): 1655–63.

Fuhrer MJ, Garber SL, Rintala DH *et al.* (1993) Pressure ulcers in community-resident persons with spinal cord injury: prevalence and risk factors. *Archives of Physical Medicine and Rehabilitation* **74**: 1172–7.

Goodall S (2001) Risk factor assessment for patients with peripheral arterial disease. *Professional Nurse* **17**(1): 27–30.

Grace P (ed.) (2006) *Leg Ulcer Guidelines: a pocket guide for practice*. National Guideline Clearinghouse. www.guideline.gov/summary/summary.aspx?doc_id=9830&nbr=5254 (last accessed 14 February 2008).

Grey JE, Lowe G, Bale S, Harding KG (1998) The use of cultured dermis in the treatment of diabetic foot ulcers. *Journal of Wound Care* **7**(7): 324–5.

Groeneveld A, Anderson M, Allen S *et al.* (2004) The prevalence of pressure ulcers in a tertiary care pediatric and adult hospital. *Journal of Wound Ostomy and Continence Nursing* **31**: 108–20.

Grocott P (1995) The palliative management of fungating malignant wounds. *Journal of Wound Care* **4**(5): 240–2.

Haisfield-Wolfe ME, Rund C (1997) Malignant cutaneous wounds: a management protocol. *Ostomy Wound Management* **43**(1): 56–66.

Ham R, Cotton L (1991) *Limb Amputation*. Chapman & Hall, London.

Hampton S, Collins F (2004) *Tissue Viability*. Whurr Publishers, London.

Harding KG (1996) Managing wound infection. *Journal of Wound Care* **5**(8): 391–2.

Hasdai D, Garratt KN, Grill DE et al. (1997) The effect of smoking status on the long term outcome after successful percutaneous revascularisation. *New England Journal of Medicine* **336**(11): 755–61.

Hawkins J, Lindsay E (2006) We listen but do we hear? The importance of patient stories. *British Journal of Community Nursing* **11**(9 suppl): S6–S14.

Healthcare A2Z (2007) *Decontamination*. www.healthcarea2z.org/stdPage.aspx/home/Decontamination/CoreContent/Skindecontamination#asepsis (last accessed 14 February 2008).

Herlihy B, Maebius N (2000) *The Human Body in Health and Illness*. WB Saunders, London.

Hinshaw J (2000) Larval therapy: a review of clinical human and veterinary studies. www.worldwidewounds.com/2000/0ct/Janet-Hinshaw/Larval-Therapy-Human-and-Veterinary.html (last accessed 20 October 2011).

Hofman D, Ryan TJ, Arnold F et al. (1997) Pain in venous leg ulcers. *Journal of Wound Care* **6**(5): 222–4.

Hopkins A (2004) Disrupted lives: investigating coping strategies for non-healing leg ulcers. *British Journal of Nursing* **13**(9): 556–63.

Housley E (1988) Treating claudication in five words. *British Medical Journal* **296**: 1483–4.

Hutchinson JJ, Lawrence JC (1991) Wound infection under occlusive dressings. *Journal of Hospital Infection* **17**(2): 83–94.

Johnston E (2007) The role of nutrition in tissue viability. *Wound Essentials* **2**: 10–21.

KCI International (2004) *VAC Recommended Guidelines for Use: physician and caregiver reference manual*. KCI International, Oxford.

Kelly J (1994) The aetiology of pressure sores. *Journal of Tissue Viability* **4**(3): 77–8.

Kindlen S, Morison M (1997) The physiology of wound healing. In: Morison M, Moffatt C, Bridel-Nixon J, Bale S (eds) *Nursing Management of Chronic Wounds*, pp. 1–26. Mosby, London.

Kingsley A (2001) A proactive approach to wound infection. *Nursing Standard* **15**(30): 50–8.

Kingsley A (2003) The wound infection continuum and its application to clinical practice. *Ostomy/Wound Management* **49**(7A): 1–7

Kingsley A, White R, Gray D (2004) *The Wound Infection Continuum: a revised perspective*. http://www.wounds-uk.com/downloads/applied_wounds_management_supplement.pdf

Kudoh A (2005) Perioperative management for chronic schizophrenic patients. *Anesthesia & Analgesia* **101**(6): 1867–72.

Kumar P, Clark M (eds) (2001) *Clinical Medicine* (4e). WB Saunders, London.

Lavery LA, Armstrong DG, Harkless LB (1996) Classification of diabetic foot wounds. *Journal of Foot and Ankle Surgery* **35**: 528–31.

Lewis B (1997) Nutrition and age in the aetiology of pressure sores. *Journal of Wound Care* **6**(1): 41–2.

Lindsay E (2004) The Lindsay Leg Club Model: a model for evidence based leg ulcer management. *British Journal of Community Nursing*. www.legclub.org/downloads/BJCN_article.pdf (last accessed 25 August 2011).

Linger F (2010) Functions of skin. www.articleinput.com/e/a/title/The-seven-basic-functions-of-human-skin/ (last accessed 3 September 2011).

Lookingbill DP, Marks JG (1993) *Principles of Dermatology*. WB Saunders, London.

Marieb EN (2006) *Essentials of Human Anatomy & Physiology* (8e). Pearson Education, San Francisco.

Marston W, Vowden K (2003) Compression therapy: a guide to safe practice. In: European Wound Management Association (EWMA) Position Document. *Understanding Compression Therapy*. Medical Education Partnerships, London. Available from http://ewma.org/fileadmin/user_upload/EWMA/pdf/Position_Documents/2003/Spring_2003__English_.pdf

Martini FH, Bartholomew EF (2000) *Essentials of Anatomy and Physiology* (2e). Prentice Hall, New Jersey.

McCaffery M, Beebe A (1993) *Pain: clinical manual for nursing practice*. Mosby, Baltimore.

McCaffery M, Beebe A (1999) *Pain: clinical manual for nursing practice* (2e). Mosby, St Louis.

McIntosh A, Peters J, Young R et al. (2003) Prevention and Management of Foot Problems in Type 2 Diabetes: clinical guidelines and evidence. University of Sheffield, Sheffield; National Institute for Clinical Excellence (NICE). Moffatt C (2001) Leg ulcers. In: *Vascular Disease Nursing and Management*, pp. 200–37. Whurr, London.

Meuleneire F (2002) Using a soft silicone-coated net dressing to manage skin tears. *Journal of Wound Care* **11**(10): 365–9.

Moffatt C (2004) Factors that affect concordance with compression therapy. *Journal of Wound Care* **13**(7): 291–4.

Moffatt CJ, O'Hare L (1995) Fundamentals in clinical practice. *Journal of Community Nursing* **9**(9): 27–31.

Moffatt C, Martin R, Smithdale R (2007) *Leg Ulcer Management*. Blackwell Publishing, Oxford.

Moody M, Grocott P (1993) Let us extend our knowledge base: assessment and management of fungating wounds. *Professional Nurse* **8**(9): 58–79.

Morgan DA (2000) *Formulary of Wound Management Products: a guide for healthcare staff* (8e). Euromed Communications, Haselmere.

Morison MJ (1989) Wound cleansing-which solution? *Professional Nurse* **4**: 220–5.

Morison M, Moffatt C (1997) Leg ulcers. In: Morison M, Moffatt C, Bridel-Nixon J, Bale S (1997) *Nursing Management of Chronic Wounds*, pp. 177–220. Mosby, London.

Morison M, Moffatt CJ, Franks PJ (2007) *Leg Ulcers: a problem-based learning approach*. Mosby, Elsevier, Edinburgh.

Mortimer P (1993) Skin problems in palliative care. In: Doyle D, Hanks G, Macdonald N (eds) *Oxford Textbook of Palliative Medicine*. Oxford Medical Publications, Oxford.

Murray J, Boulton A (1995) The pathophysiology of diabetic foot ulceration. *Clinics in Podiatriac Medicine and Surgery* **12**(1): 1–17.

National Institute for Clinical Excellence (2001) *NICE Guide on Pressure Ulcer: risk management and prevention*. NICE, London.

National Institute for Clinical Excellence (2003) *Pressure Ulcer Prevention. Clinical Guideline 7*. NICE, London.

National Institute for Health and Clinical Excellence (2004) *Type 2 Diabetes; prevention and management of foot problems.* Clinical Guideline 10. NICE, London.

National Institute for Health and Clinical Excellence (2005) *Pressure Ulcers – Prevention and Treatment.* Clinical Guideline 29. NICE, London.

National Institute for Health and Clinical Excellence (2005) *CG29 Pressure Ulcer Management: quick reference guide.* www.nice. org.uk/nicemedia/pdf/CG029quickrefguide.pdf (last accessed 7 February 2008).

National Institute for Health and Clinical Excellence (2008) *Prevention and Treatment of Surgical Site Infection.* Clinical Guideline 74. NICE, London.

National Patient Safety Agency (2010) *NHS to adopt zero tolerance approach to pressure ulcers, press release.* NPSA, London. www.npsa.nhs.uk/corporate/news/nhs-to-adopt-zero-tolerance-approach-to-pressure-ulcers

National Pressure Ulcer Advisory Panel (NPUAP) and European Ulcer Advisory Panel (EPUAP) (2009) *Prevention and Treatment of Pressure Ulcers: clinical practice guideline.* National Pressure Ulcer Advisory Panel., Washington, DC.

Naylor W (2001) Using a new foam dressing in the care of fungating wounds. *British Journal of Nursing* **10**(6): 24–31.

Naylor W, Laverty D, Mallett J (2001) *Handbook of Wound Management in Cancer Care.* Blackwell Science, Oxford.

Nemeth KA, Harrison MB, Graham ID, Banks S (2003) Pain in pure and mixed aetiology venous leg ulcer: a three-phase point prevalence survey. *Journal of Wound Care* **12**(9): 336–40.

NHS Centre for Reviews and Dissemination and Nuffield Institute for Health (1995) *Effective Health Care. The prevention and treatment of pressure sores.* NHS Centre for Reviews and Dissemination, University of York, York.

NHS London (2011) *Pressure Ulcer Reporting Framework.* NHS London, London.

Nixon J, McGough A (2001) Principles of patient assessment: screening for pressure ulcers and potential risk. In: Morison M (ed.) *The Prevention and Treatment of Pressure Ulcers,* pp. 55–74. Mosby, London.

Nyquist R, Hawthorn PJ (1987) The prevalence of pressure sores in an area health authority. *Journal of Advanced Nursing* **12**: 183–7.

Papantonio CJ, Wallop JM, Kolodner KB (1994) Sacral ulcers following cardiac surgery: incidence and risk factors. *Advances in Wound Care* **7**(2): 24–36.

Parker L (2000) Applying the principles of infection control to wound care. *British Journal of Nursing* **9**(7): 394–8.

Partsch H (2003) Understanding the pathophysiological effects of compression. In: *European Wound Management Association (EWMA) position document,* Understanding Compression Therapy. MEP, London, pp. 2–4.

Payne RL, Martin ML (1993) Defining and classifying skin tears: need for a common language. *Ostomy Wound Management* **39**(5): 16.

Persoon A, Heinen MM, van der Vleuten CJ *et al.* (2004) Leg ulcers: a review of their impact on daily life. *Journal of Clinical Nursing* **13**(3): 341–54.

Pinchkofsky-Devin G (1994) Nutritional wound healing. *Journal of Wound Care* **3**(5): 231–4.

Posnett J, Franks P (2007) The costs of skin breakdown and ulceration in the UK. In: The Smith & Nephew Foundation. *Skin Breakdown. The Silent Epidemic,* pp. 6–12. Smith & Nephew Foundation, Hull.

Price P (2005) An holistic approach to wound pain in patients with chronic wounds. *Wounds* **17**(3): 55–7.

Rainey J (2002) *A Handbook for Community Nurses. Wound Care.* Whurr Publishers, London.

Reid J, Morrison M (1994) Stirling Pressure Sore Severity Scale. Towards a consensus: classification of pressure sores. *Journal of Wound Care* **3**(3): 157–60.

Rintala DH (1995) Quality of life considerations. *Advances in Wound Care* **8**(4): 28–71.

Rowell LB (1986) *Human Circulation: regulation during physical stress.* Oxford University Press, Oxford.

Royal College of Nursing (2005) *The Management of Pressure Ulcers in Primary and Secondary Care, A Clinical Practice Guideline.* RCN, London. www.nice.org.uk/page.aspx?o= cg029fullguideline

Royal College of Nursing (2006) *Clinical Practice Guidelines/ Recommendations: the nursing management of patients with venous leg ulcers.* RCN, London.

Ruff D (2003) Doppler assessment: calculating an ankle brachial pressure index. *Nursing Times* **99**: 42–62.

Ryecroft-Malone J, McInnes E (2001) *Pressure Ulcer Risk Assessment and Prevention. Clinical Guidelines.* Royal College of Nursing, London.

Sciarra J (ed.) (2003) *Wound Care Made Incredibly Easy.* Lippincott, London.

Scottish Intercollegiate Guidelines Network (1998) *The Care of Patients with Chronic Leg Ulcers.* SIGN Publication, Edinburgh.

Scottish Intercollegiate Guidelines Network (2010) SIGN Guideline 120. *Management of Chronic Venous Leg Ulcers.* www. sign.ac.uk/guidelines/fulltext/120/index.html (last accessed 20 October 2011).

Shubert V, Heraud J (1994) The effects of pressure and shear on skin microcirculation in elderly stroke patients lying in supine or semi-recumbent positions. *Age and Aging* **23**(5): 405–10.

Sibbald RG, Orsted H, Schultz GS *et al.* (2003) Preparing the wound bed 2003: focus on infection and inflammation. *Ostomy Wound Management* **49**: 23–51.

Sieggreen MY, Kline RA (2004) Recognizing and managing venous leg ulcers. *Advances in Skin & Wound Care* **17**(6): 302–11.

Simon D A, Dix F P, McCollum C N (2004) Management of venous leg ulcers. *British Medical Journal,* **328**: 1358–1362

Sims R, Fitzgerald V (1985) *Community Nursing Management of Patients with Ulcerating/fungating Breast Disease.* Royal College of Nursing, London.

Smoker A (1999) Skin care in old age. *Nursing Standard* **13**: 47–53.

Souza Nogueira G, Zanin CR, Miyazaki MC, Pereira de Godoy JM (2009) Venous leg ulcers and emotional consequences. *International Journal of Lower Extremity Wounds* **8**(4): 194–6.

Stevens J (2004) The diagnosis and management of mixed aetiology ulcers (Wound Care Suppl). *Nursing Times* **100**(46): 65–8.

Stevens J, Franks PJ, Harrington M (1997) A community/hospital leg ulcer service. *Journal of Wound Care* **6**(2): 62–8.

Tanj LF, Phillips TJ (2001) Skin problems in the elderly. *Wounds* **13**(3): 93–7.

Thomas B, Bishop J (2007) *Manual of Dietetic Practice 4 ed*. Blackwell Publishing, Oxford.

Thomas S, Jones M (1999) *The Use of Sterile Maggots in Wound Management*. Wound Care Society Education Leaflet 6. www.woundcaresociety.com/news.html

Thomas S (1992) *Current Practices in the Management of Fungating Lesions and Radiation Damaged Skin*. The Surgical Materials Testing Laboratory, Bridgend.

Thomas S (1998) Compression bandaging in the treatment of venous leg ulcers. World Wide Wounds. www.worldwidewounds.com/1997/september/Thomas-Bandaging/bandage-paper.html (last accessed 25 August 2011).

Tortora GJ, Anagnostakos NP (1987) *Principles of Anatomy and Physiology* (5e) Harper & Row, London.

Van den Berghe G, Wouters P, Weekers F *et al.* (2001) Intensive insulin therapy in critically ill patients. *New England Journal of Medicine* **345**: 1359–67.

Vanderwee K, Grypdonck M, Defloor T (2007) Non blanchable erythema as an indicator for the need for pressure ulcer prevention: a randomized controlled trial. *Journal of Clinical Nursing* **16**(2): 325–35.

Van Rijswijk L (2001) Epidemiology. In: Morison M (ed.) *The Prevention and Treatment of Pressure Ulcers*. Mosby, London.

Vermeulen H, Ubbink DT, Schreuder SM, Lubbers MJ (2007) Inter- and intra-observer (dis)agreement among nurses and doctors to classify colour and exudation of open surgical wounds according to the Red-Yellow-Black scheme. *Journal of Clinical Nursing* **16**(7): 1270–7.

Versluysen M (1986) How elderly patients with femoral fractures develop pressure sores in hospital. *British Medical Journal* **292**: 1311–13.

Vowden KR, Vowden P (1999) Wound debridement, part 2: sharp techniques. *Journal of Wound Care* **8**(6): 291–4.

Vowden P, Vowden R (2001) Doppler assessment and ABPI: interpretation in the management of leg ulceration. World Wide Wounds. www.worldwidewounds.com/2001march/vowden/Doppler-assessment-and-ABPI.html (last accessed September 2011).

Vowden KR, Goulding V, Vowden P (1996) Hand-held Doppler assessment for peripheral arterial disease. *Journal of Wound Care* **5**(3): 125–8.

Waldrop J, Doughty D (2000) Wound healing-physiology. In: Bryant R (ed.) *Acute and Chronic Wounds. Nursing Management* (2e), pp. 17–39. Mosby, London.

Wagner FW (1987) The diabetic foot. *Orthopedics* **10**(1): 163–72.

Waterlow J (1985) Pressure sores: a risk assessment card. *Nursing Times* **81**: 49–55.

Waterlow J (1988). Prevention is cheaper than cure. *Nursing Times* **84**(25): 69–70.

Watkins PJ (2003) The diabetic foot. ABC of Diabetes. *British Medical Journal* **326**: 977–9.

West JM, Gimbel ML (2000) Acute surgical and traumatic healing. In Bryant R (ed.) *Acute and Chronic Wounds. Nursing Management* (2e). Mosby, London.

Westaby S (1985) *Wound Care*. William Heinemann Medical Books, London

Whiteing NL (2009) Skin assessment of patients at risk of pressure ulcers. *Nursing Standard* **24**(10): 40–4.

Wiersema-Bryant LA, Kraemer BA (2000) Vascular and neuropathic wounds: the diabetic wound. In: Bryant R (ed.) *Acute and Chronic Wounds. Nursing Management* (2e), pp. 301–15. Mosby, London.

Wild S, Roglic G, Green A *et al.* (2004) Global prevalence of diabetes. Estimates for the year 2000 and projections for 2030. *Diabetes Care* **27**(5): 1047–53.

Williams L, Leaper D (2000) Nutrition and wound healing. *Clinical Nutrition Update* **5**(1): 3–5.

Winter GD (1962) Formation of the scab and the rate of epithelialisation of superficial wounds in the skin of the domestic pig. *Nature* **193**: 293–4.

Wong DL, Hockenberry-Eaton M, Wilson D *et al.* (2001) *Wong's Essentials of Pediatric Nursing* (6e). Mosby, St Louis, p. 1301.

World Health Organization (2003) *Diabetes Estimates and Projections*. www.who.int/ncd/dia/databases4.htm (last accessed 28 December 2003).

World Union of Wound Healing Societies (2004) *Principles of Best Practice: Minimising Pain at Wound Dressing-Related Procedures: A Consensus Document*. Medical Education Partnerships, London.

Wounds UK (2006) *Notes and feedback from the meeting of Consultants and Specialists in Tissue Viability*. Wounds UK, Harrogate.

Wysocki AB (1992) Skin. In: Bryant R A (ed.) *Acute and Chronic Wounds. Nursing Management*, pp. 1–30. Mosby Year Book, London.

Wysocki AB (2000) Anatomy and physiology of skin and soft tissue. In: Bryant R (ed.) *Acute and Chronic Wounds. Nursing Management* (2e), pp. 1–16. Mosby, London.

Index

411

414

415